09

DATE DUE FOR RETURN

Pediatric Nephrology in the ICU

Stefan G. Kiessling · Jens Goebel
Michael J.G. Somers
Editors

Pediatric Nephrology in the ICU

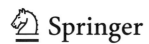 Springer

Stefan G. Kiessling, MD
Division of Pediatric Nephrology
and Renal Transplantation
Kentucky Children's Hospital
University of Kentucky
740 South Limestone Street Room J460
Lexington, KY 40536, USA
skies2@email.uky.edu

Jens Goebel, MD
Nephrology and Hypertension Division
Medical Director, Kidney Transplantation
Cincinnati Children's Hospital Medical Center
3333 Burnet Avenue
Cincinnati, OH 45229-3039, USA
Jens.Goebel@cchmc.org

Michael J.G. Somers, MD
Harvard Medical School
Children's Hospital Boston
Division of Nephrology
300 Longwood Avenue
Boston MA 02115, USA
michael.somers@childrens.harvard.edu

ISBN 978-3-540-74423-8   e-ISBN 978-3-540-74425-2

DOI: 10.1007/978-3-540-74425-2   100393930 9

Library of Congress Control Number: 2008928719

Cover design: eStudio Calamar, Spain

Printed on acid-free paper

9 8 7 6 5 4 3 2 1

springer.com

To our families and our mentors

*S.K. and J.G. would also like to dedicate this book to the memory of
Dr. Heinrich A. Werner, their late colleague, friend and role model with whom they
spent so many hours in the PICU. Heinrich, we miss you greatly.*

Preface

The responsibilities of the Pediatric Nephrologist in the critical care setting are multifaceted. Management of acute renal failure with and without renal replacement therapy, fluid and electrolyte abnormalities and hypertensive emergencies are only some of the major clinical circumstances where the renal specialist is involved in the care of children admitted to the Pediatric Intensive Care Unit. Due to the complex and specialized care required, critical care nephrology could even be considered a separate entity compared to the clinical scenarios treated in the outpatient setting or on the inpatient pediatric ward. Recently, the changing role of the Nephrologist in the ICU setting, much more expanded than the classic provision of renal replacement therapy, has been discussed in the community of providers involved in renal care, and fellowships with special emphasis on Intensive Care Pediatric Nephrology are being considered. This changing role requires coordination of care between the Pediatric Nephrologist and other teams of physicians caring for critically ill children more often than in the past.

As several providers are involved in the majority of critically ill children and many valid approaches may exist, consensus needs to be reached before making important diagnostic or therapeutic decisions. Good on-going communication between the Intensivist, the Nephrologist and other involved specialists is vital to optimize the outcome for each individual child.

In this first edition of the book, we have included chapters focused on general topics in pediatric nephrology that are most germane to the care of the critically ill child. We have tried to look at the clinical situations from the aspect of both the Pediatric Intensivist and renal specialist. We hope that this book will supply the medical providers with a framework to approach the challenges faced in practicing Pediatric Intensive Care Nephrology.

We express our thanks to all the contributing authors, all of whom have expertise in either Critical Care Pediatrics or Pediatric Nephrology and have years of experience with the care of this unique patient population. Any task as complex as the completion of a book publication requires several sets of helping hands in the background. We especially appreciate the constant help of Jodi Boyd and Jan Wilkins, as this project would not have been possible without them.

Lexington, USA   Stefan G. Kiessling
Cincinnati, USA   Jens Goebel
Boston, USA   Michael J.G. Somers
June 2008

Contents

List of Contributors

Ghazala Abuazza
Division of Pediatric Nephrology
University of Kentucky Children's Hospital
740 South Limestone Street
Lexington, KY 40536, USA

Erman Al-Khadra
Cincinnati Children's Hospital Medical Center
Critical Care
3333 Burnet Avenue
Cincinnati, OH 45229-3039, USA

Carlos Araya
University of Florida, College of Medicine
Division of Pediatric Nephrology
P.O. Box 100296, 1600 SW Archer Road
Gainesville, FL 32610-0296, USA

Philip Bernard
Division of Pediatric Critical Care
Kentucky Children's Hospital
University of Kentucky
800 Rose Street
Lexington, KY 40536, USA
Philip.bernard@uky.edu

Michael T. Bigham
Critical Care Medicine
Akron Children's Hospital
One Perkins Square
Akron, OH 44308, USA
mbigham@chmca.org

Catherine L. Dent
Division of Cardiology
Cincinnati Children's Hospital Medical Center
3333 Burnet Avenue
Cincinnati, OH 45229-3039, USA

Prasad Devarajan
University of Cincinnati College of Medicine
Cincinnati Children's Hospital Medical Center
3333 Burnet Avenue
Cincinnati, OH 45229-3039, USA

Vikas R. Dharnidharka
University of Florida College of Medicine
Division of Pediatric Nephrology
P.O. Box 100296, 1600 SW Archer Road
Gainesville, FL 32610-0296, USA
vikasmd@peds.ufl.edu

John D'Orazio
Division of Hematology-Oncology
University of Kentucky College of Medicine
Markey Cancer Center
Combs Research Building Room 204
800 Rose Street
Lexington, KY 40536-0096, USA
jdorazio@uky.edu

Jörg Dötsch
Kinder- und Jugendklinik
Universitätsklinikum Erlangen
Loschgestr 15
91054 Erlangen, Germany
Joerg.Doetsch@kinder.imed.uni-erlangen.de

Jens Goebel
Nephrology and Hypertension Division
Medical Director, Kidney Transplantation
Cincinnati Children's Hospital Medical Center
3333 Burnet Avenue
Cincinnati, OH 45229-3039, USA
Jens.Goebel@cchmc.org

Stuart L. Goldstein
Texas Children's Hospital
6621 Fannin Street, MC-3-2482
Houston, TX, 77030, USA

Dwayne Henry
University of Florida, College of Medicine
Division of Pediatric Nephrology
P.O. Box 100296, 1600 SW Archer Road
Gainesville, FL 32610-0296, USA

John T. Herrin
Division of Nephrology
Children's Hospital Boston
300 Longwood Avenue
Boston, MA 02115, USA
john.herrin@childrens.harvard.edu

Tamara K. Hutson
Divisions of Pharmacology and Critical
Care Medicine
Cincinnati Children's
Hospital Medical Center
3333 Burnet Avenue
Cincinnati OH 45229-3039, USA
tamara.hutson@cchmc.org

Mona Khurana
Department of Nephrology
Suite W.W. 1.5-100
Children's National Medical Center
111 Michigan Avenue, NW
Washington, DC 20010, USA
mkhurana@cnmc.org

Stefan G. Kiessling
Division of Pediatric Nephrology
and Renal Transplantation
Kentucky Children's Hospital
University of Kentucky
740 South Limestone Street Room J460
Lexington, KY 40536, USA
skies2@email.uky.edu

Neil W. Kooy
Division of Pediatric Critical Care Medicine
University of Minnesota School of Medicine
University of Minnesota Children's Hospital
Fairview, 420 Delaware St. SE
Minneapolis, MN 55455, USA

Vesna M. Kriss
Department of Radiology and Pediatrics
University of Kentucky
and Kentucky Children's Hospital
Lexington, KY 40536, USA
vkris0@email.uky.edu

James A. Listman
SUNY Upstate Medical University
Department of Pediatrics
750 E. Adams St
Syracuse, NY 13210, USA

Kera E. Luckritz
Division of Nephrology
Children's Hospital and Regional Medical Center
4800 Sand Point Way NE
Seattle, Washington 98105, USA
kera.luckritz@seattlechildrens.org

Elizabeth H. Mack
Division of Critical Care Medicine
Cincinnati Children's Hospital Medical Center
3333 Burnet Avenue
Cincinnati, OH 45229-3039
elizabeth.mack@cchmc.org

Kirtida Mistry
Pediatric Nephrology
University of California, San Diego
9500 Gilman Drive, MC 0634
La Jolla, CA 92093, USA
kmistry@ucsd.edu

Chris Nelson
Division of Pediatric Infectious Diseases
University of Kentucky Children's Hospital
740 South Limestone Street
Lexington, KY 40536, USA

Raymond Quigley
Department of Pediatrics
UT Southwestern Medical Center
5323 Harry Hines Blvd
Dallas, TX 75390-9063, USA
Raymond.quigley@utsouthwestern.edu

Nancy M. Rodig
Division of Nephrology
Children's Hospital Boston
300 Longwood Avenue
Boston, MA 02115, USA
nancy.rodig@childrens.harvard.edu

Dmitry Samsonov
Nephrology Division
Schneider Medical Center for Children
Kaplan 14
Petach Tikvah 49202, Israel
dmitrys@clalit.org.il
dmitry_samsonov@yahoo.com

Scott Schurman
SUNY Upstate Medical University
Department of Pediatrics
750 E. Adams St
Syracuse, NY 13210, USA

Lawrence R. Shoemaker
Division of Nephrology, Department of Pediatrics
University of Louisville
Ste 424, KCPC Building
571 S. Floyd St
Louisville, KY 40202, USA
lrshoe01@louisville.edu

Michael J.G. Somers
Harvard Medical School
Children's Hospital Boston
Division of Nephrology
300 Longwood Avenue
Boston, MA 02115, USA
michael.somers@childrens.harvard.edu

Jordan M. Symons
Division of Nephrology
Children's Hospital and
Regional Medical Center
4800 Sand Point Way NE
Seattle, WA 98105, USA
jordan.symons@seattlechildrens.org

Avram Z. Traum
Massachusetts General Hospital
Pediatric Nephrology Unit
55 Fruit Street, Yawkey 6C
Boston, MA 02114, USA
atraum@partners.org

Derek S. Wheeler
Division of Critical Care Medicine
Cincinnati Children's Hospital Medical Center
3333 Burnet Avenue
Cincinnati, OH 45229-3039, USA
derek.wheeler@cchmc.org

Michael Zappitelli
Texas Children's Hospital
6621 Fannin Street, MC-3-2482
Houston, TX 77030, USA
mzaprdr@yahoo.ca

Disorders of Salt and Water Balance

1

M. Khurana

Contents

S.G. Kiessling et al. (eds) *Pediatric Nephrology in the ICU.*
© Springer-Verlag Berlin Heidelberg 2009

Core Messages

> Dysnatremias usually reflect an imbalance in total body water (TBW) rather than a surfeit or deficit of sodium.

> At any given time in the basal state, the extracellular and intracellular osmolalities are equal. If there is a change in the solute concentration of a given fluid compartment that alters that compartment's osmolality, water will shift across the newly created osmotic gradient until the osmolality in all fluid compartments is once again equal.

> Maintenance of the extracellular volume is conducted via both volume regulation and osmoregulation through a number of afferent signals that result in effector responses.

- Because sodium is the primary extracellular solute, volume regulation of the extracellular volume is directly mediated by changes in total body sodium balance.

- Osmoregulation is mediated by changes in water balance.

> Afferent receptors that detect changes in the elasticity of the arterioles include the cardiopulmonary baroreceptors of the carotid sinus and the aortic arch as well as renal baroreceptors of the juxtaglomerular apparatus.

- Collectively, decreased perfusion of the cardiopulmonary and renal baroreceptors results in the activation of three main vasoconstrictor systems antidiuretic hormone (ADH), the sympathetic nervous system (SNS), and the renin–angiotensin–aldosterone system.

- The converse holds true in the setting of effective circulating volume expansion.

Case Vignette

A 7-month-old male infant is brought to the emergency department with a 4-day history of persistent emesis. He is lethargic and quiet during the examination. He has normal vital signs and his physical exam is remarkable for dry mucous membranes. Initial labs are most notable for a serum sodium of 115 mmol/L. Upon further questioning, the parents report that he had been exclusively breastfed for the first 6 months of his life. His parents had recently begun feeding him powdered formula mixed with filtered water. With his acute illness, he has been receiving small volumes of dilute formula as well as water.

1.1 Introduction

The plasma sodium concentration is equal to the total body sodium divided by the TBW:

$$\text{Plasma } [\text{Na}^+ \text{ (mmol / L)}] = \frac{\text{Total body sodium (mmol)}}{\text{Total body water (L)}} \quad (1.1)$$

Like any fraction, this value either decreases or increases depending on changes in the numerator relative to the denominator. While changes in the total body sodium can and do occur, changes in TBW are far more common and are more directly related to a drop in the plasma sodium concentration. Thus, dysnatremias typically reflect an imbalance in TBW.

1.2 Total Body Water

From birth onwards, the human body increases in size, and its relative proportions of bone, fat, muscle, viscera, and water change. During early gestation, nearly 90% of a fetus' body weight consists of water. Premature babies have a TBW content that is 80% of their body weight. This percentage drops to 70% in term infants, 65% in young children, and 60% in older children and adolescents [18, 28]. In adulthood, TBW content equals 60% of lean body weight in males and 50% in females.

The TBW is distributed into two major body compartments (Fig. 1.1). Two-thirds of the TBW is distributed into the intracellular compartment, and one-third is distributed into the extracellular compartment.

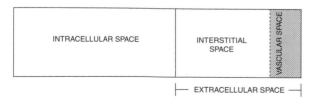

Fig. 1.1 Body fluid compartments

Water makes up almost 80% of a cell's composition [32, 34]. A notable exception is adipose tissue, which is virtually water-free. This means that individuals with excess adiposity, such as women when compared with men, have lower TBW content.

The extracellular compartment is further subdivided into the intravascular and extravascular spaces. Extravascular sites for fluid accumulation include the space surrounding cells (interstitial space) and localized cavities where fluid may potentially sequestrate such as the pericardial, peritoneal, and pleural spaces [15]. The intravascular space represents one-fourth of the extracellular compartment; the extravascular space is composed of the remaining three-fourths. It is noteworthy that the intravascular space makes up the smallest percentage of TBW.

1.2.1 Effective Osmoles

All body compartments are freely permeable to water but are not as readily permeable to all solutes. Water will move from an area of high random movement to an area of relatively lower random movement. Cohesive forces between molecules increase in the presence of a solute, leading to a reduction in the random movement of water in the body compartment containing the solute. As a result, water moves in from other body compartments until the hydrostatic pressure in the compartment containing the solute equals the forces causing the movement of water into this compartment. The hydrostatic pressure at which this occurs is called the osmotic pressure of the compartment containing the solute [10]. The osmotic pressure is directly related to the number of solutes present in the compartment. Any solute that cannot cross fluid compartments will dictate water movement into its compartment, creating an osmotic pressure. Such a solute is referred to as an effective osmole. In contrast, solutes that freely cross fluid compartments, and are therefore not restricted to any one fluid compartment, are considered to be ineffective osmoles because they do not generate an osmotic pressure.

Each body compartment contains a predominant solute that acts as an effective osmole. Potassium salts are the predominant solutes found in the intracellular space. Large proteins and inorganic phosphates are the major intracellular anions and cannot easily leave the intracellular compartment. Sodium salts are the primary solutes found in the extracellular space, where they are evenly equilibrated between the intravascular and interstitial spaces. Although both potassium and sodium are cell membrane permeable, they remain in their respective fluid compartments largely because of the actions of Na^+–K^+ ATPase that is present along the basolateral aspects of cell membranes. For this pump to remain effective, there must be a readily available supply of potassium and sodium for exchange. Within the extracellular space, sodium salts and glucose can easily move between the intravascular and interstitial spaces. Plasma proteins, however, do not readily traverse the vascular membrane separating the intra vascular and interstitial spaces because of their larger size. Thus, plasma proteins act as effective osmoles to keep water in the vascular space. The pressure exerted by plasma proteins is termed plasma oncotic pressure. In the basal state, the capillary hydrostatic pressure balances the plasma oncotic pressure. The former is the pressure of blood generated by the heart with each cardiac output. Net filtration of fluid from the vascular space to the interstitial space depends on the balance between the hydrostatic and oncotic pressures between these two spaces.

1.3 Plasma Osmolality

Sodium salts are the predominant effective osmoles found in the vascular space. Thus, the plasma ionic contribution to the osmotic pressure can be calculated as two times the plasma sodium concentration. The plasma sodium concentration is multiplied by two to account for accompanying anions such as chloride. Glucose and urea comprise the rest of the major osmoles present in the vascular space. The plasma osmolality (P_{osm}) is equal to the sum of the individual osmolalities of each solute present in the vascular space. It is defined as the number of milliosmoles of solute present per kilogram of water. One milliosmole equals 1 mmole of solute.

$$
\begin{aligned}
P_{osm} = & (2 \times plasma\ [Na^+(mmol/L)]) \\
& + \frac{(10\ [glucose\ (mg/dL)])}{180\,(mg/mmol)} \\
& + \frac{(10\ [BUN\ (mg/dL)])}{28\,(mg/mmol)} \\
= & (2 \times plasma\ [Na^+(mmol/L)]) \\
& + \frac{[glucose\ (mg/L)]}{18\,(mg/mmol)} + \frac{[BUN\ (mg/L)]}{2.8\ (mg/mmol)}. \quad (1.2)
\end{aligned}
$$

Both plasma glucose and BUN are reported in milligram per deciliter. Multiplying these values by 10 will convert the units to milligram per liter, and dividing the product by the molecular weight of each will convert the units to milliosmoles per liter. The molecular weight of glucose is 180, and the molecular weight of BUN is 28.

The majority of individuals are neither hyperglycemic nor uremic, so the osmolar contributions from glucose and BUN are often negligible. In individuals with acute renal failure and uremia, the plasma osmolality will be elevated due to a large osmolar contribution from the plasma BUN. However, urea is considered to be an ineffective osmole because it can readily cross cell membranes. As a result, the effective P_{osm} should be determined in uremic individuals.

$$
\begin{aligned}
Effective\ P_{osm} = & (2 \times plasma\ [Na^+mmol/L]) \\
& + [glucose\ mg/L]/18. \quad (1.3)
\end{aligned}
$$

Normal plasma concentrations for sodium, fasting glucose, and BUN are 135–145 mmol L^{-1}, 60–100 mg dL^{-1}, and 10–20 mg dL^{-1}, respectively. Based on these normative values, a normal plasma osmolality falls between 275 and 290 mOsm kg^{-1} [16].

Unlike solutes which are limited in their passage between fluid compartments, water is freely permeable between all fluid compartments. This ensures that, at any given time in the basal state, the extracellular and intracellular osmolalities are equal. If there is a change in the solute concentration of a given fluid compartment that alters that compartment's osmolality, water will shift across the newly created osmotic gradient until the osmolality in all fluid compartments is once again equal.

Maintaining the volume of each fluid compartment is essential to normal body functioning. Normal cell function relies on close regulation of the intracellular volume. To remain viable, cells must be able to maintain their intracellular pH and cytoplasmic ion concentration. Both of these factors rely on close regulation of the cell volume. This is because changes in cell volume will lead to variations in not only the intracellular pH but also in the concentration of key cytoplasmic components such as cofactors, enzymes, and ions such as calcium. Volume regulation in nonpolarized cells is determined by the difference in osmotic pressures between the intracellular and the extracellular spaces. Increases in cell volume in encapsulated organs that have limited compliance, such as the brain, will lead to significant changes in tissue pressure. For all of the aforementioned reasons, tight regulation of cell volume is critical to proper intracellular functioning. Polarized cells rely on a balance in transport mechanisms between the apical and basolateral cell surfaces to achieve volume regulation. Nonpolarized cells achieve volume control by adjusting the intracellular concentration of solutes [32].

Two types of solutes used by cells to adapt to changes in cell volume include electrolytes and organic molecules. Initially and overall during states of osmolar stress, ionic solutes mainly contribute to cell volume regulation. Potassium and chloride are the primary ions that either accumulate within or are removed from cells via various transport mechanisms in this regulatory process. If cell volume regulation relied only on inorganic electrolytes, this would lead to excessive changes in the cytoplasmic strengths of these various ions, which has been associated with protein denaturation.

Unlike electrolytes, osmolytes are a group of osmotically active molecules that can change their cell concentration without altering protein structure or function. Previously known as idiogenic osmoles, these osmolytes fall into three separate classes that include free amino acids, carbohydrates and polyhydric sugar alcohols, and methylamines. These solutes are typically low in molecular weight and are uncharged. They are characterized by their lack of interaction with surrounding proteins or other substrates at physiological concentrations. Some osmolytes even demonstrate a protective effect by countering the destabilizing effects introduced by the cellular entry of extracellular osmoles such as NaCl and urea. In the brain, osmolytes are primarily composed of amino acids such as taurine and glutamine followed then by myoinositol and betaine. Although osmolytes were previously thought to be derived from degradation of larger intracellular molecules or from the release of cell organelles, it is becoming increasingly clear that virtually all organic osmolytes are taken up from the extracellular space via specific Na^+-dependent cotransporters [32].

In response to the creation of a new osmotic gradient, cellular adaptive mechanisms in the brain begin with a change in the cytoplasmic electrolyte content. This begins within 12 h after the extracellular fluid osmolality has changed. Cerebral cell osmolyte content only begins to change after extracellular fluid osmolar changes have lasted for more than 24 h [32]. Thus, with acute changes in the plasma sodium concentration, there is no change in the levels of organic osmolytes in brain cells.

Just as maintenance of intracellular volume is critical to proper functioning, preservation of the extracellular volume is important for adequate tissue perfusion. The portion of the extracellular fluid that is present in the arteriolar vascular bed and directly perfuses tissue is referred to as the effective circulating volume (ECV). Preservation of adequate tissue perfusion is mandated by close regulation of the ECV at all times. Maintenance of the ECV is conducted via both volume regulation and osmoregulation through a number of afferent signals that result in effector responses. Because sodium is the primary extracellular solute, volume regulation of the ECV is directly mediated by changes in total body sodium balance. Osmoregulation, in contrast, is mediated by changes in water balance [34].

1.4 Volume Regulation

1.4.1 Afferent Signals

Both cardiac output and peripheral arterial vascular resistance primarily determine the adequacy of the ECV by directly affecting the integrity of the arterial vascular bed. Afferent receptors that detect changes in the elasticity of the arterioles include the cardiopulmonary baroreceptors of the carotid sinus and the aortic arch as well as renal baroreceptors of the juxtaglomerular apparatus [34]. A primary decrease in the ECV activates the cardiopulmonary baroreceptors to not only stimulate thirst and the release of ADH but also to stimulate the SNS to release norepinephrine. The renal baroreceptors respond by activating the renin–angiotensinogen–angiotensin system (RAAS). Collectively, decreased perfusion of the cardiopulmonary and renal baroreceptors results in the activation of three main vasoconstrictor systems – ADH, the SNS, and the RAAS. The converse holds true in the setting of ECV expansion.

1.4.2 Effector Response

When baroreceptors sense decreased arterial pressure, the baseline inhibition of afferent glossopharyngeal pathways to the central nervous system is decreased resulting in increased sympathetic adrenergic tone [34]. This increased sympathetic tone results in arteriolar vasoconstriction as well as increased afterload to raise the blood pressure. Additionally, when there is 5% depletion of the ECV, the nonosmotic release of ADH is stimulated to increase ECV. Finally, SNS activation also increases renal neural signaling, which stimulates the RAAS.

Activation of the RAAS ultimately results in the production of angiotensin II (AT II). AT II plays a number of physiological roles both within and outside the kidney to help restore ECV. AT II causes vascular smooth muscle contraction, which results in arteriolar vasoconstriction and increased blood pressure. AT II also increases proximal tubular sodium reabsorption and triggers aldosterone release from the adrenal glands. Aldosterone ultimately increases sodium reabsorption from the collecting tubules [19]. Thus, in the presence of AT II, both proximal and distal nephron segments are in a sodium and water avid state. The resultant salt and water retention serves to restore the ECV.

Atrial natriuretic factor (ANF) is a peptide that is produced by and localized to the cardiac atria. Its systemic release is stimulated by either a direct change in atrial wall tension or indirectly via an increase in atrial pressure. Increased circulating levels of ANF result in a natriuresis by causing a decrease in proximal tubular and distal tubular reabsorption of sodium [12].

1.5   Osmoregulation

1.5.1   Afferent Signals

Osmoreceptors in the hypothalamus are exquisitely sensitive to variations in the plasma osmolality, as little as 1–2% from the normal range (Fig. 1.2a). Upon activation, these osmoreceptors stimulate changes

to appropriately alter water intake and excretion to keep the plasma osmolality normal [27]. As a result, whereas volume regulation is determined by changes in sodium balance, osmoregulation is almost entirely mediated by changes in water balance.

In addition to osmotic stimuli, there are a number of nonosmotic stimuli that cause ADH secretion. In animal studies, a decrease of 5% in TBW stimulates ADH release, even in the presence of hypoosmolality [13] (Fig 1.2b). This means that, in cases of severe volume depletion that may adversely affect tissue perfusion, the volume regulatory system supercedes the osmoregulatory system, triggering ADH release to maintain ECV even if the plasma osmolality is low.

1.5.2   Effector Response

Upon activation of osmoreceptors, the synthesis and release of ADH is stimulated. Circulating ADH binds to V_2 receptors along the basolateral aspects of collecting tubular cells in the kidneys. V_2 receptor binding leads to the insertion of aquaporin 2 channels along the apical surface of renal collecting tubular cells. Increased water reabsorption then occurs via these inserted channels. The increase in urine osmolality is directly proportional to the amount of circulating ADH and subsequent water reabsorption (Fig. 1.3). Osmoreceptor activation is also a potent stimulus for thirst and intake of free water.

(a)

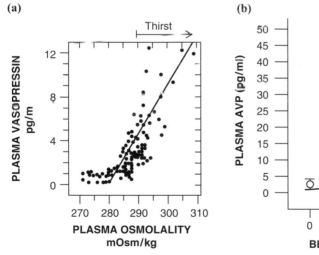

(b)

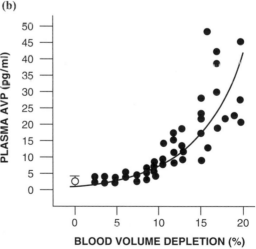

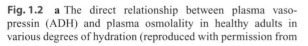

Fig. 1.2   **a** The direct relationship between plasma vasopressin (ADH) and plasma osmolality in healthy adults in various degrees of hydration (reproduced with permission from [27]). **b** Plasma vasopressin (ADH) concentration increases as the percentage of blood volume depletion begins to exceed 5% (reproduced from [13])

1.6 Diagnostic Approach to Hyponatremia

When a sample of venous blood is obtained for electrolyte analysis, it is first centrifuged to separate the cellular component from the plasma component. The plasma component consists of a layer of plasma water and a layer of plasma proteins and lipids. While in the past, sodium concentrations were generally measured in the entire plasma component using flame photometry, laboratories are now increasingly measuring the sodium concentration in only the plasma water component using ion-selective electrodes. Using the latter technique, a normal plasma sodium falls between 135 and 145 mmol L^{-1}. If the plasma sodium concentration falls below 135 mmol L^{-1}, it is important to first establish that the value is not falsely low due to a laboratory measurement technique. This can be done by checking the plasma osmolality.

1.6.1 Pseudohyponatremia

Laboratories generally measure the plasma sodium concentration as milligrams of sodium per deciliter of plasma volume but report the plasma sodium concentration as milligrams of sodium per deciliter of plasma water. This is based on the assumption that plasma volume equals plasma water. Clinical situations that can lead to a reduction in the plasma water relative to the plasma volume

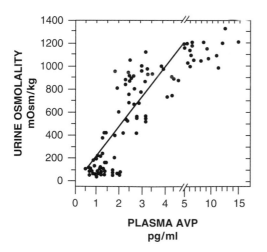

Fig. 1.3 Changes in urine osmolality are directly related to changes in the plasma vasopressin (ADH) concentration. Urine osmolality normally ranges between 50 and 1,200 mOsm kg^{-1} (reproduced with permission from [27])

include hyperproteinemia or hyperlipidemia. In these situations, if the sodium concentration is still being measured per deciliter of total plasma volume – not just per liter of plasma water – the resultant value will be falsely low [31]. Plasma osmolality, in contrast, is measured per liter of plasma water and will be normal in this scenario. In these cases, if the sodium concentration is measured per deciliter of plasma water, the plasma sodium concentration will be normal. This condition, in which the plasma sodium concentration is low but the plasma osmolality is normal, is referred to as pseudohyponatremia. Because pseudohyponatremia reflects a falsely low plasma sodium due to how it is measured in plasma components, no therapy is required for this type of hyponatremia. This illustrates the importance of obtaining a plasma osmolality in any patient with a low plasma sodium before considering any therapy, especially if the laboratory method of measuring the sodium concentration is unknown by the clinician. To avoid artifactually low plasma sodium measurements, most laboratories now use ion-selective electrodes that measure sodium concentration in only the water component of plasma (Fig. 1.4).

1.6.2 Hyponatremia with Hyperosmolality (Dilutional Effect)

If the plasma sodium concentration falls below 135 mmol L^{-1} while the plasma osmolality is increased above 290 mOsm kg^{-1}, then the presence of an effective osmole in the extracellular space should be suspected. Hyponatremia with an increased plasma osmolality is seen in the presence of any solute added to the extracellular space that is impermeable to cells. Glucose, mannitol, and maltose found in intravenous immunoglobulin are good examples of these types of solutes. Because of their cellular impermeability, when these solutes are present in the extracellular space they act as effective osmoles, causing water movement out of cells. As water leaves cells to enter the extracellular space, it causes the plasma water volume to increase and the plasma sodium concentration to decrease due to dilution.

In settings of hyperglycemia, every 100-mg dL^{-1} increase in the plasma glucose concentration is associated with a 1.6-mEq L^{-1} decrease in the plasma sodium concentration from this dilution effect. The presence of mannitol or another effective unmeasured osmole is suspected if the difference between the measured and calculated plasma osmolality

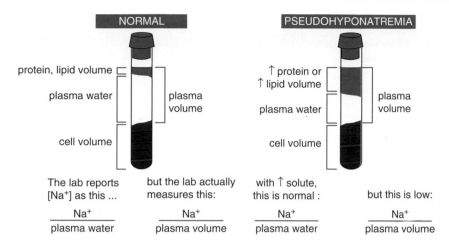

Fig. 1.4 Pseudohyponatremia is associated with a reduction in the plasma water component of the plasma volume. If the plasma sodium concentration falls below 135 mmol L^{-1} while the plasma osmolality stays in the normal range of 275–290 mOsm kg^{-1} then an increase in the size of the plasma proteins and lipid layer relative to the plasma water layer should be suspected (reproduced with permission from [31])

is greater than 10 mOsm kg^{-1} [16, 26]. In all such cases, therapy of the hyponatremia should target correction or removal of the offending solute in the extracellular space.

While uremia and the ingestion of ethanol, methanol, and ethylene glycol all lead to an increased plasma osmolality, these substances readily cross cell membranes and are, therefore, ineffective osmoles that do not lead to the translocation of water out of cells. In these cases, the plasma water volume does not increase, so the plasma sodium concentration does not change.

1.6.3 Hyponatremia with Hypoosmolality (True Hyponatremia)

If the plasma sodium concentration falls below 135 mmol L^{-1} and the plasma osmolality falls below 275 mOsm kg^{-1}, then true hyponatremia should be suspected. Interpretation of the plasma osmolality in the setting of impaired renal function must be done with caution. Individuals with renal impairment tend to have an elevated measured plasma osmolality because of their increased plasma BUN concentration. However, because urea is an ineffective osmole, the effective plasma osmolality (see (1.3)) should be determined. Individuals with renal disease who have hyponatremia and an effective plasma osmolality less than 275 mOsm kg^{-1} may be at risk for symptoms (Table 1.1).

1.7 True Hyponatremia

1.7.1 Etiology

$$\text{Plasma } [Na^+ (mmol / L)] = \frac{\text{Total body sodium (mmol)}}{\text{Total body water (L)}}$$

$$(1.4)$$

Based on (1.1), it becomes evident that hyponatremia, defined as a plasma sodium concentration less than 135 mmol L^{-1}, can only develop in one of two ways. First, if sodium-rich solute losses are replaced with relatively hypotonic fluids, total body sodium stores will slowly become depleted because they are not being adequately replenished. This will lead to a progressive decrease in the plasma sodium concentration because the numerator in (1.1) will decrease. Second, provision or retention of water in excess of sodium will lead to progressive expansion of the TBW as reflected by an increase in the denominator in (1.1). Thus, hyponatremia does not necessarily result only from total body sodium loss. Depending on the individual's TBW balance, it can actually occur in the presence of decreased, increased, or normal total body sodium (Table 1.3).

1.7.1.1 *Decreased Total Body Sodium*

Decreased ECV is associated with either a decrease in or expansion of the interstitial space. ECV depletion associated with a decrease in the interstitial

Table 1.1 Summary of the diagnostic approach to hyponatremia

	$P_{OSM} = 275–290$	$P_{OSM} > 290$	$P_{OSM} < 275$
Plasma sodium less than 135 mmol L^{-1}	Pseudohyponatremia Hyperlipidemia Hyperproteinemia	Effective osmoles Glucose Mannitol Maltose	True hyponatremia

Plasma osmolality (P_{OSM}) in mOsm kg^{-1}

Table 1.2 Electrolyte composition of body fluids

Fluid	Sodium	Electrolyte (mEq L^{-1}) Potassium	Chloride	g dL^{-1}
Gastric	20–80	5–20	100–150	–
Pancreatic	120–140	5–15	90–120	–
Small intestine	100–140	5–15	90–130	–
Bile	120–140	5–15	80–120	–
Ileostomy	45–135	3–15	20–115	–
Diarrheal	10–90	10–80	10–110	–
Sweat[a]				
Normal	10–30	3–10	10–35	–
Cystic fibrosis	50–130	5–25	50–110	–
Burns	140	5	110	3–5

Reproduced from [24]

[a] Sweat sodium concentrations progressively increase with increasing sweat flow rates

space arises from fluid losses via the gastrointestinal tract, the skin, or the kidneys that are replaced with the intake of hypotonic fluids. Pertinent aberrant gastrointestinal losses include vomiting, diarrhea, ostomy drainage, bleeding, or intestinal obstruction. Similar pathological skin losses include excess sweat from long-distance running or cystic fibrosis as well as water losses from burns.

Cardiopulmonary and renal baroreceptors sense the decreased ECV and elicit effector responses to restore the ECV. SNS and RAAS activation lead to a low absolute urine sodium concentration of <20 mmol L^{-1} and a fractional excretion of sodium of <1% as both proximal and distal nephron segments reabsorb the bulk of filtered sodium. Volume regulatory mechanisms sensing greater than a 5% deficit in TBW stimulate ADH release, even if hyponatremia and hypoosmolality are present. These individuals have concentrated urines with high urine osmolality and low daily urine volumes. The opposite urinary findings are seen with renal salt and water losses as seen with solute diuresis

secondary to diuretics, hypoaldosteronism, or renal tubulopathies.

Cerebral salt wasting is a controversial entity that is most commonly encountered in the intensive care unit setting among individuals who have sustained either central nervous system trauma or infection [30]. Increased urine output is one of the first clinical signs of this condition. The polyuria is characterized by an elevated urine sodium concentration (>20 mmol L^{-1}). The loss of urinary solutes and ECV depletion lead to an elevation in the urine osmolality. This combination of urinary findings can sometimes make it difficult to distinguish cerebral salt wasting from the syndrome of inappropriate ADH secretion (SIADH) because both conditions are associated with increased urine sodium concentration and urine osmolality. Because individuals with cerebral salt wasting have significant urinary sodium and water losses, they often appear clinically volume depleted. Those with SIADH, in contrast, actually have ECV expansion and appear clinically euvolemic. The distinction can be confirmed by central venous pressure monitoring [25]. ECV depletion stimulates the hypothalamic osmoreceptors to release ADH. Cardiopulmonary and renal baroreceptors are also activated in response to the decreased ECV. Brain natriuretic peptide, predominantly produced in the ventricles of the brain, is believed to play an important role in this entity by an as yet unclear mechanism. BNP-mediated antagonism of the effector responses elicited by the SNS, RAAS, and ADH results in the polyuria, natiuresis, and lack of thirst seen with this condition [8].

Gastrointestinal fluid losses such as vomiting and diarrhea tend to be isosmotic or equivalent to plasma in osmolality [24] (Table 1.2). Consequently, these fluid losses alone should not drop the plasma sodium concentration. However, hyponatremia will ensue in such individuals if they either drink or are administered hypotonic fluids, leading to relative water repletion when compared with solute.

Diuretic-induced hyponatremia occurs similarly via one of three mechanisms. First, diuretics-induced salt and water losses cause ECV depletion resulting in ADH release and increased thirst. Thirsty individuals will drink hypotonic fluids. In the presence of ADH, this ingested fluid will be reabsorbed by the renal collecting tubules leading to the retention of more water relative to sodium. Second, diuretic-induced urinary potassium losses lead to extracellular potassium depletion. To help restore extracellular potassium stores,

increased activity of a transcellular cation transporter will extrude intracellular potassium in exchange for extracellular sodium, leading to hyponatremia. Third, the kidneys generate less free water at the loop of Henle and distal renal tubule in the presence of either a loop diuretic or thiazide diuretic, respectively.

Interestingly, almost all cases of diuretic-induced hyponatremia are due to the thiazide – not the loop – class of diuretics. This is because, by inhibiting NaCl reabsorption in the medullary thick ascending limb of the loop of Henle, loop diuretics prevent the medullary interstitium from increasing its osmolality [10]. A hyperosmolar medullary interstitium is critical for maximal water reabsorption in the collecting tubules. As a result, individuals taking loop diuretics are unable to maximally concentrate their urine in response to ADH. In contrast, thiazide diuretics do not act in the loop of Henle so they do not directly affect the osmolality of the medullary intcrstitum and therefore do not interfere with the water reabsorption at the collecting tubule. The medullary interstitium is not disrupted in the presence of thiazide diuretics, so ingested water can be maximally reabsorbed at the collecting tubules.

Clinically, individuals with decreased total body sodium, regardless of the primary cause, present with all of the objective signs typically seen with extracellular volume depletion.

Table 1.3 Differential diagnosis of hyponatremia based on total body sodium content

Low total body sodium	High total body sodium	Normal total body sodium
GI fluid losses	Congestive heart failure	Acute renal failure
Emesis	Liver cirrhosis	ECV depletion
Diarrhea	Nephrotic syndrome	Solute diuresis
Ostomy output	Multiorgan dysfunction	SIADH
Bleeding	Pancreatitis	Adrenal insufficiency
Intestinal obstruction	Ileus	Hypothyroidism
Skin fluid losses		
Sweat		
Marathon running		
Cystic fibrosis		
Renal fluid losses		
Diuretics		
Hypoaldosteronism		
Renal tubulopathies		
Cerebral salt wasting		

1.7.1.2 Increased Total Body Sodium

Reduction in the intravascular space accompanied by expansion of the extravascular space classically arises from diseases such as congestive heart failure (CHF), cirrhosis, and nephrotic syndrome. Respectively, these conditions are associated with decreased cardiac output, peripheral vasodilatation, and decreased plasma oncotic pressure [29]. Each of these three physiological changes is associated with decreased ECV. The perceived decrease in the ECV by the cardiopulmonary and renal baroreceptors triggers afferent signals and efferent responses to increase salt and water retention to help restore the ECV. Unless the underlying problem is corrected, the ECV will remain decreased causing afferent signals to perpetuate a cycle of salt and water retention that leads to progressive expansion of the interstitial space. Similar pathophysiology is seen in ileus, multiorgan dysfunction syndrome, pancreatitis, and rhabdomyolysis where extravascular fluid sequestration occurs despite a persistently low intravascular volume.

Individuals with ECV depletion and expansion of the extravascular space are total body salt and water overloaded. They are hyponatremic because they are relatively more water than salt overloaded. Clinically, any individual with expansion of the interstitial space will present with edema.

1.7.1.3 Normal Total Body Sodium

In the vast majority of cases, hyponatremia ensues due to impaired clearance of water by the kidneys. This can develop in one of the following three clinical scenarios: (1) decreased fluid delivery to the ascending limb of the loop of Henle and the distal renal tubule, (2) excretion of an increased solute load in the urine, and (3) presence of ADH.

Decreased fluid delivery to the loop and distal nephron is seen commonly with acute renal failure when less plasma water is filtered due to overall decreased glomerular filtration. Mild to moderate decreases in the glomerular filtration rate are not associated with free water retention largely because the remaining nephrons that are functioning develop a compensatory increase in their solute and water excretion. However, severe decreases in the glomerular filtration rate below 15% of normal are associated with progressive solute and fluid retention. Volume depletion also results in less fluid delivery to distal nephron segments due to decreased glomerular filtration of plasma water with concomitantly increased water reabsorption in proximal nephron segments.

Renal free water excretion is impaired in any clinical situation where ADH release is stimulated. Once hyponatremia develops, osmoreceptor deactivation normally leads to inhibition of ADH synthesis and release, resulting in decreased water reabsorption in the collecting tubules. ADH suppression begins when plasma osmolality falls below 275 mOsm kg^{-1}. ADH suppression is complete once the serum osmolality falls below 270 mOsm kg^{-1}. The urine osmolality will decrease in a dose-dependent fashion based on how much ADH release is inhibited [13]. Those patients who have an inability to appropriately suppress ADH release in response to hypoosmolality become progressively hyponatremic.

The syndrome of inappropriate secretion of ADH (SIADH) results from a variety of causes that stimulate the nonphysiological release of ADH. Normally, in the presence of ADH, the renal collecting tubules increase water reabsorption to create an initial hyponatremia and ECV expansion. Once the ECV is expanded, the cardiopulmonary receptors are stimulated to release ANP and suppress the SNS. The renal baroreceptors are also stimulated to suppress the RAAS. Collectively, the afferent signals' responses to ECV expansion result in increased urinary sodium and water losses. With restoration of the ECV, plasma osmolality also normalizes, which should also result in ADH suppression.

In SIADH, however, circulating ADH is not suppressed despite an adequate or restored ECV. Nonosmotic stimuli associated with inappropriate ADH release include central nervous system diseases, lower respiratory tract illnesses, malignancies, physical pain, emotional stress, hypoxia, and a large number of medications (Fig. 1.5).

Overall, SIADH is clinically characterized by the following:

1. Hyponatremia (plasma [Na$^+$] < 135 mmol L^{-1})
2. Hypoosmolality (plasma osmolality < 275 mOsm kg^{-1})
3. Inappropriately elevated urine osmolality (>100 mOsm kg^{-1})
4. Clinical euvolemia or volume expansion
5. Normal kidney, adrenal, and thyroid function
6. Normal acid–base balance
7. Normal potassium balance
8. Hypouricemia from volume expansion and resultant decreased proximal tubular sodium and urate reabsorption
9. Elevated urine sodium concentration (>20 mmol L^{-1})

Malignant Diseases	Pulmonary Disorders	Disorders of the Central Nervours System	Drugs	Other Causes
Carcinoma	Infections	Infection	Drugs that stimulate release of AVP or enhance its action	Hereditary (gain-of-function mutations in the vaso-press inV$_2$ receptor)
Lung	Bacterial prieumonia	Encephalitis	Chlorpropramide	
Small-cell	Viral pneumonia	Meningitis	SSRIs	Idiopathic
Mesothelioma	Pulmonary abscess	Brain abscess	Tricyclic antidepressants	Transient
Orophary rix	Tuberculosis	Rocky mountain spotted fever	clofibrate (Atromid-s, Wyeth-Ayerst)	Endurance exercise
Gastrointestinal tract	Aspergillosis	AIDS	Carbamazepine (Epitol, Lemmon: Tegretol, Gba-Geigy)	General anesthesia
Stomach	Asthma	Bleeding and masses	Vincristine (Oncovin, Lilly: Vincasar, Pharmacia and Upjohn)	Nausea
Duodenum	Cystic fibrosis	Subdural hematoma		Pain
Pancreas	Respiratory failure associat-ed with positive-pres-sure breathing	Subarachnoid hemorrhage	Nicotine	Stress
Genitourinary tract		Cerebrovascular accident	Narcotics	
Ureter		Brain tumors	Antipsychotic drugs	
Bladder		Head trauma	Ifosfamide (Ifex, Bristol-Myers Squibb)	
Prostate		Hydrocephalus	Cyclophosphamide (Cytoxan, Bristol-Myers Squibb; Neosar, Pharmacia and Upjohn)	
Endometrium		Cavernous sinus thrombosis		
Endocrine thymoma		Other	Nonsteroidal antiinflammatory drugs	
Lymphomas		Multiple sclerosis	MDMA ("ecstasy")	
Sarcomas		Guillain-Barré syndrome	AVP analogues	
Ewing's sarcoma		Shy-Drager syndrome	Desmopressin (DDAVP, Rhone-Poulenc Rorer, Stimate, Centeon)	
		Delirium tremens		
		Acute intermittent porphyria	Oxytocin (Pitocin, Parke-Davis; Syntocinon, Novartis) Vasopressin	

AIDS denotes the acquired immunodeficiency syndrome, AVP arginine vasopressin, SSRI selective in-reuptake inhibitor, and MDMA 3,4-methylenedioxymethamphetamine.

Fig. 1.5 Non-osmotic stimuli associated with SIADH (reproduced from [14])

Although less common clinically than SIADH, certain endocrine anomalies can potentiate hyponatremia. For instance, adrenal insufficiency plays a multifactorial role in causing hyponatremia. First, the mineralocorticoid deficiency prevents sodium reabsorption in the renal collecting tubule. This leads to increased urinary salt and water losses. The ensuing ECV depletion triggers ADH release. Second, cortisol normally inhibits ADH release from the hypothalamus. With cortisol deficiency, this negative feedback loop is not working, resulting in unregulated ADH release [36].

Hypothyroidism leads to hyponatremia through unclear mechanisms. Decreased cardiac output leading to increased ADH release and decreased GFR – both mediating water retention – are suspected to play causative roles [34].

Individuals with normal total body sodium who develop hyponatremia as a result of relative water excess tend to appear clinically euvolemic. This is because the excess water is distributed into all body compartments, of which the intravascular space represents the smallest portion.

1.7.2 Signs and Symptoms

Hypoosmolality of the extracellular fluid results in the movement of water from the extracellular to the intracellular space. Because of the brain's limited capacity to tolerate fluctuations in cell volume, intracellular water movement in neurons is particularly responsible for the signs and symptoms seen with hyponatremia [33].

The severity of symptoms directly correlates with the degree of intracellular overhydration. The osmolar gradient between neurons and the extracellular fluid across the blood-brain barrier triggers water movement from the extracellular space into the neurons.

With increased water movement into the cells, the intracellular osmolality decreases. Cells then begin to extrude solutes out of the intracellular space as they attempt to reequilibrate their osmolality with that of the extracellular space. Initially, cells adapt by losing intracellular potassium and sodium via membrane channels. This occurs within minutes. Later, within hours to days, osmolytes are lost. While there is greater quantitative intracellular loss of cations such as potassium and sodium in this process, there is a much higher percentage of osmolyte loss. It appears that the severity of the hyponatremia is directly related to the degree of osmolyte loss [33]. Because the cellular adaptation to changes in extracellular osmolality takes hours to days, severe neurological symptoms can result from cellular overhydration depending on the rapidity and severity in the reduction of the plasma sodium concentration. Conversely, if hyponatremia develops slowly over a prolonged period of time, minimal symptoms are present.

Symptoms begin to develop with sequential reductions in the plasma sodium concentration. As the concentration acutely falls below 125 mmol L^{-1}, individuals begin to complain of nausea, vomiting, fever, labored respirations, and malaise. Once the concentration is between 115 and 120 mmol L^{-1}, individuals tend to develop headache, altered mental status, restlessness, lethargy, ataxia, pyschosis, weakness, cramps, and obtundation. Once the concentration falls below 110–115 mmol L^{-1}, seizures and coma are usually seen. Signs of severe cerebral edema include seizures, coma, respiratory depression, and even death [10].

1.7.3 Treatment

How rapidly the clinician should correct the hyponatremia depends largely on the duration of hyponatremia, the presence of symptoms, and the presence of preexisting risk factors for neurologic damage. Acute hyponatremia is characterized by a change in the plasma sodium concentration within 48 hours. Hyponatremia is deemed chronic if it develops over greater than a 48-h period. If the duration of the sodium balance is difficult to establish, it is prudent to assume that the hyponatremia is chronic vs acute when formulating management decisions. Those patients who appear greatest at risk for cerebral edema include children [23], postoperative menstruating females [5], elderly females particularly those taking thiazide diuretics [11], individuals with primary polydipsia [17], and those with hypoxemic injury.

Acute, symptomatic hyponatremia can more aggressively be treated. With an acute reduction in the plasma sodium concentration, brain cell volume regulatory mechanisms have not yet been activated, so cerebral swelling will occur due to water movement into the cells. There is a resultant increase in the risk of neurological sequelae if the sodium imbalance is not rapidly corrected. Experimental studies have demonstrated that rapid correction of the plasma sodium up to 130 mmol L^{-1} within 12–24 h in this context is safe [33]. Calculation of the total body sodium deficit is done as follows:

$$[\text{Desired plasma sodium (mmol/L)} - \text{current plasma sodium (mmol/L)}] \times \text{weight (kg)} \times k.$$

The plasma sodium is expressed in millimoles per liter, and weight is expressed in kilograms (kg). The constant, k, refers to the percentage of body weight that equals TBW. This value is 0.7 in term neonates, 0.65 in younger children, and 0.6 in older or pubertal children (see Sect. 1.2). The result equals the total millimoles of sodium that must be provided to the individual to raise their plasma sodium concentration to the desired value. The sodium deficit can be provided either as oral sodium salt supplementation or as an intravenous solution.

Hypertonic saline should only be administered to those individuals with symptomatic hyponatremia to rapidly reverse the clinical sequelae of cerebral edema. Hypertonic saline should be given judiciously until the individual becomes asymptomatic. Generally, this can be accomplished by increasing the serum sodium to 5 mEq L^{-1}. The risk of developing brain cell shrinkage with rapid correction is low because, without activation of cell volume regulatory mechanisms in acute hyponatremia, the cerebral osmolyte content is still at normal levels.

A loop diuretic such as furosemide can be given concurrently to promote greater free-water excretion if the cause of the hyponatremia is due to relative TBW excess. Hyponatremia will typically not be corrected unless the sum of the urinary sodium and potassium concentrations is less than the plasma sodium concentration. Other means with which increased free-water excretion can be achieved include water restriction, use of vasopressin receptor antagonists, and provision of an increased solute load.

In individuals with chronic asymptomatic hyponatremia, rapid correction of the plasma sodium is unnecessary regardless of how low the plasma concentration. In chronic hyponatremia, brain volume is ultimately restored as electrolytes and osmolytes are extruded from neurons in their attempt to regulate their cell volume. It is in this context of chronically low brain osmolyte concentration from chronic cerebral adaptation that the risk for the osmotic demyelinating syndrome is greatest if the sodium imbalance is corrected too rapidly. Those individuals suffering from alcoholism, malnutrition, and burns seem to be most vulnerable to developing this complication.

The osmotic demyelinating syndrome is characterized by a lucid period followed in 12–24 h by altered mental status, altered motor function, flaccid quadriplegia, cranial nerve abnormalities, and loss of consciousness. These clinical findings are associated with demyelinating lesions found in the pons, basal ganglia, thalamus, and internal capsule [33]. Whether the degree of hyponatremia or the rate of correction of hyponatremia is the true causative factor remains an area of controversy. In an experimental model of hyponatremia induced in rats, rapid correction of hyponatremia led to a 32% mortality.

No rats died with a correction of sodium of 1 mmol L^{-1} h^{-1}. Virtually all other similar experimental animal models demonstrate an increased incidence of neuropathological sequelae and mortality if hyponatremia is corrected faster than 0.8 mmol L^{-1} h^{-1} [3, 6, 20, 33, 35]. A precise rate of sodium correction has been difficult to unequivocally establish [1, 2, 4, 22, 33]. As a result, a cautious approach commonly used involves increasing the plasma sodium concentration by no more than 0.5 mmol L^{-1} h^{-1} or by no more than 12 mmol L^{-1} day^{-1}.

The cornerstone to management of hyponatremia should ideally focus on correction of the underlying cause. Gastrointestinal, skin, and renal losses should all be adequately replaced to restore the ECV. Diuretics and other offending agents should be dose adjusted or discontinued until the plasma sodium concentration normalizes. Hypoaldosteronism and hypothyroidism should be medically treated. Those with SIADH should be water restricted to approximately 2/3 of their daily maintenance fluid needs. Fluid restriction, alone, is usually sufficient to correct the plasma sodium in SIADH. If the hyponatremia persists, either furosemide or demeclocycline may be given to promote greater water excretion by the kidneys. Cerebral salt wasting should be treated with NaCl and water provision to restore the ECV and to keep up with ongoing urinary salt and water losses. Identification and correction of the underlying cause of the cerebral salt wasting should also be addressed.

1.8 Hypernatremia

1.8.1 Etiology

Hypernatremia is defined as a plasma sodium concentration greater than 145 mmol L^{-1}. Hypernatremia is similar to hyponatremia in that it can occur in the presence of decreased, increased, or normal total body sodium. Increases in the plasma sodium concentration reflect either a relative increase in total body sodium or a relative decrease in TBW.

1.8.1.1 Decreased Total Body Sodium

Gastrointestinal losses such as vomiting, diarrhea, and ostomy drainage as well as skin losses such as sweat from marathon running or cystic fibrosis can all lead to hypernatremia if water losses exceed sodium losses. Renal causes include excess water losses via an osmotic diuresis. Finally, individuals with limited renal concentrating ability such as infants will have increased renal water losses in the presence of high solute loads. The hypernatremia in all of these clinical scenarios will persist if the excess water losses are not adequately replaced.

1.8.1.2 Increased Total Body Sodium

Total body sodium increases with the inadvertent ingestion or iatrogenic administration of a salt load. The former has been reported when well-meaning parents administered improperly diluted formula to their infants. The latter has been reported in hospital settings when repeated infusions of sodium bicarbonate were used in cardiopulmonary resuscitation or in the treatment of refractory metabolic acidosis. Individuals admitted after a near-drowning incident in sea water often also present with hypernatremia from ingestion of salt water.

1.8.1.3 Normal Total Body Sodium

Excess free water losses relative to sodium result in hypernatremia. In the basal state, water intake must match water output. Daily water intake not only includes water consumed exogenously from dietary fluids or water containing solids but also water produced endogenously from oxidative metabolism of dietary carbohydrates, fats, and proteins [10].

Daily water output can be divided into insensible and sensible losses. Insensible losses refer to evaporative water losses from the moist surfaces of the skin and respiratory tract. Daily body metabolism generates both water and heat. The heat must be eliminated on a daily basis to prevent the development of hyperthermia [10]. Evaporative water losses play an important role in thermoregulation via radiation and convection. Collectively, insensible losses are electrolyte-free.

Hypernatremic dehydration develops from increased insensible losses that are not adequately replaced. This includes any clinical situation where evaporative water losses from the skin and respiratory tract are increased. Examples include the presence of fever, prematurity where there is often use of phototherapy or radiant warmers, tachypnea, hyperventilation, or the use of mechanical ventilation without sufficient humidified air.

An acute elevation in the plasma sodium concentration is associated with an increase in the plasma osmolality, which will activate the hypothalamic osmoreceptors to release ADH and stimulate thirst in an attempt to normalize the plasma osmolality. Hypernatremia is unusual among individuals who are cognitively intact, capable of becoming thirsty, and are physically able to obtain water or other fluids to satisfy their thirst. As a result, hypernatremia is often seen at both ends of the age spectrum, namely in infancy or small children and in geriatrics. Additionally, cognitively impaired or neurologically devastated patients who are unable to communicate their thirst are also more likely to develop iatrogenic hypernatremia unless their fluid management is not closely monitored (Table 1.4).

Individuals who are unable to release ADH or stimulate thirst in response to increases in plasma sodium concentration are also more likely to develop significant hypernatremia. Classically, this is seen with central diabetes insipidus. Similar abnormalities will develop in nephrogenic diabetes insipidus where circulating ADH is not appropriately sensed or responded to by the kidneys. Both forms of diabetes insipidus can have either congenital or acquired causes [7] (Table 1.5).

1.8.2 Signs and Symptoms

If the duration of hypernatremia is less than 4–8 h, mechanisms for cell volume regulation are not stimulated. In the absence of cellular adaptation, brain cells will diminish in size as water moves out of cells into the extracellular space. Animal studies demonstrate that cerebral hemorrhage occurs when brain cells shrink from acute, untreated hypernatremia. The brain is tethered to the overlying bony skull by membranes that contain blood vessels. Brain cell shrinkage is associated with rupture of these blood vessels that connect the brain to the dura mater. Capillary and venous congestion as well as subarachnoid bleeding with venous sinus thrombosis have been reported. Clinically, these structural changes manifest in animals as poor feeding, irritability, seizure activity, and abnormal limb movements. Infants with acute elevations in their plasma sodium concentration commonly develop emesis, fever, respiratory distress, tonic–clonic seizure activity, spasticity, and coma [33]. In cases of acute hypernatremic dehydration, because water is moving from the intracellular to the extracellular space, the volume of the extracellular space is relatively well preserved, delaying the appearance of objective signs of ECV depletion that clinicians often use to assess effective volume depletion.

1.8.3 Treatment

During correction of hypernatremia, there appears to be a lag between correction of the serum sodium concentration and normalization of the brain osmolyte content. In the presence of a compensatory increase in the brain osmolyte content, rapid correction of the hyperosmolality will lead to cerebral edema and associated neurological symptoms. This potential complication forms the theoretical basis for fluid management in affected individuals.

Table 1.4 Differential diagnosis of hypernatremia based on total body sodium content

Low total body sodium	High total body sodium	Normal total body sodi
GI fluid losses	Inadvertent ingestion	Insensible losses
Emesis	Infant formula	Skin
Diarrhea	Salt water drowning	Fever
Ostomy output	Iatrogenic administration	Prematurity
Skin fluid losses	CPR	Phototherapy
Sweat	Metabolic acidosis	Radiant warmers
Marathon running		Respiratory
Cystic fibrosis		Tachypnea
Osmotic diuresis		Hyperventilation
Glucose		Mechanical vent
Mannitol		Without humidified
Immature renal concentrating ability		Air
Infants		

Table 1.5 Congenital and acquired causes of central and nephrogenic diabetes insipidus

Central DI	Nephrogenic Di
Familial	Familial
Autosomal dominant	X linked recessive
Cerebral malformations	V_2 receptor gene defect
Septo-optic dysplasia	Autosomal recessive
Lawrence-Moon-Beidl syndrome	Aquaporin 2 gene defect
Acquired	Acquired
Trauma	Osmotic diuresis
Head injury	Metabolic
Neurosurgery	Hypercalcemia
Tumors	Hyperkalemia
Craniopharyngioma	Chronic renal disease
Germinoma	Drugs
Optic glioma	Lithium
Hypoxic/ischemic brain injury	Demeclocycline
Lymphocytic neurohypophysitis	Postobstructive uropathy
Granuloma	Renal medullary solute washout
Tuberculosis	
Sarcoidosis	
Histiocytosis	
Infections	
Congenital cytomegalovirus	
Congenital toxoplasmosis	
Encephalitis	
Meningitis	
Vascular	
Aneurysm	
Arteriovenous malformation	

Adapted form [7]

In cases of hypernatremic dehydration with hemodynamic instability, restoration of the ECV with isotonic saline to restore perfusion of vital organs is the first priority. Once hemodynamic stability is restored, subsequent correction of the hypernatremia should involve provision of hypotonic fluids to allow restoration of the free-water deficit judiciously. While the actual rate of correction remains an area of debate, data from most studies suggest that correction should take place over at least 48 h to minimize complications of cerebral edema [10, 15]. Calculation of the free-water deficit can be done as follows:

$$\text{Current plasma sodium (mmol / L)} = \frac{\text{Desired plasma sodium (mmol / L)}}{\text{New total body water}}$$

Equation (1.5) should be solved for the new TBW. This value should be subtracted from the individual's current TBW, which equals 50–70% of their body weight in kilograms depending on the size of the individual (see Sect. 1.2). The difference between the new and the current TBW represents the free-water deficit in liters. This volume of water should be provided to the individual over 48 h to provide a plasma sodium concentration reduction rate of 0.5 mmol L^{-1} h^{-1} or no more than 12 mmol L^{-1} day^{-1} [9, 21, 34].

Cases of hypernatremia from salt loading should be treated by facilitating removal of the excess total body sodium. This is typically achieved with a combination of diuretics and dietary salt restriction. Again, correction must proceed carefully in the setting of chronic hypernatremia and reassessment of serum electrolytes, urine chemistries, and findings on physical examination must be done at regular intervals.

References

1. Arieff, A.I., Hyponatremia, convulsions, respiratory arrest, and permanent brain damage after elective surgery in healthy women. N Engl J Med, 1986. **314**(24): p. 1529–35
2. Ayus, J.C., J.J. Olivero, and J.P. Frommer, Rapid correction of severe hyponatremia with intravenous hypertonic saline solution. Am J Med, 1982. **72**(1): p. 43–8
3. Ayus, J.C., R.K. Krothapalli, and D.L. Armstrong, Rapid correction of severe hyponatremia in the rat: histopathological changes in the brain. Am J Physiol, 1985. **248**(5, Part 2): p. F711–F719
4. Ayus, J.C., R.K. Krothapalli, and A.I. Arieff, Treatment of symptomatic hyponatremia and its relation to brain damage. A prospective study. N Engl J Med, 1987. **317**(19): p. 1190–5
5. Ayus, J.C., J.M. Wheeler, and A.I. Arieff, Postoperative hyponatremic encephalopathy in menstruant women. Ann Intern Med, 1992. **117**(11): p. 891–7
6. Ayus, J.C., et al., Symptomatic hyponatremia in rats: effect of treatment on mortality and brain lesions. Am J Physiol, 1989. **257**(1, Part 2): p. F18–F22
7. Baylis, P.H. and T. Cheetham, Diabetes insipidus. Arch Dis Child, 1998. **79**(1): p. 84–9
8. Berendes, E., et al., Secretion of brain natriuretic peptide in patients with aneurysmal subarachnoid haemorrhage. Lancet, 1997. **349**(9047): p. 245–9
9. Blum, D., et al., Safe oral rehydration of hypertonic dehydration. J Pediatr Gastroenterol Nutr, 1986. **5**(2): p. 232–5
10. Rose, B.D., Post, T., Rose, B., Clinical Physiology of Acid–Base and Electrolyte Disorders, Fifth Edition, 2001. New York: McGraw-Hill, p. 961
11. Chow, K.M., Kwan, B.C., and Szeto, C.C., Clinical studies of thiazide-induced hyponatremia. J Natl Med Assoc, 2004. **96**(10): p. 1305–8
12. de Zeeuw, D, Janssen, W.M., and de Jong, P.E., Atrial natriuretic factor: its (patho)physiological significance in humans. Kidney Int, 1992. **41**(5): p. 1115–33
13. Dunn, F.L., et al., The role of blood osmolality and volume in regulating vasopressin secretion in the rat. J Clin Invest, 1973. **52**(12): p. 3212–9
14. Ellison, D.H. Berl, T. Clinical Practice. The syndrome of inappropriate antidiuresis. NEJM, 2007. **356**(20): p. 2064–72
15. Feig, P.U. and McCurdy, D.K., The hypertonic state. N Engl J Med, 1977. **297**(26): p. 1444–54
16. Gennari, F.J., Current concepts. Serum osmolality. Uses and limitations. N Engl J Med, 1984. **310**(2): p. 102–5
17. Goldman, M.B., Luchins, D.J., and Robertson, G.L., Mechanisms of altered water metabolism in psychotic patients with polydipsia and hyponatremia. N Engl J Med, 1988. **318**(7): p. 397–403
18. Haschke, F., Body Composition Measurements in Infants and Children, 1989. Columbus: W.J. Klish & N. Kretchmer
19. Ichikawi, I. and Harris, R.C., Angiotensin actions in the kidney: renewed insight into the old hormone. Kidney Int, 1991. **40**(4): p. 583–96
20. Illowsky, B.P. and Laureno, R., Encephalopathy and myelinolysis after rapid correction of hyponatraemia. Brain, 1987. **110**(Part 4): p. 855–67
21. Kahn, A., Brachet, E., and Blum, D., Controlled fall in natremia and risk of seizures in hypertonic dehydration. Intensive Care Med, 1979. **5**(1): p. 27–31
22. Laureno, R. and Karp, B.I., Pontine and extrapontine myelinolysis following rapid correction of hyponatraemia. Lancet, 1988. **1**(8600): p. 1439–41
23. Moritz, M.L. and Ayus, J.C., The pathophysiology and treatment of hyponatraemic encephalopathy: an update. Nephrol Dial Transplant, 2003. **18**(12): p. 2486–91
24. Nelson, W.E. and Vaughan, V.C., III, Textbook of Pediatrics, 14th Edition, 1992. Philadelphia: W.B. Saunders
25. Palmer, B.F., Hyponatremia in patients with central nervous system disease: SIADH versus CSW. Trends Endocrinol Metab, 2003. **14**(4): p. 182–7
26. Pickett, W.J., III, et al., Measurement of plasma osmolality. N Engl J Med, 1971. **285**(6): p. 354–5
27. Robertson, G.L., Aycinena, P., and Zerbe, R.L., Neurogenic disorders of osmoregulation. Am J Med, 1982. **72**(2): p. 339–53
28. Ruth, J.L. and Wassner, S.J., Body composition: salt and water. Pediatr Rev, 2006. **27**(5): p. 181–7; quiz 188
29. Schrier, R.W., Pathogenesis of sodium and water retention in high-output and low-output cardiac failure, nephrotic syndrome, cirrhosis, and pregnancy (2). N Engl J Med, 1988. **319**(17): p. 1127–34
30. Sherlock, M., et al., The incidence and pathophysiology of hyponatraemia after subarachnoid haemorrhage. Clin Endocrinol, 2006. **64**(3): p. 250–4
31. Topf, J., Faubel, S., The Fluid, Electrolyte, and Acid–Base Companion, 1999. San Diego: Alert and Oriented, p. 591

32. Trachtman, H., Cell volume regulation: a review of cerebral adaptive mechanisms and implications for clinical treatment of osmolal disturbances. I. Pediatr Nephrol, 1991. **5**(6): p. 743–50

33. Trachtman, H., Cell volume regulation: a review of cerebral adaptive mechanisms and implications for clinical treatment of osmolal disturbances. II. Pediatr Nephrol, 1992. **6**(1): p. 104–12

34. Trachtman, H., Sodium and water homeostasis. Pediatr Clin North Am, 1995. **42**(6): p. 1343–63

35. Verbalis, J.G. and Martinez, A.J., Neurological and neuropathological sequelae of correction of chronic hyponatremia. Kidney Int, 1991. **39**(6): p. 1274–82

36. Zimmerman, E.A., Ma, L.Y., and Nilaver, G., Anatomical basis of thirst and vasopressin secretion. Kidney Int Suppl, 1987. **21**: p. S14–S19

Disorders of the Acid–Base Status

2

E. Al-Khadra

Contents

Core Messages

> Essentially all pediatric disorders, if severe enough, can lead to acid–base disturbances directly, as a result of therapy, or both.

> Acid–base disorders need to be anticipated in all critically ill patients. Proactive monitoring of the acid–base status will allow the early recognition of derangements and the prevention of what could become a life-threatening state.

> Acidosis is the most common acid–base derangement in the intensive care unit (ICU), with metabolic acidosis potentially indicating a more severe course and worse outcome.

> A pH of <7.2 merely indicates a primary acidosis-inducing disorder. Further assessment of the type of acidosis and the presence of a mixed acid–base disorder requires measurement of pCO_2, serum bicarbonate, albumin, and calculation of the anion gap.

> The most commonly encountered causes of metabolic acidoses in the ICU are renal insufficiency, sepsis, and DKA, while acute respiratory distress syndrome (ARDS) and severe status asthmaticus are the *usual suspects* in respiratory acidoses.

> Alkalosis, on the other hand, is less common in the ICU. Fluid status derangements and, especially, gastric fluid depletion are the usual underlying causes of metabolic alkaloses, whereas rapid respiration secondary to lung diseases, excessive mechanical ventilation, pain, or central nervous system processes are the common causes of respiratory alkaloses.

> In the ICU, identification of acid–base derangements is followed by timely stabilization of the patient irrespective of the underlying cause. Depending on the severity of the derangement and the patient's response to the stabilizing interventions, the underlying cause might also need to be aggressively sought and emergently reversed.

> Identification of the underlying cause(s) of the acid–base disorder at hand may be the final step in the management of these patients, but plays an important role both in the prevention of worsening of the derangement and other complications as well as in the determination of the patient's overall prognosis.

S.G. Kiessling et al. (eds) *Pediatric Nephrology in the ICU.*
© Springer-Verlag Berlin Heidelberg 2009

Case Vignette 1

An 11-year-old girl with a history of mild bronchial asthma presented with fever and increased work of breathing refractory to repeated albuterol treatments at her pediatrician's office. Status asthmaticus was diagnosed, and an ABG was obtained upon arrival to the emergency room, showing a pH of 7.22, a pCO_2 of 38 mmHg, and a serum bicarbonate level of 15 meq L^{-1}. Her serum sodium and chloride were 141 and 110 meq L^{-1}, respectively; her serum lactate concentration was 11 mmol L^{-1}, and her serum albumin level was 1 g dL^{-1}. What is your interpretation of her ABG?

The ABG is consistent with acidosis, given the low pH of 7.22. The bicarbonate level is low at 15 meq L^{-1} whereas pCO_2 is almost normal, rendering the primary disorder a metabolic acidosis. Following the rule of 1:1 compensation, pCO_2 would be expected to be 30–32. Thus, this patient also has an element of pCO_2 retention and thus a mixed acid–base disorder, namely primary metabolic acidosis and acute respiratory acidosis. The metabolic component is secondary to an AG acidosis, with the AG measuring 16 prior to the required adjustment as follows:

Corrected albumin (4 g dL^{-1} expected – 1 g dL^{-1} observed) of $3 \times 2.5 = 7.5$. Hence, adjusted AG 16 measured + 7.5 = 23 with a delta/delta of 1, indicating no other underlying type of metabolic acidosis. Treatment to target lower airway obstruction with bronchodilators and steroids will assist in resolving both the respiratory and the metabolic defect. The latter will also be alleviated with judicious use of hydration. Lastly, the cause of severe hypoalbuminemia needs to be sought.

Case Vignette 2

A 2-year-old child was found unconscious and with increased work of breathing. An ABG showed a pH of 7.38, a pCO_2 of 28 mmHg, and a serum bicarbonate of 16 meq L^{-1}. What is your interpretation?

This is a typical ABG of a patient with salicylate poisoning. Depending on further clinical and laboratory evaluations, this patient might need intubation, gastric lavage, dialysis, or simple hydration and supportive care.

Acid–base disorders are among the most commonly encountered medical problems in critically ill patients. Departure of blood acidity from the normal range can result in a spectrum of adverse consequences and, when severe, can be life-threatening. Identifying acid–base derangements, correcting the pH, and arriving at the correct underlying cause for each derangement are of paramount importance for caring for patients in the intensive care unit. This chapter will address physiology of acid–base status, interpretation of blood gas measurements, common causes of derangements, and approach to reestablishing normalcy.

2.1 Introduction

The human organs and tissues function under a tightly controlled pH in the range of 7.35–7.45. Depending on the degree of the deviation of pH outside this narrow range, several homeostatic responses are activated in an effort to restore normal acid–base status. Initially, reactions by chemical buffers will attempt to neutralize the derangement, followed by ventilatory adjustments by the lungs and, finally, alterations in acid excretion by the kidneys.

Several factors impact the prognosis of patients with acid–base disturbances:

1. Severity of acidemia or alkalemia.
2. Acuity and duration of the derangement.
3. Functional status of the lungs and kidneys.
4. Underlying cause: This factor is what ultimately defines the patient's outcome.

A plasma pH of 7.10 can be inconsequential when caused by diabetic ketoacidosis, but it portends a poorer outcome if it is secondary to septic shock and poor organ perfusion. Likewise, a plasma pH of 7.60 caused by anxiety-hyperventilation syndrome is inconsequential, whereas it signals a worse prognosis if it is secondary to a brain tumor.

To manage patients with serious acid–base disturbances appropriately, accurate history taking, precise interpretation of blood gas results, and arriving at the correct cause underlying the disorder are critical. Even though our management in the ICU is centered on stabilizing patients' cardiopulmonary status and correcting derangements, including acid–base disorders, knowing the underlying etiology of these disturbances and addressing it with the proper interventions, if deemed necessary, can expedite a patient's recovery and reverse the pathologic process.

2.2 Physiology of Acid–Base Balance

Hydrogen ion (H^+) is much more precisely regulated in the extracellular fluid in order to achieve a concentration of $0.00004\,meq\,L^{-1}$ ($40\,neq\,L^{-1}$) compared with sodium, for example, which is maintained at $135–145\,meq\,L^{-1}$. This precision with which H^+ is regulated emphasizes this ion's critical impact on cellular unctions.

By definition, an acid is a substance that has at least one H^+ and can donate H^+ ions when in a solution, and a base is a substance that can accept H^+ ions [65]. A strong acid rapidly dissociates and releases large amounts of H^+, such as hydrochloric acid, whereas a weak acid, such as carbonic acid, releases H^+ with less vigor. Similarly, hydroxides are strong bases, while bicarbonate (HCO_3^-), phosphate, and proteins are weak bases. Most acids and bases in the extracellular space are weak, but they constitute the body's principal buffers.

The two classes of physiologically produced acids are volatile acids, also known as carbonic acid (H_2CO_3), and fixed acids, also known as noncarbonic acids. The metabolism of carbohydrates and fats generates approximately $10{,}000–15{,}000\,meq$ of CO_2 daily (~$300\,meq$ of $CO_2\,kg^{-1}\,day^{-1}$), which in turn results in increased carbonic acid. The lung is the main organ charged with the elimination of volatile acids. The metabolism of proteins, on the other hand, generates fixed acids. Approximately $100\,meq$ of fixed acids are generated daily from ingestion and metabolism (~$1–2\,meq\,kg^{-1}\,day^{-1}$) [48]. The kidneys are the only organs capable of eliminating fixed acids through excretion in the urine. The resulting extracellular level of H^+ is approximately $40\,neq\,L^{-1}$ ($30–60\,neq\,L^{-1}$). As a result of this disproportionate degree of production of volatile acids compared with fixed acids, the lung plays a profound role in acid base status. Acute respiratory failure and inability to eliminate CO_2 as a result of airway obstruction or severe ARDS would result in a significant rise of pCO_2 and corresponding drop in pH that would overwhelm the cellular buffers and the kidneys' acute compensatory capabilities. On the other hand, acute renal failure and consequent inability to eliminate fixed acids, in the absence of pathological sources of noncarbonic acids, would result in a much milder and less acute derangement.

2.2.1   Henderson–Hasselbalch Equation

The pH of a solution is the negative logarithm of H^+ concentration as defined by

$$pH = -\log\,[H^+].$$

As CO_2 dissolves in a solution, it dissociates into carbonic acid following the Henderson–Hasselbalch equation:

$$H_2CO_3 <\Rightarrow H^+ + HCO_3^-.$$

The dissociation constant of carbonic acid follows the law of mass action and is as follows:

$$Ka = [H^+] \times [HCO_3^-]/[H_2CO_3]$$

Given that the concentration of H_2CO_3 is proportional to that of dissolved CO_2

$$Ka = [H^+] \times [HCO_3^-]/[CO_2$$

After logarithmic transformation into $\log Ka = \log [H^+] + \log[HCO_3^-]/[CO_2]$ and rearrangement into $-\log [H^+] = -\log Ka + \log[HCO_3^-]/[CO_2]$, it follows that

$$pH = pKa + \log[base]/[acid],$$

given that pH is the negative logarithm of H^+ concentration.

Normal acid–base status is maintained by the pulmonary excretion of carbonic acids and by the renal excretion of noncarbonic, fixed acids, and formation of bicarbonate. Hence, the last equation could be envisioned to be as follows: pH is proportionate to kidney $[HCO_3^-]$ over pulmonary $[pCO_2]$. Therefore, pH increases with increasing HCO_3^-, the numerator, and declines with increasing levels of pCO_2, the denominator.

2.2.2   Homeostatic Resposnses

Once derangement occurs, H^+ concentration is corrected in a timely and stepwise approach starting with chemical buffers, followed by pulmonary ventilation and finally renal control of acid–base excretion.

2.2.2.1   Chemical Acid–Base Buffers

Chemical buffers are available in both extracellular and intracellular compartments. They respond within minutes to neutralize derangements. Chemical buffers are naturally occurring weak acids and bases. They impart their correction on systemic pH by converting strong acids or bases into weak acids or bases, thus minimizing alterations in pH.

There are three buffering systems that are recognized:

1. The bicarbonate system constituted of plasma sodium bicarbonate ($NaHCO_3$) and carbonic acid (H_2CO_3) and cellular H_2CO_3 and potassium bicarbonate ($KHCO_3$)
2. The phosphate system found in renal tubular fluid and intracellularly
3. Proteins

The bicarbonate buffer system is the most powerful of all the three systems in the extracellular space, while proteins dominate the intracellular buffering compartment.

Depending on the severity of the derangement and its chronicity, the limited amount of chemical buffers may not be capable of completely ameliorating the derangements and correcting the pH.

2.2.2.2 Pulmonary Regulation

The lungs respond to deviations in pH by altering the rate and depth of ventilation. The lungs can only eliminate or retain CO_2. Peripheral chemoreceptors in the carotid and aortic bodies respond within minutes to changes in pO_2, pCO_2, and pH. On the other hand, central chemoreceptors in the cerebral medulla are sensitive only to pCO_2 with a slower but stronger and more predominant response [74]. Arterial pCO_2, therefore, is the most important factor in altering ventilation. These pulmonary responses typically begin in the first hour and are fully established by 24 h [61]. Pulmonary regulation, however, is only 50–75% effective in restoring H^+ concentration all the way back to normal when the primary process is metabolic, as the lung is only capable of eliminating CO_2 and not fixed acids. Nevertheless, the pulmonary buffering system is at least as effective as the chemical buffering system.

2.2.2.3 Renal Acid Regulation

The kidneys correct extracellular pH by controlling serum bicarbonate concentration through the regulation of H^+ excretion, bicarbonate reabsorption, and the production of new bicarbonate. The kidneys excrete H^+ in combination with phosphate ($HPO_4^{2-} + H^+ \rightarrow H_2PO_4^-$), other acids, or with ammonia to form ammonium [68]. When blood acidity is significantly increased, glutamine is proportionately metabolized into ammonia. Ammonia, in turn, serves as the recipient of H^+. Whereas the lungs can eliminate or retain only volatile acid, namely pCO_2, the kidneys can eliminate or retain both acids and bases and are the primary removal site for fixed acids. Renal compensation is the last process to join other buffering forces but insures complete correction over time. Renal compensation typically begins in the first day and is fully established in 3–5 days.

2.3 Acid–Base Monitoring

Acid–base status can be monitored intermittently or continuously. Arterial blood gas (ABG) analysis remains the gold standard in assessing for acid–base disorders. In the ICU, ABGs can be obtained by arterial puncture or through an indwelling arterial catheter.

2.3.1 Blood Gas Measurement

Blood gas measurements provide data on the acidity of the blood as reflected by pH, pCO_2, and serum bicarbonate level, all at a single point in time. After sterilizing and subcutaneously anesthetizing the skin overlying a palpable arterial site, typically the radial artery, with 2% lidocaine, arterial blood is obtained by percutaneous needle puncture utilizing a 22- or 24-gauge needle. The brachial, axillary, posterior tibial, dorsalis pedis, and femoral arteries are all potential alternatives that are commonly used in the ICU. The umbilical artery is typically cannulated in neonates within the first week of life.

Several factors affect the accuracy of blood gas measurements. First, the type of syringe can introduce diffusion errors if the sample was left longer than 15 min prior to analyzing it. This error is most appreciated when utilizing plastic syringes as compared with glass syringes and can be minimized by placing the sample on ice [11, 24, 34]. Second, the presence of air bubbles in the blood sample, especially if they constituted more than 1–2% of the blood volume, could result in underestimation of pCO_2 [75]. This error is further magnified if the sample was agitated, increasing the surface area of the blood exposed to the air, especially the longer the sample was left before analysis [34, 57]. Third, the use of heparin as an anticoagulant would lower the measured pH slightly, but more importantly can result in lowering pCO_2 secondary to a dilutional effect [11, 33]. Given that most samples are now analyzed almost immediately, the utilization of heparin for the purpose of measuring ABGs has mostly dropped out of favor.

2.3.2 Sample Analysis

In a whole-blood ABG analysis, oxygen saturation and bicarbonate are calculated numbers based on the measured pH, pO_2, and pCO_2, respectively. A measured bicarbonate level is readily available from a serum sample instead, typically, as part of an electrolyte panel.

2.3.3 Temperature Correction

Even though the amount of carbon dioxide in the blood does not change, changes in temperature result in a predictable deviation pattern of the pH and pCO_2.

Table 2.1 The effect of temperature on blood gas measurements

Temperature			
°C	°F	pH	pCO_2
20	68	7.65	19
30	86	7.50	30
35	95	7.43	37
36	97	7.41	38
37	98	7.40	40
38	100	7.39	42
40	104	7.36	45

Adapted from [70]

As temperature drops, pCO_2 decreases while pH increases and vise versa (Table 2.1). Contemporary blood gas analyzers are capable of measuring all blood gas elements at either 37°C or any alternative temperature that is entered corresponding to the patient's body temperature. The current recommendation is to utilize uncorrected values measured at 37°C to guide management while keeping in mind the expected values that would correspond to the patient's temperature [64]. This becomes important when interpreting blood gas measurements in hypothermic patients.

2.4 Interpretation of Blood Gas Measurements

Interpretation of blood gas measurements is one of the easy mathematical exercises that, when done correctly and correlated with the patient's history and clinical presentation, yields immediate and rapid insight into the underlying process causing the acid–base status disturbance.

2.4.1 Definitions

Keeping in mind that CO_2 is an acid and the respiratory system is the main organ in charge of its homeostasis, while bicarbonate is an alkali with the kidneys being the organ in charge of its homeostasis, the following definitions would become easy to follow:

Acidosis is a disorder that predisposes to low systemic pH. Utilizing the Henderson–Hasselbalch equation, this can be caused by a fall in systemic bicarbonate concentration or by an elevation in the pCO_2. Acidosis can exist whether the pH became low or was restored by compensatory mechanisms. It basically defines a process that continues to risk derangement and lower pH. *Acidemia*, on the other hand, is a state of low plasma pH.

Alkalosis is a disorder that predisposes to high systemic pH. This is usually caused either by an increase in systemic bicarbonate concentration or by a fall in the pCO_2.

Alkalemia, on the other hand, is the state of high plasma pH.

Metabolic acidosis is a disorder that predisposes to low pH and is induced by a low serum bicarbonate concentration.

Metabolic alkalosis is a disorder that predisposes to high pH and is induced by a high bicarbonate concentration.

Respiratory acidosis is a disorder that predisposes to low pH and is induced by high pCO_2.

Respiratory alkalosis is a disorder that predisposes to high pH and is induced by low pCO_2.

Respiratory derangements are either acute, reflecting a disorder of a few hours duration, or chronic, i.e., resulting from a process that is ongoing for longer than a few days.

2.4.2 Compensatory Responses

For every acid–base deviation, there is an appropriate compensatory response that follows a very predictable pattern. As was shown earlier, pH is determined by the ratio between the HCO_3 concentration and pCO_2 and not by either value in isolation. As such, processes that result in deviation in serum bicarbonate are compensated for by the lungs, which control pCO_2, and processes that result in deviation in pCO_2 are corrected by the kidneys, which regulate bicarbonate.

In metabolic acidosis, for example, a low HCO_2^-/pCO_2 ratio causes a decline in pH, resulting in stimulation of peripheral chemoreceptors, which, in turn, increase ventilation to decrease pCO_2. Given that CO_2 is an acid, its fall causes the pH to increase back toward normal. In metabolic alkalosis, on the other hand, a high pH induces hypoventilation through peripheral chemoreceptors, resulting in a rise in pCO_2, which, in turn, lowers the pH. This latter response is limited by the degree of the resulting hypoxemia induced by hypoventilation, rendering pulmonary compensation for an increased pH not nearly as effective as for a reduced pH.

A very convenient approach to recall the appropriate compensatory mechanisms to the primary disorders is that bicarbonate and CO_2 vary in the *same direction* (e.g., a fall in bicarbonate is compensated for by a fall in pCO_2 and vice versa), as one is an acid and the other is an alkali, each with biologically equivalent potential to neutralize the primary derangement.

In metabolic acidosis, the expected pulmonary compensation is a ~1 mmHg fall in pCO_2 for every 1 meq L^{-1} reduction in bicarbonate concentration [14].

In metabolic alkalosis, on the other hand, the pulmonary compensation raises pCO_2 by 7 mmHg for every 10 meq L^{-1} elevation in bicarbonate concentration [39, 40].

In *respiratory disorders*, the compensatory mechanisms are biphasic: The first phase is *acute* and dominated by chemical buffering mechanisms, while the second, *chronic* phase is dominated by renal responses. In *acute respiratory acidosis*, the serum bicarbonate concentration rises 1 meq L^{-1} for every 10 mmHg increase in pCO_2, whereas this ratio increases to 4 meq L^{-1} per 10 mmHg in *chronic respiratory acidosis*. This latter renal compensation is the result of neutralization of H^+, initially by phosphate and subsequently by ammonium excretion [62, 73]. It is essential to recognize that the renal response is tightly regulated, in that the provision of medical bicarbonate results in the urinary excretion of the excess alkali with no change in the plasma HCO_3 or pH [62].

In *acute respiratory alkalosis,* bicarbonate concentration falls by 2 meq L^{-1} for every 10 mmHg decrease in the pCO_2, whereas this ratio becomes 5 meq L^{-1} per 10 mmHg in *chronic respiratory alkalosis* [9, 45]. This serum bicarbonate decline is achieved by decreased urinary bicarbonate reabsorption and ammonium excretion [31]. The compensatory responses outlined earlier are summarized in mnemonic form in Table 2.2.

Table 2.2 Mnemonic version of expected compensatory responses to acid–base disturbances

	For every	Expect
Metabolic acidosis	1 ↓ HCO_3	1 ↓ pCO_2
Metabolic alkalosis	10 ↑ HCO_3	7 ↑ pCO_2
Respiratory acidosis, acute	10 ↑ pCO_2	1 ↑ HCO_3
Respiratory acidosis chronic	10 ↑ pCO_2	4 ↑ HCO_3
Respiratory alkalosis, acute	10 ↓ pCO_2	2 ↓ HCO_3
Respiratory alkalosis, chronic	10 ↓ pCO_2	5 ↓ HCO_3

Assuming a normal ABG of pH 7.4, pCO_2 40, HCO_3^- 24, and utilizing meq L^{-1} or mmol L^{-1} for bicarbonate and mmHg for pCO_2, the mnemonic is 1 for 1, 10 for 7, 1, 4, 2, 5

2.4.3 Mixed Acid–Base Disorders

In the ICU, it is not infrequent to encounter patients with two or more acid–base disorders. This type of complex presentation is easily recognized whenever the measured compensatory values of either bicarbonate or pCO_2 differ significantly from what would be expected [21, 54]. For example, in a patient with primary metabolic acidosis, a bicarbonate level of 14 meq L^{-1} should be adequately compensated by hyperventilation that decreases pCO_2 to 30 mmHg (for every 1 meq decline of bicarbonate, pCO_2 declines by 1 mmHg in compensation).

2.4.4 Guidelines for Interpretation

There are several methods utilized to assess the acid–base status; they include the following:

1. Measurement of base deficit (or excess)
2. Comprehensive interpretation of the pH, pCO_2, and bicarbonate utilizing the Henderson–Hasselbalch principles
3. The recently developed Stewart-Fencl approach
4. Normograms

The simple measurement of serum bicarbonate and base deficit is the least accurate of the mentioned methods, because it depends on the presence of conditions that rarely exist in severely ill patients in the ICU, namely normal electrolyte, water, and albumin levels. The Steward-Fencl method is a comprehensive method that employs the concepts of strong ions and weak acids in calculating *strong-ion difference* (*SID*) when assessing acid–base status [26]. Accuracy of this method is superior to the base deficit method and equivalent to the simple interpretation of pH, pCO_2, and bicarbonate utilizing the Henderson–Hasselbalch method, provided the latter is augmented by calculation of the anion gap (AG) and adjustment for the serum albumin level [12]. Blood gas measurements can also be directly assessed utilizing a Davenport diagram or an acid–base normogram in which the acid–base status of the patient is identified by plotting pH, pCO_2, and HCO_3^- measurements. Generally, however, these methods do not take into account AG, delta/delta, or any adjustment based on albumin level, rendering them less accurate than the methods described earlier. For the purpose of providing an accurate, comprehensive, and widely utilized method of ABG interpretation, the Henderson–Hasselbalch method will therefore be discussed in more detail later.

The first step in interpreting acid–base measurements accurately is the assessment of pH. Normal pH ranges between 7.35 and 7.45. For simplicity, in ICU patients with abnormal pCO_2 or bicarbonate levels, an arterial pH of less than 7.4 is indicative of acidosis while a pH higher than 7.4 indicates alkalosis.

The second step is to evaluate the primary type of derangement, whether respiratory or metabolic. In acidosis, low bicarbonate indicates a primary metabolic acidosis, while an elevated pCO_2 corresponds to a primary respiratory acidosis. Likewise, in alkalosis, high bicarbonate indicates a primary metabolic alkalosis, whereas a low pCO_2 is consistent with a primary respiratory alkalosis.

Once the primary change is established, the third step is to assess the extent of compensation. Metabolic derangements are corrected quickly; hence, any significant deviation from the expected compensation is indicative of a mixed acid–base disorder regardless of chronicity. Primary metabolic acidosis with superimposed respiratory acidosis is a common presentation in patients with severe status asthmaticus and respiratory failure. The goal of this third step is twofold: to identify mixed acid–base disorders, and to define the acuity of the disorder in the case of respiratory derangements.

If metabolic acidosis is noted, three additional steps are usually executed prior to determining whether the patient has a simple or a mixed acid–base derangement. A fourth step identifies the type of metabolic acidosis present, i.e., whether it is secondary to an anion that creates an AG on electrolyte measurement or not. The AG is a diagnostic tool to uncover the actual anions elevated in the blood but not routinely included in our measurements under normal conditions. It is calculated as follows:

AG = serum sodium − serum chloride − serum bicarbonate.

A normal anion gap is <12 mmol L^{-1}.

The fifth step in interpreting metabolic acidosis is adjusting for factors that would falsely lower the anion gap if one existed, e.g., hypoalbuminemia and lithium or bromide ingestion [22]:

Adjusted AG in hypoalbuminemia = observed AG + [2.5(normal albumin − observed albumin)].

The sixth step is the comparison of the degree of change in AG with the change in serum bicarbonate, aiming to assess the extent of contribution of the AG-producing process to the actual acidosis. This measurement is called delta/delta:

delta/delta= ΔAG/ ΔHCO$^-$ =(AG -12) / (24 - HCO$_3^-$).

Obviously, clinical correlation is very important throughout this process. For example, a blood gas measurement indicating an acute primary respiratory acidosis mixed with metabolic alkalosis out of proportion to the expected compensation could be seen in severe asthma with vomiting caused by theophylline toxicity, or it could reflect acute respiratory failure superimposed on chronic respiratory insufficiency in a patient with advanced cystic fibrosis and chronic CO_2 retention (also see Tables 2.3 and 2.4).

2.5 Causes of Acidosis

Acidosis is the predominant acid–base derangement encountered in critically ill pediatric ICU patients [37].

2.5.1 Respiratory Acidosis

Respiratory acidosis is caused by elevated pCO_2, whether acutely or over time [4]. This could be secondary to hypoventilation, airway obstruction, severe impairment of diffusion (e.g., pulmonary fibrosis), ventilation–perfusion mismatch (as observed in pneumonia, pulmonary edema, or ARDS), or excessive production of CO_2 to an extent that overwhelms even increased respiratory elimination. Common disorders causing hypoventilation in children are congenital central hypoventilation, drugs and toxins, for example, narcotic overdose, or severe restriction caused by either neuromuscular disorders or splinting secondary to rib fractures, e.g., in flail chest [10, 17]. The most common causes of airway obstruction in children include croup, foreign body aspiration, asthma, and bronchiolitis. In the ICU, ARDS is a frequent cause of respiratory failure secondary to ventilation–perfusion inequality

Table 2.3 Steps in interpreting blood gas measurements

Define whether the primary process is acidosis vs. alkalosis (pH)
Identify the source of the primary acid–base derangement (metabolic vs. respiratory)
Assess extent of compensation (acute vs. chronic respiratory disorders)
In metabolic acidosis: calculate anion gap
In metabolic acidosis: adjust for hypoalbuminemia
In anion gap metabolic acidosis: calculate delta/delta
Identify mixed acid–base disorders
Investigate possible underlying causes

Table 2.4 Algorithm for the interpretation of ABGs

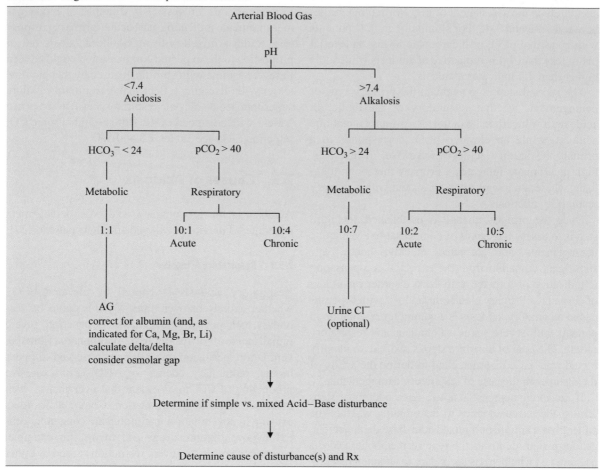

leading to CO_2 retention. Disorders of increased CO_2 production are uncommon but can impart an ominous prognosis if not detected timely, for example, in malignant hyperthermia. CO_2 production can also be elevated by increased carbohydrate intake, especially in parenteral nutrition.

Chemical buffering mechanisms are promptly elicited with elevated pCO_2, resulting in an acute rise in serum bicarbonate [2, 17, 50]. This process becomes further bolstered by the renal alkalinization process [13, 20, 51]. The rise in pCO_2 corresponds to a decline in pO_2 as determined by the alveolar gas equation. In severe respiratory acidosis, hypoxemia becomes the principal determinant of mortality, and treating it with prompt and adequate provision of oxygen is critical for patients' survival. Diagnosing the underlying cause of the respiratory acidosis is usually the key in reversing the acidosis in these patients.

Treatment: Depending on the severity of acidosis, endotracheal intubation, mechanical ventilation (whether noninvasive through a mask or invasive through an endotracheal tube or tracheostomy cannula), or in very severe cases, extracorporeal membrane CO_2 removal with or without oxygenation (ECOR vs ECMO, respectively) might be needed [3, 10, 17].

In patients with chronic pCO_2 retention, acute decompensation from infection, cardiopulmonary edema, narcotics, or excessive oxygen therapy can all result in exacerbations, given these patients' limited reserve. Antibiotics, bronchodilator therapy, diuretics, and removal of secretions are important interventions to implement timely. Naloxone therapy should be considered in suspected narcotic overdose (titrating $1–5\,\mu g\ kg^{-1}\ dose^{-1}$ until recovery of adequate respiratory effort). Treatment of a superimposed metabolic alkalosis with carbonic anhydrase inhibitors can also be helpful in restoring ventilatory drive.

Conservative institution of mechanical ventilatory assistance in chronic respiratory failure is driven by the concern about the difficulty in weaning affected patients off the ventilator.

Increasing minute ventilation by increasing the respiratory rate is the mainstay in ventilatory treatment of severe respiratory acidosis secondary to parenchymal lung disease. In obstructive pulmonary disease, decreasing the respiratory rate will likely allow for adequate exhalation of CO_2 and is usually implemented in patients with status asthmaticus or severe bronchiolitis. The current standard of care utilizes *lung protective strategy* in mechanical ventilation in which the tidal volume is limited to ~5–7 mL kg^{-1} ideal body weight while maintaining a plateau pressure below 35 cm of H_2O in order to avert large swings in alveolar volume that in turn results in increased microvascular permeability and ventilator-induced lung injury [25, 78]. Such a lung-protective strategy was found to impart better survival rates on patients mechanically ventilated for parenchymal lung disease. Additionally, current practice employs *permissive hypercapnia* in which there is no therapeutic pCO$_2$ target level but, rather, a pII goal that should be maintained above 7.25 in order to ensure adequate myocardial and cellular function. The combination of low tidal volume ventilation with permissive hypercapnia results in patient discomfort and necessitates judicious use of sedation and, at times, neuromuscular paralysis. It is prudent to provide patients with an adequate respiratory rate to achieve the intended gas exchange, especially if paralyzed or oversedated. As CO_2 decreases, excess bicarbonate is excreted by the kidneys (assuming the serum chloride level has normalized, as patients with respiratory acidosis are usually hypochloremic) [3, 10].

Of note, alkali therapy has a very limited role in the treatment of respiratory acidosis. Mixed metabolic and respiratory acidosis or severe respiratory acidosis are potential indications of alkali therapy. Alkali therapy can be of special benefit in patients with severe bronchospasm by directly resulting in smooth muscle relaxation and by indirectly restoring their responsiveness to beta-adrenergic agonists [3, 10]. Moreover, alkali use to raise pH is especially beneficial in patients with severe component of pulmonary hypertension resulting in pulmonary smooth muscle relaxation. In general, however, alkali therapy can also result in pH-mediated ventilatory failure, in a further increase in pCO$_2$ from bicarbonate decomposition, and in volume expansion from sodium provision.

2.5.2 Metabolic Acidosis

Causes of metabolic acidosis are categorized into two groups: AG acidoses and non-AG acidoses.

2.5.2.1 AG Acidoses

Causes of AG acidosis can be summarized by the acronym KUSMALE: ketones, uremia, salicylates, methanol, alcohols, lactate, and ethylene glycol. Lactic acid and the ketoacids are organic acids generated from incomplete metabolism of carbohydrate or fat. When accumulating in large quantities, they result in severe acidosis that can be life-threatening. Under normal conditions and when these organic acids are only mildly elevated, the kidneys increase the excretion rate of these organic acids and restore homeostasis. As the amount of organic acids increases and exceeds the renal excretion capacity, lactic acidosis or ketoacidosis develops.

1. Diabetic Ketoacidosis

Diabetic ketoacidosis is not uncommon in pediatric patients. It occurs in patients with insulin-dependent diabetes mellitus and is the result of severe insulin deficiency in the setting of increased metabolic demand, as would occur in the setting of a concurrent infection. As a result of insulin deficiency and depletion of glycogen stores, lipolysis ensues with increased production of ketoacids. Insulin is integral to the metabolism of ketoacids, and its relative or complete deficiency in the setting of increased ketoacid production results in severe keto-, i.e., AG acidosis.

Treatment: Intravenous insulin is the most important therapy for patients with diabetic ketoacidosis [47]. Fluid, potassium, and phosphorous should be judiciously replaced. Insulin therapy induces the metabolism of ketones and results in the generation of alkali, hence obviating the need for sodium bicarbonate administration [43]. Indeed, sodium bicarbonate treatment that can delay the metabolic recovery by stimulating ketogenesis [56, 58] was found to be of no benefit for patients with severe DKA (as defined by a pH of 6.9–7.14), and was associated with an increased risk of cerebral edema in children [32, 56]. Therefore, sodium bicarbonate therapy is currently reserved for severe acidemia (pH < 6.9 in our practice) in order to avoid myocardial and cellular functional impairment at such an extremely low pH.

2. Uremia

While mild chronic renal failure can be associated with a non-AG, i.e., renal tubular acidosis (RTA) (see later), more advanced renal failure also results in an

AG metabolic acidosis secondary to the accumulation of sulfates and other ions. Dialysis is the cornerstone intervention in treating this type of acidosis.

3. Salicylate

Aspirin intoxication is becoming uncommon since aspirin use has been discouraged in febrile children because of concerns about Reye syndrome. Nonetheless, it continues to occur, and prompt recognition is a key in recovering these patients. The anions in salicylate intoxication include salicylate as well as lactic acid and ketoacids [28]. These organic acids are likely to be excessively produced as a result of respiratory alkalosis, as it has been shown that salicylate-induced acidosis can be ameliorated by controlling hypocapnia in animals [28].

Therefore, aspirin toxicity typically results in mixed respiratory alkalosis and metabolic acidosis. Initially, central hyperventilation results in early respiratory alkalosis. As time progresses and as lactic acid and ketoacids accumulate, metabolic acidosis ensures. Prognosis in aspirin toxicity is highly dependent on aspirin concentration; hence, limiting further drug absorption is a key in treating these patients. Activated charcoal and blood and urinary alkalinization are two common practices that aid in eliminating aspirin from the CNS and the blood, respectively [35]. Sodium bicarbonate can be administered in order to reach a pH of 7.45–7.50 [16]. In severe cases, and when the presentation is complicated by renal insufficiency, hemodialysis is used [30]. Finally, hydration typically aids in aspirin excretion and lactate and ketone clearance.

4. Methanol, Alcohols, and Ethylene Glycol

Alcohol toxicity, with either methanol, ethanol, or ethylene glycol, can result in profound AG acidosis secondary to the accumulation of ketoacids and lactic acid [19, 27]. Ketoacidosis is very common in alcohol intoxication. It generally ensues after large ingestions, especially if combined with limited food intake or protracted vomiting. Hepatic ketogenesis can be enhanced by superimposed alkalosis induced by vomiting, dehydration (contraction alkalosis), or hyperventilation [19].

Treatment: Discontinuing alcohol intake and provision of hydration and dextrose typically result in prompt recovery unless the acidosis is very severe enough to cause complications, especially myocardial depression [76]. Dextrose stimulates insulin secretion, thereby promoting the generation of bicarbonate from ketoacid metabolism. Hydration, on the other hand, will correct fluid deficits and lactic acidosis.

Additional therapeutic measures include gastric lavage, oral charcoal, as well as, in the case of ethylene glycol toxicity, intravenous or oral ethanol (which occupies alcohol dehydrogenase, rendering it unavailable for further metabolite production from the ingested ethylene glycol) and, when very severe, hemodialysis [30].

5. Lactate

Lactic acidosis is commonly encountered in the pediatric ICU. It is caused by either increased lactate production or decreased hepatic metabolism. Tissue hypoxia secondary to hypotension with or without sepsis is the main cause. In sepsis, similar to other causes of circulatory failure, severe lactic acidosis, sets of a vicious cycle of further circulatory failure, worsening tissue perfusion, more lactate production, and decreased consumption by the liver and kidneys [36, 49, 53]. Either lactate itself or the ensuing acidosis can result in myocardial depression and hypotension [46, 77]. In patients with severe status asthmaticus, lactic acidosis occurs secondary to increased work of breathing with elevated skeletal muscular oxygen demand.

Treatment: Management of lactic acidosis should center on reestablishing tissue perfusion while identifying and reversing the underlying disease [18, 36, 49, 53]. Restoring intravascular volume and effective circulation is the cornerstone in treating patients with lactic acidosis, and reversing the underlying cause promptly can be lifesaving. Specifically, management includes the provision of antibiotics in sepsis, operative repair of tissue ischemia or intestinal perforation, insulin for patients with diabetic ketoacidosis, and dextrose infusion (and possibly dialysis) in alcohol toxicity and congenital lactic acidosis [49, 52, 53].

Alkali therapy is not considered a standard intervention in lactic acidosis and carries a real risk of increased lactate production [18, 71, 72]. Nevertheless, it is our practice to utilize sodium bicarbonate in lactic acidosis when blood pH falls below 7.1, predominantly for concerns about hemodynamic compromise.

6. Other

Sniffing hydrocarbon (toluene in glue) is increasingly recognized as a cause of rapidly developing, profound AG acidosis secondary to the production of benzoic acid and hippuric acid during toluene metabolism. With normal renal function, this acidosis is typically transformed to a non-AG acidosis following the rapid renal excretion of hippurate anion [15].

2.5.2.2 Non-AG Acidoses

Non-AG acidosis, also described as *hyperchloremic metabolic acidosis* results from a decrease in serum bicarbonate secondary to its either absolute or relative extracellular depletion (Table 2.5).

1. Decline in extracellular bicarbonate content (bicarbonate loss)

Whereas hydrochloric acid is the major chemical lost in vomiting (resulting in metabolic alkalosis), bicarbonate is the main chemical lost from the digestive tract distal to the stomach, whether secondary to diarrhea or any form to enterocutaneous or uroenteric fistula. If profuse diarrhea results in dehydration serious enough to decrease tissue perfusion, a picture of mixed metabolic acidosis ensues with non-AG acidosis (secondary to the bicarbonate loss) as well as an AG acidosis (secondary to lactic acidosis, acute renal failure, or hyperproteinemia) [6, 44].

Treatment: Even though the kidneys are capable of generating bicarbonate through ammonium production, severe losses require timely provision of exogenous bicarbonate to correct acid–base status. Restoring hydration and electrolyte homeostasis is also an essential part of treatment.

2. Saline

Aggressive resuscitation and generous intraoperative hydration are the two most common causes of saline-induced, dilutional acidosis.

Treatment: Provision of sodium bicarbonate in cases of severe acidosis corrects the derangement promptly.

3. Early renal insufficiency and RTA

Patients with RTA can maintain a stable acid–base status by decreasing production of endogenous fixed acids [41], but more severe renal insufficiency or RTA can lead to profound hypobicarbonatemia.

Treatment: Severe cases necessitate treatment with sodium bicarbonate (e.g., RTA type I) [69]. Mixed acidosis can occur in these patients as a result of hypokalemia-induced muscle weakness and consequent

Table 2.5 Causes of non-AG acidosis

Ureterosigmoidostomy/fistulae
Saline
Early renal insufficiency
Diarrhea
Carbonic anhydrase inhibitors
Amino acids
Renal tubular acidosis
Supplements

Mnemonic: USED CARS

hypoventilation-related respiratory acidosis; hence, correcting electrolyte levels is especially important in these patients.

4. Other

Carbonic anyhydrase inhibitors (e.g., acetazolamide and topiramate) are known to cause a non-AG acidosis that is typically mild and does not require aggressive intervention. Total parenteral nutrition and excessive arginine supplementation are additional causes of non-AG acidosis.

2.6 Causes of Alkalosis

2.6.1 Respiratory Alkalosis

Respiratory alkalosis is caused by increased elimination of CO_2 or decreased production [5]. The latter can occur in moderate to severe hypothermic states. Increased CO_2 elimination, on the other hand, can occur under any of the circumstances listed in Table 2.6.

2.6.2 Metabolic Alkalosis

There are very few conditions that can lead to metabolic alkalosis, and a careful assessment of the clinical presentation is typically most helpful in their recognition. Additionally, the urinary chloride level is a useful discriminating marker, with a low level suggesting either vomiting, diuretic therapy, or a posthypercapnic state as likely underlying causes and a high urinary chloride level pointing toward steroid excess.

Table 2.6 Clinical scenarios predisposing to respiratory alkalosis

Primary pulmonary disease
Early asthma
Pneumonia
Central nervous system disease
Pain
Infection
Tumors
Metabolic acidosis
Psychogenic hyperventilation
Iatrogenic causes
Excessive mechanical ventilatory rate or tidal volume (high minute ventilation)
Swift CO_2 removal through an extracorporeal circuit

2.7 Complications of Severe Acidemia

While the prognosis of acidosis as a process is largely driven by its underlying cause as long as blood pH is maintained within the normal range through adequate compensation, acidemia (defined as pH < 7.2), on the other hand, has a set of detrimental effects warranting corrective intervention (also see Table 2.7). Acid–base homeostasis affects cellular and tissue performance through its influence on protein structure and function: Hydrogen ions, for example, are highly reactive when they interact with proteins [29, 66]. Upon either net gain or loss of H^+, proteins accordingly undergo major changes in their charge distribution, structural configuration, and, ultimately, their function.

Even though metabolic acidemia is generally more deleterious than respiratory acidemia, either type of acidosis will result in severe tissue injury if the pH continues to decline. Cardiovascular consequences of acidemia are the most significant complications in critically ill patients and include dysrhythmias and catecholamine-refractory shock, causing systemic hypoperfusion and ultimately multiorgan-system failure [42, 49, 59, 60]. Of note, hyperkalemia resulting from acidosis-induced potassium shifts out of cells is most prominent in nonorganic acidoses and carries the risk of fatal dysrhythmia [1, 7].

Acidemia is characteristically associated with a significant mismatch between the increased metabolic demands caused by the concomitant sympathetic surge and the decreased tissue uptake and anaerobic utilization of glucose induced by insulin resistance [8, 38]. Patients, consequently, enter a hypercatabolic state with significant protein breakdown [23, 55, 63]. Additionally, hepatic lactate uptake is impaired, resulting in lactic acidosis that further aggravates acidemia [49]. These metabolic complications are proportionate to the severity of acidosis and are further compounded by hypoxemia.

2.8 Complications of Severe Alkalemia

Alkalemia is defined as a blood pH above 7.60 and is seldom encountered in the ICU (also see Table 2.7). However, in its most severe forms, respiratory alkalemia can impair cerebral and coronary perfusion and result in fatal infarctions [17, 67]. This is partly the result of the decline of CO_2, a potent cerebral and coronary vasodilator.

Table 2.7 Consequences of acid–base disturbance by organ system

Organ	Acidosis	Alkalosis
Cardiac	Impaired myocardial contractility with decreased cardiac output and hypotension	Reduction in ischemia threshold
	Reentrant dysrhythmias and ventricular fibrillation	Refractory dysrhythmias
	Catecholamine insensitivity	
Peripheral vasculature	Arteriolar dilation	Arteriolar constriction
	Venoconstriction	Reduction in coronary blood flow
	Centralization of blood volume	Reduction in PVR
	Increased pulmonary vascular resistance (PVR)	
Respiratory	Hyperventilation	Hypoventilation
	Skeletal muscle weakness	Impaired hypoxic pulmonary vasoconstriction and worsened ventilation–perfusion mismatch
	Shift of the oxygen–hemoglobin dissociation curve to the right (resulting in desaturation)	Increased hemoglobin affinity for oxygen
Metabolic	Increased metabolic demands	Stimulation of organic acid production
	Insulin resistance	Decreased plasma electrolyte levels: hypokalemia, hypocalcemia (ionized), hypomagnesemia, and hypophosphatemia)
	Hyperkalemia	
	Increased protein degradation	
Central nervous system	Altered mental status and depressed level of consciousness	Reduction in cerebral blood flow if respiratory in origin
		Reduced seizure threshold
		Altered mental status and depressed level of consciousness

Hypokalemia is another characteristic complication of alkalemic disorders, more prominently those of metabolic origin. Shift into the cells at least partly account for the decline in extracellular potassium. The remainder of potassium deficit is attributable to renal and extrarenal losses [17, 67]. Hypokalemia can result in weakness, dysrhythmias, polyuria, and increased ammonia production. Other electrolyte abnormalities occurring during alkalemia can also result in severe complications commensurate to the severity of the particular electrolyte derangement: hypocalcemia and hypomagnesemia can lead to tetany, seizures, and altered mental status. As mentioned previously in this chapter, alkalemia stimulates the generation of lactic acid and ketoacids through the induction of anaerobic glycolysis. Additionally, acute alkalemia shifts the oxygen–hemoglobin dissociation curve to the left, resulting in increased oxygen affinity of hemoglobin and consequent relative tissue hypoxia. This effect is eventually ameliorated in persistent alkalemic states by the induction of 2,3-diphosphoglyceric acid production in red cells.

2.9 Summary

Acid–base derangements are encountered in almost every critically ill patient. A stepwise approach of recognizing the derangements, accurately defining their type and severity, actively intervening to restore cardiopulmonary and hemodynamic stability, and, whenever possible, reversing the underlying cause can be lifesaving.

Take-Home Pearls

> Any pediatric disease when severe can result in an acid-base disturbance, directly, as a result of therapy or both.
> Acid-base disorders should be anticipated in all critically ill patients and proactively monitored. This will allow the early recognition of derangements and the prevention of what could become a life-threatening state.
> Acidosis is the most common acid-base derangement in the ICU with metabolic acidosis signaling a more severe course and worse outcome.
> A pH of < 7.2 merely indicates a primary acidosis-inducing disorder. Further assessment of the type of acidosis and the presence of a mixed acid-base disorders requires measurement of PCO_2, serum bicarbonate, albumin and calculation of the anion gap.
> The most commonly encountered causes of metabolic acidoses in the ICU are renal insufficiency, sepsis and DKA, while ARDS and severe status asthmaticus are the usual suspects in respiratory acidoses.

> Alkalosis, on the other hand, is less encountered in the ICU. Fluid status and gastric fluid depletion are the common underlying causes of metabolic alkaloses. Whereas rapid respiration secondary to lung diseases, excessive mechanical ventilation, pain or central nervous system process are the common causes of respiratory alkaloses.
> When caring for critically ill patients, identifying derangements are followed by timely stabilization of the patient irrespective of the underlying cause of the derangement. Depending on the severity of the derangement and the patient's response to the stabilizing interventions, the underlying cause might need to be aggressively sought and emergently reversed.
> Identifying the underlying cause(s) of the acid-base disorder at hand is the final step in the management of these patients and plays an important in preventing further derangement, worsening of the derangement and defining the patient's overall prognosis.

References

1. Adrogue HJ, Madias NE (1981) Changes in plasma potassium concentration during acute acid–base disturbances. Am J Med 71(3):456–67
2. Adrogue HJ, Madias NE (1985) Influence of chronic respiratory acid–base disorders on acute CO2 titration curve. J Appl Physiol 58(4):1231–8
3. Adrogue HJ, Tobin MJ (1997) Respiratory failure. Blackwell's basics of medicine. Cambridge, MA: Blackwell Science, xii, 560 p
4. Adrogue HJ, Madias NE (1998) Management of life-threatening acid–base disorders. First of two parts. N Engl J Med 338(1):26–34
5. Adrogue HJ, Madias NE (1998) Management of life-threatening acid–base disorders. Second of two parts. N Engl J Med 338(2):107–11
6. Adrogue HJ, Brensilver J, Madias NE (1978) Changes in the plasma anion gap during chronic metabolic acid–base disturbances. Am J Physiol 235(4):F291–F297
7. Adrogue HJ, Lederer E, Suki W, et al. (1986) Determinants of plasma potassium levels in diabetic ketoacidosis. Medicine 65(3):163–72
8. Adrogue HJ, Chap Z, Okuda Y, et al. (1988) Acidosis-induced glucose intolerance is not prevented by adrenergic blockade. Am J Physiol 255(6, Part 1):E812–E823
9. Arbus GS, Hebert LA, Levesque PR, et al. (1969) Potassium depletion and hypercapnia. N Engl J Med 280(12):670
10. Arieff AI, DeFronzo RA (1985) Fluid, electrolyte, and acid–base disorders. New York: Churchill Livingstone, 2 vols. (xxi 1246, 44 p)
11. Bageant R (1975) Variations in arterial blood gas measurements due to sampling techniques. Respiratory Care 20:565
12. Balasubramanyan N, Havens PL, Hoffman GM (1999) Unmeasured anions identified by the Fencl-Stewart method predict mortality better than base excess, anion gap, and

lactate in patients in the pediatric intensive care unit. Crit Care Med 27(8):1577–81

13. Batlle DC, Downer M, Gutterman C, et al. (1985) Relationship of urinary and blood carbon dioxide tension during hypercapnia in the rat. Its significance in the evaluation of collecting duct hydrogen ion secretion. J Clin Invest 75(5):1517–30

14. Bushinsky DA, Coe FL, Katzenberg C, et al. (1982) Arterial pCO2 in chronic metabolic acidosis. Kidney Int 22(3):311–14

15. Carlisle EJ, Donnelly SM, Vasuvattakul S, et al. (1991) Glue-sniffing and distal renal tubular acidosis: sticking to the facts. J Am Soc Nephrol 1(8):1019–27

16. Chatton JY, Bessighir K, Roch-Ramel F (1990) Salicylic acid permeability properties of the rabbit cortical collecting duct. Am J Physiol 259(4, Part 2):F613–F618

17. Cohen JJ, Kassirer JP (1982) Acid–base, 1st ed. Boston: Little, Brown, xxii, 510 p

18. Cooper DJ, Walley KR, Wiggs BR, et al. (1990) Bicarbonate does not improve hemodynamics in critically ill patients who have lactic acidosis. A prospective, controlled clinical study. Ann Intern Med 112(7):492–8

19. Cusi K, Consoli A (1994) Alcoholic ketoacidosis and lactic acidosis. Diabetes Rev 2:195–208.

20. Da Silva Junior JC, Perrone RD, Johns CA, et al. (1991) Rat kidney band 3 mRNA modulation in chronic respiratory acidosis. Am J Physiol 260(2, Part 2):F204–F209

21. DuBose TD, Jr (1983) Clinical approach to patients with acid–base disorders. Med Clin North Am 67(4): 799–813

22. Durward A, Mayer A, Skellett S, et al. (2003) Hypo-albuminaemia in critically ill children: incidence, prognosis, and influence on the anion gap. Arch Dis Child 88(5):419–22

23. England BK, Chastain JL, Mitch WE (1991) Abnormalities in protein synthesis and degradation induced by extracellular pH in BC3H1 myocytes. Am J Physiol 260(2, Part 1): C277–C282

24. Evers W, Racz GB, Levy, AA (1972) A comparative study of plastic (polypropylene) and glass syringes in blood-gas analysis. Anesth Analg 51(1):92–7

25. Feihl F, Perret C (1994) Permissive hypercapnia. How permissive should we be? Am J Respir Crit Care Med 150(6, Part 1):1722–37

26. Figge J, Rossing TH, Fencl V (1991) The role of serum proteins in acid–base equilibria. J Lab Clin Med 117(6):453–67

27. Fulop M, Hoberman HD (1975) Alcoholic ketosis. Diabetes 24(9):785–90

28. Gabow PA, Anderson RJ, Potts DE, et al. (1978) Acid–base disturbances in the salicylate-intoxicated adult. Arch Intern Med 138(10):1481–4

29. Ganapathy V, Leibach FH (1991) Protons and regulation of biological functions. Kidney Int Suppl 33:S4–S10

30. Garella S (1988) Extracorporeal techniques in the treatment of exogenous intoxications. Kidney Int 33(3):735–54

31. Gennari FJ, Goldstein MB, Schwartz WB (1972) The nature of the renal adaptation to chronic hypocapnia. J Clin Invest 51(7):1722–30

32. Glaser N, Barnett P, McCaslin I, et al. (2001) Risk factors for cerebral edema in children with diabetic ketoacidosis. The Pediatric Emergency Medicine Collaborative Research Committee of the American Academy of Pediatrics. N Engl J Med 344(4):264–9

33. Hansen JE, Simmons DH (1977) A systematic error in the determination of blood pCO2. Am Rev Respir Dis 115(6):1061–3

34. Harsten A, Berg B, Inerot S, et al. (1988) Importance of correct handling of samples for the results of blood gas analysis. Acta Anaesthesiol Scand 32(5):365–8

35. Hill JB (1973) Salicylate intoxication. N Engl J Med 288(21):1110–13

36. Hindman BJ (1990) Sodium bicarbonate in the treatment of subtypes of acute lactic acidosis: physiologic considerations. Anesthesiology 72(6):1064–76

37. Hood VL, Tannen RL (1998) Protection of acid–base balance by pH regulation of acid production. N Engl J Med 339(12):819–26

38. Hood VL, Tannen RL (1994) Maintenance of acid base homeostasis during ketoacidosis and lactic acidosis: implications for therapy. Diabetes Rev 2:177–94

39. Javaheri S, Kazemi H (1987) Metabolic alkalosis and hypoventilation in humans. Am Rev Respir Dis 136(4): 1011–16

40. Javaheri S, Shore NS, Rose B, et al. (1982) Compensatory hypoventilation in metabolic alkalosis. Chest 81(3):296–301

41. Kamel K, Gowrishankar M, Cheema-Dhadli S, et al. (1996) How is acid–base balance maintained in patients with renal tubular acidosis. J Am Soc Nephrol 7:1350

42. Kerber RE, Pandian NG, Hoyt R, et al. (1983) Effect of ischemia, hypertrophy, hypoxia, acidosis, and alkalosis on canine defibrillation. Am J Physiol 244(6): H825–H831

43. Kokko JP, Tannen RL (1996) Fluids and electrolytes, 3rd ed. Philadelphia: Saunders, xii, 899 p

44. Kowalchuk JM, Heigenhauser GJ, Jones NL (1984) Effect of pH on metabolic and cardiorespiratory responses during progressive exercise. J Appl Physiol 57(5):1558–63

45. Krapf R, Beeler I, Hertner D, et al. (1991) Chronic respiratory alkalosis. The effect of sustained hyperventilation on renal regulation of acid–base equilibrium. N Engl J Med 324(20):1394–401

46. Landry DW, Oliver JA (1992) The ATP-sensitive K+ channel mediates hypotension in endotoxemia and hypoxic lactic acidosis in dog. J Clin Invest 89(6):2071–4

47. Lebovitz HE (1995) Diabetic ketoacidosis. Lancet 345(8952):767–72

48. Lennon EJ, Lemann J, Jr, Litzow JR (1966) The effects of diet and stool composition on the net external acid balance of normal subjects. J Clin Invest 45(10):1601–7

49. Madias NE (1986) Lactic acidosis. Kidney Int 29(3):752–74

50. Madias NE, Adrogue HJ (1983) Influence of chronic metabolic acid–base disorders on the acute CO2 titration curve. J Appl Physiol 55(4):1187–95

51. Madias NE, Wolf CJ, Cohen JJ (1985) Regulation of acid–base equilibrium in chronic hypercapnia. Kidney Int 27(3):538–43

52. Madias NE, Goorno WE, Herson S (1987) Severe lactic acidosis as a presenting feature of pheochromocytoma. Am J Kidney Dis 10(3):250–3

53. Massry SG, Glassock RJ (2001) Massry & Glassock's textbook of nephrology, 4th ed. Philadelphia: Lippincott Williams & Wilkins, xl, 2072 p

54. Maxwell MH, Kleeman CR, Narins RG (1987) Clinical disorders of fluid and electrolyte metabolism, 4th ed. New York: McGraw-Hill, xiii, 1268 p

55. Mitch WE, Medina R, Grieber S, et al. (1994) Metabolic acidosis stimulates muscle protein degradation by activating the adenosine triphosphate-dependent pathway involving ubiquitin and proteasomes. J Clin Invest 93(5):2127–33

56. Morris LR, Murphy MB, Kitabchi AE (1986) Bicarbonate therapy in severe diabetic ketoacidosis. Ann Intern Med 105(6):836–40

57. Mueller RG, Lang GE, Beam JM (1976) Bubbles in samples for blood gas determinations. A potential source of error. Am J Clin Pathol 65(2):242–9

58. Okuda Y, Adrogue HJ, Field JB, et al. (1996) Counterproductive effects of sodium bicarbonate in diabetic ketoacidosis. J Clin Endocrinol Metab 81(1):314–20

59. Orchard CH, Kentish JC (1990) Effects of changes of pH on the contractile function of cardiac muscle. Am J Physiol 258(6, Part 1):C967–C981

60. Orchard CH, Cingolani HE (1994) Acidosis and arrhythmias in cardiac muscle. Cardiovasc Res 28(9):1312–19

61. Pierce NF, Fedson DS, Brigham KL, et al. (1970) The ventilatory response to acute base deficit in humans. Time course during development and correction of metabolic acidosis. Ann Intern Med 72(5): 633–40

62. Polak A, Haynie GD, Hays RM, et al. (1961) Effects of chronic hypercapnia on electrolyte and acid–base equilibrium. I. Adaptation. J Clin Invest 40:1223–37

63. Reaich D, Channon SM, Scrimgeour CM, et al. (1992) Ammonium chloride-induced acidosis increases protein breakdown and amino acid oxidation in humans. Am J Physiol 263(4, Part 1):E735–E739

64. Ream AK, Reitz BA, Silverberg GB (1982) Temperature correction of pCO2 and pH in estimating acid–base status: an example of the emperor's new clothes? Anesthesiology 56(1):41–4

65. Relman AS (1954) What are acids and bases? Am J Med 17(4):435–7

66. Relman AS (1972) Metabolic consequences of acid–base disorders. Kidney Int 1(5):347–59

67. Rimmer JM, Gennari FJ (1987) Metabolic alkalosis. J Intensive Care Med 2:137–50

68. Rose BD (2001) Clinical physiology of acid–base and electrolyte disorders, 5th ed. New York: McGraw-Hill, x, 992 p

69. Schrier RW (2007) Diseases of the kidney and urinary tract, 8th ed. Philadelphia: Wolters Kluwer Health/Lippincott Williams & Wilkins

70. Shapiro et al. (1994) Clinical application of blood gases, 5th ed. St. Louis: Mosby-Year Book, p. 128

71. Spriet LL, Lindinger MI, Heigenhauser GJ, et al. (1986) Effects of alkalosis on skeletal muscle metabolism and performance during exercise. Am J Physiol 251(5, Part 2): R833–R839

72. Sutton JR, Jones NS, Toews CJ (1981) Effect of PH on muscle glycolysis during exercise. Clin Sci 61(3):331–8

73. Van Yperselle de S, Brasseur L, DeConick JD (1966) The "carbon dioxide response curve" for chronic hypercapnia in man. N Engl J Med 275(3):117–22

74. West JB (2005) Respiratory physiology: the essentials, 7th ed. Philadelphia: Lippincott Williams & Wilkins, ix, 186

75. Williams AJ (1998) ABC of oxygen: assessing and interpreting arterial blood gases and acid–base balance. BMJ 317(7167):1213–16

76. Wrenn KD, Slovis CM, Minion GE, et al. (1991) The syndrome of alcoholic ketoacidosis. Am J Med 91(2):119–28

77. Yatani A, Fujino T, Kinoshita K, et al. (1981) Excess lactate modulates ionic currents and tension components in frog atrial muscle. J Mol Cell Cardiol 3(2):147–61

78. Ventilation with lower tidal volumes as compared with traditional tidal volumes for acute lung injury and the acute respiratory distress syndrome. The Acute Respiratory Distress Syndrome Network (2000) N Engl J Med 342(18):1301–8

Dyskalemias

3

E.H. Mack and L.R. Shoemaker

Contents

Core Messages

> ❭ Potassium chloride has been identified by The Joint Commission on the Accreditation of Healthcare Organizations (JCAHO) as the drug that causes the most sentinel events; therefore, particular attention should be paid to potassium balance in the PICU.
> ❭ Many drugs commonly used in the PICU contribute to hypokalemia and hyperkalemia.
> ❭ Hypokalemia can lead to cardiovascular, neurologic, endocrine, metabolic, and renal dysfunction.
> ❭ In the case of hyperkalemia, sources of potassium that should be discontinued include enteral and parenteral nutrition, enteral and parenteral supplementation, and drugs.

Case Vignette

A 2-month-old infant with respiratory syncytial virus and acute respiratory distress syndrome was receiving a furosemide infusion to facilitate weaning from ventilatory support. Overnight he developed mild hypotension and the house staff discontinued the furosemide. This morning he develops cardiovascular collapse associated with ventricular fibrillation. The suspect? *Hyperkalemia due to exogenous load.* His parenteral nutrition contains abundant potassium chloride that was previously necessary to achieve normal K^+ levels, because of prior renal losses attributable to the furosemide. In addition, relative hypovolemia has exacerbated the situation.

S.G. Kiessling et al. (eds) *Pediatric Nephrology in the ICU.*
© Springer-Verlag Berlin Heidelberg 2009

3.1 Potassium

Potassium (K$^+$) is the most abundant intracellular cation in the body. Only 2% of total body stores resides in the extracellular space under normal circumstances. Therefore a high intracellular K$^+$ concentration (100–150 meqL^{-1}) and a steep transcellular gradient must be maintained [45, 55, 103, 116]. The homeostatic mechanisms responsible to maintain these gradients are influenced by a variety of physiologic factors that are frequently altered in children hospitalized in the ICU. It is not surprising, then, that moderate deviation of plasma K$^+$ outside the normal range is commonly seen in these patients. It is perhaps due to the redundancy of these homeostatic mechanisms and the presence of adaptive responses that extreme deviation in the plasma K$^+$ concentration is fortunately rare.

3.2 Potassium Homeostasis

3.2.1 Intracellular

The K$^+$ concentrations in the intracellular and extracellular space are regulated by conceptually separate homeostatic mechanisms. A high cytosolic K$^+$ concentration is required for growth, metabolism, cell division, protein synthesis, and many other normal cellular functions. In specialized cells, such as nerve and muscle, the large transcellular K$^+$ gradient must fluctuate upon appropriate stimulation, and this is tightly regulated for normal tissue function [103, 125].

All mechanisms responsible for maintaining the high cytosolic K$^+$ concentration and the transcellular K$^+$ gradient do so through their effects on the basolateral cell membrane enzyme, Na$^+$–K$^+$–ATPase, which pumps Na$^+$ out of and K$^+$ into the cell in a 3:2 ratio and consumes ATP [30, 44, 70]. This enzyme, and hence intracellular K$^+$ homeostasis, is physiologically regulated by insulin, thyroid hormone, catecholamines, and aldosterone [18, 30, 31, 39, 41, 42, 52, 109, 133, 152]. Secretion of these hormones is influenced by a variety of other stimuli, including dietary intake, plasma volume, and plasma K$^+$ concentration, which in turn is affected by numerous physiologic factors [18, 52, 55, 78, 127, 151, 152]. Hormonal dysregulation may result from pathologic conditions present in critically ill children, such as the systemic inflammatory response syndrome. Independent of these hormones, Na$^+$–K$^+$–ATPase activity, and hence intracellular K$^+$ concentration, is also affected directly by plasma K$^+$ and cytosolic ATP

concentrations [37, 41, 42, 78]. Lastly, certain pathologic states may promote rapid K$^+$ release from cells, faster than that which Na$^+$–K$^+$–ATPase can rectify, usually resulting from cell lysis. Examples include tumor lysis, rhabdomyolysis, and hemolysis [40, 67].

3.2.2 Extracellular

Mean age-related values and standard deviations for plasma potassium concentration decline with children's age, from 5.2 ± 0.8 meq L^{-1} in the first 4 months of life to 4.3 ± 0.3 meq L^{-1} between 11 and 20 years [114]. These values are dependent upon the maintenance of external and internal K$^+$ balance. External balance is primarily determined by the rate of extracellular fluid (ECF) K$^+$ uptake (GI absorption or IV input) and renal excretion. Unlike adults, whose external balance must equal zero, in children this balance is adjusted for accretion commensurate with their growth rate [129]. Sweat and gastrointestinal K$^+$ losses are usually minor; however, severe diarrhea, such as due to rotavirus, may occasionally result in significant negative balance [149]. Gastrointestinal losses may increase up to threefold following adaptation to chronic hyperkalemia, as may be seen in patients with renal failure [13, 18]. The kidneys are primarily responsible for K$^+$ excretion, but this is delayed after an oral load, with only about one-half excreted during the first 4–6 h [41, 42, 109]. Internal balance is therefore necessary to maintain relative constancy of plasma K$^+$ concentration during entry of K$^+$ into the ECF. This is achieved within minutes, by hormonally mediated temporary translocation of K$^+$ into cells: primarily muscle, and to a lesser extent in liver, red cells, and bone [18, 41, 42, 109]. Since the vast majority of total body K$^+$ is intracellular, several physiologic and pathologic factors (independent of hormones) that may have minor effects on cytosolic K$^+$ have a significant influence on plasma K$^+$ concentration. These include acid–base balance, transcellular osmolar gradients, and cytosolic ATP depletion as well as excessive membrane depolarization in muscle, as may be seen with depolarizing paralytic agents or following strenuous exercise [116].

The kidneys reabsorb about 90% of filtered K$^+$ in the proximal tubules and ascending limb of the loop of Henle, and the remaining distal nephron segments have variable reabsorptive capacity linked to hydrogen ion secretion [54, 81]. External K$^+$ homeostasis, however, is maintained by regulation of K$^+$ secretion along the distal nephron, primarily in the cortical collecting duct [54, 55, 140]. Here, principal cells secrete K$^+$ and absorb sodium ions (Na^+) [55, 70]. The cortical collecting duct K^+ secretory rate is positively affected by tubular flow rate, cytosolic K^+ concentration, luminal Na^+ concentration, and luminal nonreabsorbable anions such as bicarbonate, sulfate, and β-hydroxybutyrate [26, 47, 73, 92]. Acute metabolic and respiratory alkalosis promote renal K^+ excretion, whereas acute metabolic acidosis decreases it [77, 116, 117, 124]. Chronic metabolic acidosis and organic acidemia both stimulate net distal renal K^+ secretion [110, 116, 124]. Aldosterone, glucocorticoids, and antidiuretic hormone stimulate net renal K^+ excretion and Na^+ absorption [12, 48, 49, 117], whereas catecholamines and β-agonists reduce renal K^+ secretion [39, 66]. Adaptive responses may result in very high rates of K^+ excretion, even exceeding the filtered load, as may be seen in patients with renal insufficiency or on long-term, high K^+ diets [53, 80, 138].

3.3   Hypokalemia

Hypokalemia is defined as a serum K^+ concentration below 3.5 meq/L. It results from total body K^+ deficit, transcellular shift of K^+ from extracellular to cytosolic space (with normal total body K^+ stores), or a combination of both processes [53, 95, 116].

3.3.1   Hypokalemia vs Pseudohypokalemia

Rarely, a low plasma K^+ level may result from uptake of K^+ by metabolically active white blood cells *ex vivo* in blood specimens collected from a patient with a truly normal extracellular K^+ concentration. This occurs when there is marked leukocytosis and procedural delay in refrigerating or separating the plasma. In such cases, the pseudohypokalemia is not associated with clinical features of hypokalemia [53, 95, 111, 116].

3.3.2   Clinical Features Associated with Hypokalemia

Hypokalemia hyperpolarizes cell membranes by increasing the magnitude of the membrane potential. Its effects vary depending on the speed with which hypokalemia develops and the concentration of other electrolytes including calcium, magnesium, sodium, and hydrogen ions. Whereas a rapid fall in plasma K^+ concentration typically results in marked symptoms, a stable and chronic K^+ loss to the same concentration is usually well tolerated [53, 111, 116]. Table 3.1 outlines the major clinical manifestations of hypokalemia.

Cardiovascular effects of hypokalemia include disturbances in electrical conduction and blood pressure

Table 3.1 Clinical features associated with hypokalemia

Cardiovascular	Renal/electrolytes/fluid status
Electrocardiogram abnormalities	Renal concentrating defect
Low-amplitude T waves	Metabolic alkalosis
Sagging ST segment, widened QRS	Renal tubule dilation and atrophy
Prolonged PR segment	Interstitial fibrosis
Enlarged U waves	Proximal tubule vacuolization
Increased risk of digitalis toxicity	Renal medullary cysts
Supraventricular and ventricular dysrrhythmias	Reduced glomerular filtration
Hypertension	ECV expansion or contraction[a]
Neuromuscular	Endocrine/metabolic
Weakness	Growth retardation
Hypokalemic paralysis	Reduced insulin secretion
Enhanced aminoglycoside toxicity	Carbohydrate intolerance
Cramps/tetany/rhabdomyolysis	Exacerbation of hepatic encephalopathy
Nausea/vomiting	
Constipation/ileus	
Voiding dysfunction	
Postural hypotension	

[a] *Expansion* if extrarenal or endocrine cause of hypokalemia; *contraction* if primary renal cause of hypokalemia

regulation. Mild hypokalemia is usually not associated with either symptoms or EKG changes [111]. As the plasma K^+ drops below 3.0 meq L^{-1}, the T-wave amplitude declines and U waves develop voltages that equal or exceed that of the T waves. At lower K^+ concentrations, near 2.5 meq L^{-1}, sagging of the ST segment and further flattening of the T waves, with prominent U waves are seen. With more severe hypokalemia, the QRS complex may widen slightly, and the PR interval is often prolonged [4, 53, 95, 111]. Supraventricular and ventricular dysrhythmias are prone to develop, especially in patients who take digitalis, have congestive heart failure, or experience cardiac ischemia [4, 51]. Particular attention should also be given to avoid hypokalemia in children with the long QT syndrome. This syndrome may be inherited or acquired, and is caused by malfunction of ion channels responsible for ventricular repolarization [141]. The resulting dysrhythmia is *torsades de pointes*, which may present as syncope or cardiac arrest. Immediate treatment includes correction of hypokalemia and administration of intravenous magnesium sulfate [4, 141].

Hypokalemia is associated with chronic hypertension in several disorders related to aberrant adrenal hormone metabolism [11, 93, 135]. In the presence of a high salt diet, low K^+ intake has also been implicated in causing hypertension [2].

Neuromuscular dysfunction typically manifests as skeletal muscle weakness, usually in an ascending fashion, with worsening hypokalemia. Lower extremity muscles are initially affected, followed by the quadriceps, the trunk, upper extremity muscles, and later those involved with respiration [116, 145]. Reduced skeletal muscle blood flow may also result [2, 116]. Under such conditions, exercise may lead to ischemia and result in cramps, tetany, and rhabdomyolysis [53, 75, 95, 116]. Smooth muscle dysfunction related to hypokalemia typically includes nausea, vomiting, constipation, postural hypotension, and bladder dysfunction associated with urinary retention [53, 95, 116]. Aminoglycoside neurotoxicity is enhanced during hypokalemia [36].

Endocrine and metabolic perturbations associated with hypokalemia include glucose intolerance, growth restriction, and protein catabolism [53, 95, 116]. Insulin release from the pancreatic beta cell is dependent on K^+ influx through specific channels, and this process is dampened by K^+ depletion [2, 33]. Hypokalemia- related impairment in glucose metabolism is mild and usually subclinical in normal individuals. However, this effect may be significant in those with subclinical diabetes, and marked in those with overt diabetes, in whom hypokalemia impairs both insulin release and end-organ sensitivity [116]. Growth is often impeded in children with chronic hypokalemia associated with K^+ depletion. This is partly explained by the associated intracellular acidosis and stimulated protein catabolism [53, 95, 116, 145]. This may also account for the greater severity of hepatic encephalopathy associated with hypokalemia [143].

Renal physiology is significantly altered by prolonged hypokalemia, which may lead to a chronic nephropathy associated with microscopic structural abnormalities as well [2, 53, 95, 116]. The most common functional disorder that develops is a urinary concentrating defect that is associated with increased renal prostaglandin synthesis and is resistant to exogenous vasopressin and prolonged water deprivation [84, 118]. In individuals with extrarenal causes of hypokalemia, this feature does not lead to ECF depletion. This is because there is concurrent stimulation of renin release and angiotensin II production, which stimulates the central thirst center. Also, chronic hypokalemia stimulates proximal tubular Na^+ reabsorption, which leads to isotonic Na^+ retention, expansion of the ECF, and occasionally edema [53, 116, 145]. Intracellular acidosis within renal tubular cells due to chronic K^+ depletion also leads to H^+ secretion and ammonia production [53, 116, 131]. The combined effect of these processes that result from chronic K^+ depletion is fluid expansion with aldosterone suppression, and mild metabolic alkalosis with acid urine, polyuria, and polydipsia [53, 116]. Interestingly, K^+ conservation is not affected [106, 116, 145].

The microscopic structural abnormalities reported to result from chronic K^+ depletion include interstitial fibrosis, tubular dilation and atrophy, and medullary cyst formation [53, 95, 116]. This is associated with reduced renal flow and glomerular filtration. A reversible lesion of the proximal tubular cells, characterized by the presence of intracytoplasmic vacuoles, is also seen [53, 116, 136].

Renal mineral handling is abnormal in several inherited syndromes associated with severe hypokalemia and K^+ wasting, although not as a direct consequence of hypokalemia. These disorders are included in Table 3.2. Marked hypercalciuria and nephrocalcinosis may be seen in certain children with Bartter's syndrome and Dent's disease. Severe hypomagnesemia is often associated with exacerbations of Gitelman's syndrome. Excessive phosphate wasting may be observed in children with Dent's disease and proximal tubular disorders, collectively referred to as the Fanconi syndrome.

Table 3.2 Inherited disorders associated with renal K⁺ wasting

Disease	Nephron segment affected
Fanconi syndrome	Proximal tubule
Cystinosis	
Tyrosinemia type 1	
Dent's disease	
Wilson's disease	
Fructosemia	
Mitochondrial disorders	
Glycogen storage disease (types 1 & 11)	
Oculocerbral (Lowe's) syndrome	
Fanconi–Bickel syndrome	
Proximal RTA (type II)	Proximal tubule
Bartter syndromes	Ascending limb, loop of Henle
Familial hypocalcemia (CaSR activating mutation)	Ascending limb, loop of Henle
Gitelman syndrome	Distal tubule
Distal RTA (type I)	Collecting duct
Stimulated mineralocorticoid activity syndromes	Collecting duct
Adrenal enzymopathies	
11-β hydroxylase	
17-α hydroxylase	
11-β hydroxysteroid dehydrogenase deficiency (AME)	
Familial hyperaldosteronism I (GRA)	
Familial hyperaldosteronism II	
Epithelial sodium channel activation (Liddle's syndrome, PA-I)	
Mineralocorticoid receptor activation (PA-II)	
Glucocorticoid receptor inactivation	

Correction of phosphate and magnesium deficiency when present, concurrent with adequate K⁺ replacement, is necessary to achieve optimal care [116].

3.3.3 Causes of Hypokalemia

The causes of hypokalemia are numerous and can be categorized mechanistically as due to the following: (1) *insufficient K⁺ or Cl⁻ intake*, (2) *increased cellular uptake of K⁺*, and (3) *excessive K⁺ loss* (Table 3.3). Insufficient intake of K⁺ or Cl⁻ as an isolated phenomenon is an exceedingly rare cause of hypokalemia, which is of primarily historical and research interest. Deficient K⁺ intake is not apt to be a relevant clinical consideration with the current care of hospitalized children who manifest hypokalemia, which typically includes intravenous fluids that provide at least 20 meq m⁻² day⁻¹ of K⁺ and much more chloride.

In the absence of K⁺ loss, this degree of intravenous supplementation is sufficient. Studies suggest that obligatory kaliuria persists at a level near 10 meq day⁻¹ in adults who underwent prolonged K⁺ deprivation [123]. Hence, unless patients are placed on K⁺-free intravenous fluids for prolonged periods along with dietary K⁺ restriction, insufficient intake is unlikely to be a primary cause of hypokalemia.

The causes of increased cellular uptake are outlined in Table 3.4. In most of these conditions, concurrent volume contraction may exacerbate hypokalemia due to secondary hyperaldosteronism [53, 116]. Either nonselective or β₂-selective adrenergic agonists promote intracellular uptake of K⁺ [31]. Hypokalemic periodic paralysis is rare and occurs more often in males. It may be sporadic or familial, usually with autosomal dominant inheritance, and typically presents in late childhood or during teenage years.

Table 3.3 Causes of low and high serum potassium concentrations

Low potassium level	High potassium level
Pseudohypokalemia	Pseudohyperkalemia
Insufficient intake of K^+ or Cl^-	Exogenous load
Increased cellular uptake (Table 3.4)	$\quad$ K^+-containing IVF/TPN
Excessive loss	$\quad$ K^+ supplementation
$\quad$ Low or normal BP (Table 3.5)	$\quad$ Blood or platelet transfusion
$\quad$ Hypertension and metabolic alkalosis (Table 3.6)	$\quad$ Penicillin potassium salts
	$\quad$ Dietary/herbal sources
	Endogenous release
	$\quad$ Rhabdomyolysis
	$\quad$ Burns
	$\quad$ Tumor lysis syndrome
	$\quad$ Hemolysis
	$\quad$ Exercise
	$\quad$ Prolonged seizure
	$\quad$ Infection
	$\quad$ Trauma
	$\quad$ Intravascular coagulopathy
	$\quad$ Starvation
	$\quad$ Resorption of hematoma
	$\quad$ Gastrointestinal bleeding
	Extracellular shift
	$\quad$ Metabolic acidosis
	$\quad$ Hyperosmolarity
	$\quad$ Insulinopenia
	$\quad$ Drugs (Table 3.9)
	Impaired renal excretion
	$\quad$ Extremely premature neonates
	$\quad$ Renal failure
	$\quad$ Drugs (Table 3.9)
	$\quad$ Mineralocorticoid deficiency (Table 3.10)
	$\quad$ Mineralocorticoid resistance (Table 3.10)
	$\quad$ Primary renal secretory defect (Table 3.10)

There is weakness of the limbs and thorax, which may lead to flaccid paralysis that may last 6–24 h. Attacks often occur at night, after events that stimulate Na^+–K^+–ATPase via insulin or epinephrine release, such as a high carbohydrate meal, after exercise, or following stressful events. Hyperthyroidism may also trigger episodes through its effect on Na^+–K^+–ATPase, driving K^+ into cells. During periodic paralysis, K^+ is sequestered in myocytes, and a diminished sarcolemmal ATP-sensitive K^+ current impedes propagation of the muscle action potential, leading to paralysis. After attacks, K^+ is released from cells and K^+ levels return to normal [104, 116, 120, 126]. Barium leads to hypokalemia by reducing cellular K^+ conductance, thereby impairing outward diffusion of K^+ from myocytes and resulting in intracellular K^+ accumulation [62, 113].

The list of causes associated with ongoing body loss of K^+ is lengthy, and is categorized into those that result

Table 3.4   Causes of hypokalemia: cellular uptake of K^+

Acute alkalosis (metabolic or respiratory)
Insulin therapy
Increased β-adrenergic activity
Hypokalemic periodic paralysis
Increased bone marrow cell production
Barium poisoning

in extrarenal K^+ loss, via the skin and gastrointestinal system, and those with primary renal wasting [53, 95, 116]. These conditions may alternatively be classified into those that are associated with low or normal blood pressures, usually with mild hypovolemia, and those with hypertension. All extrarenal causes of hypokalemia fall in the first category, as well as many primary *Renal* K^+ wasting conditions. The conditions in this group with low-normal blood pressure are associated with secondary aldosteronism, which enhances kaliuresis. These are itemized in Table 3.5.

Patients with increased blood pressure and hypokalemia, especially with metabolic alkalosis, may be categorized depending on the status of their plasma renin concentration or activity to screen for low-renin disorders [11, 93, 95, 135]. Conditions associated with low-renin activity are uncommon and are associated with salt-water retention (Table 3.6). They may be further classified based upon concentrations of the patient's endogenous mineralocorticoids, aldosterone, and deoxycorticosterone (DOC) [119].

3.3.4   Diagnostic Approach to Hypokalemia

A detailed history and review of medical records is necessary to clarify whether hypokalemia is due to a chronic condition that preceded admission to the intensive care unit. Important areas to investigate include growth parameters, medicine list (diuretics, chemotherapeutic agents, antibiotics, etc.), unusual diets, excessive sweating, polyuria, nighttime thirst, blood pressures, and chronic constipation or diarrhea. A family history of hypokalemia or unusual inherited conditions is helpful. Important findings on physical examination include evidence of growth restriction, adenopathy or abdominal mass, edema, weakness or abnormal neurologic findings, and either high or low blood pressure and heart rate, and evidence of gastrointestinal or urologic surgery.

Simple blood tests, such as a CBC, blood gas analysis, and basic chemistry panel, in conjunction with a review of the medical and dietary history and the physical examination, are sufficient to assess for the presence or absence of pseudohypokalemia or intracellular shifts of K^+. These tests also help to categorize the cause of hypokalemia among those with excessive renal K^+ loss.

It is often difficult to distinguish primary renal from extrarenal causes of K^+ loss in ICU patients who are receiving intravenous fluids containing sodium and potassium salts. This is because the conditions in Table 3.5 are often associated with mild hypovolemia and secondary aldosteronism-induced kaliuresis. While intravenous fluids may reduce this phenomenon, the salt replacement may mask the primary cause as well. If hypokalemia persists despite intravenous sodium and potassium supplementation in patients without large gastrointestinal losses, then a primary renal K^+ wasting condition is almost certain. This issue may be further analyzed by measuring urinary electrolytes, urinary osmolality, and concurrent plasma osmolality. In the absence of diuretic use, extrarenal K^+ depletion is strongly suggested by a urinary profile characterized by K^+ concentration $\leq 15\,meqL^{-1}$, in the setting of adequate distal nephron sodium delivery (urine Na^+ concentration > 25 meq L^{-1}) [53, 95, 116]. If the patient's urine is not dilute relative to plasma, then the transtubular potassium gradient (TTKG) may also distinguish renal from extrarenal K^+ loss. This ratio is calculated as follows: TTKG = $(K_u/K_p) \times (O_p/O_u)$, where urine potassium (K_u) and plasma potassium (K_p) concentrations are in milliequivalents/liter, and urine osmolality (O_u) and plasma osmolality (O_p) are in milliosmolality per kilogram [146]. The use of this ratio is only valid if $O_u \geq O_p$ and adequate distal nephron sodium delivery is assured (urine Na^+ concentration >25 meq L^{-1}). Renal K^+ wasting is suggested by a TTKG > 4 in a child with hypokalemia [116, 146].

Hypokalemic disorders associated with excessive kaliuresis may best be classified by the concomitant acid–base status, as depicted in Table 3.5. Those with hypokalemic metabolic alkalosis are further tested for urinary chloride concentration and by assessing volume status with pulse and blood pressure [95]. Systemic chloride depletion, such as from protracted vomiting, may lead to renal K^+ loss [116]. In these cases the urinary chloride concentration is low (≤ 15 meq L^{-1}) and the exam suggests hypovolemia or normal volume status. Disorders responsible for hypokalemic metabolic alkalosis associated with elevated urinary chloride concentration (≤ 15 meq L^{-1}) include those associated with fluid retention and hypertension (Table 3.6), or those

Table 3.5 Causes of hypokalemia: excessive K$^+$ loss and low-normal blood pressure

Renal loss	Extrarenal loss
Metabolic acidosis	Sweat loss
Renal tubular acidosis (I and II)	Ostomies and fistulas
Use of carbonic anhydrase inhibitors	VIPoma
Ureterosigmoid diversion	Dialysis
Diabetic ketoacidosis	GI loss
Variable acid–base status	Diarrhea
Polyuric states (concentrating defect, hypercalcemia)	Laxatives
Prolonged (K$^+$-free) saline resuscitation/diuresis	Pica/geophagia
Magnesium depletion	K$^+$ binders
Congenital K$^+$ wasting	
Acquired K$^+$ wasting	
Leukemia	
Thyrotoxicosis	
Edematous states	
Drugs (carbenicillin, gentamicin, amphotericin B, cis-platinum)	
Metabolic alkalosis with low urine Cl$^-$ concentration ($\leq$15 meq L^{-1})	
Cl$^-$ deficient diet	
Gastric Cl$^-$ loss (vomiting, NG tube to suction)	
Sweat Cl$^-$ loss	
Congenital chloridorrhea	
Cl$^-$ secreting villous adenomas (colon and rectum)	
Posthypercapnea	
Postdiuretic effect	
Metabolic alkalosis with normal–high urine Cl$^-$ concentration (>15 meq L^{-1})	
Recent diuretic effect	
Bartter's syndrome	
Gitelman's syndrome	
Congenital K$^+$ wasting	
Severe hypercalcemia	
Familial hypocalcemia (activating CaSR mutation)	
Hypovolemia (and secondary aldosteronism)	

with signs of hypovolemia or normal (compensated) volume status, resulting from excessive renal electrolyte and fluid loss, such as from diuretic therapy or Bartter's syndrome (Table 3.5) [95, 119].

The evaluation of hypokalemic metabolic alkalosis and hypertension (Table 3.6) is best performed when the patient is off intravenous fluids, and is facilitated by testing for plasma renin activity (PRA) or the newer direct renin (DR) assay [61, 76], prior to treatment with diuretics or antihypertensives.

The finding of a very low PRA ($\leq$0.65 ng mL^{-1} h^{-1}) or DR ($\leq$15 mU L^{-1}) is indicative of intravascular fluid expansion, and in the absence of excessive fluid administration, suggests stimulated renal salt-water retention due to an endocrine cause [61]. The causes of low-renin hypertension and hypokalemic alkalosis may be further evaluated by measuring plasma aldosterone, desoxycorticosterone (DOC), and 17-hydroxyprogesterone (17-OHP), according to Table 3.6 [95, 119].

Table 3.6   Causes of hypokalemia: excessive (renal) K^+ loss, high blood pressure, and metabolic alkalosis

Low rennin	Normal or high renin
High aldosterone; low/normal DOC	Renal parenchymal disease
Adrenal tumors	Renal compression
Adrenal hyperplasia	Renal tumors
Dexamethasone-suppressible hyperaldosteronism (FH-I)	Pheochromocytoma
Familial hyperaldosteronism II (FH-II)	Prolonged high ACTH/glucocorticoid exposure
Low aldosterone; low/normal DOC	
Prolonged exposure to licorice, carbenoxolone, grapefruit juice	
Prolonged high ACTH/glucocorticoid exposure	
Exogenous mineralocorticoid exposure	
Apparent mineralocorticoid excess	
Liddle's syndrome (pseudoaldosteronism type 1, PA-I)	
Minereralocorticoid receptor (MR) activating mutation (PA-II)	
L810 mutation of MR (pregnancy-associated PA-II)	
High DOC; variable aldosterone	
11- β hydroxylase deficiency	
17- α hydroxylase deficiency	
Glucocorticoid receptor resistance	
DOC-secreting tumors	

3.3.5   Therapy of Hypokalemia

K^+ replacement is the cornerstone of treatment in the intensive care unit, with the goal to expeditiously raise the K^+ level above $3.0\,meq\,L^{-1}$ and thereby avoid cardiac and neuromuscular dysfunction. Additionally, removal or minimizing exposure to offending agents that cause hypokalemia, and treating underlying medical conditions (adrenal tumors, leukemia, hyperthyroidism, diabetic ketoacidosis, etc.) should be pursued. Plasma magnesium concentration should be monitored, and replacement provided when needed. Additional specific therapies should also be instituted for specific conditions [4].

The choice of K^+ replacement will depend on the severity of hypokalemia, cardiac and renal stability, and the ability of the patient to take enteral K^+ salts. Oral therapy is safer and preferable. Doses are given every 3–4h, and titrated as needed or until gastrointestinal irritation develops. Potassium chloride is most often used, but gluconate, bicarbonate, or citrate salts are preferred in the absence of cardiac rhythm disturbances, for hypokalemia associated with chronic acidosis, hypercalciuria, or lithiasis (Table 3.7) [143]. Oral potassium phosphate is less commonly used, but

can be very effective for hypokalemic disorders associated with marked hypophosphatemia, which usually result from disorders or use of medications associated with proximal renal tubular injury.

Intravenous therapy requires continuous EKG monitoring and frequent measurments of plasma K^+ concentrations, and should be reserved for severe hypokalemia associated with cardiac or neuromuscular dysfunction, digitalis toxicity, diabetic ketoacidosis, or in those who are unable to receive it enterally. It should be provided as a dextrose-free solution of potassium chloride or phosphate, at a total K^+ concentration not exceeding $40\,meq\,L^{-1}$, and infused at a rate not exceeding $1\,meq\,kg^{-1}\,h^{-1}$ in children, or at a maximum of $40\,meq\,h^{-1}$ [116, 143]. The use of intravenous potassium phosphate is limited primarily to treatment of diabetic ketoacidosis, and in cases of documented severe hypophosphatemia.

Additional therapy should be considered in certain cases of hypokalemia. For example, either or both sodium chloride and sodium bicarbonate supplementation may be necessary to minimize hypovolemia associated with salt wasting and to correct acid–base abnormalities characteristic of several conditions outlined in Table 3.5. Phosphate salts are required

Table 3.7 Oral potassium supplements

Supplements
Potassium chloride
Solution: 10, 15, and 20% (15% = 10 meq/5 mL)
Sustained-release tabs: 8, 10, 15, 20 meq
Sustained-release caps: 8, 10 meq
Powder: 15, 20, 25 meq per packet
Potassium gluconate
Solution: 20 meq/15 mL
Tabs: 500 mg (2.15 meq), 595 mg (2.56 meq)
Potassium bicarbonate and citrate
Effervescent tab (to make solution): 25 meq
Potassium citrate
Polycitra-K solution: 10 meq K/5 mL
Polycitra or Polycitra-LC solution: 5 meq K and 5 meq Na/5 mL[a]
Urocit tabs: 5 meq, 10 meq
Potassium phosphate[a]
Neutra-Phos-K caps, powder: 250 mg (14.25 meq K, 8 mM P)
Neutra-Phos caps, powder: 250 mg (7.125 meq K, 7.125 meq Na, 8 mM P)[b]

[a] Supplement contains both sodium and potassium
[b] Other preparations are available with less potassium and more sodium

to correct hypophosphatemia in patients with proximal tubular dysfunction. Magnesium supplementation is necessary to correct hypokalemia associated with hypomagnesemia, and it is a primary treatment for *torsades des pointes*, as intravenous magnesium sulfate [141]. Nonselective β-blockers and acetazolamide are helpful for hypokalemic periodic paralysis, in addition to infusion of potassium salts [126]. Surgical correction, angiotensin converting enzyme inhibitors, spironolactone, α- and β-adrenergic receptor blockers, and other antihypertensives are effective treatments for many causes of high-renin hypertension and hypokalemia. Diuretic-dependent children with hypokalemia may benefit from adding spironolactone, amiloride, or triamterene. The endocrine causes of hypokalemia should be managed in conjunction with experienced subspecialists. The range of therapy for this group includes surgical tumor removal, institution of replacement glucocorticoid therapy, and treatment with spironolactone, amiloride, or triamterene.

3.4 Hyperkalemia

Hyperkalemia is defined as serum K^+ exceeding 6.0 meq L^{-1} in neonates or 5.5 meq L^{-1} in older children and adults. Plasma K^+ concentrations are as much as 0.5 meq L^{-1} less than serum values in normal individuals, due to K^+ release from cells during clotting of the specimen [53, 116]. The clinical disorders associated with hyperkalemia may be categorized as due to (1) *excessive K^+ load*, (2) *transcellular K^+ shift*, and (3) *impaired renal K^+ excretion* (Table 3.3). PICU patients are at increased risk for hyperkalemia due to frequent comorbid conditions (including sepsis, acidosis, trauma, and renal failure), transfusion requirements for blood components, and exposure to multiple medications.

3.4.1 Hypokalemia vs Pseudohyperkalemia

Pseudohyperkalemia should be entertained when high K^+ measurements are encountered without clinical evidence of hyperkalemia, and results from the egress of K^+ from cells and platelets *ex vivo*, during phlebotomy or later (prior to separation from the cellular elements). The artifactual elevation of the K^+ concentration may be dramatic. This is typically seen from hemolysis associated with a difficult or traumatic (heel stick) capillary blood collection in neonates, and often in children whose illness results in markedly increased numbers of circulating leukocytes, red cells, or platelets [4, 53, 116]. It may also result from prolonged tourniquet use, as a consequence of local muscle ischemia and K^+ release [43, 144]. Less often, pseudohyperkalemia may be associated with disorders of erythrocyte membrane permeability [64].

3.4.2 Clinical Features Associated with Hyperkalemia

Clinical features of hyperkalemia predominantly involve cardiac, skeletal muscle, and peripheral nerve tissue, and are a consequence of altered cellular transmembrane K^+ gradients. Hyperkalemia reduces the resting membrane potential, thereby increasing tissue excitability initially. However, this is followed by a sustained reduction in excitability.

Cardiac dysrrhythmias are the most serious consequences of hyperkalemia, and their presentation is influenced not only by K^+ concentration, but also by its rate of rise, concurrent acid–base status, and sodium and calcium concentration. Toxicity is exacerbated by a rapid rise in K^+ concentration, acidosis, hyponatremia, and hypocalcemia [3, 4, 112]. Early EKG changes develop at K^+ levels above 6.5 meq L^{-1}, and are characteristic of more rapid repolarization. These include narrow peaked T waves, shortened QT interval, and prolonged PR interval. Once K^+ reaches 7–8 meq L^{-1}, EKG changes characteristic of delayed depolarization occur, such as widened QRS, progressive loss of P-wave amplitude, and eventually a sine-wave pattern when the QRS merges with the T wave. This is typically followed by ventricular fibrillation or asystole [130, 142].

Neuromuscular effects of hyperkalemia are rarely evident until K^+ levels exceed 8 meq L^{-1}, and include skeletal muscle weakness, ascending flaccid paralysis, and paresthesias. Reduced excitability is a consequence of inactivated cell membrane sodium channels, which result from excessive depolarization. Respiratory muscles as well as head and trunk muscles are usually spared [50, 112].

3.4.3   Causes of Hyperkalemia

3.4.3.1   *Excessive K^+ Load*

Exogenous K^+ loads are frequently administered to ICU patients and rarely result in life-threatening hyperkalemia. This is due to adequate disposal by initial cellular uptake, and later by renal excretion. Hence, hyperkalemia is more likely to develop following a load in patients with impaired hormonal activity that is necessary for cellular uptake, or in those who have renal impairment.

Clinically significant hyperkalemia has resulted from large volume PRBC transfusions, often given for trauma or during operative procedures [20–23, 29, 60, 99, 115]. With better blood bank storage and cross-matching practices, the use of in-line leukofilters to replace blood product radiation, and increased use of loop diuretic with transfusions, hyperkalemia is not a common complication from blood cell transfusion seen in the PICU [9, 16, 27, 100, 101, 105, 148]. Medicines with a large K^+ load, such as Penicillin G potassium (1.7 meq K^+ per 1 million units) [87, 139], are administered less often than before, but intravenous KCl is still commonly used, and errors in its administration still result in significant mortality [153–156]. Less obvious is the significant enteral K^+ load provided in

many liquid nutritional formulas and foods (Table 3.8), from salt substitutes (50–65 meq per level teaspoon) [68, 122] and less common herbal remedies such as Noni juice, alfalfa, dandelion, horsetail, and nettle [65, 89, 97].

Endogenous sources of K^+, typically associated with a permanent cell damage and release of K^+, should also be considered as a K^+ load. Examples of causes include burns, trauma, intravascular hemolysis, gastrointestinal bleeding, resorption of hematomas, rhabdomyolysis, and tumor lysis.

3.4.3.2   *Transcellular K^+ Shift*

Clinical scenarios associated with extracellular shifts of K^+ that are common in the PICU include acidosis, hyperosmolarity, and deficiency or interference of the activities of hormones that regulate Na^+–K^+–ATPase, including insulinopenia and the use of β-adrenergic receptor blockers as well as other inhibitors of the renin–angiotensin–aldosterone system. K^+ moves from the intracellular space to the extracellular space in the setting of acidosis. Metabolic acidosis due to mineral acids such as hydrochloric acid and ammonium chloride has a greater hyperkalemic effect than respiratory acidosis or organic acidosis due to lactic and ketoacids [1, 24]. Hyperosmolality leads to extracellular shift of K^+, as the cation follows the fluid transit out of the cell. This may be seen following the administration of mannitol or hypertonic saline [34, 88], or in children with diabetic ketoacidosis, although in these children insulin deficiency is also a contributing factor [127]. Familial hyperkalemic periodic paralysis is a rare autosomal dominant disorder, which is the cause of muscle weakness associated with hyperkalemia. Attacks usually occur during rest, after strenuous exercise. These patients have a mutation in the α subunit of the voltage-gated sodium channel of human skeletal muscle (SkM1), that leads to increased sodium entry, myocyte depolarization, and subsequent exit of K^+ from the cytosol [25, 108]. Therapies aimed to abort the periodic paralysis attacks include albuterol, thiazide diuretics, mineralocorticoids, carbonic anhydrase inhibitors, limiting exercise, and use of a low-K^+, high- carbohydrate diet.

Several drugs commonly used in the PICU are associated with extracellular shifts of K^+ (Table 3.9). Nonspecific β_2-blockers, particularly in the setting of exposure to a K^+ load or in children with renal

Table 3.8 Common high-potassium-containing foods (mg/serving) and enteral formulas [157]

Food	mg K$^+$/100 g food	mg K$^+$/serving size
Standard infant formulas		131–187/8 oz; 14–20 meq L^{-1}
Toddler formulas		281–375/8 oz; 30–40 meq L^{-1}
Chicken	259	220/3 oz
Beef, round	266	226/3 oz
Unsweetened chocolate	1,033	310/1 oz
Salmon	375	319/3 oz
Pork (loin)	421	358/3 oz
Peanuts	656	374/2 oz
Milk, nonfat	153	376/cup
Almonds	723	412/2 oz
Banana	396	467/1 medium
Tuna, yellowfin	569	484/3 oz
Cantaloupe	309	494/cup
Orange juice	200	496/cup
Yogurt, low-fat	234	531/cup
Avocado	635	540/3 oz
Dates	653	542/10 dates
Figs, dried	713	542/4 figs
Raisins	745	544/½ cup
Black-eyed peas	418	690/cup
Prune juice	276	707/cup
Kidney beans	403	713/cup
Lentils	369	731/cup
Baked beans	296	752/cup
Pinto beans	468	800/cup
Spinach	466	839/cup
Soybeans	515	886/cup
Lima beans	508	955/cup
Potatoes with skin	535	1,081/1 potato
White beans	454	1,189/cup

insufficiency, may lead to hyperkalemia by blocking catecholamine-induced cellular uptake [72, 134, 150]. They also inhibit both renin release and aldosterone synthesis. Pure β_1-adrenergic blockers may be safer in this setting [28]. Vasoconstrictive α-adrenergic agonists promote a mild extracellular K$^+$ shift and reduce muscle uptake [72, 134]. Spironolactone, ACE inhibitors, and ARBs inhibit the renin–angiotensin–aldosterone system and are commonly prescribed. They impede both intracellular K$^+$ uptake and renal excretion, thereby increasing the risk of hyperkalemia. Although the cardiac toxicity of digitalis is enhanced in patients with hypokalemia, high digoxin

levels tend to promote hyperkalemia through inhibition of Na$^+$–K$^+$–ATPase [19, 102]. Several herbal remedies are available that have similar digitalis-like effect, including milkweed, lily of the valley, and Siberian ginseng. The depolarizing neuromuscular blocking agent succinylcholine typically raises plasma K$^+$ levels about 0.5 meq L^{-1}. By stimulating the acetylcholine receptor, it increases the ionic permeability of muscle and allows efflux of K$^+$ [59]. PICU patients with certain comorbid conditions are susceptible to develop severe hyperkalemia with this agent. Succinylcholine-induced hyperkalemia has been reported in patients with burns,

Table 3.9 Drugs (potassium-free) associated with hyperkalemia

Extracellular release of K+	Impaired renal excretion
Propranolol	NSAIDs (Ibuprofen, etc.)
Phenylephrine	Drospirenone
Spironolactone	Spironolactone
ACE inhibitors	Amiloride
ARBs	Triamterene
Digitalis	Trimethoprim
Succinylcholine	Pentamidine
Sodium fluoride	Azole antifungals
Epsilon-amino caproic acid	ACE inhibitors
HCl, lysine HCl	Arginine
	ARBs
	Cyclosporine
	Tacrolimus
	Heparin

spinal cord injury, rhabdomyolysis, traumatic brain injury, renal failure, and progressive neuromuscular disorders such as Friedrich's ataxia, Duchenne's muscular dystrophy, and central core disease [35, 102]. Sodium fluoride may cause hyperkalemia by shifting K+ extracellularly, particularly in chronic renal failure patients who drink highly fluorinated water. Lastly, cationic amino acids (in parenteral nutrition or other forms of supplementation) such as lysine and arginine, or epsilon-aminocaproic acid, a fibrinolysis inhibitor, are small molecules that can contribute to hyperkalemia by entering the cytosol in exchange for K+. Arginine HCl should be used with caution in patients with renal or hepatic failure [24, 63].

3.4.3.3 Decreased Renal Excretion

Reduced renal K+ excretion may result from any combination of several clinical perturbations, some of which are frequently encountered in the PICU: (1) mineralocorticoid deficiency exclusive of renal disease, (2) acute or chronic renal insufficiency, (3) inherited or acquired renal tubular dysfunction (with normal GFR and mineralocorticoid sufficiency), (4) hypovolemia, and (5) drug effects.

Mineralocorticoids stimulate cellular K+ uptake, as well as colonic and renal K+ excretion; thus, their deficiency from any cause may lead to hyperkalemia. Examples include adrenal suppression from prolonged glucocorticoid use, primary adrenal insufficiency;

secondary adrenal insufficiency from Addison's disease, infiltrative disease, or hemorrhage; congenital adrenal enzymopathies, and hyporeninemic hypoaldosteronism (Table 3.10).

Renal insufficiency is associated with decreased glomerular filtration rate, decreased filtrate flow at the distal nephron (where K+ secretion is flow-dependent), impaired cellular K+ uptake, and metabolic acidosis, which all contribute to hyperkalemia. Despite this, adaptive mechanisms exist in stable patients with chronic renal failure to prevent hyperkalemia. Such patients have markedly increased renal tubular and colonic K+ excretion, but virtually no excretory reserve, and therefore poorly tolerate K+ loads, even from their diet.

Despite normal kidney and adrenal function, isolated distal nephron tubular dysfunction may result from inherited or acquired causes (Table 3.10). These conditions result in sodium wasting, acidosis, impaired K+ secretion, and hyperkalemia. This can also occur transiently in otherwise normal, extremely low-birth weight premature neonates [38, 128]. *Inherited* causes seen primarily in neonates and infants and lasting into early childhood (symptoms usually resolve by age 10) include pseudohypoaldosteronism (PHA) types I and II. PHA I is autosomal recessive, more severe, and is often associated with respiratory distress. Type II follows autosomal dominant inheritance and is milder. Both are managed with sodium chloride and sodium bicarbonate supplementation, and by avoiding dehydration. Rarely, fludrocortisone may be beneficial. Occasionally a premature infant will present similar to PHA I with salt wasting, hyperkalemia, and acidosis, but after a month will develop alkalosis and hypokalemia. Genetic studies typically confirm a diagnosis of the ROMK form of antenatal Bartter syndrome. *Acquired* causes of hyperkalemia due to renal tubular dysfunction are also itemized in Table 3.10, and are associated with distal nephron injury. Type 4 renal tubular acidosis is characterized by hyperkalemia and salt wasting, associated with a normal plasma aldosterone level. Impaired distal Na+ absorption impedes K+ secretion; this condition is typically seen in children with obstructive uropathy [15] and sickle cell disease [14]. Familial hyperkalemia and hypertension differ from PHA I and II in that these children have increased effective circulating volume, hypertension, suppressed PRA and aldosterone concentrations, and require lifelong therapy. Like PHA, they have metabolic acidosis and are often short.

Hypovolemia increases the risk of hyperkalemia through several mechanisms. Reduced extracellular

Table 3.10 Disorders associated with hyperkalemia, impaired K^+ excretion, and adequate renal function

	Inherited	Acquired
Mineralocorticoid deficiency	21-Hydroxylase deficiency	Primary adrenal insufficiency
	3 β-Hydroxysteroid-dehydrogenase deficiency	Secondary adrenal insufficiency
	Congenital lipoid hyperplasia (StAR)	Aldosterone synthase deficiency
		Hyporeninemic hypoaldosteronism
Impaired renal excretion, mineralocorticoid sufficient	Pseudohypoaldosteronism I	Obstructive uropathy
	Pseudohypoaldosteronism II	Lead nephropathy
	Antenatal Bartter syndrome (ROMK)	Sickle cell disease
	Familial hyperkalemia with hypertension	Papillary necrosis
		Systemic lupus erythematosis
		Type 4 distal RTA
		Renal transplant tubular dysfunction

volume will lead to hemoconcentration, while reduced effective circulating volume tends to lower glomerular filtration and increase proximal tubular reabsorption of filtrate Na^+ and water. Distal nephron flow is therefore reduced, and despite secondary aldosterone stimulation, net K^+ secretion is impaired.

Many drugs commonly used in the PICU may inhibit K^+ excretion and result in hyperkalemia (Table 3.9). Potassium sparing diuretics, such as spironolactone or its analogue drospirenone, block mineralocorticoid receptors in the distal nephron. Amiloride and triamterene block epithelial sodium channel function, thereby reducing the cytosol–lumen electrical gradient necessary for principal cell K^+ secretion. Trimethoprim [46, 57, 58] and pentamidine have similar effects [74]. Prolonged heparin use may result in hyperkalemia in predisposed children with renal impairment, through reversible suppression of aldosterone synthesis [96]. Prostaglandin synthase inhibitors, such as the nonsteroidal anti-inflammatory drugs (NSAIDs) ibuprofen and indomethacin, impair K^+ excretion by reducing glomerular filtration (from afferent arteriolar constriction) and distal nephron flow, as well as suppressing renin and aldosterone secretion [17, 72]. The calcineurin inhibitors cyclosporine and tacrolimus may cause hyperkalemia by suppressing renin release and subsequent aldosterone synthesis [86]. Azole antifungals inhibit adrenal steroid synthesis, which can lead to mineralocorticoid deficiency. ACE inhibitors block the conversion of angiotensin I to angiotensin II, which is a physiologic stimulus for aldosterone release [132]. They also reduce glomerular filtration and may provoke the generation of bradykinin, which may cause a dry cough and hypotension. Most ACE inhibitors are excreted by the kidneys, and hence may have a prolonged effect in children with renal insufficiency. ARBs block AT1 receptors and have similar physiologic effects as ACE inhibitors, but hyperkalemia is less severe. They do not lead to bradykinin generation and are primarily excreted by the liver.

3.4.4 Diagnostic Approach to Hyperkalemia

The basic diagnostic workup of hyperkalemia should include a complete medical history including medication exposure, assessment of intravascular volume status, and a complete physical examination. An electrocardiogram should be obtained immediately to exclude cardiac toxicity. A plasma chemistry panel, including electrolytes, calcium, BUN, and creatinine is necessary, as well as the urinalysis, which often provides insight about distal tubular function and the presence or absence of significant nephropathy. Depending on the clinical situation, other studies that may be considered include urine electrolytes, osmoles, and creatinine; plasma osmoles; uric acid; complete blood count; creatine phosphokinase; lactate dehydrogenase; and concurrent 8 A.M. PRA or direct renin assay, aldosterone, and cortisol level.

Reduced effective circulating volume or renal failure is usually recognized quickly. The other major cause of hyperkalemia in children is hypoaldosteronism, and like the less common causes associated with mineralocorticoid resistance, it typically presents with hypovolemia and poses a greater challenge to evaluate. 8 A.M. levels of PRA (or the newer direct renin assay), aldosterone, and cortisol are often necessary. Calculation of the TTKG (see "Diagnostic Approach to Hypokalemia") provides complementary information, which is helpful to assess distal nephron response to hyperkalemia. A TTKG less than 5 in a child with hyperkalemia suggests impaired excretion, either from mineralocorticoid deficiency or from resistance. Higher values are consistent with appropriate renal excretion of a K^+ load.

3.4.5 Therapy of Hyperkalemia

Adrenal insufficiency due to abrupt glucocorticoid withdrawal should be recognized and appropriately treated with hydrocortisone replacement and volume resuscitation if clinically indicated. Patients with aldosterone resistance will require salt supplements, usually both chloride and bicarbonate salts, and rarely may benefit from fludrocortisone.

Urgent treatment is required when plasma K^+ concentration exceeds $7\,meq\,L^{-1}$, or in the presence of ECG changes (Table 3.11). Although easily overlooked, it is imperative to immediately discontinue ongoing K^+ input. This may include K^+ intake in intravenous fluids, parenteral or enteral nutrition, or parenteral or enteral K^+ supplementation. Available therapies for management of acute hyperkalemia target four strategies to prevent complications: (1) removing K^+ from the body, (2) shifting K^+ intracellularly, (3) antagonizing the effects of K^+ at cell membranes, and (4) diluting the ECF. Because all but the first maneuver are temporizing and because the onset and duration of each therapy varies, several therapies should be employed simultaneously. If hyperkalemia is asymptomatic, sole treatment with sodium polystyrene sulfonate is appropriate. If widening of the QRS or other dysrhythmias is observed, calcium chloride (20–$25\,mg\,kg^{-1}$ IV over 2–$5\,min$) should be given immediately.

Removal of K^+ from the body is often necessary, but it is a slower process, often taking several hours. Sodium polystyrene sulfonate (Kayexalate), an ion exchange resin, binds K^+ in exchange for sodium within the intestinal lumen and is very effective for K^+ removal. Kayexalate in sorbitol or dextrose should be given 0.5–$2.0\,g\,kg^{-1}$ PO/NG/PR every 4 hours as needed. The resin binds $1\,meq$ of K^+ in exchange for $1\,meq$ of sodium, and $1\,g\,kg^{-1}$ can be expected to reduce plasma K^+ by $1\,meq\,L^{-1}$. Oral doses may be given in up to 70% sorbitol or 10% dextrose with 3–$4\,mL$ of water per $1\,g$ of resin. Rectal doses may be given without sorbitol, and in concentrations not greater than 20% to avoid colonic damage [107]. Rectal doses must be retained for 15–$30\,min$ in order to be efficacious. Electrolytes should be monitored frequently because the resin is not specific for K^+. Furosemide should be considered, in doses of $1\,mg\,kg^{-1}$, to facilitate distal nephron excretion of K^+; a higher dose is necessary in patients with renal insufficiency. In those with impaired renal function, hemodialysis and peritoneal dialysis are effective modalities to lower plasma K^+. Hemodialysis provides more rapid clearance, but peritoneal dialysis may be more practical in cardiovascularly unstable neonates and infants, or children in whom hyperkalemia is not at a life-threatening level [69, 94].

Several therapies lower K^+ levels through redistribution from the extracellular to the intracellular compartment; as such, the following therapies are not definitive and often provide only transient benefit. Sodium bicarbonate may be given 1–$2\,meq\,kg^{-1}$ IV over 5–$15\,min$ if metabolic acidosis is demonstrated. Nebulized albuterol, a β_2 agonist, has been shown to rapidly lower K^+ in premature neonates [121], children [71, 85, 90], and adults [5–8, 83] with hyperkalemia. This effect is mediated by stimulation of Na^+–K^+–ATPase, which drives K^+ intracellularly [10, 32, 56], and can result in a decrease in plasma K^+ of $0.5\,meq\,L^{-1}$ [5, 85]. Insulin, which also shifts K^+ intracellularly, should be given 0.1–0.2 units kg^{-1} IV or SQ following administration of glucose 0.5–$1.0\,g\,kg^{-1}$ IV. Serum glucose should be monitored closely. The shift effect of insulin begins in $1\,h$ and has a transient duration.

To antagonize the adverse effect of hyperkalemia on cardiac conduction, calcium chloride 10–$25\,mg\,kg^{-1}$ IV (or 10% calcium gluconate 50–$100\,mg\,kg^{-1}$ IV) should be given over 1–$5\,min$ with ECG monitoring. Cardiology consultation should be sought in patients taking digitalis, as this therapy may provoke other dysrhythmias. Treatment with calcium salts should also be considered as a temporary measure, since it does not reduce plasma K^+ levels.

The use of isotonic saline as a therapy of hyperkalemia is supported by observational data, which demonstrate that fluid resuscitation results in hypokalemia [82]. This is particularly helpful in patients with hypovolemia and tenuous renal perfusion, in whom the use of diuretics along with vascular volume expansion facilitates K^+ excretion and lowers the K^+ concentration. In cases of mineralocorticoid deficiency or resistance, fludrocortisone should be considered, as well as saline expansion and diuresis.

Table 3.11 Treatment of hyperkalemia

Therapy	Dose	Mechanism	Onset	Duration	Comments
Kayexalate	0.5–2.0 g kg^{-1} dose^{-1} PO/NG/PR	Removal	1–2 h	4–6 h	Rectal route faster
Calcium chloride	20–25 mg kg^{-1} dose^{-1} IV	Antagonism; protects myocardium	Immediate	30 min	Push over 2–5 min; caution bradycardia; may worsen digitalis toxicity
10% Calcium gluconate	100 mg kg^{-1} dose^{-1} IV	Antagonism	Immediate	30 min	Same as above
Insulin (regular)	0.1–0.3 Units kg^{-1}	Redistribution	15–30 min	2–6 h	During or after dextrose 0.5–2.0 g kg^{-1} is administered; monitor blood glucoses
Sodium bicarbonate	1–2 meq kg^{-1}	Dilution, antagonism, redistribution	30–60 min	2 h	Give over 5–15 min
Sodium chloride (0.9%)	10 mL kg^{-1} IV	Dilution, antagonism			Especially for hyponatremic patients
Albuterol	2.5–5.0 mg nebulized	Redistribution	15–30 min	2–4 h	May be given continuously
Furosemide	1 mg kg^{-1} dose^{-1}	Removal	15–60 min	4–6 h	Give with saline if hypovolemic
Dialysis	Per nephrology	Removal			HD, PD, or CRRT

3.5   Other Issues

3.5.1   Point-of-Care Testing

The i-STAT Portable Clinical Analyzer, a point-of-care testing system for blood gases and electrolytes using the EG7+ and EG8+ cartridges, has been shown to yield accurate and rapid K$^+$ values compared with traditional laboratory testing in neonatal and pediatric populations [91, 98].

3.5.2   Morbidity/Mortality from Hyperkalemia: Prescribing K$^+$ Salts in the PICU

In light of the Institute of Medicine's report *To Err is Human* and national attention directed at the prevention of medical errors, PICUs have begun to focus on patient safety initiatives. Leape et al. reported in a retrospective review of over 30,000 charts a 4% incidence of medical errors, many of which were preventable [79]. Mistakes in the ordering or administration of K$^+$ may lead to ominous outcomes, particularly in the critically ill population [153, 156]. KCl has been named one of the five *high-alert medications* by the National Patient Safety Goals of the Joint Commission of

Accreditation of Healthcare Organizations (JCAHO) because of the high risk of injury when misused [154]. In addition, KCl has been implicated by JCAHO as the drug contributing to the most sentinel events [155]. In a review of the literature evaluating best practices for the administration of K$^+$, Tubman et al. published a set of recommendations regarding storage, packaging, preparation, and prescribing of KCl [137]. Many PICUs have protocols and policies for the administration of supplemental K$^+$; for example, orders for a KCl dose greater than 0.3–0.5 mEq kg^{-1} h^{-1} must often be cosigned by a fellow or attending physician [147].

When insulin or furosemide infusions are decreased or discontinued, practitioners must also consider decreasing supplemental K$^+$. White et al. introduced an intervention requiring the clinician ordering K$^+$ to consider whether the patient is symptomatic from hypokalemia, had a recent cardiac repair, is on digoxin, is receiving other sources of K$^+$ (IVF, TPN, oral supplements), has renal failure, recently had increase in K$^+$ content of IVFs, had dialysis discontinued recently, had mannitol or furosemide infusions discontinued recently, and the lab values for the most recent K$^+$ and creatinine [147]. Such interventions are designed to reduced proximal causes of error, and in this case resulted in statistically significant reduction in postinfusion elevation of serum K^+ (7.7% to 0%) [147].

Take-Home Pearls

> The TTKG is often useful to evaluate renal potassium handling for both hyper and hypokalemia.

> If hyperkalemic changes are present on electrocardiogram, calcium should be given, realizing that this measure is temporizing and does not facilitate K^+ removal or redistribution. In addition, several therapies should be employed simultaneously to remove, redistribute, dilute, and antagonize K^+.

References

1. Adrogue HJ, Madias NE (1981) Changes in plasma potassium concentration during acute acid–base disturbances. Am J Med 71(3):456–67
2. Adrogue HJ, Madias NE (2007) Sodium and potassium in the pathogenesis of hypertension. N Engl J Med 356(19):1966–78
3. Ahmed J, Weisberg LS (2001) Hyperkalemia in dialysis patients. Semin Dial 14(5):348–56
4. Alfonzo AV, Isles C, Geddes C, et al. (2006) Potassium disorders – clinical spectrum and emergency management. Resuscitation 70(1):10–25
5. Allon M (1995) Hyperkalemia in end-stage renal disease: Mechanisms and management. J Am Soc Nephrol 6(4):1134–42
6. Allon M, Shanklin N (1995) Effect of albuterol treatment on subsequent dialytic potassium removal. Am J Kidney Dis 26(4):607–13
7. Allon M, Shanklin N (1996) Effect of bicarbonate administration on plasma potassium in dialysis patients: Interactions with insulin and albuterol. Am J Kidney Dis 28(4):508–14
8. Allon M, Dunlay R, Copkney C (1989) Nebulized albuterol for acute hyperkalemia in patients on hemodialysis. Ann Intern Med 110(6):426–9
9. Andriessen P, Kollee LA, van Dijk BA (1993) Effect of age of erythrocyte concentration administered to premature infants: A retrospective study. Tijdschr Kindergeneeskd 61(3):82–7
10. Angelopoulous M, Leitz H, Lambert G, et al. (1996) In vitro analysis of the Na(+)-K + ATPase activity in neonatal and adult red blood cells. Biol Neonate 69(3):140–5
11. Armanini D, Calo L, Semplicini A (2003) Pseudohyperaldosteronism: Pathogenetic mechanisms. Crit Rev Clin Lab Sci 40(3):295–335
12. Barraclough MA, Jones NF (1970) The effect of vasopressin on the reabsorption of sodium, potassium and urea by the renal tubules in man. Clin Sci 39(4):517–27
13. Bastl C, Hayslett JP, Binder HJ (1977) Increased large intestinal secretion of potassium in renal insufficiency. Kidney Int 12(1):9–16
14. Batlle D, Itsarayoungyuen K, Arruda JA, et al. (1982) Hyperkalemic hyperchloremic metabolic acidosis in sickle cell hemoglobinopathies. Am J Med 72(2): 188–92
15. Batlle DC, Arruda JA, Kurtzman NA (1981) Hyperkalemic distal renal tubular acidosis associated with obstructive uropathy. N Engl J Med 304(7):373–80
16. Batton DG, Maisels MJ, Shulman G (1983) Serum potassium changes following packed red cell transfusions in newborn infants. Transfusion 23(2):163–4
17. Bennett WM, Henrich WL, Stoff JS (1996) The renal effects of nonsteroidal anti-inflammatory drugs: Summary and recommendations. Am J Kidney Dis 28(1, Suppl 1): S56–S62
18. Bia MJ, DeFronzo RA (1996) Extrarenal potassium homeostasis. Am J Physiol 240(4):F257–F268
19. Bismuth C, Gaultier M, Conso F, et al. (1973) Hyperkalemia in acute digitalis poisoning: Prognostic significance and therapeutic implications. Clin Toxicol 6(2):153–62
20. Bolton DT (2000) Hyperkalaemia, donor blood and cardiac arrest associated with ECMO priming. Anaesthesia 55(8):825–6
21. Bostic O, Duvernoy WF (1972) Hyperkalemic cardiac arrest during transfusion of stored blood. J Electrocardiol 5(4):407–9
22. Brown KA, Bissonnette B, McIntyre B (1990) Hyperkalaemia during rapid blood transfusion and hypovolaemic cardiac arrest in children. Can J Anaesth 37(7):747–54
23. Buntain SG, Pabari M (1999) Massive transfusion and hyperkalaemic cardiac arrest in craniofacial surgery in a child. Anaesth Intensive Care 27(5):530–3
24. Bushinsky DA, Gennari FJ (1978) Life-threatening hyperkalemia induced by arginine. Ann Intern Med 89(5, Part 1): 632–4
25. Cannon SC (1997) From mutation to myotonia in sodium channel disorders. Neuromuscul Disord 7(4):241–9
26. Carlisle EJ, Donnelly SM, Ethier JH, et al. (1991) Modulation of the secretion of potassium by accompanying anions in humans. Kidney Int 39(6):1206–12
27. Carmichael D, Hosty T, Kastl D, et al. (1984) Hypokalemia and massive transfusion. South Med J 77(3):315–17
28. Castellino P, Bia MJ, DeFronzo RA (1990) Adrenergic modulation of potassium metabolism in uremia. Kidney Int 37(2):793–8
29. Chen CH, Hong CL, Kau YC, et al. (1999) Fatal hyperkalemia during rapid and massive blood transfusion in a child undergoing hip surgery – A case report. Acta Anaesthesiol Sin 37(3):163–6
30. Clausen T, Everts ME (1989) Regulation of the Na, K-pump in skeletal muscle. Kidney Int 35(1):1–13
31. Clausen T, Flatman JA (1987) Effects of insulin and epinephrine on Na^+–K^+ and glucose transport in soleus muscle. Am J Physiol 252(4, Part 1):E492–E499
32. Clausen T, Flatman JA (1977) The effect of catecholamines on Na–K transport and membrane potential in rat soleus muscle. J Physiol 270(2):383–414
33. Conn JW (1965) Hypertension, the potassium ion and impaired carbohydrate tolerance. N Engl J Med 273(21):1135–43

34. Conte G, Dal Canton A, Imperatore P, et al. (1990) Acute increase in plasma osmolality as a cause of hyperkalemia in patients with renal failure. Kidney Int 38(2):301–7

35. Cooperman LH (1970) Succinylcholine-induced hyperkalemia in neuromuscular disease. JAMA 213(11):1867–71

36. Cronin RE, Thompson JR (1991) Role of potassium in the pathogenesis of acute renal failure. Miner Electrolyte Metab 17(2):100–5

37. Daut J, Maier-Rudolph W, von Beckerath N, et al. (1990) Hypoxic dilation of coronary arteries is mediated by ATP-sensitive potassium channels. Science 247(4948): 1341–4

38. Day GM, Radde IC, Balfe JW, et al. (1976) Electrolyte abnormalities in very low birthweight infants. Pediatr Res 10(5):522–6

39. DeFronzo RA, Bia M, Birkhead G (1981) Epinephrine and potassium homeostasis. Kidney Int 20(1):83–91

40. DeFronzo RA, Bia M, Smith D (1982) Clinical disorders of hyperkalemia. Annu Rev Med 33:521–54

41. DeFronzo RA, Lee R, Jones A, et al. (1980) Effect of insulinopenia and adrenal hormone deficiency on acute potassium tolerance. Kidney Int 17(5):586–94

42. DeFronzo RA, Sherwin RS, Dillingham M, et al. (1978) Influence of basal insulin and glucagon secretion on potassium and sodium metabolism. Studies with somatostatin in normal dogs and in normal and diabetic human beings. J Clin Invest 61(2):472–9

43. Don BR, Sebastian A, Cheitlin M, et al. (1990) Pseudohyperkalemia caused by fist clenching during phlebotomy. N Engl J Med 322(18):1290–2

44. Doucet A (1988) Function and control of Na–K–ATPase in single nephron segments of the mammalian kidney. Kidney Int 34(6):749–60

45. Edelman IS, Leibman J (1959) Anatomy of body water and electrolytes. Am J Med 27:256–77

46. Ellison DH (1997) Hyperkalemia and trimethoprim-sulfamethoxazole. Am J Kidney Dis 29(6):959–62; discussion 962–5

47. Engbretson BG, Stoner LC (1987) Flow-dependent potassium secretion by rabbit cortical collecting tubule in vitro. Am J Physiol 253(5, Part 2):F896–F903

48. Field MJ, Giebisch GJ (1985) Hormonal control of renal potassium excretion. Kidney Int 27(2):379–87

49. Field MJ, Stanton BA, Giebisch GH (1984) Differential acute effects of aldosterone, dexamethasone, and hyperkalemia on distal tubular potassium secretion in the rat kidney. J Clin Invest 74(5):1792–802

50. Finch CA, Sawyer CG, Flynn JM (1946) Clinical syndrome of potassium intoxication. Am J Med 1:337–352

51. Fisch C (1973) Relation of electrolyte disturbances to cardiac arrhythmias. Circulation 47(2):408–19

52. Funder JW, Blair-West JR, Coghlan JP, et al. (1969) Effect of (K+) on the secretion of aldosterone. Endocrinology 85(2):381–4

53. Gennari FJ (1998) Hypokalemia. N Engl J Med 339(7): 451–8

54. Giebisch G (1998) Renal potassium transport: Mechanisms and regulation. Am J Physiol 274(5, Part 2):F817–F833

55. Giebisch G, Malnic G, Berliner RW (2005) Control of renal potassium excretion. In: Brenner BM, Rector FCJ (eds) The Kidney, 5th edn. WB Saunders, Philadelphia, pp. 371–407

56. Gillzan KM, Stewart AG (1997) The role of potassium channels in the inhibitory effects of beta 2-adrenoceptor agonists on DNA synthesis in human cultured airway smooth muscle. Pulm Pharmacol Ther 10(2):71–9

57. Greenberg S, Reiser IW, Chou SY, et al. (1993) Trimethoprim-sulfamethoxazole induces reversible hyperkalemia. Ann Intern Med 119(4):291–5

58. Greenberg S, Reiser IW, Chou SY (1993) Hyperkalemia with high-dose trimethoprim-sulfamethoxazole therapy. Am J Kidney Dis 22(4):603–6

59. Gronert GA, Theye RA (1975) Pathophysiology of hyperkalemia induced by succinylcholine. Anesthesiology 43(1):89–99

60. Hall TL, Barnes A, Miller JR, et al. (1993) Neonatal mortality following transfusion of red cells with high plasma potassium levels. Transfusion 33(7):606–9

61. Hartman D, Sagnella GA, Chesters CA, et al. (2004) Direct renin assay and plasma renin activity assay compared. Clin Chem 50(11):2159–61

62. Hermsmeyer K, Sperelakis N (1970) Decrease in K^+ conductance and depolarization of frog cardiac muscle produced by Ba^{++}. Am J Physiol 219(4):1108–14

63. Hertz P, Richardson JA (1972) Arginine-induced hyperkalemia in renal failure patients. Arch Intern Med 130(5):778–80

64. Iolascon A, Stewart GW, Ajetunmobi JF, et al. (1999) Familial pseudohyperkalemia maps to the same locus as dehydrated hereditary stomatocytosis (hereditary xerocytosis). Blood 93(9):3120–3

65. Isnard Bagnis C, Deray G, Baumelou A, et al. (2004) Herbs and the kidney. Am J Kidney Dis 44(1):1–11

66. Johnson MD, Barger AC (1981) Circulating catecholamines in control of renal electrolyte and water excretion. Am J Physiol 240(3):F192–F199

67. Jones DP, Mahmoud H, Chesney RW (1995) Tumor lysis syndrome: Pathogenesis and management. Pediatr Nephrol 9(2):206–12

68. Kallen RJ, Rieger CH, Cohen HS, et al. (1976) Near-fatal hyperkalemia due to ingestion of salt substitute by an infant. JAMA 235(19):2125–6

69. Karnik JA, Young BS, Lew NL, et al. (2001) Cardiac arrest and sudden death in dialysis units. Kidney Int 60(1):350–7

70. Katz AI (1982) Renal Na–K–ATPase: Its role in tubular sodium and potassium transport. Am J Physiol 242(3): F207–F219

71. Kemper MJ, Harps E, Hellwege HH, et al. (1996) Effective treatment of acute hyperkalaemia in childhood by short-term infusion of salbutamol. Eur J Pediatr 155(6):495–7

72. Khilnani P (1992) Electrolyte abnormalities in critically ill children. Crit Care Med 20(2):241–50

73. Khuri RN, Strieder N, Wiederholt M, et al. (1975) Effects of graded solute diuresis on renal tubular sodium transport in the rat. Am J Physiol 228(4):1262–8

74. Kleyman TR, Roberts C, Ling BN (1995) A mechanism for pentamidine-induced hyperkalemia: Inhibition of distal nephron sodium transport. Ann Intern Med 122(2):103–6

75. Knochel JP, Dotin LN, Hamburger RJ (1972) Pathophysiology of intense physical conditioning in a hot climate. I. Mechanisms of potassium depletion. J Clin Invest 51(2):242–55

76. Kruger C, Hoper K, Weissortel R, et al. (1996) Value of direct measurement of active renin concentrations in congenital adrenal hyperplasia due to 21-hydroxylase deficiency. Eur J Pediatr 155(10):858–61

77. Kubota T, Biagi BA, Giebisch G (1983) Effects of acid base disturbances on basolateral membrane potential and intracellular potassium activity in the proximal tubule of necturus. J Membr Biol 73(1):61–8

78. Laragh JH, Capeci NE (1955) Effect of administration of potassium chloride on serum sodium and potassium concentration. Am J Physiol 180(3):539–44

79. Leape LL, Brennan TA, Laird N, et al. (1991) The nature of adverse events in hospitalized patients. Results of the harvard medical practice study II. N Engl J Med 324(6):377–84

80. Lorenz JM, Kleinman LI, Disney TA (1986) Renal response of newborn dog to potassium loading. Am J Physiol 251(3, Part 2):F513–F519

81. Malnic G, Klose RM, Giebisch G (1966) Micropuncture study of distal tubular potassium and sodium transport in rat nephron. Am J Physiol 211(3):529–47

82. Malone DR, McNamara RM, Malone RS, et al. (1990) Hypokalemia complicating emergency fluid resuscitation in children. Pediatr Emerg Care 6(1):13–16

83. Mandelberg A, Krupnik Z, Houri S, et al. (1999) Salbutamol metered-dose inhaler with spacer for hyperkalemia: How fast? How safe? Chest 115(3):617–22

84. Manitius A, Levitin H, Beck D, et al. (1960) On the mechanism of impairment of renal concentrating ability in potassium deficiency. J Clin Invest 39:684–92

85. McClure RJ, Prasad VK, Brocklebank JT (1994) Treatment of hyperkalaemia using intravenous and nebulised salbutamol. Arch Dis Child 70(2):126–8

86. Mentser M, Bunchman T (1998) Nephrology in the pediatric intensive care unit. Semin Nephrol 18(3):330–40

87. Mercer CW, Logic JR (1973) Cardiac arrest due to hyperkalemia following intravenous penicillin administration. Chest 64(3):358–9

88. Moreno M, Murphy C, Goldsmith C (1969) Increase in serum potassium resulting from the administration of hypertonic mannitol and other solutions. J Lab Clin Med 73(2):291–8

89. Mueller BA, Scott MK, Sowinski KM, et al. (2000) Noni juice (Morinda citrifolia): Hidden potential for hyperkalemia? Am J Kidney Dis 35(2):310–12

90. Murdoch IA, Dos Anjos R, Haycock GB (1991) Treatment of hyperkalaemia with intravenous salbutamol. Arch Dis Child 66(4):527–8

91. Murthy JN, Hicks JM, Soldin SJ (1997) Evaluation of i-STAT portable clinical analyzer in a neonatal and pediatric intensive care unit. Clin Biochem 30(5):385–9

92. Muto S, Giebisch G, Sansom S (1988) An acute increase of peritubular K stimulates K transport through cell pathways of CCT. Am J Physiol 255(1, Part 2):F108–F114

93. New MI, Geller DS, Fallo F, et al. (2005) Monogenic low renin hypertension. Trends Endocrinol Metab 16(3):92–7

94. Nolph KD, Popovich RP, Ghods AJ, et al. (1978) Determinants of low clearances of small solutes during peritoneal dialysis. Kidney Int 13(2):117–23

95. Osorio FV, Linas SL (1999) Woodard disorders of potassium metabolism. In: Schrier RW, Berl T, Bonventre JV (eds) Atlas of Diseases of the Kidney, Vol. 1: Disorders of Water, Electrolytes, and Acid–Base, 1st edn. Current Medicine, Philadelphia, pp. 3.5–3.12

96. Oster JR, Singer I, Fishman LM (1995) Heparin-induced aldosterone suppression and hyperkalemia. Am J Med 98(6):575–86

97. Pantanowitz L (2002) Drug-induced hyperkalemia. Am J Med 112(4):334–5

98. Papadea C, Foster J, Grant S, et al. (2002) Evaluation of the i-STAT portable clinical analyzer for point-of-care blood testing in the intensive care units of a university children's hospital. Ann Clin Lab Sci 32(3):231–43

99. Parshuram CS, Cox PN (2002) Neonatal hyperkalemic-hypocalcemic cardiac arrest associated with initiation of blood-primed continuous venovenous hemofiltration. Pediatr Crit Care Med 3(1):67–9

100. Parshuram CS, Joffe AR (2003) Prospective study of potassium-associated acute transfusion events in pediatric intensive care. Pediatr Crit Care Med 4(1):65–8

101. Patten E, Robbins M, Vincent J, et al. (1991) Use of red blood cells older than five days for neonatal transfusion. J Perinatol 11(1):37–40

102. Perazella MA (2000) Drug-induced hyperkalemia: Old culprits and new offenders. Am J Med 109(4):307–14

103. Pierson RN, Jr, Lin DH, Phillips RA (1974) Total-body potassium in health: Effects of age, sex, height, and fat. Am J Physiol 226(1):206–12

104. Ptacek LJ, Tawil R, Griggs RC, et al. (1994) Dihydropyridine receptor mutations cause hypokalemic periodic paralysis. Cell 77(6):863–8

105. Ramirez AM, Woodfield DG, Scott R, et al. (1987) High potassium levels in stored irradiated blood. Transfusion 27(5):444–5

106. Relman AS, Schwartz WB (1956) The nephropathy of potassium depletion; a clinical and pathological entity. N Engl J Med 255(5):195–203

107. Rogers FB, Li SC (2001) Acute colonic necrosis associated with sodium polystyrene sulfonate (kayexalate) enemas in a critically ill patient: Case report and review of the literature. J Trauma 51(2):395–7

108. Rojas CV, Wang JZ, Schwartz LS, et al. (1991) A met-to-val mutation in the skeletal muscle Na$^+$ channel alpha-subunit in hyperkalaemic periodic paralysis. Nature 354(6352):387–9

109. Rosa RM, Silva P, Young JB, et al. (1980) Adrenergic modulation of extrarenal potassium disposal. N Engl J Med 302(8):431–4

110. Rose BD (1994) Clinical Physiology of Acid–Base and Electrolyte Disorders. McGraw-Hill, New York

111. Rose BD, Post TW, Hypokalemia (2001) In: Wonsciewicz M, McCullough K, Davis K (eds) Clinical Physiology of Acid–Base and Electrolyte Disorders, 5th edn. McGraw-Hill, New York, pp. 836–87

112. Rose BD, Post TW (2001) Hyperkalemia. In: Wonsciewicz M, McCullough K, Davis K (eds) Clinical Physiology of Acid–Base and Electrolyte Disorders, 5th edn. McGraw-Hill, New York, pp. 888–930

113. Roza O, Berman LB (1971) The pathophysiology of barium: Hypokalemic and cardiovascular effects. J Pharmacol Exp Ther 177(2):433–9

114. Satlin LM, Schwartz GJ (1990) Metabolism of potassium. In: Ichikawa I (ed) Pediatric Textbook of Fluids and Electrolytes, 1st edn. Williams & Wilkins, Baltimore, pp. 89–98

115. Scanlon JW, Krakaur R (1980) Hyperkalemia following exchange transfusion. J Pediatr 96(1):108–10

116. Schwartz GJ, Potassium (2004) In: Avner ED, Harmon WE, Niaudet P (eds) Pediatric Nephrology, 5th edn. Lippincott Williams & Williams, Philadelphia, pp. 147–188

117. Schwartz GJ, Burg MB (1978) Mineralocorticoid effects on cation transport by cortical collecting tubules in vitro. Am J Physiol 235(6):F576–F585.

118. Schwartz WB, Relman AS (1967) Effects of electrolyte disorders on renal structure and function. N Engl J Med 276(7):383–9 contd

119. Shoemaker L, Eaton B, Buchino J (2007) A three-year-old with persistent hypokalemia. J Pediatr 151:696–699

120. Sillen A, Sorensen T, Kantola I, et al. (1997) Identification of mutations in the *CACNL1A3* gene in 13 families of Scandinavian origin having hypokalemic periodic paralysis and evidence of a founder effect in Danish families. Am J Med Genet 69(1):102–6

121. Singh BS, Sadiq HF, Noguchi A, et al. (2002) Efficacy of albuterol inhalation in treatment of hyperkalemia in premature neonates. J Pediatr 141(1):16–20

122. Sopko JA, Freeman RM (1977) Salt substitutes as a source of potassium. JAMA 238(7):608–10

123. Squires RD, Huth EJ (1959) Experimental potassium depletion in normal human subjects. I. Relation of ionic intakes to the renal conservation of potassium. J Clin Invest 38(7):1134–48

124. Stanton BA, Giebisch G (1982) Effects of pH on potassium transport by renal distal tubule. Am J Physiol 242(5): F544–F551

125. Stanton BA, Giebisch GH (1992) Renal potassium transport. In: Windhager EE (ed) Handbook of Physiology, 1st edn. Oxford University Press, New York, pp. 813–74

126. Stedwell RE, Allen KM, Binder LS (1992) Hypokalemic paralyses: A review of the etiologies, pathophysiology, presentation, and therapy. Am J Emerg Med 10(2):143–8

127. Sterns RH, Cox M, Feig PU, et al. (1981) Internal potassium balance and the control of the plasma potassium concentration. Med Baltimore 60(5):339–54

128. Sulyok E (1971) The relationship between electrolyte and acid–base balance in the premature infant during early postnatal life. Biol Neonate 17(3):227–37

129. Sulyok E, Nemeth M, Tenyi I, et al. (1979) Relationship between maturity, electrolyte balance and the function of the renin–angiotensin–aldosterone system in newborn infants. Biol Neonate 35(1–2):60–5

130. Surawicz B (1967) Relationship between electrocardiogram and electrolytes. Am Heart J 73(6):814–34

131. Tannen RL (1977) Relationship of renal ammonia production and potassium homeostasis. Kidney Int 11(6):453–65

132. Textor SC, Bravo EL, Fouad FM, et al. (1982) Hyperkalemia in azotemic patients during angiotensin-converting enzyme inhibition and aldosterone reduction with captopril. Am J Med 73(5):719–25

133. Therien AG, Blostein R (2000) Mechanisms of sodium pump regulation. Am J Physiol Cell Physiol 279(3):C541–C566

134. Todd EP, Vick RL (1971) Kalemotropic effect of epinephrine: Analysis with adrenergic agonists and antagonists. Am J Physiol 220(6):1964–9

135. Torpy DJ, Stratakis CA, Chrousos GP (1999) Hyper- and hypoaldosteronism. Vitam Horm 57:177–216

136. Torres VE, Young WF, Jr, Offord KP, et al. (1990) Association of hypokalemia, aldosteronism, and renal cysts. N Engl J Med 322(6):345–51

137. Tubman M, Majumdar SR, Lee D, et al. (2005) Best practices for safe handling of products containing concentrated potassium. BMJ 331(7511):274–7

138. Tudvad F, McNamara H, Barnett HL (1954) Renal response of premature infants to administration of bicarbonate and potassium. Pediatrics 13(1):4–16

139. Tullett GL (1970) Sudden death occurring during "massive-dose" potassium penicillin G therapy. An argument implicating potassium intoxication. Wis Med J 69(9):216–17

140. Velazquez H, Ellison DH, Wright FS (1987) Chloride-dependent potassium secretion in early and late renal distal tubules. Am J Physiol 253(3, Part 2):F555–F562

141. Viskin S (1999) Long QT syndromes and torsade de pointes. Lancet 354(9190):1625–33

142. Weidner NJ, Gaum WE, Chou TC, et al. (1978) Hyperkalemia-electrocardiographic abnormalities. J Pediatr 93(3):462–4

143. Weiner ID, Wingo CS (1997) Hypokalemia–Consequences, causes, and correction. J Am Soc Nephrol 8(7):1179–88

144. Weiner ID, Wingo CS (1998) Hyperkalemia: A potential silent killer. J Am Soc Nephrol 9(8):1535–43

145. Welt LG, Hollander W, Jr, Blythe WB (1960) The consequences of potassium depletion. J Chronic Dis 11:213–54

146. West ML, Marsden PA, Richardson RM, et al. (1986) New clinical approach to evaluate disorders of potassium excretion. Miner Electrolyte Metab 12(4):234–8

147. White JR, Veltri MA, Fackler JC (2005) Preventing adverse events in the pediatric intensive care unit: Prospectively targeting factors that lead to intravenous potassium chloride order errors. Pediatr Crit Care Med 6(1):25–32

148. Wiley JF, Koepke JA (1985) Changes in serum potassium in premature infants receiving packed red blood cells. Clin Lab Haematol 7(1):27–31

149. Woodard JP, Chen W, Keku EO, et al. (1993) Altered jejunal potassium (rb+) transport in piglet rotavirus enteritis. Am J Physiol 265(2, Part 1):G388–G393

150. Yang WC, Huang TP, Ho LT, et al. (1986) Beta-adrenergic-mediated extrarenal potassium disposal in patients with end-stage renal disease: Effect of propranolol. Miner Electrolyte Metab 12(3):186 93

151. Young DB, Paulsen AW (1983) Interrelated effects of aldosterone and plasma potassium on potassium excretion. Am J Physiol 244(1):F28–F34

152. Young DB, Smith MJ, Jr, Jackson TE, et al. (1984) Multiplicative interaction between angiotensin II and K concentration in stimulation of aldosterone. Am J Physiol 247(3, Part 1):E328–E335

153. Intravenous potassium predicament (1997) Clin J Oncol Nurs 1(2):45–9

154. Joint commission IDs five high-alert meds (2000) ED Manag 12(2):21–2

155. Medication error prevention: Potassium chloride (2001) Int J Qual Health Care 13(2):155

156. Medication error prevention – Potassium chloride (1998) Sentinel Event Alert (1):1–2

157. USDA national nutrient reference for standard reference, release 17. Available at http://www.nal.usda.gov/fnic/foodcomp/Data/SR17/wtrank/sr17a306.pdf

Disorders of Calcium and Phosphate Regulation

4

Raymond Quigley

Contents

Core Messages

› Intracellular calcium concentrations are very low compared to blood concentrations.
› Treatment of calcium disorders requires an understanding of the distribution of calcium in the body fluids, primarily the extracellular fluid.
› The skeletal system acts as a reservoir for calcium and can buffer many changes in the blood calcium concentration.
› Long term regulation of serum calcium involves the coordinated function of several organs.
› While hypocalcemia is common in the intensive care setting, aggressive treatment is not always indicated.
› Phosphate regulation is primarily achieved by the kidneys.
› Treatment of severe hyperphosphatemia usually requires renal replacement therapy.

4.1 Calcium

4.1.1 Regulation of Calcium Homeostasis

Figure 4.1 outlines the overall homeostasis of calcium in the adult human. Calcium is both absorbed and secreted in the gastrointestinal tract for a net gain of about 200 mg day^{-1}. The daily turnover of bone calcium is about 500 mg. The kidneys handle a large quantity of calcium in the process of filtration and reabsorption and serve as the final regulator of homeostasis for the body. In patients with normal calcium balance, the kidneys will excrete the 200 mg that were absorbed by the GI tract. The extracellular pool of calcium serves as the medium for the exchange of calcium from these various pools. We will review

S.G. Kiessling et al. (eds) *Pediatric Nephrology in the ICU*.
© Springer-Verlag Berlin Heidelberg 2009

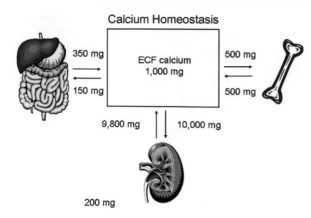

Table 4.1 Conversion of units of measure for calcium (atomic weight is 40.06)

	mg dl^{-1}	mmol l^{-1}	mEq l^{-1}
mg dl^{-1}	×1	×0.25	×0.5
mmol l^{-1}	×4	×1	×2
mEq l^{-1}	×2	×0.5	×1

Conversion is from the units in the left hand column to the column in the table. For example, to convert 10 mg dl^{-1} of calcium into mmol l^{-1}, the multiplication factor would be 0.25 so that the result would be 2.5 mmol l^{-1}. This would also correspond to 5 mEq l^{-1}.

Fig. 4.1 Calcium homeostasis. Dietary intake of calcium is approximately 1,000 mg. About 350 mg is absorbed into the blood stream while 150 mg is secreted into the gastrointestinal tract for a net absorption of 200 mg. There is constant turn over of 500 mg day^{-1} of calcium in the bones. The ionized fraction of calcium is filtered in the kidney. The tubules then reabsorb the bulk of the calcium so that the urinary excretion is 200 mg

the distribution of calcium in these pools and then discuss the regulation of the absorption and excretion of calcium as well as the regulation of the turnover of calcium in the bones.

4.1.1.1 Calcium Distribution in Body Fluids

Calcium is the most abundant cation in the adult body, making up about 2% of the total body weight [1–3]. Most of the body's calcium (~99%) is in the skeleton in the form of hydroxyapatite ($Ca_{10}(PO_4)_6(OH)_2$). Only a small fraction is in the soft tissues where it plays a critical role in the regulation of cellular processes. The remaining calcium is in the extracellular fluid compartment (ECF; ~1,000 mg in the adult). This includes the blood space from which we measure calcium. Calcium measurements are reported in various units depending on the laboratory. Conversion from one unit of measurement to another is outlined in Table 4.1. These calculations are based on the atomic weight of calcium, 40.06 Da, which for all practical purposes can be rounded to 40 Da.

The ECF calcium is approximately 40% bound to plasma proteins, 48% free or ionized, and 12% complexed with other ions such as phosphate, citrate, and bicarbonate [3, 4]. Because a large percentage of the calcium in the ECF is protein bound, variations in the blood protein concentration will affect the measured total calcium concentration. For example, patients with a low serum albumin from nephrotic syndrome will have a low total calcium concentration; however, their

ionized calcium concentration is usually normal. There have been several rules of thumb for correcting the total calcium concentration for the altered albumin concentration. Usually, for every g dl^{-1} decrease in albumin, the total calcium concentration will decrease by about 0.8 g dl^{-1}. However, studies have indicated that these rules can be misleading [5–9]. As a result, it is much safer to measure the ionized calcium concentration directly and not rely on estimates of the ionized calcium based on the albumin concentration. Most hospital laboratories routinely measure ionized calcium, so this should not be a problem.

The ionized fraction of calcium is the portion that exerts physiologic effects and is the concentration that is regulated by the body. The fraction of calcium that is protein bound is determined to some degree by the blood pH. As the pH decreases, hydrogen ions will displace calcium from proteins and increase the ionized calcium concentration. Alkalosis has the opposite effect. As the pH increases, more binding sites on the proteins for calcium will be available and the ionized calcium concentration will decrease. The general rule of thumb is that every 0.1 change in the pH will change the ionized calcium by approximately 0.12 g dl^{-1} [3, 4]. The fraction of calcium binding to serum proteins is also influenced by the concentration of protein. At lower concentrations of albumin, the fraction of bound calcium is higher than when the albumin concentration is in the normal range [10]. This is one of the main reasons that estimating the ionized calcium from the albumin concentration can be misleading.

4.1.1.2 Calcium Homeostasis

The physiologic regulation of calcium involves the coordination of three primary organ systems (Fig. 4.1). The intestines are involved in the absorption of calcium from the diet. The kidneys filter and excrete calcium. The kidneys, as well as the skin and the liver, are involved in the production of vitamin D which in turn affects the intestinal absorption of calcium and the bone turnover rate. The skeletal system serves as a large storehouse for calcium. The endocrine control of calcium is performed by the parathyroid gland which secretes parathyroid hormone (PTH) and the thyroid gland which secretes calcitonin. We will discuss basic principles of cellular calcium homeostasis and transepithelial calcium transport and then discuss the functions and coordination of these organ systems in more detail.

4.1.1.3 Cellular Calcium Homeostasis

The concentration of ionized calcium in the blood is approximately 5 mg dl^{-1} ($\sim$1.25 mmol l^{-1}) [1–3]. The concentration of ionized calcium in the intracellular space is several orders of magnitude lower ($\sim$10^{-7} mol l^{-1}) It is critical for the cell to maintain a low intracellular calcium concentration because of its toxicity. This concentration gradient is maintained by the function of a calcium ATPase located in the plasma membrane that actively transports calcium from the cellular compartment to the extracellular compartment [11, 12]. Some cells have another transport system that exchanges calcium for sodium to help maintain a low intracellular calcium concentration [13, 14]. In addition, most of the intracellular calcium is sequestered in organelles that have higher concentrations of calcium that can be released upon activation. This system is used as a signal transduction mechanism for many hormonal signals and for secretion of compounds from the cell such as insulin or acetylcholine [15]. This is a complex system and the details are beyond the scope of this chapter [15–17].

Striated muscle cells use a similar compartmentalized pool of calcium for electromechanical coupling. Calcium is stored in the sarcoplasmic reticulum until the action potential reaches the myocyte. This electrical signal stimulates release of calcium that is then used in the actin–myosin contraction coupling. This system requires a calcium ATPase in the membrane of the sarcoplasmic reticulum to move the calcium from the cytoplasmic compartment back into the storage pool in the sarcoplasmic reticulum. This system is also responsible for electromechanical coupling in the cardiac myocytes [18].

Smooth muscle cells also use calcium to cause contraction. This is a slower process since there are no action potentials to create a rapid synchronized depolarization of the smooth muscle bed. Instead, signals that are delivered to the smooth muscle cell (e.g. from hormones or endothelial cells) cause calcium channels in the plasma membrane to open and allow the influx of calcium. There are other intracellular pools of calcium that play a role in the regulation of smooth muscle contraction [19, 20].

Specialized epithelial cells in the intestine and kidney that transport calcium across an epithelium must do so in a fashion that does not expose the cytoplasmic compartment to a high ionized calcium concentration. This is accomplished by proteins in the cell, known as calbindins, which bind calcium and transport the calcium ions through the cell [21]. These proteins are found in high abundance in the cells that are responsible for the transport of calcium. This will be discussed in detail below.

4.1.1.4 Epithelial Transport of Calcium

We will next review the general principles involved in the transepithelial transport of calcium [22]. Fig. 4.2 shows a generic epithelial cell that transports calcium. This could represent a cell in the small intestine that reabsorbs calcium from the diet or a renal epithelial cell transporting calcium from the filtered fluid back into the blood stream. The cell has a luminal membrane and a basolateral membrane. In addition, the cells of the epithelium also have attachments to their neighboring cells. These junctions make up the paracellular pathway.

Epithelial transport can be transcellular or paracellular. Transcellular transport requires energy input but has the advantage of being highly regulated. It is also necessary for the transport of solutes against a concentration

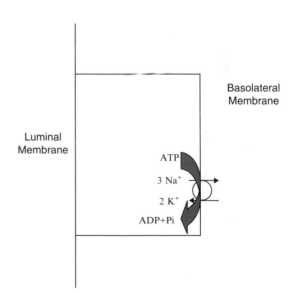

Fig. 4.2 Generic epithelial cell. Transport across the epithelium can occur by way of the paracellular pathway or the transcellular pathway

gradient. Paracellular transport has the advantage of being passive so that the energy requirements are minimal. While this form of transport can be regulated, it is not as tightly regulated as the transcellular transport.

The orientation of these epithelial cells ascertains that calcium will be transported into the cell across the luminal membrane and subsequently into the blood stream by crossing the basolateral membrane. As discussed above, the intracellular concentration of calcium is very low, usually about 10^{-7} mol l^{-1}. The calcium concentration in the luminal fluid is much higher, which provides a driving force for calcium entry into the cell. The simplest way to allow for calcium entry into the cell is through a channel. This channel is known as the Epithelial Calcium Channel (ECaC). There is evidence for at least two isoforms of ECaC, ECaC1, and ECaC2. These channels are members of the transient receptor potential (TRP) channel family (TRPV5 and TRPV6) [23–25]. The exit step across the basolateral membrane is not as well defined. Some cells utilize a sodium–calcium exchanger while other cells rely on the plasma membrane Ca-ATPase.

While calcium is traversing the cytoplasmic compartment, it is bound to a calbindin (calbindin-D) [21]. This class of proteins is found in the tissues that transport calcium, primarily the kidney and the intestines, and plays a critical role in maintaining a low intracellular ionized calcium concentration in these cells. The predominant isoform in the kidney is calbindin-D_{28K}, and the predominant isoform in the intestine is calbindin-D_{9K}.

4.1.2 Gastrointestinal System

The intestine is responsible for absorption of calcium from the diet [26]. About 90% of the calcium is absorbed in the small intestine. The fraction of the calcium that is transported via the transcellular versus the paracellular route depends on the amount of calcium in the diet. When the dietary calcium is low, the active transcellular route is stimulated by vitamin D to help maintain the body's calcium balance. If dietary calcium intake is high, then the bulk of the absorbed calcium is transported via the paracellular route. Since this is not as tightly controlled, excess dietary intake can lead to hypercalcemia. This is especially true if the patient takes vitamin D supplements.

Vitamin D has several effects on the intestinal handling of calcium [27, 28]. It upregulates the expression of ECaC as well as the expression of calbindin-D_{9K}. Studies indicate that the expression of calbindin-D_{9K} directly correlates with the transport rate of calcium

[27]. In addition, the expression of calbindin-D_{9K} is tightly controlled by vitamin D [28]. Thus, calbindin-D_{9K} appears to be one of the primary targets of vitamin D and a key regulator of intestinal absorption of calcium.

The expression of these transport molecules in the intestinal tract correlates with data on the location of active and passive transport of calcium. The duodenum has been shown to be the site for active transport of calcium. When calcium in the diet is limited, the expression of TRPV6 (ECaC2) and calbindin-D_{9K} in the duodenum increase in response to vitamin D. This enhances the duodenum's ability to absorb calcium actively from the intestinal lumen. The jejunum and ileum appear to have more passive transport of calcium. The regulation of calcium transport in these segments is not tightly regulated and does not respond as well to vitamin D.

4.1.3.   Renal Transport of Calcium

The fraction of calcium that is protein bound is not available for filtration at the glomerulus [29]. Thus, only the 60% that is ionized or complexed is filterable. In the adult, this is approximately 10,000 mg day^{-1} (Fig. 4.1). The renal tubules are then responsible for reabsorbing the bulk of the calcium and regulating the final excretion of the amount necessary to keep the body in balance. We will briefly discuss the role of the nephron segments involved in the reabsorption of calcium.

The proximal tubule is responsible for reabsorbing the bulk of the glomerular ultrafiltrate. This is accomplished primarily by active transport of sodium. Transport of other solutes such as glucose and amino acids are then coupled to the transport of sodium. Transport of phosphate is also coupled to sodium and will be discussed in greater detail in the section on phosphorus regulation. These transport processes result in bulk fluid reabsorption due to the high water permeability in the proximal tubule. This will increase the luminal concentration of calcium and allow for passive paracellular transport to occur, resulting in the reabsorption of 60–70% of the filtered load of calcium [3, 29].

The descending and ascending thin limbs of Henle do not appear to transport calcium to any significant degree. The thick ascending limb of Henle, however, is responsible for reabsorbing about 20% of the filtered load of calcium [29]. It is important to understand the mechanism of transport in this segment since loop diuretics have a large effect on calcium transport. Figure 4.3 illustrates transport in the thick ascending limb. The sodium–potassium ATPase on the basolateral membrane provides the energy for transport by maintaining a low intracellular sodium concentration. On the luminal membrane, the sodium–potassium-2 chloride co-transporter (NKCC2) uses the sodium gradient to transport these ions into the cell. The potassium channel (ROMK) on the luminal membrane will recycle the potassium back into the lumen of the tubule which makes the tubule lumen electrically positive. This will then provide the driving force for passive absorption of cations such as calcium across the paracellular pathway. Loop diuretics such as furosemide will inhibit NKCC2 and will abolish the lumen positive voltage. This then inhibits the reabsorption of calcium as well as other cations.

The distal convoluted tubule actively reabsorbs calcium in a manner that is similar to the small intestine [29, 30]. As shown in Fig. 4.4, the apical membrane has a calcium channel, TRPV5 (ECaC1) that regulates the entry of calcium into the cell. Calcium is then bound to calbindin-D_{28K} and is transported to the basolateral membrane where it then exits the cell by way of the plasma membrane Ca-ATPase. There is evidence for a sodium–calcium exchanger that also serves to transport calcium out of the cell and into the blood stream. These processes may also be regulated by vitamin D, but this remains unclear. It is clear, however, that PTH will upregulate this process to help conserve calcium.

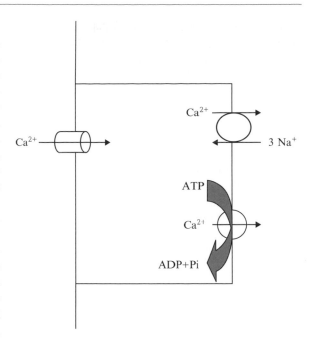

Fig. 4.4 Distal convoluted tubule cell. The apical membrane calcium channel is TRPV5 (also known as ECaC1). The basolateral exit step is a plasma membrane calcium pump as well as the sodium calcium exchanger

4.1.4 Bone Turnover

In addition to serving as a framework for our body, the skeletal system also serves as a reservoir for calcium. This is accomplished by a complex interplay of PTH, vitamin D, and calcitonin. In addition, the blood pH and other factors can alter the bones' metabolism of calcium. When the ionized calcium concentration in the blood falls, the parathyroid gland will release PTH which then activates the osteoclasts to release calcium from the bone. The mechanism for sensing the calcium concentration will be discussed in the next section on the parathyroid gland.

Formation of bone is a complex process [3]. The osteoblasts will begin the formation of bone by secreting osteoid. This is a cartilaginous substance that provides the framework for the mineral, hydroxyapatite, to be deposited on. Vitamin D activates calcification of osteoid and is thus a key player in the formation of new bone. When the body is deficient in vitamin D as the bone is growing, the patient will develop rickets. Calcitonin can also stimulate the movement of calcium into the bone [31]. Another factor in the calcification of bone is the abundance of phosphate. If the patient is phosphate deficient, the osteoblasts will be unable to form hydroxyapatitie and will not be able to

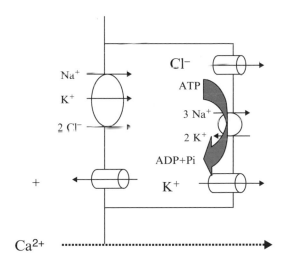

Fig. 4.3 Thick ascending limb cell. The thick ascending limb of Henle is a key regulator of calcium transport. The lumen positive potential is created by the potassium channel in the luminal membrane. Inhibition of transport by loop diuretics will abolish this potential and lead to an increase in calcium excretion

mineralize the bone in the presence of vitamin D. Other factors that will cause difficulty in calcifying the bone are acidosis, aluminum toxicity, and immobilization. These conditions will enhance the release of calcium from the bone and will lead to hypercalcemia.

4.1.5 Parathyroid Gland

The parathyroid gland, four small glands attached to the thyroid, is responsible for the minute to minute regulation of the serum ionized calcium concentration. The parathyroid gland monitors the serum ionized calcium concentration through the calcium sensing receptor (CaSR) [32]. This receptor is a G-protein coupled receptor that binds calcium and other divalent ions. When the receptor is activated by high calcium concentrations, it inhibits the secretion of PTH. When the calcium concentration is low, the receptor then triggers a cascade of events that results in the secretion of PTH which will then help to increase the serum calcium. A complete discussion of the function of the CaSR is beyond the scope of this chapter, but the intensivist and nephrologist should be aware that mutations in the CaSR can be responsible for chronic alterations in the patient's serum calcium concentration [32, 33].

Primary hyperparathyroidism is very rare in pediatric patients. Secondary hyperparathyroidism is commonly seen in patients with chronic renal failure. This occurs because the kidney can no longer activate vitamin D because of decreased 1-α-hydroxylase activity. The patient then becomes hypocalcemic which then activates the release of PTH. The serum calcium concentration can be maintained in the normal range until the bones are depleted of their stores which results in renal osteodystrophy. In the extreme case, the patient can develop osteitis firbrosis cystica (fibrosis of the bone marrow) or can develop brown tumors. In most patients, treatment with vitamin D analogs will correct the serum calcium and will then suppress the secretion of PTH. In addition, medications that directly stimulate the CaSR have been developed and can be used to suppress the secretion of PTH. Rarely, the patient could develop tertiary hyperparathyroidism, where the parathyroid gland has hypertrophied to the point of escape from control by the usual factors, allowing autonomous PTH secretion.

4.1.6 Calcitonin

Calcitonin is produced by parafollicular C cells in the thyroid gland and promotes movement of calcium

from the blood into the bone cells by mechanisms that are not completely understood.

4.2 Phosphorus

4.2.1 Regulation of Phosphorus Homeostasis

Figure 4.5 illustrates the overall metabolism of phosphorus in the adult human. The intestines absorb about 1,100 mg and secrete about 200 mg for a net gain of 900 mg. There is a daily turnover of 350 mg in the bones. The kidneys will filter 7,000 mg of phosphorus and then reabsorb 6,100 mg so that the kidneys excrete the 900 mg that was absorbed in the intestines. We will first briefly review the cellular metabolism of phosphate, and then will review the regulation of total body phosphate.

4.2.2 Distribution of Phosphorus

In the adult human, phosphorus accounts for about 1% of the body weight, or roughly 700 g. Most of the phosphorus (85%) is located in the skeleton and teeth with the remaining 15% in soft tissues [3]. In the blood stream, phosphate is found as phospholipids, phosphate esters, and inorganic phosphate. The primary forms of inorganic phosphate are HPO_4^{2-} and $H_2PO_4^-$ and at a pH of 7.4 are in a 4:1 ratio. Thus, 1 mmol of phosphate at

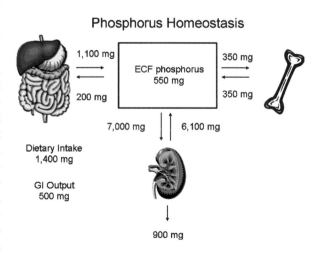

Fig. 4.5 Phosphorus homeostasis. Dietary intake of phosphorus averages about 1,400 mg day^{-1}. Of this, 1,100 mg is absorbed into the blood stream. About 200 mg is secreted by the gastrointestinal tract so that 500 mg is excreted in the stool. Daily turn over in the bones is about 350 mg. Phosphate is filtered in the kidney and the bulk is reabsorbed by the tubules so that 900 mg is excreted in the urine

pH 7.4 is 1.8 mEq of phosphate. Laboratory measurements of phosphate are generally reported as mg dl^{-1} of phosphorus. Since the atomic weight of phosphorus is 30.9 Da, 1 mmol l^{-1} of phosphate is approximately 3.1 mg dl^{-1} of phosphorus.

4.2.3   Cellular Metabolism of Phosphorus

Inside the cell, most of the phosphate is in the form of organic molecules such as DNA, RNA, and phospholipids or nucleotides such as ATP or ADP. The cell utilizes a ubiquitous sodium phosphate transporter for constant uptake of phosphate to ensure its availability for these metabolic processes [34].

4.2.4   Intestinal Transport of Phosphate

Phosphate absorption in the intestines occurs primarily in the duodenum and jejunum [3]. As with calcium, the transepithelial transport of phosphate can be paracellular or transcellular. When dietary phosphate is high, most of the phosphate is absorbed passively by the paracellular route. During periods of low phosphate intake, the active transport route increases and will ensure absorption of the necessary phosphate. The active transport of phosphate is mediated by an apically located sodium-phosphate co-transporter termed NaPi IIb. This transport protein is regulated by vitamin D. There is very little absorption of phosphate in the large bowel, but there is some secretion of phosphate by the intestinal tract.

4.2.5   Renal Transport of Phosphate

About 90% of the inorganic phosphate in the blood is freely filtered at the glomerulus. The proximal tubule is responsible for the reabsorption of phosphate and is the primary regulator of phosphate balance in the body. Thus, understanding of proximal tubule transport of phosphate is critical to the understanding of phosphate metabolism by the body.

Transport in the proximal tubule is driven primarily by the sodium–potassium ATPase which is located in the basolateral membrane of the cell [35, 36]. This pump maintains a low intracellular sodium concentration which can then be used by transporters located in the apical membrane for secondary active transport (Fig. 4.6). Most of the active transport processes in the proximal tubule are driven by this low intracellular sodium concentration by way of sodium coupled transporters. This includes mechanisms involved in the reabsorption of phosphate.

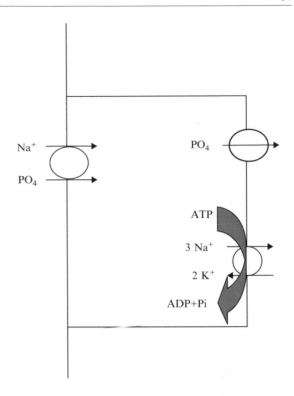

Fig. 4.6   Proximal tubule cell. Phosphate is taken up into the cell across the apical membrane due to the driving force of the sodium concentration gradient. The high intracellular concentration of phosphate then allows for passive diffusion across the basolateral membrane via a facilitative transporter. PTH causes the sodium-phosphate cotransporter to be endocytosed so that reabsorption of phosphate will be inhibited

Under normal conditions about 85% of the filtered phosphate is reabsorbed by the proximal tubule using the sodium–phosphate co-transporter (NaPi2a) [37]. This can be significantly increased under conditions of low phosphate intake so that the body will conserve phosphate. In the setting of a high phosphate intake the tubule will reabsorb less of the filtered phosphate so that a larger fraction will be excreted. PTH is one of the most potent hormonal regulators of phosphate transport and promotes renal excretion of phosphate. It has now become clear that the mechanism of action of PTH is to stimulate endocytosis of the NaPi2a co-transporters from the apical membrane of the proximal tubule cells [37, 38]. The PTH receptor is a G-protein coupled receptor that stimulates the production of cAMP. Activation of PKA by cAMP then causes internalization of NaPi2a. The mechanism by which this occurs serves as a paradigm for regulation of transport in the proximal tubule and has revealed the coordinated interaction of scaffolding proteins in the apical membrane of the tubule [39–42].

4.2.6 Phosphotonins

Phosphotonins are another recently discovered class of regulators for phosphate transport [43]. Briefly, these factors result in inhibition of phosphate transport and, therefore, promote phosphate excretion independently from PTH. They play a role in tumor induced osteomalacia and X-linked and autosomal dominant forms of hypophosphatemic rickets and will be discussed in the section on hypophosphatemia [43].

4.3 Dysregulation of Calcium and Phosphate

Having reviewed the normal regulation and physiology of calcium and phosphate, we will now review conditions where there are alterations in calcium and phosphate.

4.3.1 Hypercalcemia

4.3.1.1 Signs and Symptoms

Hypercalcemia is associated with a number of signs and symptoms depending on the severity and duration of the hypercalcemia [4, 44]. One of the first symptoms is anorexia. As the hypercalcemia worsens, the patients can develop headache, irritability, abdominal pain, nausea and vomiting, and muscle cramps. They may also become constipated. In the kidney, hypercalcemia leads to nephrocalcinosis and can eventually cause renal failure. Early on, the patients develop a concentrating defect which can become frank nephrogenic diabetes insipidus. Because of the nausea and vomiting in combination with the diabetes insipidus, the patients can become very dehydrated.

The common causes of hypercalcemia are listed in Table 4.2 [45–47]. The frequency of causes in the pediatric population is different from that in the adult population, but many of the same principles apply to the differential diagnosis of hypercalcemia. The problem can be related to increased resorption of calcium from the bones due to an increase in PTH or acidosis, an increase in gastrointestinal absorption of calcium due to excess vitamin D or intake of calcium, or decreased excretion of calcium from the kidneys. We will discuss briefly some of the more common causes of hypercalcemia that are seen in the ICU.

Table 4.2 Disorders leading to hypercalcemia

1. Increased intestinal absorption
   a. Vitamin D excess
   b. Granulomatous diseases
2. Increased bone reabsorption
   a. Hyperparathyroidism
   b. Hypercalcemia of malignancy
   c. Immobilization
   d. Hypophosphatemia
   e. Aluminum toxicity
3. Excess calcium intake
   a. Total peripheral nutrition
   b. Milk-alkali syndrome
4. Other causes
   a. William's syndrome
   b. Thyroid disease
   c. Pheochromocytoma

Many cases of sustained hypercalcemia are due to hyperparathyroidism, so one of the first diagnostic studies to do is to check the serum PTH concentration. PTH is secreted as a full length peptide of 81 amino acids. It then undergoes degradation to N-terminal and C-terminal fragments. These peptides each have different activities in the body. The full length (81-amino acid) peptide is the most important to measure in the long-term care of patients with secondary hyperparathyroidism from end stage renal disease. Tumors can also produce a PTH related protein (PTHrp) that will act like PTH and cause hypercalcemia.

Acidosis can also lead to hypercalcemia via the following mechanisms. First, acidosis will cause the ionized calcium fraction to increase. As discussed above, this is due to displacement of calcium by hydrogen ions from binding sites on albumin. Secondly, with time, hydroxyapatite in the bones will be used to buffer the hydrogen ions. The hydroxyapatite releases calcium and phosphate into the blood as it releases the hydroxyl group to neutralize the acid. If this process continues for a protracted period of time, the bone will become demineralized and will be easily fractured.

Long-term immobilization will also lead to hypercalcemia [48–50]. It is unclear what the initiating events are in the sequence, but it appears to be related to activation of osteoclasts. This can be a severe problem in patients who are in the intensive care unit for a prolonged course of time and is often compounded by concomitant chronic acidosis.

Excess intake of calcium with or without excess vitamin D can also cause hypercalcemia. The gastrointestinal absorption of calcium is mostly paracellular when the intake of calcium is high which means that the absorptive rate is not well regulated under these conditions. If there is excessive vitamin D activity in parallel with the high calcium intake, absorption both via the transcellular and paracellular routes will be increased. Excess vitamin D could be from an exogenous source (oral forms of vitamin D) or from tumor production of vitamin D or granulomatous diseases such as sarcoidosis. The milk-alkali syndrome has been reported in adults as high oral intake of calcium leading to hypercalcemia.

Decreased excretion of calcium by the kidneys occurs in an inherited condition known as familial hypocalciuric hypercalcemia. This condition is caused by a mutation in the CaSR [33]. Thiazide diuretics inhibit the excretion of calcium and may lead to hypercalcemia.

4.3.1.2   *Treatment*

Of course, the ultimate treatment of hypercalcemia will depend on the cause of the hypercalcemia [46, 47]. Thus, it is crucial to determine the etiology of the disorder for the best long term treatment. While the workup is being done, the patient will need to be treated empirically to avoid any short term or long term consequences of hypercalcemia.

In patients with normal renal function, saline diuresis will be the best treatment for reducing the calcium concentration [47]. The calcium excretion can be enhanced by giving the patient a loop diuretic such as furosemide. As discussed above, this will inhibit the reabsorption of calcium in the thick ascending limb and will promote calcium excretion.

If the patient does not have good renal function, another therapeutic approach is administration of calcitonin [31]. This is a temporary treatment option because many patients will quickly develop resistance to calcitonin because of the generation of antibodies. Commercially available calcitonin is derived from salmon and is therefore a foreign protein. However, it can usually be used for a long enough period of time to bring the calcium into the normal range.

Another option is to use a bisphosphonate [51, 52]. These compounds act by inhibiting the osteoclast from reabsorbing calcium from the bones. Since many of the causes of hypercalcemia are due to calcium reabsorption from the bones, these compounds tend to work very well. The problem with them is that they are very long acting. Thus, it is possible that the patient will quickly become hypocalcemic and can remain hypocalcemic for a prolonged period of time [53]. Because of the extremely long half-life of these compounds, their administration to girls may even pose a risk of subsequent teratogenicity [54]. Biphosphonates have also been associated with necrosis of the mandible [55]. Lastly, and of special nephrological importance, these agents can not only induce acute renal failure [56], but their dose may also need to be adjusted when used for the treatment of patients with chronic kidney disease [57].

4.3.2   Hypocalcemia

A number of studies have shown that hypocalcemia is very common in the intensive care unit [58–60]. Many septic patients have low ionized calcium concentrations. The exact mechanism for this is unclear and might be related to dysregulation of PTH or calcitonin. The precursor molecule of calcitonin (procalcitonin) has been shown to be elevated in septic patients and might be a good indicator of significant infection [61–63].

While the mechanism of hypocalcemia in this setting is not clear, it is becoming clearer that treatment of hypocalcemia in the ICU must be judicious, as there is evidence from animal studies that aggressive treatment of hypocalcemia could lead to problems: in a rat study of sepsis, administration of calcium correlated with a higher mortality rate [64], and another model utilizing pigs also demonstrated no improvement in blood pressure and tissue perfusion with the administration of calcium [65].

Hypocalcemia is also common in patients with renal failure. As mentioned earlier, the kidneys perform the 1-α-hydroxylase step in the activation of vitamin D. In renal failure, this step is impaired, potentially leading to profound hypocalcemia. Treatment should be aimed at providing renal replacement therapy and activated vitamin D.

Other causes of hypocalcemia are found in association with hyperphosphatemia. These include tumor lysis syndrome and rhabdomyolysis. These will be discussed in detail in the next section on hyperphosphatemia. It should be pointed out though that in the setting of hyperphosphatemia, hypocalcemia cannot be treated with excess calcium infusion. With an elevated calcium–phosphate cross product, there will be precipitation of calcium and phosphate in the tissues. In patients with end stage renal disease, this has led to a condition known as calciphylaxis that can be fatal.

4.3.3 Hyperphosphatemia

In general, sustained hyperphosphatemia is a result of renal failure. Since the kidneys are responsible for the regulation and excretion of phosphate, renal failure results in the retention of phosphate. Patients with chronic renal failure are usually placed on low phosphate diets as well as phosphate binders to reduce the amount of phosphate absorbed from their diet. Nevertheless, hyperphosphatemia and its consequences can often be a major problem in the long-term management of these patients.

Acute hyperphosphatemia can occur when cells break down and release their intracellular stores of phosphate. As mentioned earlier, the intracellular forms of phosphate are organic in nature and include DNA, RNA, phospholipids, and other nucleotides. The two primary conditions featuring significant release of phosphate form cells are tumor lysis syndrome and rhabdomyolysis. Both of these conditions can also lead to acute renal failure which will exacerbate the hyperphosphatemia. Therefore, hemodialysis should be initiated promptly if patients develop renal failure and severe hyperphosphatemia.

Tumor lysis syndrome is most commonly associated with rapidly expanding tumors such as Burkitt's lymphoma [66–68]. The tumor either outgrows its blood supply and begins to break down on its own or will begin to break down when chemotherapy is begun. Acute renal failure develops as a result of uric acid nephropathy or in some cases as a result of calcium–phosphate precipitation in the kidneys. Recently, uricase has become available for the treatment of hyperuricemia and has greatly reduced the incidence of renal failure as a result of tumor lysis [69]. Consequently, it might now be feasible to reduce the efforts to alkalinize the urine if the serum uric acid concentration is minimal to avoid precipitating calcium and phosphate.

Rhabdomyolysis can result from infections, usually influenza, or from excessive exercise [70, 71]. In addition, a number of medications as well as hypokalemia or hypophosphatemia can result in rhabdomyolysis [72]. Myoglobin released from the muscle cells can damage the kidneys and result in acute renal failure. Therapy is usually aimed at hydrating the patient and attempting to alkalinize the urine to prevent the heme moiety of the myoglobin from causing damage to the renal epithelium. When rhabdomyolysis occurs, a tremendous amount of phosphate is released from the muscle cells. When the cell membrane breaks down, calcium can furthermore enter and lead to hypocalcemia as well as soft tissue calcification. Recommendations for the treatment of rhabdomyolysis, therefore, include treating hypocalcemia only when it is symptomatic and not attempting to normalize the serum calcium concentration. Moreover, and after taking up large amounts of calcium, muscle cells will eventually release it back, possibly causing at times severe hypercalcemia during recovery from rhabdomyolysis.

4.3.4 Hypophosphatemia

Acute hypophosphatemia can occur as a result of shifting phosphate from the extracellular fluid space to the intracellular space [73]. This is most often seen in the treatment of diabetic ketoacidosis when insulin therapy is initiated, but it can also result from respiratory alkalosis. The refeeding syndrome is probably also related to suddenly increased secretion of insulin and can be a devastating cause of hypophosphatemia [73].

Chronic hypophosphatemia usually occurs from renal wasting of phosphate or from long-term starvation. To determine whether or not the kidneys are wasting phosphate, the fractional excretion of phosphate should be determined. This is done by measuring urinary phosphate and creatinine as well as serum phosphate and creatinine and using the following equation:

$$\mathrm{FE}_{\mathrm{Phos}} = \frac{U_{\mathrm{Phos}} / S_{\mathrm{Phos}}}{U_{\mathrm{Phos}} / S_{\mathrm{Creat}}}$$

where U_{Phos} represents the urinary phosphate concentration, U_{Creat} the urinary creatinine concentration, S_{Phos} the serum phosphate concentration, and S_{Creat} the serum creatinine concentration. Although the $\mathrm{FE}_{\mathrm{Phos}}$ varies with diet, it is usually less than 0.15 (15%). Thus, a patient with hypophosphatemia and $\mathrm{FE}_{\mathrm{Phos}}$ greater than 0.15 likely has a renal phosphate wasting syndrome. If the $\mathrm{FE}_{\mathrm{Phos}}$ is very low (far less than 0.15), the patient most likely has dietary phosphate depletion.

Causes of renal phosphate wasting include the Fanconi syndrome, X-linked hypophosphatemia, autosomal dominant hypophosphatemic rickets, and tumor induced osteomalacia. The Fanconi syndrome is a generalized defect of the proximal tubule that leads to wasting of phosphate as well as glucose, bicarbonate, and amino acids [74]. The other conditions are caused by an increase in activity of phosphotonins [43, 73]. This class of hormones causes renal wasting of phosphate through various mechanisms. In X-linked hypophosphatemia, the enzyme PHEX (phosphate regulating gene with homologies to endopeptidase on X chromosome) can no longer metabolize fibroblast growth factor-23 (FGF-23), leading to increased circulating levels of this growth factor and consequent phosphate wasting. The autosomal dominant form of the disease is due to a mutation in FGF-23 that prevents it from being degraded. Tumor induced osteomalacia is a result of phosphotonins that are secreted by the tumor.

4.4   Conclusions

Our understanding of the regulation of calcium and phosphorus has increased dramatically over the past 10 years. Growing knowledge about the molecular biology of ECaCs, the CaSR, the vitamin D receptor and PTH translates into our improved ability to diagnose and treat disorders of calcium regulation. Similarly, the key molecules in phosphate regulation that have been recently uncovered are the phosphotonins. As our understanding of these molecules expands, treatment strategies for hypophosphatemia and osteomalacia should also improve.

Take-Home Pearls

> The ionized calcium concentration should be directly measured and not estimated from total calcium and albumin concentrations.
> Correction of calcium concentrations requires a thorough understanding of the factors regulating the extracellular fluid calcium concentration.
> In particular, acidosis should not be corrected if the patient has a low ionized calcium concentration.
> Hypocalcemia cannot be safely corrected by administration of calcium if the patient also has severe hyperphosphatemia.
> Because the kidneys are the primary regulator of serum phosphorus concentrations, treatment of acute hyperphosphatemia often involves renal replacement therapy

4.4.1   Illustrative Cases

4.4.1.1   Hypercalcemia

A 2-week-old infant has been evaluated by the cardiologist for a murmur. On examination, the infant is somewhat jittery and is very irritable. The blood pressure is normal and the physical exam reveals an infant with elfin shaped ears and a harsh 4/6 systolic murmur. On laboratory examination, the electrolytes and creatinine were all normal except for the serum calcium which was found to be $14.8\,\mathrm{mg\,dl^{-1}}$. The infant is admitted and the next day the calcium is $15.2\,\mathrm{mg\,dl^{-1}}$ and the infant continues to be very irritable and not feed well. Salmon calcitonin is administered over the next 2 days and the serum calcium decreases to $11.3\,\mathrm{mg\,dl^{-1}}$. The infant is much more consolable and is feeding well. A dose of bisphosphonate is given and the calcium becomes stable at $10.6\,\mathrm{mg\,dl^{-1}}$. The infant is discharged home and on follow up at 2 weeks, the calcium was found to be $10.8\,\mathrm{mg\,dl^{-1}}$.

4.4.1.2   Hyperphosphatemia

A 10-year-old male is admitted with a diagnosis of T-cell ALL and has a white blood cell count of 1 million mm^{-3}. His initial laboratory studies revealed a phosphorus concentration of $8.3\,\mathrm{mg\,dl^{-1}}$, creatinine of $0.8\,\mathrm{mg\,dl^{-1}}$, and uric acid of $12.5\,\mathrm{mg\,dl^{-1}}$. He was receiving intravenous fluids at a rate of 1.5 times the maintenance rate when his urine output was noted to have decreased to less than $1\,\mathrm{ml\,kg^{-1}\,h^{-1}}$. His serum chemistries were repeated and his creatinine was found to be $2.3\,\mathrm{mg\,dl^{-1}}$ and his phosphorus had increased to $14.6\,\mathrm{mg\,dl^{-1}}$. At this time a central venous catheter was inserted and hemodialysis was initiated. After 3 h of treatment, his phosphorus was $5.5\,\mathrm{mg\,dl^{-1}}$ and the dialysis treatment was discontinued. Twelve hours later, his phosphorus had increased again to $12.3\,\mathrm{mg\,dl^{-1}}$ and he underwent a second treatment of hemodialysis for 3 h. Subsequent to this treatment, his phosphorus became stable at $8.6\,\mathrm{mg\,dl^{-1}}$ and his creatinine at $1.2\,\mathrm{mg\,dl^{-1}}$. He was then able to undergo the necessary chemotherapy for treatment of his T-cell ALL.

References

1. Bushinsky, D.A. and Monk, R.D. (1998) Electrolyte quintet: calcium. Lancet 352:306–311
2. Ariyan, C.E. and Sosa, J.A. (2004) Assessment and management of patients with abnormal calcium. Crit. Care Med. 32:S146–S154
3. Portale, A.A. (2004) Calcium and Phosphorus. 5:209–236

4. Milliner, D.S. and Stickler, G.B. (1992) Hypercalcemia, Hypercalciuria, and Renal Disease. 2:1661–1685

5. Pain, R.W., Rowland, K.M., Phillips, P.J. et al (1975) Current "corrected" calcium concept challenged. Br. Med. J. 4:617–619

6. Pain, R.W., Phillips, P.J., and Duncan, B.M. (1980) Corrected calcium conflict continues. J. Clin. Pathol. 33:413

7. Slomp, J., van der Voort, P.H., Gerritsen, R.T. et al (2003) Albumin-adjusted calcium is not suitable for diagnosis of hyper- and hypocalcemia in the critically ill. Crit. Care Med. 31:1389–1393

8. Goransson, L.G., Skadberg, O., and Bergrem, H. (2005) Albumin-corrected or ionized calcium in renal failure? What to measure? Nephrol. Dial. Transplant. 20:2126–2129

9. Byrnes, M.C., Huynh, K., Helmer, S.D. et al (2005) A comparison of corrected serum calcium levels to ionized calcium levels among critically ill surgical patients. Am. J. Surg. 189:310–314

10. Besarab, A. and Caro, J.F. (1981) Increased absolute calcium binding to albumin in hypoalbuminaemia. J. Clin. Pathol. 34:1368–1374

11. Guerini, D., Coletto, L., and Carafoli, E. (2005) Exporting calcium from cells. Cell Calcium 38:281–289

12. Guerini, D., Garcia-Martin, E., Zecca, A. et al (1998) The calcium pump of the plasma membrane: membrane targeting, calcium binding sites, tissue-specific isoform expression. Acta Physiol Scand. Suppl. 643:265–273

13. Dipolo, R. and Beauge, L. (2006) Sodium/calcium exchanger: influence of metabolic regulation on ion carrier interactions. Physiol Rev. 86:155–203

14. Dipolo, R. and Beauge, L. (1991) Regulation of Na-Ca exchange. An overview. Ann. N.Y. Acad. Sci. 639:100–111

15. Bootman, M.D., Collins, T.J., Peppiatt, C.M. et al (2001) Calcium signalling–an overview. Semin. Cell Dev. Biol. 12:3–10

16. Berridge, M.J., Lipp, P., and Bootman, M.D. (2000) The versatility and universality of calcium signalling. Nat. Rev. Mol. Cell Biol. 1:11–21

17. Berridge, M.J., Lipp, P., and Bootman, M.D. (2000) Signal transduction. The calcium entry pas de deux. Science 287:1604–1605

18. Diaz, M.E., Graham, H.K., O'Neill, S.C. et al (2005) The control of sarcoplasmic reticulum Ca content in cardiac muscle. Cell Calcium 38:391–396

19. Wellman, G.C. and Nelson, M.T. (2003) Signaling between SR and plasmalemma in smooth muscle: sparks and the activation of Ca^{2+}-sensitive ion channels. Cell Calcium 34:211–229

20. Wray, S., Burdyga, T., and Noble, K. (2005) Calcium signalling in smooth muscle. Cell Calcium 38:397–407

21. Sooy, K., Kohut, J., and Christakos, S. (2000) The role of calbindin and 1,25dihydroxyvitamin D3 in the kidney. Curr. Opin. Nephrol. Hypertens. 9:341–347

22. Hoenderop, J.G., Nilius, B., and Bindels, R.J. (2005) Calcium absorption across epithelia. Physiol Rev. 85:373–422

23. Nilius, B., Owsianik, G., Voets, T. et al (2007) Transient receptor potential cation channels in disease. Physiol Rev. 87:165–217

24. Nilius, B., Voets, T., and Peters, J. (2005) TRP channels in disease. Sci. STKE. 2005:

25. van Abel, M., Hoenderop, J.G., and Bindels, R.J. (2005) The epithelial calcium channels TRPV5 and TRPV6: regulation and implications for disease. Naunyn Schmiedebergs Arch. Pharmacol. 371:295–306

26. Bronner, F. (2003) Mechanisms of intestinal calcium absorption. J. Cell Biochem. 88:387–393

27. Bouillon, R., Van Cromphaut, S., and Carmeliet, G. (2003) Intestinal calcium absorption: molecular vitamin D mediated mechanisms. J. Cell Biochem. 88:332–339

28. Christakos, S., Barletta, F., Huening, M. et al (2003) Vitamin D target proteins: function and regulation. J. Cell Biochem. 88:238–244

29. Friedman, P.A. (1999) Calcium transport in the kidney. Curr. Opin. Nephrol. Hypertens. 8:589–595

30. Hoenderop, J.G., Nilius, B., and Bindels, R.J. (2002) Molecular mechanism of active Ca2+ reabsorption in the distal nephron. Annu. Rev. Physiol 64:529–549

31. Zaidi, M., Inzerillo, A.M., Moonga, B.S. et al (2002) Forty years of calcitonin–where are we now? A tribute to the work of Iain Macintyre, FRS. Bone 30:655–663

32. Raue, F., Haag, C., Schulze, E. et al (2006) The role of the extracellular calcium-sensing receptor in health and disease. Exp. Clin. Endocrinol. Diabetes 114:397–405

33. Hendy, G.N., D'Souza-Li, L., Yang, B. et al (2000) Mutations of the calcium-sensing receptor (CASR) in familial hypocalciuric hypercalcemia, neonatal severe hyperparathyroidism, and autosomal dominant hypocalcemia. Hum. Mutat. 16:281–296

34. Kavanaugh, M.P., Miller, D.G., Zhang, W. et al (1994) Cell-surface receptors for gibbon ape leukemia virus and amphotropic murine retrovirus are inducible sodium-dependent phosphate symporters. Proc. Natl. Acad. Sci. U.S.A 91:7071–7075

35. Hamm, L.L. and Alpern, R.J. (2000) Cellular Mechanisms of Renal Tubular Acidification. 3:1935–1979

36. Rector, F.C. (1983) Sodium, bicarbonate, and chloride absorption by the proximal tubule. Am. J. Physiol Renal Physiol 244:F461–F471

37. Forster, I.C., Hernando, N., Biber, J. et al (2006) Proximal tubular handling of phosphate: a molecular perspective. Kidney Int. 70:1548–1559

38. Biber, J., Hernando, N., Traebcrt, M. et al (2000) Parathyroid hormone-mediated regulation of renal phosphate reabsorption. Nephrol. Dial. Transplant. 15 (Suppl 6):29–30

39. Moe, O.W. (2003) Scaffolds: Orchestrating proteins to achieve concerted function. Kidney Int. 64:1916–1917

40. Gisler, S.M., Pribanic, S., Bacic, D. et al (2003) PDZK1: I. a major scaffolder in brush borders of proximal tubular cells. Kidney Int. 64:1733–1745

41. Biber, J., Gisler, S.M., Hernando, N. et al (2004) PDZ interactions and proximal tubular phosphate reabsorption. Am. J. Physiol Renal Physiol 287:F871–F875

42. Biber, J., Gisler, S.M., Hernando, N. et al (2005) Protein/protein interactions (PDZ) in proximal tubules. J. Membr. Biol. 203:111–118

43. Schiavi, S.C. and Moe, O.W. (2002) Phosphatonins: a new class of phosphate-regulating proteins. Curr. Opin. Nephrol. Hypertens. 11:423–430

44. Bajorunas, D.R. (1990) Clinical manifestations of cancer-related hypercalcemia. Semin. Oncol. 17:16–25

45. Lee, C.T., Yang, C.C., Lam, K.K. et al (2006) Hypercalcemia in the emergency department. Am. J. Med. Sci. 331:119–123

46. Body, J.J. and Bouillon, R. (2003) Emergencies of calcium homeostasis. Rev. Endocr. Metab. Disord. 4:167–175

47. Ralston, S.H., Coleman, R., Fraser, W.D. et al (2004) Medical management of hypercalcemia. Calcif. Tissue Int. 74:1–11

48. Buchs, B., Rizzoli, R., and Bonjour, J.P. (1991) Evaluation of bone resorption and renal tubular reabsorption of calcium and phosphate in malignant and nonmalignant hypercalcemia. Bone 12:47–56

49. Stewart, A.F., Adler, M., Byers, C.M. et al (1982) Calcium homeostasis in immobilization: an example of resorptive hypercalciuria. N. Engl. J. Med. 306:1136–1140

50. Hyman, L.R., Boner, G., Thomas, J.C. et al (1972) Immobiliza-tion hypercalcemia. Am. J. Dis. Child 124:723–727

51. Ross, J.R., Saunders, Y., Edmonds, P.M. et al (2004) A systematic review of the role of bisphosphonates in metastatic disease. Health Technol. Assess. 8:1–176

52. Saunders, Y., Ross, J.R., Broadley, K.E. et al (2004) Systematic review of bisphosphonates for hypercalcaemia of malignancy. Palliat. Med. 18:418–431

53. Whitson, H.E., Lobaugh, B., and Lyles, K.W. (2006) Severe hypocalcemia following bisphosphonate treatment in a patient with Paget's disease of bone. Bone 39:954–958

54. Marini, J.C. (2003) Do bisphosphonates make children's bones better or brittle? N. Engl. J Med. 349:423–426

55. Woo, S.B., Hellstein, J.W., and Kalmar, J.R. (2006) Narrative [corrected] review: bisphosphonates and osteonecrosis of the jaws. Ann. Intern. Med. 144:753–761

56. Strampel, W., Emkey, R., and Civitelli, R. (2007) Safety considerations with bisphosphonates for the treatment of osteoporosis. Drug Saf. 30:755–763

57. Miller, P.D. (2007) Is there a role for bisphosphonates in chronic kidney disease? Semin. Dial. 20:186–190

58. Singhi, S.C., Singh, J., and Prasad, R. (2003) Hypocalcaemia in a paediatric intensive care unit. J. Trop. Pediatr. 49: 298–302

59. Carlstedt, F. and Lind, L. (2001) Hypocalcemic syndromes. Crit. Care Clin. 17:139–viii

60. Cardenas-Rivero, N., Chernow, B., Stoiko, M.A. et al (1989) Hypocalcemia in critically ill children. J. Pediatr. 114:946–951

61. Clec'h, C., Ferriere, F., Karoubi, P. et al (2004) Diagnostic and prognostic value of procalcitonin in patients with septic shock. Crit. Care Med. 32:1166–1169

62. Jensen, J.U., Heslet, L., Jensen, T.H. et al (2006) Procalcitonin increase in early identification of critically ill patients at high risk of mortality. Crit. Care Med. 34:2596–2602

63. Russwurm, S. and Reinhart, K. (2004) Procalcitonin mode of action: new pieces in a complex puzzle. Crit. Care Med. 32:1801–1802

64. Zaloga, G.P., Sager, A., Black, K.W. et al (1992) Low dose calcium administration increases mortality during septic peritonitis in rats. Circ. Shock 37:226–229

65. Carlstedt, F., Eriksson, M., Kiiski, R. et al (2000) Hypocalcemia during porcine endotoxemic shock: effects of calcium administration. Crit. Care Med. 28:2909–2914

66. Sakarcan, A. and Quigley, R. (1994) Hyperphosphatemia in tumor lysis syndrome: the role of hemodialysis and continuous veno-venous hemofiltration. Pediatr. Nephrol. 8:351–353

67. Haller, C. and Dhadly, M. (1991) The tumor lysis syndrome. Ann. Intern. Med. 114:808–809

68. Tiu, R.V., Mountantonakis, S.E., Dunbar, A.J. et al (2007) Tumor lysis syndrome. Semin. Thromb. Hemost. 33:397–407

69. Cammalleri, L. and Malaguarnera, M. (2007) Rasburicase represents a new tool for hyperuricemia in tumor lysis syndrome and in gout. Int. J. Med. Sci. 4:83–93

70. Huerta-Alardin, A.L., Varon, J., and Marik, P.E. (2005) Bench-to-bedside review: rhabdomyolysis – an overview for clinicians. Crit. Care 9:158–169

71. Allison, R.C. and Bedsole, D.L. (2003) The other medical causes of rhabdomyolysis. Am. J. Med. Sci. 326:79–88

72. Coco, T.J. and Klasner, A.E. (2004) Drug-induced rhabdomyolysis. Curr. Opin. Pediatr. 16:206–210

73. Amanzadeh, J. and Reilly, R.F., Jr. (2006) Hypophosphatemia: an evidence-based approach to its clinical consequences and management. Nat. Clin. Pract. Nephrol. 2:136–148

74. Baum, M. (1993) The cellular basis of Fanconi syndrome. Hosp. Pract. (Off Ed) 28:137–138

Abnormalities in Magnesium Metabolism

5

D. Samsonov

Contents

Case Vignette

A 6-day-old baby was admitted to the Pediatric Cardiac ICU after surgery for complex congenital heart disease. During the operation, the patient was on cardiopulmonary bypass for 4 h. The early postoperative admission was complicated by cardiac

S.G. Kiessling et al. (eds) *Pediatric Nephrology in the ICU*.
© Springer-Verlag Berlin Heidelberg 2009

Core Messages

> Magnesium physiology depends on a balance between intestinal absorption and renal excretion.
> Magnesium is the major regulator of its own homeostasis. Hypomagnesemia stimulates and hypermagnesemia inhibits the reabsorption of Mg^{2+} in the loop of Henle.
> Magnesium is a cofactor in all reactions that require adenosine triphosphate (ATP), and it is essential for the activity of Na^+–K^+–ATPase.
> Symptomatic magnesium depletion needs repletion via oral or parenteral route. Extracellular magnesium does not readily equilibrate with intracellular stores; therefore, fast infusion rapidly increases the plasma concentration but does not correct the total body magnesium.
> Hypermagnesemia usually occurs in two clinical settings: compromised renal function or excessive magnesium intake.
> Hypomagnesemia induces hypocalcemia via multiple mechanisms including both decreased secretion and peripheral resistance to parathyroid hormone (PTH) and Vitamin D; thus, low, normal, or slightly elevated levels of PTH can be seen in the presence of laboratory picture of hypoparathyroidism.
> As soon as the diagnosis of hypomagnesemia is confirmed, treatment with enteral magnesium for at least 7–10 days is necessary for normalization of magnesium stores.

instability, pulmonary edema, and mild ATN necessitating ionotropic support and daily furosemide administration. The patient was on IV fluids and minimal enteral feeding. Laboratory evaluation on day 6 postoperation showed hypocalcemia (ca. 7.3 mg dL^{-1}, ionized calcium 3.5 mg dL^{-1}, albumin level 3.4 mg dL^{-1}), and treatment with oral calcium and vitamin D supplementation was started. Labs consistently showed hypocalcemia, hyperphosphatemia, and hypercalciuria suggesting hypoparathyroidism. However, serum

PTH level returned slightly elevated (116 ng L⁻¹; normal range 10–65 ng L⁻¹). 1, 25 VitD level, which was drawn after treatment with vitamin D was initiated, was normal. Despite treatment, calcium levels remained low and furosemide treatment was discontinued. On postoperative day 8, laboratory evaluation showed significant hypomagnesemia (1.1 mg dL⁻¹) treated with intravenous magnesium sulfate. For the next 2 days, magnesium and calcium levels remained low despite repeated daily magnesium infusions and continuous treatment with calcium and vitamin D. Following consultation with Pediatric Nephrology, enteral magnesium replacement was started on day 11 postoperation. After 4 days of enteral magnesium treatment calcium levels normalized, and calcium and magnesium supplementation was subsequently decreased and discontinued.

5.1 Introduction

Magnesium is the second most common intracellular cation after potassium, and the fourth most common cation in the body. Magnesium is a cofactor in more than 300 enzymatic reactions and is involved in multiple processes including hormone receptor binding, calcium channel gating, regulation of adenylate cyclase, muscle contraction, neuronal activity, cardiac excitability, and others [14, 37]. Under physiological conditions, serum magnesium concentration is maintained in a narrow range. Magnesium homeostasis depends on intestinal absorption and renal excretion. Interestingly, magnesium itself is the major regulator of its own homeostasis. Magnesium deficiency can result from low intake, reduced intestinal absorption, and/or renal loss. Magnesium excess is usually a consequence of decreased excretion in acute or chronic renal failure. For the clinician, a complete understanding of the normal magnesium physiology, knowledge of signs and symptoms of magnesium deficiency or excess, and basic principles of therapy are important for the treatment of a critically ill child.

5.2 Units of Measurement and Normal Plasma Concentration

Most laboratories in the United States report the results of body fluid magnesium concentration in units of milliequivalents per liter or milligrams per deciliter, while other countries use also millomoles per liter. The relationship among these units can be expressed by the following equations:

$$1 \text{ mg dL}^{-1} = [1 \text{ mmol L}^{-1} \times 10]/\text{mol wt.,}$$
$$1 \text{ meq L}^{-1} = 1 \text{ mmol L}^{-1}/\text{valence}$$

Since the molecular weight of magnesium is 24.3 and the valence is +2, 1 meq L⁻¹ is equivalent to 0.50 mmol L⁻¹ and to 1.2 mg dL⁻¹. The normal range of plasma magnesium concentration of 1.2–1.9 meq L⁻¹ is equivalent to 0.60–0.95 mmol L⁻¹ and 1.5–2.3 mg dL⁻¹.

5.3 Magnesium Physiology

5.3.1 Overview

Magnesium is predominantly stored in bone (53%), the intracellular compartment of muscle (27%), and soft tissues (19%). Serum magnesium comprises less than 1% of total body magnesium and presents in three states: ionized (62%), protein bound (33%), mainly to albumin, and bound to anions (5%) such as phosphate and citrate [44, 47].

The average daily dietary intake of magnesium is about 300–400 mg in adults and about 5–10 mg kg⁻¹ in children. The main sources of magnesium are green vegetables, soybeans, seafood, and whole grain cereals [27, 49]. Thirty percent to fifty percent of the dietary magnesium is absorbed, but this can vary from 10–20% in a high-magnesium diet to 65–75% in a low-magnesium diet. Absorption of magnesium in the GI tract occurs mainly in the small intestine via two different mechanisms: a saturable active transcellular transport and a nonsaturable paracellular passive transport [16, 19, 23]. At low intraluminal concentrations, magnesium is absorbed primarily via the active transcellular route, whereas at higher concentrations, paracellular passive route becomes significant (Fig. 5.1). The major identified epithelial transcellular magnesium transporter (TRPM6) belongs to the transient receptor potential family of cation channels and accounts for both intestinal absorption and renal tubular transcellular reabsorption of magnesium [38, 45].

About 70% of serum magnesium (not protein bound) is freely filtered at the glomerulus to the Bowman space [23, 47]. In contrast to other ions, only a small fraction of filtered magnesium (15–20%) is reabsorbed in the proximal tubule (Fig. 5.2). In immature animals, the proximal tubule accounts for 60–70% of magnesium ions (Mg²⁺) reabsorption [26]. The mechanism of this phenomenon remains unknown. The majority

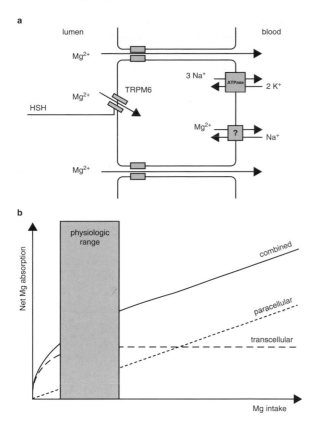

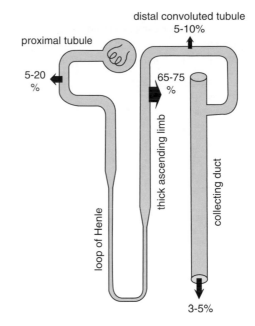

Fig. 5.2 Magnesium reabsorption along the nephron (from [39], with permission)

Fig. 5.1 a Schematic model of intestinal magnesium absorption via two independent pathways: passive absorption via the paracellular pathway and active, transcellular transport consisting of an apical entry through a putative magnesium channel and a basolateral exit mediated by a putative sodium-coupled exchange. **b** Kinetics of human intestinal magnesium absorption. Paracellular transport lineary rising with intraluminal concentrations (*dotted line*) and saturable active transcellular transport (*dashed line*) together yield a curvilinear function for net magnesium absorption (*solid line*). HSH hypomagnesemia with secondary hypocalcemia, TRPM6 epithelial transcellular magnesium transporter (from [39], with permission)

of magnesium (70%) is reabsorbed in the loop of Henle, especially in the cortical thick ascending limb (TAL) [23, 36]. Transport in this segment appears to be passive and paracellular, driven by the favorable electrical gradient resulting from the reabsorption of sodium chloride (Fig. 5.3a). Paracellular magnesium reabsorption is facilitated by the tight junction protein paracellin-1, which also serves as a main route for calcium reabsorption in this segment. The remaining 5–10% of the filtered magnesium is reabsorbed in the distal convoluted tubule (DCT). Magnesium transport in the DCT is active and transcellular [23]. The proposed model of magnesium absorption in DCT includes apical entry via TRPM6 and extrusion via unidentified sodium–magnesium exchanger (Fig. 5.3b).

5.3.2   Regulation of Renal Magnesium Handling

In contrast to other body cations, no single hormone has been identified as an important regulator of magnesium intestinal absorption or kidney excretion [36]. Serum magnesium concentration appears to be the major factor determining renal magnesium handling. Most of the filtered Mg^{2+} ions are reabsorbed passively in the TAL (Fig. 5.3a). Mg^{2+} reabsorption in the TAL is driven by a transepithelial voltage generated by apical Na^+–K^+–$2Cl^-$ cotransporter (NKCC2) concominant with apical K^+ recycling via potassium channel ROMK (rat outer medulla K^+ channel), basolateral Cl^- exit through the chloride channel, and basolateral Na^+ exit via Na^+–K^+–ATPase. The resulting lumen positive (under normal circumstances) voltage is expected to drive the Mg^{2+} reabsorption even against the concentration gradient. Factors controlling Mg^{2+} reabsorption in the TAL include transepithelial voltage and permeability of the paracellular pathway. Factors diminishing the voltage will decrease Mg^{2+} transport in the TAL. For example, loop diuretics inhibit Na^+–K^+–$2Cl^-$ cotransporter NKCC2 and prevent establishment of transepithelial voltage gradient in TAL, thus reducing Mg^{2+} reabsorption [36, 47]. Volume expansion results in decreased Na^+ and Cl^- reabsorption in TAL and subsequent reduction of Mg^{2+} reabsorption. Permeability of the

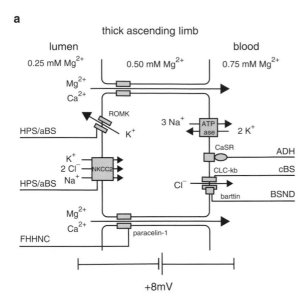

a

thick ascending limb

lumen   blood

0.25 mM Mg^{2+} 0.50 mM Mg^{2+} 0.75 mM Mg^{2+}

Mg^{2+}
Ca^{2+}

ROMK   3 Na$^+$ ATP ase 2 K$^+$
HPS/aBS   K$^+$
                                              CaSR   ADH
K$^+$
2 Cl$^-$ NKCC2   CLC-kb   cBS
HPS/aBS Na$^+$ Cl$^-$
                                              barttin BSND

Mg^{2+}
Ca^{2+}
FHHNC   paracelin-1

+8mV

b

distal convoluted tubule

lumen   blood

0.25 mM Mg^{2+} 0.50 mM Mg^{2+} 0.75 mM Mg^{2+}

                     Mg^{2+} ?   Na$^+$
Mg^{2+} TRPM6
HSH   3 Na$^+$ ATP ase 2 K$^+$

Na$^+$ γ-subunit IDH
Cl$^-$ NCCT   CaSR   ADH
GS   CLC-Kb   cBS
Ca^{2+} Cl$^-$
ECaC   barttin   BSND

−10mV

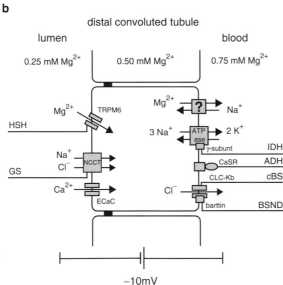

Fig. 5.3 a Magnesium reabsorption in the thick ascending limb (TAL) of Henle's loop. Paracellular reabsorption of magnesium and calcium is driven by lumen-positive transcellular reabsorption of NaCl. **b** Magnesium reabsorption in the distal convoluted tubule (DCT). Magnesium is reabsorbed actively via the transcellular pathway involving an apical entry step through a magnesium-selective ion channel and a basolateral exit, presumably mediated by a sodium-coupled exchange mechanism. *ADH* autosomal dominant hypoparathyroidism, *BSND* Bartter syndrome with sensorineural deafness, *CaSR* calcium sensing receptor, *cBS* classic Bartter syndrome, *CLC-Kb* chloride channel, *ECaC* epithelium calcium channel, *FHHNC* familial hypomagnesemia with hypercalciuria and nephrocalcinosis, *GS* Gitelman syndrome, *HPS/aBS* hyperprostaglandin E syndrome/antenatal Bartter syndrome variant, *IDH* isolated dominant hypomagnesemia, NKCC2 Na$^+$–K$^+$–2Cl$^-$ cotransporter, *ROMK* rat outer medulla K$^+$ channel, *TRPM6* epithelial transcellular magnesium transporter (from [39], with permission)

paracellular pathway can be diminished as a result of paracellin-1 mutations (see Sect. 5.4.4.2) [39]. The major factor regulating Mg^{2+} transport in the TAL is Mg^{2+} serum concentration, whereas hypomagnesemia stimulates and hypermagnesemia inhibits the reabsorption of Mg^{2+} [36]. The proposed mechanism involves binding of Mg^{2+} to calcium sensing receptor (CaSR) on the basolateral membrane with subsequent modulation of adenylate cyclase activity and activation of phospholipase C, which results in the inhibition of apical (luminal) potassium channels [21]. This in turn reduces K$^+$ recycling and decreases activity of Na$^+$–K$^+$–2Cl$^-$ cotransporter NKCC2, preventing establishment of positive lumen voltage. Obviously, binding of Ca^{2+} to basolateral CaSR should have similar effect on Mg^{2+} handling. Thus, hypercalcemia also inhibits Mg^{2+} and Ca^{2+} reabsorption in the TAL resulting in hypercalciuria and hypermagnesuria [47]. The role of magnesium feedback loop via CaSR is debated because the affinity of the receptor for magnesium is quite low. In experimental studies, a number of hormones including PTH, calcitonin, glucagons, and vasopressin have been shown to increase magnesium transport in the TAL but none has a primary importance. All of them work through adenylate cyclase activity and activation of phospholipase C. Metabolic acidosis, hypokalemia, and phosphate depletion inhibit magnesium reabsorption in the TAL [36]; however, the mechanism remains unknown (Table 5.1).

The distal tubule reabsorbs 5–10% of filtered Mg^{2+} (Fig. 5.2). Mg^{2+} enters the tubular cell via a recently identified membrane protein TRPM6, which

Table 5.1 Factors affecting magnesium tubular reabsorption

Factor	TAL	DT	Total effect
Volume expansion	↓	?	↓
Hypomagnesemia	↑	No change	↑
Hypermagnesemia	↓	No change	↓
Hypercalcemia	↓	No change	↓
Hypocalcemia	↑	No change	↑
Phosphate depletion	↓	↓	↓
Metabolic acidosis	↓?	↓	↓?
Metabolic alkalosis	?	?	↑?
PTH	↑	↑?	↑
Loop diuretics	↓	No change	↓
Thiazide diuretics	↑?	↓?	No change

TAL thick ascending limb of Henle, *DT* distal tubule, *PTH* parathyroid hormone functions as a Mg^{2+} channel (Fig 5.3b). Mutation of TRPM6 is responsible for familial hypomagnesemia with secondary hypocalcemia, an autosomal recessive disorder characterized primarily by intestinal malabsorption of Mg^{2+} (see Sect. 5.4.4.1) [38, 45]. TRPM6 is expressed in intestine and highly expressed in the distal tubule. Evaluation of these patients reveals additional defect of magnesium renal handling. Compared with normal individuals these patients have lower threshold for magnesium urinary wasting during magnesium sulfate infusion [38, 39]. Some data suggest that Mg^{2+} exits the basolateral membrane via not identified Na^+–Mg^{2+} exchanger. The driving force for the exchange is a high-sodium concentration gradient between extracellular (140 meq L^{-1}) and intracellular (10–15 meq L^{-1}) compartments, which favors Na^+ entry and Mg^{2+} exit. Because Mg^{2+} transport in the distal tubule operates close to its maximal capacity, it is believed that the DCT plays minor role in regulating Mg^{2+} homeostasis. However, some evidence suggests that this segment regulates the final urine magnesium excretion. Both phosphate depletion and metabolic acidosis increase magnesium urinary losses, which were localized to the TAL and the DCT (Table 5.1). Amiloride, a potassium and magnesium sparing diuretic, causes hyperpolarization of the membrane voltage that increases the driving force for Mg^{2+} entry. The result is increased Mg^{2+} reabsorption in the DCT. Interestingly, thiazide-type diuretics have little effect on Mg^{2+} handling. Thiazide diuretics primarily act on the Na^+–K^+–$2Cl^-$ cotransporter NKCC2, which is located in the DCT. The resulting decrease in transmembrane voltage diminishes Mg^{2+} reabsorption in this segment [13, 36]. However, both human studies and animal micropuncture studies fail to demonstrate increase in Mg^{2+} excretion after treatment with thiazide diuretics [47]. These findings are puzzling when compared with evaluation of patients with Gitelman syndrome, who have inactivating mutation of NCCT and most universally show renal magnesium wasting. One possible explanation to this discrepancy could be the modest impairment of Na^+ transport in proximal tubule caused by some thiazide diuretics due to partial inhibition of carbonic anhydrase [48]. This effect is not clinically important and does not contribute to net diuresis since the excess fluid and sodium delivered out of the proximal tubule are reabsorbed in the TAL. This may account for mild increase of Mg^{2+} reabsorption in the TAL counterbalancing Mg^{2+} wasting in the distal segment.

5.3.3 Regulation of Magnesium Serum Concentration

In contrast to other ions, serum Mg^{2+} concentration is not under tight hormonal regulation. Bone, the major intracellular Mg reservoir, does not readily exchange with extracellular Mg^{2+}, and equilibration with bone stores may take several weeks [41]. These physiological observations have very important clinical implications. First, negative magnesium balance due to low intake or decreased intestinal absorption can be compensated only by increased renal reabsorption. Fractional excretion of Mg^{2+}, which is normally between 3 and 5%, may decrease to 0.5% with magnesium depletion due to extrarenal losses. Thus, patients treated with intravenous fluids containing dextrose and sodium chloride may develop hypomagnesemia rather quickly, especially in the presence of tubular damage and the inability to conserve Mg^{2+}. Second, the human body has no good protection against hypermagnesemia in the presence of impaired renal function.

5.4 Magnesium Deficiency and Hypomagnesemia

Hypomagnesemia is a common problem occurring in 7–11% of hospitalized patients and in as many as 60% of intensive care unit (ICU) patients. Magnesium deficiency can be demonstrated in up to 40% of patients with other electrolyte and acid–base abnormalities, especially hypokalemia, hypophosphatemia, hypocalcemia, and metabolic alkalosis. Hypomagnesemia in ICU patients is associated with a higher mortality [44, 46]. Hypomagnesemia may cause multiple cardiac, neuromuscular, and metabolic abnormalities; however, cardiac and neurological symptoms can also frequently be attributed to coexisting metabolic abnormalities such as hypokalemia or hypocalcemia. Also, many patients with significant hypomagnesemia remain completely asymptomatic. Thus, the clinical significance of mild hypomagnesemia remains somewhat controversial. Table 5.2 summarizes the clinical signs of hypomagnesemia and their proposed mechanisms. Magnesium is a cofactor in all reactions that require ATP, and it is essential for the activity of Na^+–K^+–ATPase. The impaired function of Na^+–K^+–ATPase activity with secondary intracellular hypokalemia is the major effect of hypomagnesemia [1, 44].

Because extracellular magnesium accounts for only 1% of total body magnesium, serum Mg^{2+} concentration may not reflect the overall magnesium status. Unfortunately,

Table 5.2 Clinical signs of magnesium deficiency and proposed mechanism

Clinical sign	Mechanism
Metabolic	
Hypokalemia	↓ Na⁺–K⁺–ATPase activity, renal K⁺ wasting
Hypocalcemia	↓ PTH, ↓ 1.25(OH)$_2$D, end-organ resistance to PTH, and 1,25(OH)$_2$D
Cardiac	
Electrocardiographic abnormalities (nonspecific T-wave abnormalities, U waves, prolonged QT, and QU intervals)	↓ Na⁺–K⁺–ATPase activity, Intracellular hypokalemia
Arrhythmias (ventricular ectopy, ventricular tachycardia, Torsdaes de pointes, ventricular fibrillation)	↓ Na⁺–K⁺–ATPase activity, Intracellular hypokalemia, especially in presence of myocardial hypoxic damage
Neuromuscular system	
Muscle tremor and twitching	Hypomagnesemia-induced excitation of glutamate-sensitive NMDA receptors
Tetany	
Positive Trousseau and Chvostec signs	
Seizures	
Paresthesias	
Muscle weakness	

PTH parathyroid hormone, *1.25(OH)$_2$D* active vitamin D, *NMDA* N-methyl-D-aspartate-type glutamate receptors

no simple clinical test is available to measure body magnesium stores. The magnesium tolerance test has been used for many years and is thought to be the most accurate way to assess magnesium status. The test is performed by collecting twice 24-h urine for magnesium – one collected before and second after the administration of 2.0 mg kg⁻¹ of parenteral Mg²⁺. Retention of more than 20% of the administered Mg²⁺ is suggestive of magnesium depletion. Even though clinical studies show good correlation between the results of the test and magnesium status assessed by skeletal and muscle magnesium content, the test's clinical use remains limited [34, 44]. The test is invalid in patients with impaired renal function or in presence of diuretics affecting magnesium renal handling. The duration of the test is another limiting factor in the ICU setting.

5.4.1 Metabolic Abnormalities in Hypomagnesemia

Hypokalemia is a frequent finding in hypomagnesemic patients. Some conditions may result in simultaneous loss of potassium and magnesium; however, hypomagnesemia by itself can induce hypokalemia via two mechanisms: intracellular potassium depletion and renal potassium wasting. Hypomagnesemia induces impairment of Na⁺–K⁺–ATPase function, which causes K⁺ leakage from cells with subsequent K⁺ loss

in the urine. The exact mechanism of renal K⁺ wasting in hypomagnesemia remains unknown; some data suggest a defect in the TAL [1, 34].

Hypocalcemia is present in about half of the patients with severe hypomagnesemia. Multiple mechanisms, contributing to hypocalcemia, have been identified. The first identified cause is a suppression of PTH secretion by hypomagnesemia. Most hypomagnesemic–hypocalcemic patients have either low or normal (inappropriately low for low calcium concentration) PTH levels, which increase rapidly following magnesium supplementation. A second observation suggests end-organ resistance to PTH. PTH-induced calcium release from isolated bone is impaired when Mg²⁺ concentration falls below 1 mg dL⁻¹. Several studies suggest that this effect may be even of greater importance than reduced PTH secretion, because last effect requires more severe hypomagnesemia. Hypomagnesemia also impairs secretion of active vitamin D (1.25(OH)$_2$D) and causes end-organ resistance to this hormone [1, 34, 44]. The exact mechanisms for these effects are unknown.

5.4.2 Effect of Hypomagnesemia on the Cardiovascular System

One of the major effects of magnesium depletion is an impaired function of Na⁺–K⁺–ATPase with subsequent intracellular hypokalemia. The intracellular hypokalemia may potentially produce depolarized resting membrane potential predisposing to ectopic excitation and tachyarrhythmias. A reduced outward K^+ gradient diminishes K^+ efflux during repolarization that is needed to terminate cardiac action potential. As a result, the most common electrocardiographic (ECG) abnormalities seen in hypomagnesemia reflect abnormal cardiac repolarization and include nonspecific T-wave abnormalities, U waves, and prolonged QT interval. Association of hypomagnesemia with ventricular arrhythmias, especially during myocardial ischemia, is of great clinical importance and is reviewed extensively in the literature [2, 34, 44].

5.4.3 Effect of Hypomagnesemia on Neuromuscular System

Isolated magnesium depletion may induce multiple symptoms of neuromuscular irritability including tetany, muscle twitching, tremor, and positive Chvostec and Trousseau signs. Tonic–clonic generalized convulsions were described as a first manifestation of hypomagnesemia and sometimes can be triggered by noise. Data from animal studies suggest that effect of magnesium deficiency on brain neuronal excitability is mediated via N-methyl-D-aspartate (NMDA)-type glutamate receptors. Glutamate is a major excitatory neurotransmitter in the brain acting as an agonist at NMDA receptors. Extracellular Mg^{2+} normally blocks NMDA receptors, thus hypomagnesemia may release the inhibition of NMDA receptor with subsequent glutamate-mediated depolarization of the postsynaptic membrane and enhancement of epileptiform electrical activity [1, 34, 44].

5.4.4 Causes of Hypomagnesemia

Magnesium deficiency can be induced by either decreased intake or increased losses. Because bone magnesium reservoir does not readily exchange magnesium with plasma pool, negative magnesium balance can cause hypomagnesemia rather quickly. This is in contrast to calcium metabolism, where negative balance is compensated by PTH-induced Ca^{2+} release from bone. Decreased intake of magnesium can be secondary to diminished amount of enteric Mg^{2+} delivery or reduced absorption (Table 5.3). Magnesium wasting can be via gastrointestinal or renal route. Approach to the differential diagnosis of hypomagnesemia will be discussed in the Sect. 5.4.4.3.

5.4.4.1 Extrarenal Causes of Hypomagnesemia

Nutritional Deficiency

Since magnesium is present in almost all foods in significant amounts, hypomagnesemia is almost never observed in normal individuals even on a strict diet. In clinical practice, hypomagnesemia can be found in circumstances of severe protein-calorie malnutrition, pure magnesium-free parenteral feeding, and alcoholism [34]. Patients receiving pure parenteral nutrition without magnesium supplementation are at risk for developing hypomagnesemia. This is particularly true in ICU patients as those patients are sicker and often have additional risk factors for hypomagnesemia, including renal magnesium wasting secondary to nephrotoxin-induced tubulopathy.

Intestinal Malabsorption

Different malabsorption syndromes including celiac and inflammatory bowel disease can be associated with hypomagnesemia. In case of fat malabsorption, free fatty acids in the intestinal lumen combine with cations (saponification) and form nonabsorbable soaps. This process can interfere with Mg^{2+} absorption [25, 34].

Congenital defect of magnesium absorption has been recently described. This condition manifests as hypomagnesemia with secondary hypocalcemia, which usually responds to magnesium repletion. Both X-linked recessive and autosomal recessive inheritances were described. Affected patients were found to have mutation in TRMP6 gene that encodes a new protein involved in transcellular transport of Mg^{2+} in the intestinal lumen and the DCT (Figs. 5.1 and 5.3b). The major reason of hypomagnesemia in these patients is intestinal malabsorption; however, additional tubular defect in Mg^{2+} renal reabsorption has also been confirmed. The hypomagnesemia is usually severe and can manifest with seizures in infants. High doses of enteral magnesium are required to keep serum magnesium and calcium levels close to normal range [38, 45].

Intestinal Losses

Generally, secretions from the lower gastrointestinal tract have much higher magnesium concentrations (up to 16 mg dL^{-1}) than from the upper gastrointestinal tract. As a result, patients with biliary or pancreatic fistulas, iliostomy or gastric drainage rarely develop hypomagnesemia. In contrast, chronic diarrhea and short bowel syndrome can be associated with hypomagnesemia [30, 34, 44].

Table 5.3 Causes and proposed mechanisms of magnesium deficiency

Mechanism of magnesium deficiency	Disorder
Low intake	No magnesium in intravenous fluids
	Starvation
	Anorexia
Malabsorption: saponification by fat	Fat malabsorption syndromes
	Pancreatitis
Malabsorption: congenital defect due to TRMP6 mutation	Congenital hypomagnesemia with hypocalcemia
Increased gastrointestinal losses	Nasogastric suction
	Vomiting
	Short bowel syndrome
	Diarrhea
	Laxative abuse
Increased cutaneous loss	Extensive burns
Increased renal losses	Volume expansion (hyperaldosteronism)
	Osmotic diuresis (glucose, mannitol, urea)
	Diuretics (loop diuretics, mannitol)
	Polyuric phase of ATN including kidney transplant
	Postobstructive diuresis
	Drugs (cisplatin, carboplatin, amphotericin B, cyclosporine, tacrolimus, pentamidine, foscarnet, aminoglycosides)
	Inborn defects:
	Gitelman's syndrome
	Isolated familial hypomagnesemia
	Familial hypomagnesemia with hypercalciuria and nephrocalcinosis
	Autosomal dominant hypocalcemia
Electrolyte imbalance	Hypercalcemia
Increased cellular uptake of magnesium	Hungry bone syndrome

Cutaneous Losses

Sweat Mg^{2+} concentration does not exceed 0.5 mg dL^{-1}; therefore, contribution of cutaneous magnesium loss during exertion is not significant. Observed decrease in Mg^{2+} concentration most likely is secondary to intracellular shift of magnesium. Patients with severe burns can be prone to develop hypomagnesemia due to losses with cutaneous exudates [34].

Redistribution to the Intracellular Compartment

Rarely refeeding syndrome can cause hypomagnesemia. In this condition, rapid cellular uptake of water, glucose, potassium, phosphorus, and magnesium may result in electrolyte abnormalities including hypomagnesemia [7].

Hungry Bone Syndrome

Some patients with hyperparathyroidism develop hypocalcemia and hypomagnesemia after parathyroidectomy. Cessation of high bone turnover state due to PTH-induced bone resorption results in high rate of bone formation, which is thought to be responsible for Ca^{2+} and Mg^{2+} sequestration into bone tissue [17].

5.4.4.2 Renal Causes of Hypomagnesemia

Since 60% of filtered magnesium is reabsorbed passively in the TAL, any factor that blocks reabsorption of sodium and chloride in this segment promotes urinary loss of magnesium. In the ICU setting, magnesium renal losses can be especially hazardous in patients with low magnesium intake. Expansion of extracellular fluid volume as a result of hyperaldosteronism or inappropriate antidiuretic hormone secretion can result in mild hypomagnesemia. Hypermagnesuria can occur during polyuric phase of acute tubular necrosis (ATN), postobstructive, osmotic diuresis, and recovery from postischemic injury of transplanted kidney [1].

Hypercalcemia

Hypercalcemia directly induces renal Mg^{2+} wasting, the effect that is clearly observed in patients with malignant bone metastases [5]. Hypercalcemia results in increased glomerular filtration of Ca^{2+} and increased Ca^{2+} reabsorption in the TAL. Most likely, since Mg^{2+} and Ca^{2+} share the same paracellular transporter for their reabsorption in the TAL, increased delivery and reabsorption of Ca^{2+} results in decreased uptake of Mg^{2+}. In primary hyperparathyroidism, direct effect of PTH-induced increase in Mg^{2+} reabsorption is counterbalanced by the hypercalcemia-induced Mg^{2+} wasting. The net result is usually normal magnesium handling in this clinical situation [34, 47].

Diuretics

Loop diuretics block chloride and sodium reabsorption in the TAL and when used in large amounts can cause profound hypomagnesemia. Hypomagnesemia can also be associated with osmotic diuretics (mannitol, glucose in diabetic hyperglycemia). Interestingly, thiazide diuretics that block NCCT and mimic Gitelman syndrome do not cause significant hypermagnesuria and hypomagnesemia (see Sect. 5.3.2).

Other Medications

Medication-induced tubular damage may cause hypermagnesuria in a polyuric phase of ATN. Some medications can induce specific tubular defect resulting in hypermagnesuria.

Aminoglycosides cause tubular damage that typically presents with hypokalemia, hypocalcemia, and hypomagnesemia [11, 24, 34, 40]. Hypomagnesemia can also be an isolated finding in patients receiving aminoglycosides and can occur few weeks after discontinuation of the antibiotic treatment and persist for several months. Most reported adult patients who were treated with high total dose of aminoglycosides had normal therapeutic levels suggesting that cumulative dose of aminoglycosides is a predictor of development of magnesuria. However, normal cumulative dose does not exclude development of Bartter-like syndrome. Importantly, no correlation has been found between aminoglycoside-induced ATN and hypomagnesemia

in both preclinical and clinical studies. All clinically available aminoglycosides including gentamicin, amikacin, and tobramycin can cause similar tubular defect. Also topically administered for extensive burn injury, neomycin can cause classical metabolic triad of hypokalemia, hypocalcemia, and hypomagnesemia presenting with seizures in children [4, 34]. Even symptomatic hypomagnesemia as a complication of accepted 3–5 mg kg^{-1} day^{-1} standard dose regimen is relatively rare; asymptomatic hypomagnesemia can be observed in up to 30% of adult patients. For our knowledge, all reported pediatric cases, who developed Bartter-like syndrome during the treatment with aminoglycosides, had complete recovery of the tubular function after cessation of antibiotic treatment [24, 40]. The exact mechanism of gentamicin-induced Bartter-like syndrome is unknown. Low PTH levels despite hypocalcemia suggest possibility that gentamicin may activate calcium-sensing receptor on the TAL and the DCT [11].

Cisplatin is a widely used antineoplastic agent for solid tumors. Nephrotoxicity is a well-appreciated complication of cisplatin toxicity [3]. Hypomagnesemia is observed in more than 50% of patients receiving monthly cycles of cisplatin and does not correlate with the incidence of cisplatin-induced acute renal failure. Renal magnesuria can manifest during treatment and continue for months or even years after cessation of cisplatin treatment. Some patients may develop permanent tubular damage manifesting with hypokalemic metabolic acidosis, hypermagnesuria, and hypocalciuria [32]. Close resemblance to Gitelman syndrome suggests distal tubular defect; however, exact mechanism of cisplatin-induced tubulopathy remains unknown. Carboplatin, an analog of cisplatin, appears to be less nephrotoxic and rarely causes acute renal failure in adults [34]. Prospective study of 651 pediatric patients treated with either cisplatin or carboplatin in combination with ifosfamide demonstrated hypomagnesemia in 12.5 and 15.6% of patients receiving cisplatin or carboplatin, respectively, and was significantly higher than in control group. In all groups, the frequency of hypomagnesemia was decreasing during the follow-up period of 2 years, but serum magnesium remained lower in platinum-treated patients in the end of the study [43].

Amphotericin B-induced nephrotoxicity is the major side effect of this potent antifungal medication. Nephrotoxicity can present with acute renal failure due to tubular necrosis, potassium wasting, distal renal tubular acidosis, or magnesium wasting. Interestingly, amphotericin-induced hypermagnesuria is usually accompanied by hypocalciuria suggesting distal tubular defect somewhat similar to cisplatin toxicity. Hypocalciuria prevents hypomagnesemia-induced hypocalcemia; the resulting serum calcium levels are usually normal [6, 18].

Calcineurin inhibitors may induce renal Mg^{2+} wasting and hypomagnesemia in posttransplant patients. Mg^{2+} loss does not correlate with trough cyclosporine levels [34], most likely, because of poor correlation between cyclosporine trough levels and area under the curve [12]. In contrast, tacrolimus trough level is a good predictor of the drug area under the curve [15], and tacrolimus-induced magnesium urine loss correlates well with tacrolimus levels [31]. Interestingly, retrospective analysis of patients with biopsy proven cyclosporine nephrotoxicity shows that hypomagnesemia is an additional risk factor for fast decline of renal function [22]. It has been proposed that some of the neurological symptoms that were always attributed to cyclosporine toxicity can actually be a consequence of the drug-induced hypomagnesemia [34].

Intravenous pentamidine and foscarnet can cause Mg^{2+} renal wasting and hypomagnesemia, which is often accompanied by hypocalcemia [34].

Inherited Tubular Defects of Magnesium Handling

Bartter syndrome includes a group of inherited disorders characterized by chloride wasting, hypo-kalemic metabolic alkalosis, and usually hypercalciuria. Affected children usually present with failure to thrive in infancy or early childhood. Classic Bartter syndrome is caused by inactivation mutation of gene coding for the chloride channel CLC-Kb (Fig. 5.3) in the TAL and the DCT. Hypomagnesemia can be detected in up to 50% of patients with this mutation. Neonatal forms of Bartter syndrome, resulting from abnormal $Na^+–K^+–2Cl^-$ cotransporter NKCC2, potassium channel ROMK, or Barttin, are rarely associated with disturbances of magnesium homeostasis [33, 39].

Gitelman's syndrome is a variant of Bartter syndrome characterized by potassium and magnesium urine loss and hypocalciuria. Patients with Gitelman's syndrome usually have milder symptoms than Bartter patients and present after the age of 6 years with metabolic abnormalities including mild hypokalemic metabolic alkalosis, hypomagnesemia, and hypocalciuria. Some patients can be asymptomatic and others complain of transient episodes of weakness, tetany, abdominal pains, and salt craving. The defect in most studied families is a result of inactivating mutation of

thiazide-sensitive $Na^+–Cl^-$ cotransporter (NCCT) that is mainly located in the DCT (Fig. 5.3b) [33, 39]. The exact mechanisms responsible for hypocalciuria and hypermagnesuria remain poorly understood.

Isolated hypomagnesemia is a rare congenital disorder with either autosomal dominant or autosomal recessive mode of inheritance. Clinical presentation may vary from asymptomatic cases to generalized convulsions in early childhood. Laboratory findings include hypermagnesuria, hypomagnesemia, and hypocalciuria without any other electrolyte abnormalities. Whereas a genetic locus in the autosomal recessive form has not been yet identified, in the autosomal dominant form a locus was mapped to chromosome 11q23. The identified gene FXYD2 encodes the $Na^+–K^+–ATPase$ g-subunit localized in the distal tubule. The mechanism by which FXYD2 mutations cause hypermagnesuria remains unclear [29, 39].

Familial hypomagnesemia with hypercalciuria and nephrocalcinosis (FHHNC) is distinguished from other congenital hypomagnesemic syndromes by the presence of significant calcium, in addition to magnesium, renal wasting. Most FHHNC patients present in early childhood with nephrocalcinosis and/or renal stones, failure to thrive, polyuria, and polydipsia. Nephrocalcinosis and renal stones resulting from hypercalciuria are the major clinical findings. Nephrocalcinosis-related renal insufficiency, distal acidification, and concentrating defects have been also described. Some patients may develop symptomatic hypocalcemia. This syndrome is also associated with frequent ocular abnormalities including corneal calcifications, choreoretinitis, keratoconus, and macular coloboma. The association of hypercalciuria and hypermagnesuria was suggestive of the TAL reabsorptive defect. Indeed, genetic analysis revealed a locus on chromosome 3q and determined that mutated gene is responsible for paracellin-1 protein (Fig. 5.3a). Paracellin-1 is a member of the claudin family of tight junction proteins, which is expressed only in the TAL and distal tubule. Paracellin-1 is also known as claudin-16; both names are used in the literature that can be confusing. This protein plays a critical role in the paracellular Ca^{2+} and Mg^{2+} reabsorption in the TAL. Paracellin-1 gene expression is also shown in cornea and retinal epithelium in animals explaining the link with ocular abnormalities observed in some patients [34, 39, 42].

Autosomal dominant hypocalcemia results from activating mutation of calcium-sensing receptor. CaSR is expressed in the parathyroid gland and the TAL. Activation of CaSR causes a clinical picture resembling primary hypoparathyroidism including hypocalcemia and inadequately low PTH levels. In the parathyroid gland activation of the CaSR results in diminished PTH secretion, whereas in the kidney activation of the CaSR contributes to decreased reabsorption of Ca^{2+} and Mg^{2+} in the TAL. Resulting hypomagnesemia helps to differentiate these patients from primary hypoparathyroidism [39].

5.4.4.3   Clinical Approach to the Diagnosis of Hypomagnesemia

The serum Mg^{2+} concentration remains the most practical clinical test to assess magnesium deficit. In contrast to other electrolytes, the plasma magnesium concentration is not always a routine screening blood test. The presence of hypomagnesemia should be suspected in pediatric patients with chronic diarrhea, hypocalcemia, and unexplained neurological or muscular symptoms. It is reasonable to perform serum magnesium screening in most ICU patients on admission. Hypomagnesemia is defined as a decrease in serum Mg^{2+} concentration to levels less than 1.5 mg dL^{-1}. If hypomagnesemia is confirmed on two consecutive blood draws, the diagnosis can often be obtained from careful medical history and clinical picture (Table 5.3). ICU patients are prone to develop hypomagnesemia due to coexistence of two or more factors as, for example, due to low intake and increased gastrointestinal or renal loss. If the cause of hypomagnesemia remains unclear, the differential diagnosis between renal and extrarenal losses can be performed using 24-h urinary magnesium excretion, fractional excretion of Mg^{2+} (FEMg), or urine magnesium to creatinine ratio. The latter two tests are easier to perform since they do not necessitate 24-h urine collection. FEMg can be calculated from the following formula:

$$FEMg = (UMg \times PCr) \times 100/(0.7 \times PMg \times UCr),$$

where UMg and UCr are urine concentrations and PMg and PCr are plasma concentrations of magnesium and creatinine, respectively. The plasma concentration of magnesium is multiplied by 0.7 to estimate the free (not bound to albumin) concentration of magnesium,

since only free magnesium is available for glomerular filtration.

The normal renal response is to diminish magnesium excretion in the presence of hypomagnesemia to very low levels. In adults, 24-h urine magnesium excretion falls to lower than 20 mg and FEMg to less than 1–2%. Urine excretion of more than 20–30 mg and fractional excretion above 2% are suggestive of renal magnesium loss. Normal values of urine magnesium to creatinine ratio in different age groups are summarized in Table 5.4 [1, 28].

5.4.4.4   Treatment of Hypomagnesemia

Monitoring of magnesium status becomes a routine screening test in severely sick children. It is of primary importance in ICU pediatric patients maintained with parenteral nutrition for a long time. Parenteral nutrition should contain magnesium; otherwise, these patients are prone to develop hypomagnesemia. In most patients, hypomagnesemia can be prevented by sufficient daily magnesium supplementation (Table 5.5 [49]).

If hypomagnesemia develops, the treating physician should try to answer the following questions to optimize the treatment:

1. What is the etiology of magnesium deficit? Can the etiologic factor(s) be withdrawn or ameliorated?
2. Is the patient symptomatic with regard to magnesium depletion?
3. Does the patient need magnesium repletion? If he does, what is the best route for the repletion and what is the appropriate dosage?

If hypomagnesemia is attributed to loop diuretic or tubular-toxic medication, then the possibility of switching to another medication should be considered. Patients with renal magnesium wasting may benefit from the addition of potassium-sparing diuretics, such as amiloride or triamterene, which decrease magnesium renal losses in the distal tubule.

The second question is not always easy to answer. Most hypomagnesemic pediatric patients do not present

Table 5.4 Urine magnesium to creatinine ratio (mg mg^{-1}) limits (5th and 95th percentile) by age groups [28]

Age (years)	0.1–1	1–2	2–3	3–5	5–7	7–10	10–14	14–17
5th percentile	0.1	0.09	0.07	0.07	0.06	0.05	0.05	0.05
95th percentile	0.48	0.37	0.34	0.29	0.21	0.18	0.15	0.13

Magnesium concentration measured using colorimetric reaction with xylidil blue (from [28], with permission)

Table 5.5 Dietary reference intake of magnesium by age [49]

0–6 months	50 mg
6–12 months	70 mg
1–10 years	150–250 mg
11–18 years	300–400 mg
>18 years	300–400 mg
Pregnant/lactating	+150 mg

with neurological, muscular, or cardiac symptoms. However, other electrolyte abnormalities frequently coexist in these patients. It can be difficult to differentiate if these electrolyte abnormalities result from magnesium deficit or independent of magnesium renal wasting. For example, hypokalemia is often associated with hypomagnesemia and can result from the tubular wasting. On other hand, hypomagnesemia by itself causes hypokalemia due to impaired Na^+–K^+–ATPase function and loss in the urine. Thus, in some cases differentiation may be practically impossible.

Obviously, symptomatic magnesium depletion needs repletion. The importance of treating asymptomatic hypomagnesemia remains controversial. Most authors recommend to replete any hypomagnesemic patient with significant underlying cardiac disease, convulsive disorder, or concurrent hypokalemia or hypocalcemia. Also severe asymptomatic magnesium depletion (<1.2–1.4 mg dL^{-1}) should be corrected [1, 34, 44]. In asymptomatic patients with mild hypomagnesemia, we suggest to assess, if possible, magnesium balance, and in case of negative balance provide sufficient magnesium supplementation.

The route of magnesium repletion depends on the urgency of the clinical situation. Obviously, the seizing patient should be given magnesium intravenously (2–5 mg kg^{-1} of elemental magnesium) over 8–24 h. Small bolus of 1–2 mg kg^{-1} can be given over 5 min in the beginning (Table 5.6). Because extracellular

magnesium does not readily equilibrate with intracellular stores, fast infusion rapidly increases the plasma concentration but does not correct the total body magnesium. Furthermore, since plasma magnesium concentration is the major regulator of magnesium renal handling, acute rise in magnesium concentration results in hypermagnesuria with loss of up to 50% of infused magnesium [1]. Therefore, slow continuous intravenous infusion over 24 h is effective and safe. The dose may be repeated or adjusted to maintain serum Mg^{2+} concentration above 1–1.2 mg dL^{-1}. As mentioned, magnesium uptake by cells is very slow and days may be needed to correct intracellular magnesium deficit. Thus, once started magnesium repletion should be continued for 3–7 days despite normal blood magnesium concentration [1, 34]. The main adverse effects of fast magnesium repletion are due to development of hypermagnesemia. These side effects include facial flushing, hypotension, loss of deep tendon reflexes, and atrioventricular block. Monitoring of deep tendon reflexes can be used in nonparalyzed ICU patients. In addition, intravenous administration of magnesium sulfate results in decrease in plasma Ca^{2+} concentration due to binding of Ca^{2+} and sulfate ions. Therefore, in case of concurrent hypocalcemia calcium replacement should precede the magnesium repletion. Another disadvantage of magnesium sulfate salt is the fact that sulfate cannot be reabsorbed in the distal tubule; the resulting negative luminal potential increases potassium renal loss [34].

Oral magnesium replacement is usually used either in mild cases or for continued replacement after initial intravenous repletion (Table 5.6). The advantage of oral replacement is a slow elevation in magnesium serum concentration preventing hypermagnesemia and its side effects. Multiple oral Mg^{2+} salts are available. Bioavailability of oral magnesium preparations is assumed to approximately 33% in patients with normal intestinal function. Side effects include diarrhea in high doses and metabolic abnormalities. Mg^{2+} hydroxide and

Table 5.6 Magnesium preparations and dosages

Preparation	Amount of elemental magnesium	Route and forms	Dosage (mg elemental magnesium per kg)
Sol magnesium sulfate 50%	50 mg/1 mL	IV	2–5 mg kg^{-1} (0.05–0.1 mL kg^{-1}) over 8–24 h, repeat if needed
Magnesium sulfate granules	10 mg/100 mg (50 mg/5 g)	PO granules	10–20 mg kg^{-1} dose^{-1} 3–4 times daily
Magnesium oxide	60 mg/100 mg	PO tablets, capsules	10–20 mg kg^{-1} dose^{-1} 3–4 times daily
Magnesium gluconate	5.4 mg/100 mg	PO tablets	10–20 mg kg^{-1} dose^{-1} 3–4 times daily

Mg^{2+} oxide can exaggerate metabolic alkalosis, whereas Mg^{2+} sulfate and gluconate may potentially worsen K^+ wasting. Patients on magnesium replacement therapy should be monitored for magnesium, potassium, calcium, and bicarbonate levels [34].

5.5 Hypermagnesemia

In normal individuals most of the filtered magnesium load is reabsorbed in the TAL; the process is regulated mainly by magnesium serum concentration. Increased magnesium load results in decreased Mg^{2+} reabsorption and excretion of the excess Mg^{2+} in the urine. This mechanism is so efficient that hypermagnesemia usually is not seen in the presence of normal kidney function. In clinical practice, hypermagnesemia usually occurs in two settings: compromised renal function or excessive magnesium intake.

5.5.1 Causes of Hypermagnesemia

5.5.1.1 Renal Failure

In chronic renal failure, the remaining nephrons adapt to the decreased filtered magnesium load by increasing their fractional excretion of magnesium. This adaptive mechanism preserves normal magnesium serum concentration even in the presence of advanced renal failure. In patients with creatinine clearance below 15 mL min^{-1} mild hypermagnesemia can be observed. Severe hypermagnesemia can be seen in patients who receive exogenous magnesium as antacids or laxatives [8, 34].

5.5.1.2 Excessive Magnesium Intake

Hypermagnesemia can be seen in patients with normal kidney function when magnesium intake exceeds the renal excretory capacity. It is rarely observed in children, but is a well-appreciated complication of large magnesium infusions in pregnant women with preeclampsia. Severe hypermagnesemia has been described in children with Epsom salt (containing Mg^{2+} sulfate) poisoning, in laxative abusers, or in patients receiving magnesium as a cathartic [8, 20]. Hypermagnesemia from oral magnesium salts is more common in patients with bowel inflammatory disease, obstruction, or perforation [34]. Extreme hypermagnesemia with hypercalcemia has been described in pediatric and adult patients with Dead Sea water poisoning, since the ingested water contains very high concentrations of both calcium and magnesium [35].

5.5.1.3 Miscellaneous

Mild to moderate hypermagnesemia can be occasionally observed in patients with familial hypocalciuric hypercalcemia, tumor lysis syndrome, milk-alkali syndrome, hypothyroidism, Addison disease, lithium therapy, and theophylline intoxication [34]. Neonates born prematurely with asphyxia or hypotonia are often hypermagnesemic. Spontaneous return to normal values occurs within 72 h. Whether hypermagnesemia plays a pathophysiological role in asphyxic child remains unknown. Hypermagnesemia can be dangerous in neonates born from magnesium-treated eclamptic mothers [9]. Low glomerular filtration rate observed in neonates may slow the normalization of serum magnesium level.

5.5.2 Symptoms of Hypermagnesemia

Symptoms of hypermagnesemia usually correlate well with plasma magnesium concentration. Mild hypermagnesemia is usually asymptomatic, whereas severe hypermagnesemia can potentially be a fatal condition. Initial manifestations are seen when magnesium concentration exceeds 4–5 mg dL^{-1} and include nausea, vomiting, flushing, headache, drowsiness, and diminished deep tendon reflexes. Plasma magnesium concentrations between 7 and 12 mg dL^{-1} are often associated with somnolence, hypocalcemia, absent deep tendon reflexes, hypotension, bradycardia, ileus, urinary retention, and ECG changes. Further elevation of magnesium concentration above 12 mg dL^{-1} may result in flaccid muscular paralysis, respiratory depression, AV heart block, and cardiac arrest (Table 5.7).

5.5.2.1 Cardiovascular System

Hypotension usually appears when magnesium concentration exceeds 5–6 mg dL^{-1} and is thought to be the result of peripheral vasodilatation. Mg^{2+} is an effective calcium-channel blocker both intracellular and extracellular; it also modulates the function of K^+ channels in cardiac muscle and aortic smooth muscle cells [2]. ECG changes are common with magnesium concentrations above 8 mg dL^{-1} but nonspecific. Sinus or junctional bradycardia, AV and His bundle conduction block, prolonged QRS duration, and Q-T intervals can be observed [34]. Complete heart block and cardiac arrest may occur at plasma concentrations above 18 mg dL^{-1}.

Table 5.7 Clinical manifestations and treatment of hypermagnesemia

Plasma magnesium concentration (mg dL^{-1})	Clinical signs	Treatment
2.5–4	Usually asymptomatic	Cessation of magnesium supplements
4–6	Nausea, vomiting, flushing, headache, drowsiness, and diminished deep tendon reflexes	As above Forced diuresis with normal saline and loop diuretics
6–12	Somnolence, hypocalcemia, absent deep tendon reflexes, hypotension, bradycardia, ileus, urinary retention, and ECG changes (prolongation of the P-R interval, increased duration of the QRS complex and Q-T interval, increased height of the T waves)	As above IV calcium gluconate 10% 0.2–0.3 mL kg^{-1} by slow infusion Fluid resuscitation Dialysis in the presence of renal failure or ineffectiveness of forced diuresis to decrease magnesium levels
>12	Flaccid muscular paralysis, respiratory depression, coma, AV heart block, and cardiac arrest (>18 mg dL^{-1})	As above Respiratory support

5.5.2.2 Neuromuscular System

Increased concentrations of extracellular Mg^{2+} produce curare-like effect by inhibition of acetylcholine release and decreased impulse transmission across the neuromuscular junction [2]. Clinical manifestations progress from hyporeflexia to flaccid muscle paralysis, respiratory depression, smooth muscle paralysis with urinary retention, and ileus. Central nervous system depression manifests with somnolence, lethargy, and coma in severe hypermagnesemia [34].

5.5.2.3 Hypocalcemia

Hypermagnesemia can suppress the PTH secretion [10]. Resulting mild hypocalcemia is usually asymptomatic and thought not to be clinically important.

5.5.3 Treatment of Hypermagnesemia

Most cases of hypermagnesemia can be prevented by avoidance of magnesium-containing preparations in patients with advanced renal failure (Table 5.7). Mild hypermagnesemia in the presence of preserved renal function usually requires only discontinuation of magnesium supplementation. The next step of treatment is forced diuresis using normal saline infusion and loop diuretics, which results in increased magnesium wasting. In cases of severe symptoms, especially cardiac toxicity, intravenous calcium is given as a magnesium antagonist. In patients with renal failure, dialysis is the only way to clear the magnesium excess. Both hemodialysis and peritoneal dialysis have been successfully used for this application. Hemodialysis provides higher KT/V and thus is more effective in magnesium clearance. The typical dialysate for hemodialysis contains 0.6–1.2 mg dL^{-1} of magnesium; however, Mg^{2+}-free dialysate can also be used [20, 34].

> **Take-Home Pearls**
>
> › About 70% of serum magnesium (not protein bound) is freely filtered at the glomerulus to the Bowman space. The majority of filtered magnesium is reabsorbed in the loop of Henle via paracellular passive transport, which is facilitated by a tight junction protein paracellin-1 and is driven by the transepithelial voltage. A small amount of filtered magnesium is reabsorbed in the distal tubule via transcellular active transport.
>
> › Hypokalemia, hypocalcemia, cardiac and neurological abnormalities are clinical signs of hypomagnesemia.
>
> › Secretions from the lower gastrointestinal tract have much higher magnesium concentrations (up to 16 mg dL^{-1}) than from the upper gastrointestinal tract, thus chronic diarrhea can result in hypomagnesemia.
>
> › Renal loss of magnesium can occur during polyuric phase of ATN, postobstructive and osmotic diuresis, recovery from postischemic injury of transplanted kidney, and treatment with loop diuretics, amphotericin, calcineurin inhibitors, and cisplatin.
>
> › Rare inherited tubular defects of magnesium handling include Gitelman syndrome, isolated familial hypomagnesemia, familial hypomagnesemia with hypercalciuria and nephrocalcinosis as well as autosomal dominant hypocalcemia.
>
> › 7–10 day course of magnesium supplementation is necessary to correct a symptomatic hypomagnesemia.

References

1. Agus ZS (1999) Hypomagnesemia. J Am Soc Nephrol 10(7):1616–22
2. Agus ZS, Morad M (1991) Modulation of cardiac ion channels by magnesium. Annu Rev Physiol 53:299–307
3. Arany I, Safirstein RL (2003) Cisplatin nephrotoxicity. Semin Nephrol 23(5):460–4.
4. Bamford MF, Jones LF (1978) Deafness and biochemical imbalance after burns treatment with topical antibiotics in young children. Report of 6 cases. Arch Dis Child 53(4):326–9
5. Barri YM, Knochel JP (1996) Hypercalcemia and electrolyte disturbances in malignancy. Hematol Oncol Clin North Am 10(4):775–90
6. Barton CH, Pahl M, Vaziri ND, Cesario T (1984) Renal magnesium wasting associated with amphotericin B therapy. Am J Med 77(3):471–4
7. Birmingham CL, Puddicombe D, Hlynsky J (2004) Hypomagnesemia during refeeding in anorexia nervosa. Eat Weight Disord 9(3):236–7
8. Birrer RB, Shallash AJ, Totten V (2002) Hypermagnesemia-induced fatality following epsom salt gargles(1). J Emerg Med 22(2):185–8
9. Caddell JL (1991–1992) Magnesium in perinatal care and infant health. Magnes Trace Elem 10(2–4):229–50
10. Cholst IN, Steinberg SF, Tropper PJ, et al. (1984) The influence of hypermagnesemia on serum calcium and parathyroid hormone levels in human subjects. N Engl J Med 310(19):1221–5
11. Chou CL, Chen YH, Chau T, et al. (2005) Acquired Bartter-like syndrome associated with gentamicin administration. Am J Med Sci 329(3):144–9
12. Citterio F (2004) Evolution of the therapeutic drug monitoring of cyclosporine. Transplant Proc 36(2 Suppl):420S–425S
13. Dai LJ, Ritchie G, Kerstan D, et al. (2001) Magnesium transport in the renal distal convoluted tubule. Physiol Rev 81(1):51–84
14. Fawcett WJ, Haxby EJ, Male DA (1999) Magnesium: physiology and pharmacology. Br J Anaesth 83(2):302–20
15. Filler G, Grygas R, Mai I, et al. (1997) Pharmacokinetics of tacrolimus (FK 506) in children and adolescents with renal transplants. Nephrol Dial Transplant 12(8):1668–71
16. Fine KD, Santa Ana CA, Porter JL, Fordtran JS (1991) Intestinal absorption of magnesium from food and supplements. J Clin Invest 88(2):396–402
17. Frisch LS, Mimouni F (1993) Hypomagnesemia following correction of metabolic acidosis: a case of hungry bones. J Am Coll Nutr 12(6):710–13
18. Goldman RD, Koren G (2004) Amphotericin B nephrotoxicity in children. J Pediatr Hematol Oncol 26(7):421–6
19. Graham LA, Caesar JJ, Burgen AS (1960) Gastrointestinal absorption and excretion of Mg^{2+} in man. Metabolism 9:646–59
20. Harker HE, Majcher TA (2000) Hypermagnesemia in a pediatric patient. Anesth Analg 91(5):1160–2
21. Hebert SC (1996) Extracellular calcium-sensing receptor: implications for calcium and magnesium handling in the kidney. Kidney Int 50(6):2129–39
22. Holzmacher R, Kendziorski C, Michael Hofman R, et al. (2005) Low serum magnesium is associated with decreased graft survival in patients with chronic cyclosporin nephrotoxicity. Nephrol Dial Transplant 20(7):1456–62
23. Konrad M, Schlingmann KP, Gudermann T (2004) Insights into the molecular nature of magnesium homeostasis. Am J Physiol Renal Physiol 286(4):F599–F605
24. Landau D, Kher KK (1997) Gentamicin-induced Bartter-like syndrome. Pediatr Nephrol 11(6):737–40
25. LaSala MA, Lifshitz F, Silverberg M, et al. (1985) Magnesium metabolism studies in children with chronic inflammatory disease of the bowel. J Pediatr Gastroenterol Nutr 4(1):75–81
26. Lelievre-Pegorier M, Merlet-Benichou C, Roinel N, et al. (1983) Developmental pattern of water and electrolyte transport in rat superficial nephrons. Am J Physiol 245(1): F15–F21
27. Marier JR (1986) Magnesium content of the food supply in the modern-day world. Magnesium 5(1):1–8
28. Matos V, van Melle G, Boulat O, et al. (1997) Urinary phosphate/creatinine, calcium/creatinine, and magnesium/creatinine ratios in a healthy pediatric population. J Pediatr 131(2):252–7
29. Meij IC, Koenderink JB, van Bokhoven H, et al. (2000) Dominant isolated renal magnesium loss is caused by misrouting of the Na$(^+)$,K$(^+)$-ATPase gamma-subunit. Nat Genet 26(3):265–6
30. Miranda SC, Ribeiro ML, Ferriolli E, et al. (2000) Hypomagnesemia in short bowel syndrome patients. Sao Paulo Med J 118(6):169–72
31. Navaneethan SD, Sankarasubbaiyan S, Gross MD, et al. (2006) Tacrolimus-associated hypomagnesemia in renal transplant recipients. Transplant Proc 38(5):1320–2
32. Panichpisal K, Angulo-Pernett F, Selhi S, et al. (2006) Gitelman-like syndrome after cisplatin therapy: a case report and literature review. BMC Nephrol 7:10–13
33. Peters M, Jeck N, Reinalter S, et al. (2002) Clinical presentation of genetically defined patients with hypokalemic salt-losing tubulopathies. Am J Med 112(3): 183–90
34. Polak MR, Yu ASL (2004) Clinical disturbances of calcium, magnesium and phosphate metabolism. In: Brenner BM (ed) Brenner & Rector's The Kidney, 7th edn. Saunders, Philadelphia
35. Porath A, Mosseri M, Harman I, et al. (1989) Dead Sea water poisoning. Ann Emerg Med 18(2):187–91
36. Quamme GA (1997) Renal magnesium handling: new insights in understanding old problems. Kidney Int 52(5):1180–95
37. Rude RK (2000) Minerals-magnesium. In: Stipanuk MH (ed) Biochemical and Physiological Basis of Human Nutrition. Saunders, Philadelphia
38. Schlingmann KP, Weber S, Peters M, et al. (2002) Hypomagnesemia with secondary hypocalcemia is caused by mutations in TRPM6, a new member of the TRPM gene family. Nat Genet 31(2):166–70
39. Schlingmann KP, Konrad M, Seyberth HW (2004) Genetics of hereditary disorders of magnesium homeostasis. Pediatr Nephrol 19(1):13–25
40. Shetty AK, Rogers NL, Mannick EE, et al. (2000) Syndrome of hypokalemic metabolic alkalosis and hypomagnesemia associated with gentamicin therapy: case reports. Clin Pediatr 39(9):529–33
41. Shils ME (1969) Experimental human magnesium depletion. Medicine 48(1):61–85
42. Simon DB, Lu Y, Choate KA, et al. (1999) Paracellin-1, a renal tight junction protein required for paracellular Mg^{2+} resorption. Science 285(5424):103–6

43. Stohr W, Paulides M, Bielack S, et al. (2007) Nephrotoxicity of cisplatin and carboplatin in sarcoma patients: a report from the late effects surveillance system. Pediatr Blood Cancer 48(2):140–7

44. Tong GM, Rude RK (2005) Magnesium deficiency in critical illness. J Intensive Care Med 20(1):3–17

45. Walder RY, Landau D, Meyer P, et al. (2002) Mutation of TRPM6 causes familial hypomagnesemia with secondary hypocalcemia. Nat Genet 31(2):171–4

46. Whang R, Oei TO, Aikawa JK, et al. (1984) Predictors of clinical hypomagnesemia: Hypokalemia, hypophosphatemia, hyponatremia, and hypocalcemia. Arch Intern Med 144(9):1794–6

47. Yu ASL (2004) Renal Transport of calcium, magnesium, and phosphate. In: Brenner BM (ed) Brenner & Rector's The Kidney, 7th edn. Saunders, Philadelphia

48. Rose BD, Post TW (2001) Clinical physiology of acid–base and electrolyte disorders. McGraw-Hill Medical, New York Chapter 15. Clinical use of diuretics. p 449–450

49. Dietary reference intakes for calcium, phosphorus, magnesium, vitamin D and fluoride. (1997) Standing Committee on the Scientific Evaluation of Dietary Reference Intakes, Food and Nutrition Board, Institute of Medicine. National Academy Press, Washington, DC

6

Acute Kidney Injury: General Aspects

M. Zappitelli and S.L. Goldstein

Contents

Core Messages

> Acute kidney injury (AKI) complicates the course of many children admitted to the ICU. The etiology is usually multifactorial, and ischemic, hypoxic, and nephrotoxic insults are all common.

> The evaluation of AKI should be sequential. A careful history identifies risk factors for kidney injury and potential causes of acute dysfunction. Physical findings, laboratory assessment, and diagnostic imaging are aimed at both elucidating the cause of AKI and determining the extent of its severity.

> Treatment of AKI ranges from supportive care to dialysis therapies. The decision to begin dialysis in the ICU should be made collaboratively between the intensivist and the nephrologist. Choice of dialysis modality depends on clinical factors and local resources.

> Mortality rates for children requiring dialysis in the ICU for AKI are high, especially in children who develop multiorgan system dysfunction. Children who survive AKI in the ICU are at risk for long-term renal dysfunction.

> The creation of specific pediatric criteria to define AKI may facilitate further clinical research, including the identification of useful biomarkers for AKI and the response of kidney injury to specific directed therapies.

Case Vignette

A 10-year-old boy with Williams syndrome presents for assessment of dehydration. He is usually in good health and has been followed since infancy for supravalvular aortic stenosis and is status post a patch repair of his ascending aorta. He does have some residual aortic coarctation and has also been found to have mild narrowing of his left renal artery. He is maintained on enalapril and atenolol with blood pressure readings of 120/80 and had a normal CBC and chemistry panel 4 months ago. Over the last 2 months, he has developed increasing dysphagia and has been treated for gastroesophageal reflux and erosive esophagitis with proton pump inhibitors. He has had significant decrease in oral intake because of

S.G. Kiessling et al. (eds) *Pediatric Nephrology in the ICU.*
© Springer-Verlag Berlin Heidelberg 2009

his dysphagia, and his mother estimates that he has gone down from taking in 1.5 L daily to only ½ L of bottled water. He has had vomiting 3–4 times daily and visible blood in his stools over the last week. His blood pressures at home have dropped to the 90–100 range systolic but he has continued to take his antihypertensive therapy each day. His mother has noticed that he is not urinating regularly. On examination, he is pale, has a resting pulse of 70, a blood pressure of 90/50 while sitting, and a standing blood pressure cannot be done because he feels too weak. The remainder of his examination is nonfocal and unchanged from his last clinic visit. Diagnostic evaluation includes a CBC noteworthy for hemoglobin of 5 g dL^{-1} with a low reticulocyte count, electrolytes with serum bicarbonate of 18 meq L^{-1}, normal calcium levels, a mildly elevated serum phosphorus level to 6 mg dL^{-1}, a BUN of 120 mg dL^{-1}, and a serum creatinine (SCR) of 6 mg dL^{-1}. He receives an initial bolus infusion of normal saline and a transfusion of packed red blood cells. His antihypertensive therapy is held. Repeat chemistries 12 h later show that the BUN has fallen to 90 mg dL^{-1} and the creatinine is now 5.2 mg dL^{-1}, and he has begun to produce urine more regularly. The patient continues to vomit clear fluid and then develops hematemesis accompanied by blood pressure instability. He is transferred to the pediatric ICU where he requires significant volume resuscitation and the initiation of a dopamine drip to maintain a systolic pressure greater than 90 mmHg. He develops oliguria and his BUN and creatinine steadily increase with each laboratory assessment. Plans are made to initiate continuous veno-venous hemodialysis.

6.1 Introduction

Acute renal failure denotes the abrupt onset of renal dysfunction leading to the inability to regulate acid and electrolyte balance and excrete wastes and fluid [4]. Increased understanding of the pathophysiology and clinical spectrum of acute renal failure has led to a change in nomenclature of this condition to acute kidney injury (AKI), acknowledging that acute renal dysfunction occurs due to injurious endogenous or exogenous disease processes.

Glomerular filtration rate (GFR) decreases in AKI and is characterized clinically by an increase in the measured SCR and often a concomitant decrease in urine output. The clinical spectrum of AKI ranges

from mild, where effects on outcome are still unclear, to severe, a life-threatening condition mostly affecting severely ill, hospitalized patients [31, 62]. While much has been learned about the cellular and molecular pathways of AKI [11, 22, 32, 46, 48, 49], study with respect to pediatric AKI epidemiology has only recently received focus.

Diagnosis and management of AKI constitutes one of the most important roles of the pediatric nephrologist in an intensive care unit. Proper management of pediatric AKI requires understanding the multiple pathophysiologic and clinical events that lead to renal injury, the life-threatening and nonlife-threatening effects of AKI, and when conservative or supportive care is indicated vs. more invasive maneuvers. This chapter will provide an overview of the epidemiology, pathophysiology, risk factors and causes, clinical presentation, and diagnosis of AKI in the pediatric intensive care units. Management of AKI complications and acute dialysis for AKI will be covered in other chapters and only briefly reviewed here.

6.2 AKI Epidemiology

The epidemiologic importance of AKI as a public health problem is underscored by evidence showing that even a small reduction (0.3 mg dL^{-1} SCr increase) in the renal function of hospitalized adult and pediatric patients is a risk factor for morbidity and mortality [15, 45]. Although little data exist to describe the incidence of pediatric AKI, the prevalence of hospital and PICU-acquired AKI appears to be increasing [60], which may result from changes in diagnostic profiles over the last 10–20 years and increasing use of more invasive management to support critically ill children and higher illness severity of these patients. Studies have defined AKI using differing definitions, ranging from varying increases in SCr to decreases in urine output to dialysis requirement [9]. When requirement for some form of renal replacement therapy (RRT) as the strictest definition of AKI is used, its incidence in the PICU ranges from less than 1–2% [7, 39, 60]. When less strict AKI definitions are used, such as doubling of SCr, the incidence of AKI ranges from 1–21%, depending on population characteristics [3, 7, 24, 39, 60, 62]. Infants undergoing cardiopulmonary bypass (CPB) procedures have been studied more extensively than other groups of children, and the AKI incidence is fairly consistent in the range of 10–25% [14, 41, 54]. Patients receiving stem cell transplants are also at higher risk than general PICU patients, with an incidence of AKI, defined by SCr doubling, of approximately 20% [33].

In 2004, a consensus definition for AKI was proposed by the Acute Dialysis Quality Initiative: the RIFLE criteria (risk, injury, failure, loss, end-stage renal disease) [9]. The adult-derived RIFLE definition was modified, and then applied and validated in pediatric patients and renamed as the pediatric RIFLE (pRIFLE) criteria. pRIFLE stratifies AKI from mild (RIFLE R, *risk*) to severe (RIFLE F, *failure*) based on *changes* in SCR or estimated creatinine clearance (eCCl) and urine output (Table 6.1). The first study that defined AKI using the pRIFLE criteria found that AKI occurred in 82% of the most critically ill children admitted to a PICU [3]. Similar to adult studies [2, 30, 34, 37, 59], AKI defined by these criteria was an independent risk factor for both increased hospital length of stay and mortality. While the pRIFLE criteria are not currently applicable in the clinical setting for medical decision making, they provide a multidimensional research tool to assist with AKI descriptive and outcome studies. Further epidemiologic research utilizing this common definition will contribute to understanding the true incidence of mild to severe AKI in a wide range of geographic and diagnostic patient populations.

Table 6.1 Pediatric RIFLE criteria definition of acute kidney injury

	Pediatric RIFLE criteria[a]	
	Estimated CCl (eCCl)[b]	Urine output
Risk	eCCl decrease by 25%	<0.5 mL kg^{-1} h^{-1} for 8 h
Injury	eCCl decrease by 50%	<0.5 mL kg^{-1} h^{-1} for 16 h
Failure	eCCl decrease by 75% or eCCl <35 mL min^{-1} per 1.73 m^2	<0.3 mL kg^{-1} h^{-1} for 24 h or anuric for 12 h
Loss	Persistent failure >4 weeks	
End stage	End stage renal disease (persistent failure >3 months)	

[a] Patients are classified as having acute kidney injury if they attain either eCCl or urine output criteria
[b] Estimated creatinine clearance (mL min^{-1} per 1.73 m^2) is calculated using the Schwartz formula: k × height in centimeters/SCr [50]

6.3   Etiology, Classification, and Pathophysiology of AKI

The etiology of AKI has changed over the last 10–20 years from primary renal disease (e.g., hemolytic uremic syndrome, glomerulonephritis) to the renal complications of systemic illness or its treatment (postoperative cardiac surgery, oncologic diseases). Sepsis also remains an important etiologic factor of AKI [3, 7, 28, 31, 38, 43, 60, 62]. Table 6.2 lists AKI causes commonly seen in the PICU.

A recent pediatric retrospective epidemiologic study revealed that the most common causes of AKI in a tertiary health care center were renal ischemia, nephrotoxic medication use, and sepsis [31]. While each of these conditions cause AKI via different mechanisms, they lead to a final common pathway of acute tubular necrosis (ATN), characterized by renal tubular epithelial cell death. ATN is the most common cause of severe AKI in critically ill children. The remainder of this section will provide an overview of how AKI is classified and how this classification is linked to AKI pathophysiology.

6.3.1   Prerenal AKI

AKI is traditionally classified as being of *prerenal, renal* (intrinsic renal disease), or *postrenal* (obstructive) origin (Table 6.2). Prerenal AKI refers to the abrupt decrease in GFR following renal hypoperfusion, either from intravascular volume depletion or from reduced effective circulating volume. Intravascular volume depletion can occur from dehydration, in which total body water is reduced, or from fluid shifts outside the intravascular space, such as in the setting of severe hypoalbuminemia (nephrotic syndrome, severe liver disease) or capillary leak, as seen with systemic inflammatory response syndrome (SIRS). Low effective circulating volume occurs with poor cardiac output or systemic vasodilation. Prerenal AKI can also more rarely occur due to renal artery stenosis or compression (bilateral with two kidneys or unilateral with a single kidney). In either case, the common final pathway for all these processes is decreased effective perfusion of the kidney parenchyma.

In the setting of this decreased renal perfusion, several adaptive responses come into play, all aimed at maintaining GFR and restoring intravascular volume via neurohormonal mechanisms (Fig. 6.1). Decreased renal perfusion leads to increase in adrenergic activity and stimulation of the renin–angiotensin–aldosterone

Table 6.2 Causes of pediatric acute kidney injury in the intensive care unit

Prerenal (renal hypoperfusion)

Low intravascular volume

  Hemorrhage/bleeding: postoperative, trauma

  Severe dehydration: vomiting/diarrhea, nasogastric drainage, chest tube/abdominal drain losses, urinary losses (diabetes insipidus, Bartter's syndrome, adrenal disorders), diuresis (diuretic-induced or osmotic)

  Third-space losses: sepsis and capillary leak, burns, trauma, hypoalbuminemia (nephrotic syndrome/liver disease)

Decreased effective circulating volume

  Cardiac dysfunction: congestive heart failure, cardiac tamponade/pericarditis, sepsis-associated cardiac dysfunction

  Renal artery obstruction: stenosis, mass

  Sepsis-associated diffuse vasodilation

Renal (intrinsic)

Glomerular

  Glomerulonephritis: rapidly progressive (pauci-immune, immune-mediated, goodpasture's syndrome), immune-mediated diseases (lupus, post-infectious, IgA nephropathy, membranoproliferative, vasculitis).

Vascular

  Hemolytic uremic syndrome: Eschericia coli ingestion, drug – induced (calcineurin inhibitors), streptococcus pneumoniae, genetic.

  Vascular injury: cortical necrosis, renal vein/artery thrombosis, disseminated intravascular coaggulation, thrombotic disease, malignant hypertension.

Interstitial

  Acute interstitial nephritis: drug-induced, post-infectious, immune-mediated.

  Infection/pyelonephritis.

Tubular

  Acute tubular necrosis: hypoxic/ischemic injury, drug-induced, exogenous toxins (metals, venom, illicit drugs (mushrooms), ethylene glycol, methanol), endogenous toxins (rhabdomyolysis, hemolysis, tumor lysis syndrome).

  Tumor lysis syndrome

Postrenal (obstruction of urinary tract)

  Urethral obstruction: posterior urethral valves in neonates; urinary catheter obstruction

  Obstruction of solitary kidney urinary tract: congenital (ureteral–pelvic junction, ureteral stenosis, uretero–vesical junction, mass), stones, mass

  Bilateral ureteral obstruction: mass, stones

(RAA) axis and antidiuretic hormone (ADH) release [10, 22]. The increase in adrenergic activity leads to systemic vasoconstriction, thereby increasing blood pressure. Stimulation of the RAA system leads to reabsorption of salt and water through angiotensin II (proximal tubule) and aldosterone (distal tubule). Increase in systemic ADH leads to retention of water by the collecting tubule. While each of these mechanisms favors the maintenance of intravascular volume and systemic blood pressure, other mechanisms also act simultaneously to maintain GFR. Elevated angiotensin II causes preferential vasoconstriction of the glomerular efferent arteriole (distal to the glomerulus) while vasodilators such as prostaglandins and nitric oxide cause afferent arteriolar vasodilation, leading to increase in glomerular pressure and thus GFR [5, 35].

If renal hypoperfusion is ameliorated promptly, such as when intravascular fluid volume is rapidly optimized, GFR may be restored quickly. If renal hypoperfusion is severe or prolonged, however, acute tubular necrosis (ATN) can occur (Fig. 6.1) [35, 53]. Once ATN ensues, restoration of intravascular volume will not restore GFR, as the pathophysiologic process of ischemic renal injury has been triggered. Clinically, it

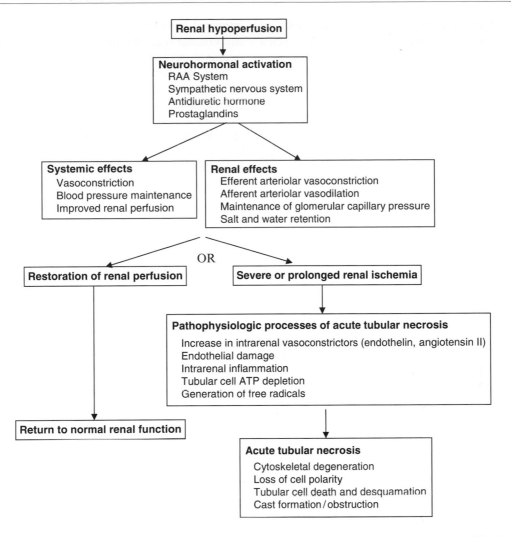

Fig. 6.1 Relationship between prerenal acute kidney injury (AKI) and ischemic acute tubular necrosis. RAA renin–anigiotensin–aldosterone, ATP adenosine triphosphate

is not difficult to recognize the presence of dehydration that may be correctable with fluid provision. It is equally important, however, to recognize clinical scenarios where effective circulating volume is reduced or when fluid shifts are the cause of intravascular depletion, sometimes in the setting of apparent total body volume overload. In the critical care setting, when faced with patients who often manifest reduced cardiac output, capillary leak (SIRS, inflammatory/infectious diseases), severe hypoalbuminemia, and third-space losses, this contradistinction between effective volume and total body volume is common. Because of the underlying disease process, compensatory salt and water retention may not actually improve effective perfusion but lead to progressive fluid overload

and resultant complications. Management should be aimed toward correcting the underlying cause of renal hypoperfusion (provision of albumin, improvement of cardiac function, and treatment of sepsis), while minimizing the effect of excessive fluid overload.

6.3.2 Intrinsic AKI

Intrinsic renal causes of AKI refer to any acute reduction in GFR secondary to direct damage to renal tissue, be it from vascular, tubular, interstitial, or glomerular causes (Table 6.2). In the critical care setting, however, ATN is by far the most common cause of intrinsic AKI, and has been the focus of ongoing research. ATN occurs via many mechanisms, including ischemic, toxic, vascular insults and inflammation [53]. Critically ill patients are at high risk for all these processes.

6.3.2.1 Hypoxic/Ischemic Acute Tubular Necrosis

Hypoxic/ischemic AKI is the most common cause of ATN. The pathophysiology of ischemic ATN involves a series of intrarenal vascular and tubular cell-mediated events. ATN is associated with profound intrarenal vasoconstriction particularly in the low oxygen tension regions of the outer medulla, leading to tubular cell necrosis of the S3 segment of the proximal tubule and the medullary thick ascending limb [22]. Endothelial injury leads to release and activation of both vasodilators such as nitric oxide (NO) and vasoconstrictors such as endothelin, although vasoconstrictive factors are favored [5, 35]. Endothelial and tubular injury also cause intrarenal inflammation, independent of systemic inflammation, causing further injury [5, 22, 27, 35]. Leukocyte recruitment occurs and intrarenal inflammatory cytokines are released, including interleukin-6 and 8 and tumor necrosis factor-alpha. Tubular cell abnormalities result from ischemic injury, but also contribute to ongoing injury [22]. Prolonged ischemia leads to reduction in tubular intracellular ATP, protease activation, and tubular cytoskeletal degradation. With reperfusion, reactive oxygen molecules are released that then moderate further injury.

Damage to the renal tubular epithelial cells ultimately leads to loss of the brush border and cell polarity, cell death, and sloughing of cellular debris into the tubular lumen, contributing to tubular obstruction and further nephron injury [22]. The process of healing is characterized by tubular cell dedifferentiation and proliferation into normal epithelial layers. While much has been learned about the molecular mechanisms of ischemic ATN, ongoing research is likely to elucidate therapeutic strategies.

6.3.2.2 Other Mechanisms of Acute Tubular Necrosis

Other common causes of ATN in the PICU are sepsis and nephrotoxin injury (Table 6.2). Sepsis causes cytokine-mediated systemic vasodilation and capillary leak, leading to renal hypoperfusion and similar processes associated with prerenal AKI and ischemic ATN [49]. However, sepsis also causes direct renal injury via multiple complex mechanisms, including intrarenal vasoconstriction, inflammation, glomerular and vascular microthrombi, and endotoxin-stimulated release of oxygen-free radicals [49].

While the pathophysiology of nephrotoxin-induced ATN is beyond the scope of this chapter, there are several pathways leading to renal cell injury, including direct tubular damage with resultant free-radical release, mitochondrial damage, as well as changes in glomerular and intrarenal hemodynamics – all leading to cell death [16]. Many antibiotics, particularly aminoglycosides, cause direct tubular injury, often characterized by tubular functional defects with resultant losses of fluids and electrolytes rather than an oliguric state. Aminoglycoside nephrotoxicity is frequently related to high serum levels and lengthy duration of treatment, and may only become apparent after cessation of therapy [57]. The antifungal agent amphotericin B also causes direct distal tubular injury as well as afferent arteriolar vasoconstriction. Amphotericin nephrotoxicity is characterized by acute reduction in GFR, distal renal tubular acidosis, salt wasting, polyuria, and significant losses of potassium and magnesium [21, 57]. Several chemotherapeutic agents also lead to ATN. Table 6.3 displays many drugs that lead to renal injury.

Other forms of intrinsic renal diseases cause AKI in the critical care unit. Acute glomerulonephritis can occur as a result of several immune-mediated or primary glomerular diseases. Vascular insults include macrovascular events, such as renal vein thrombosis, and microvascular events, such as hemolytic–uremic syndrome. These diseases are usually clinically apparent. Acute interstitial nephritis, leading to widespread interstitial inflammation, tubular damage, and reduced GFR, can occur due to infectious or autoimmune illnesses, but more commonly secondary to drug reaction, such as seen with nonsteroidal anti-inflammatory agents and several types of antibiotics (Table 6.3).

6.3.3 Postrenal Causes of AKI

Postrenal AKI refers to reduced GFR occurring as a result of obstruction of the urinary tract. In the pediatric critical care setting, such obstruction is a fairly rare cause of AKI and generally is related to tumors or bilateral ureteral obstruction from mass effect, stones, or blood clots. In children with indwelling Foley catheters, unappreciated catheter obstruction may also contribute to postrenal AKI. In neonates, congenital obstructive uropathies such as posterior urethral valves may contribute to AKI, especially when such anomalies have not been appreciated prenatally.

6.3.4   Risk Factors for AKI

From the earlier discussion of epidemiology, classification, and pathophysiology of AKI, it is clear that the most important risk factors for AKI in the PICU are clinical conditions predisposing to renal hypoperfusion or to direct renal injury.

Illness severity in itself is a risk factor for developing AKI. For example, with the critically ill patient who is intubated and receiving vasoactive medications, AKI incidence may exceed 80%, compared with levels approximating 5% in general PICU patients [3, 7].

Patients receiving stem cell transplants are at substantial risk of developing AKI. This risk is a result of several factors including the extensive use of nephrotoxic medications, veno-occlusive disease in association with hepatorenal syndrome, the high incidence of sepsis, and tumor lysis syndrome [33, 40, 61]. Because of the large amounts of fluid received during their treatment, these patients are also at particularly high risk of developing substantial fluid overload.

Patients undergoing cardiopulmonary bypass are at risk of postoperative AKI. The pathophysiology of AKI in this setting is mostly ischemic. With such patients, it is important to note preoperative renal function, intraoperative details such as ischemic time, periods of severe hypotension, bypass pump time, as well as any perioperative hypoperfusion event. Depending on the case series and AKI definition used, the incidence of AKI in the cardiopulmonary bypass population approximates 10–25% [41, 54]. In a more recent report, nearly 30% of infants undergoing cardiopulmonary bypass had at least a 50% rise in SCr postoperatively, equivalent to RIFLE R AKI [41]. Some centers perform peritoneal dialysis catheter insertion at the time of cardiac surgery given the risk of AKI; there is no evidence, however, suggesting benefit or harm to this practice vs. later catheter placement if indicated [25, 55].

6.4   Clinical Features of AKI

6.4.1   Clinical History

In the critical care unit, it is unlikely to identify a single cause of AKI. The goal of the history is to identify all potential causes and risk factors of AKI to direct appropriate management and avoid further renal injury. Renal hypoperfusion events will be extremely common, resulting from excessive blood

Table 6.3   Common nephrotoxic medications encountered in the pediatric intensive care unit [16]

Nephrotoxins primarily causing tubular dysfunction
Aminoglycosides
Beta-lactam antibiotics (cephalosporins, carbapenem)
Contrast media
Cisplatin
Ifosfamide
Nonsteroidal anti-inflammatory drugs
Acetaminophen
Amphotericin B
Acyclovir
Foscarnet
Cidofovir
Calcineurin inhibitors
Nephrotoxins directly causing decreased GFR
Amphotericin B
Angiotensin-converting enzyme inhibitors
Nonsteroidal anti-inflammatory drugs
Foscarnet
Calcineurin inhibitors
Vasoconstrictor pressor medications
Nephrotoxins causing acute interstitial nephritis
Beta-lactam antibiotics (methicillin, penicillin, cephalosporins)
Tetracyclines

loss, sepsis with SIRS and capillary leak, cardiac dysfunction, vomiting, inadequate fluid replacement, and burns. A detailed fluid balance history is necessary. A negative balance may suggest effective volume depletion and renal hypoperfusion, whereas a positive balance may suggest a defect with water excretion. If available, serial weights are invaluable for the assessment of fluid balance. Actual urine output alone is not useful without knowing contemporaneous fluid intake. Urine output may seem adequate; however, if this output coupled with other sensible and insensible losses is less than the fluid input, and leads to progressive increases in positive fluid balance, then it is likely that there is a defect in water excretion, either due to significant AKI or increased ADH.

A detailed medication history assesses for drug-induced nephrotoxicity (e.g., aminoglycosides, amphotericin-B, chemotherapeutic agents, angiotensin converting enzyme inhibitors, or calcineurin inhibitors). Serum levels of pertinent medications must be reviewed for supratherapeutic levels that may have contributed to AKI.

An understanding of baseline renal function is important, moreover, to determine the extent of renal injury and put into context any decline in GFR. Reviewing SCR values that may have been obtained prior to any AKI and comparing with more recent values will clarify the degree of acute dysfunction. Using SCR values and height measurements in the Schwartz formula will allow more specific estimation of GFR [50].

6.4.2 Physical Examination

The physical examination serves two purposes. First, it may provide the clues as to the cause of AKI. Patients with nephritis may reveal signs of vasculitis with rashes or arthritis. The patient with severe liver disease and hepatorenal syndrome may have remarkable ascites, abdominal vascular anomalies, or even jaundice. Labile blood pressure and poor peripheral perfusion will strongly suggest hypoxic–ischemic ATN as an AKI etiology.

Second, the physical examination allows some determination of the extent that the effects of either the primary renal disease or AKI are having on the patient, particularly with relation to fluid overload. A patient with glomerulonephritis may have severe volume overload with hypertension, requiring immediate management with diuretics or antihypertensive medication. Alternatively, the patient with sepsis and severe capillary leak syndrome may have severe total body volume overload and edema, but decreased effective volume and renal perfusion, better addressed by judicious ultrafiltration. Correlating changes in oxygen requirement and ventilatory support with changes in fluid balance may help determine the extent to which fluid overload is impeding respiratory status.

6.4.3 Laboratory Investigation

Focused laboratory investigation serves to elucidate the cause of AKI and helps determine the extent of its severity. A urinalysis must be performed (Table 6.4). Urine specific gravity may be very high in patients who are severely volume-depleted. However, if ATN is established, specific gravity may be low or normal due to the presence of tubular dysfunction and limitations in urinary concentration. Glycosuria may suggest tubular dysfunction or could point toward an osmotic diuresis with resultant hypovolemia. The presence of leukocytes and positive nitrites on urine dipstick suggests urinary tract infection. If blood on urine dipstick is strongly positive with no or only few red blood cells seen on microscopic examination, myoglobin (as seen with rhabdomyolysis) or free hemoglobin (severe hemolysis) in the urine must be suspected. Proteinuria may be a nonspecific marker of renal injury or can point toward significant intrinsic glomerular injury with nephrosis. Patients with ATN may have granular or muddy brown casts, and their presence may be helpful in recognizing renal injury in patients with hypovolemia as a primary cause of AKI who may not yet manifest profound alterations in SCR.

Review of urine chemistries is also useful. The fractional excretion of filtered sodium and urea can be used to help differentiate between AKI of prerenal origin and ATN (Table 6.4). The fractional excretion of sodium is calculated by the following formula:

(Urine sodium × serum creatinine/serum sodium × urine creatinine) × 100.

The fractional excretion of urea is similarly calculated by concomitant measurements of urinary and serum urea nitrogen and creatinine. With prerenal AKI, sodium and urea reabsorption will be increased, leading to low fractional excretion (<1% for sodium and <35% for urea), whereas with ATN and tubular dysfunction, fractional excretion will be higher (>2% for sodium and >35% for urea). When diuretics are used, the fractional excretion of sodium may not be reliable. The fractional excretion of urea is, however, much less affected by diuretic use [35].

Blood tests that should be drawn include creatinine, urea nitrogen, electrolytes, sodium, potassium, bicarbonate or total carbon dioxide, phosphorous, calcium, glucose, albumin, hemoglobin, and platelets. Other tests may be required in specific clinical settings. Unlike urinalysis, many of these tests are relatively nonspecific in determining the cause of AKI, but are useful in determining the extent of AKI severity. On occasion, specific laboratory assessments may be useful in pinpointing AKI etiology. For example, with hypovolemia BUN may be elevated out of proportion to creatinine, and hematocrit and platelet counts may be higher than expected.

Hyponatremia is very common in AKI and is usually dilutional due to decreased free-water clearance or secondary to states of inappropriate ADH

Table 6.4   Laboratory investigation of acute kidney injury

Urine

    Urinalysis dipstick: Infection (nitrites or leukocyte esterase reaction), diabetes mellitus (glucose or ketones positive), concentrating defect with ATN or interstitial nephritis (specific gravity ≤ 1.01), nephritis (hematuria), nephrotic syndrome (proteinuria)

    Urinalysis microscopy: Nephritis (red blood cell or white blood cell casts), ATN (granular casts), acute interstitial nephritis (eosinophiluria)

    Fractional excretion of sodium: <1% with prerenal AKI, >2% with ATN or other tubular disease

    Fractional excretion of urea: <35% with prerenal AKI, >35% with ATN

Serum/blood

    SCr: To establish AKI, compared with previous baseline

    Blood urea nitrogen: Much higher relative to increase in SCr with prerenal AKI

    Electrolytes: Hyperkalemia, hypocalcemia, hyperphosphatemia, hyponatremia, hypernatremia if hypernatremic dehydration; with tubular dysfunction/fanconi syndrome, hypokalemia, hypophosphatemia

    Blood gas: Metabolic acidosis, compensated or not

    Hemoglobin and platelets: Both low with hemolytic uremic syndrome or other microangiopathy, both elevated with intravascular depletion

    Albumin: Low with nephrotic syndrome or liver disease/hepatorenal syndrome

    Liver enzymes: Elevated with severe hepatic disease

    Medication serum levels: Aminoglycosides, calcineurin inhibitors

    Coagulation profile: Abnormal with disseminated intravascular coaagulation, prerenal biopsy assessment

    Creatinine kinase: Elevated with rhabdomyolysis

    Autoimmune work-up: antinuclear antibody, antinuclear cytoplasmic antibody, complements 3 and 4 for evaluation of glomerulonephritis

Imaging

    Renal ultrasound: Increased echogenicity and loss of corticomedullary differentiation with ATN, glomerulomegaly with glomerulonephritis, urinary tract dilation with obstruction, determine anatomy/rule out dysplasia or congenital abnormalities

    Renal vessel doppler study: Increased resistive indices with ATN and thrombosis

    Computed tomography/magnetic resonance: Assessment of renal vasculature

    Radionucleotide scan: Lack of blood flow with cortical necrosis (neonates), rule out/determine level of obstruction with neonatal congenital obstructive uropathy

    Voiding cystourethrogram: Diagnose posterior urethral valves

Renal biopsy: Diagnose glomerulonephritis, acute interstitial nephritis

secretion. AKI-associated hyponatremia is not usually severe (<120 meq L^{-1}), unless associated with severe hyponatremic dehydration or inappropriately dilute fluid administration. Conversely, hypernatremia may also be seen in the setting of severe dehydration, hypertonic solution administration such as the septic patient receiving sodium bicarbonate boluses, or in diseases with severe urinary losses of water such as Bartter's syndrome.

Hyperkalemia occurs in AKI due to reduced renal excretion of potassium and can be life-threatening at levels greater than approximately 6.5 meq L^{-1}. Hypokalemia may be seen in patients who have polyuric AKI and is particularly common in patients with Amphotericin B and aminoglycoside nephrotoxicity. Metabolic acidosis, hypocalcemia, and hyperphosphatemia may also manifest with AKI, and these perturbations should be corrected as they exacerbate.

Other laboratory tests that should be considered will be directed by the clinical presentation of the patient, for example, antinuclear antibody and antinuclear cytoplasmic antibody for patients with rapidly progressive glomerulonephritis or creatine kinase concentrations in patients with suspected rhabdomyolysis.

6.4.4 Imaging

Urinary tract imaging helps diagnose conditions such as acquired or congenital obstruction of the urinary tract, renal dysplasia, or renal cystic disease. Doppler examination of renal vessels is a useful adjunct if vascular perfusion anomalies are suspected, although more specialized imaging such as computed tomography or magnetic resonance imaging may be needed to make a more definitive diagnosis. In general, however, ultrasound examination is routinely performed in any child with AKI to document normal genitourinary anatomy and normal-sized kidneys.

6.5 Treatment of AKI

Current management of AKI in the pediatric intensive care unit is largely supportive and aimed at preventing life-threatening fluid or electrolyte complications, avoiding or minimizing further renal injury, and providing appropriate nutrition to allow recovery from acute illness and renal dysfunction (Table 6.5). Severe AKI or milder AKI in association with severe fluid overload or solute imbalance may require renal replacement therapy (RRT). One of the most important roles of the pediatric nephrologist in the ICU is to help decide in collaboration with the pediatric intensivist when RRT is indicated and the optimal RRT modality. This decision will be based upon specific patient characteristics as well as local expertise with specific dialysis techniques.

Attention to fluid and electrolyte abnormalities is essential in managing the patient with AKI. Prevention of fluid overload is extremely important, but often difficult to achieve. Many patients suffer from hemodynamic instability requiring repeated fluid boluses. Patients with stem cell transplant often require large volumes of fluids and blood products with their chemotherapy regimen or just with supportive care. ICU patients often require multiple medication infusions, vasopresor drips, and parenteral nutrition in the face of declining GFR and urine output. The negative effects of fluid overload on patient survival in the ICU have become apparent in recent years. One suggested method to assess fluid overload status is to express the difference in fluid output from fluid intake since PICU admission as a percentage of the patient's estimated dry weight, using the following formula:

$$(\text{Fluid input liters} - \text{fluid output liters}) / \text{weight in kg} \times 100 \text{ [40]}$$

Children receiving stem cell transplants with greater than 10% fluid overload had a higher mortality than those with less than 10% fluid overload [40]. Increased fluid overload is also associated with increased mortality in children receiving continuous renal replacement therapy [26, 29]. Frequent calculation of fluid balance and reassessment of fluid provision should be part of the care of the AKI patient, with a low threshold to employ diuretics or ultrafiltration to assist with volume balance.

Avoidance of further renal injury is also a necessary focus of care but difficult to achieve in the critically ill patient with multiple organ dysfunction. Serum levels of nephrotoxic medication should be followed closely, and drugs that are renally excreted should be dosed to estimated GFR. When GFR is estimated to be less than 50% of normal, most drugs that are excreted by the kidney will require modifications in scheduled dosing. Use of nonnephrotoxic medication as alternatives to more traditional nephrotoxic medication should be considered. Hypotensive episodes, medications known to further reduce GFR (such as nonsteroidal anti-inflammatories and angiotensin-converting enzyme inhibitors), and radiocontrast agents should be avoided.

Specific therapeutic interventions for AKI have eluded researchers attempting to learn how to treat and prevent extensive renal injury. The use of furosemide and *renal* dose dopamine (ranging from 1 to 5 µg kg^{-1} min^{-1}) for critically ill oliguric patients is prevalent in the ICU, but does not improve renal outcome or patient survival when studied [36, 52, 58]. Moreover, dopamine infusion has also been associated with other potentially adverse physiologic effects in critically ill patients [5].

Other drugs, such as calcium channel-blockers and *N*-acetyl cysteine have been studied in adults with AKI but have shown no substantial beneficial effect on mortality or renal outcomes [13, 44]. The selective dopamine A-1 antagonist fenoldapam has been suggested to improve urine output in children undergoing cardiopulmonary bypass surgery [19]. Some studies suggest that the human natriuretic peptide nesiritide may have favorable renal hemodynamic effects and can increase urine output after cardiac

Table 6.5 Overview of the general concepts of managing acute kidney injury

Treatment of underlying disease: sepsis, cardiac dysfunction, correction of dehydration

Correction of electrolyte abnormalities

  Acidosis: Enteral or parenteral sodium bicarbonate (monitor serum calcium and sodium)

  Hyperkalemia: Sodium bicarbonate, calcium gluconate, insulin and glucose, beta-agonists for severe hyperkalemia; sodium polystyrene sulfonate for moderate hyperkalemia; potassium restriction

  Hypocalcemia: Intravenous calcium gluconate or enteral calcium salts

  Hyponatremia: Removal of excess fluid or fluid restriction, calculate sodium deficit and replace ($<125\,meq\,L^{-1}$), hypertonic saline ($<120\,meq\,L^{-1}$ with neurologic deficits)

  Hyperphosphatemia: Phosphorous restriction; calcium salts

Management of fluids

  Restriction of fluids if fluid overloaded (provide insensible losses and urine output to maintain equal balance, if desired)

  Diuretics for fluid overload prevention or volume associated hypertension (avoid excessive use if severe AKI)

  Closely follow daily fluid balance and weights with daily calculation of % fluid overload

Avoidance of further renal injury

  Maintain blood pressure, avoid nephrotoxic medication/agents, follow serum aminoglycoside levels

Nutritional management

  Encourage enteral feeding and use of parenteral nutrition if necessary to achieve target nutrition; use of renal disease-sepcific formulas if high potassium and phosphorous, provide at least basal metabolic needs for calories; provide at least $2\,g\,kg^{-1}\,day^{-1}$ protein; daily recommended intake for vitamins and minerals

Appropriate drug dosing

  Calculation of estimated GFR; review all medications that require adjusted dosing, with frequent reassessment of changes in GFR

Renal replacement therapy when indicated

The table provides an overview of AKI management. Each item is described in more detail in other chapters

surgery [8, 17, 18]. Randomized controlled trials are lacking in children, however, for both fenoldapam and nesiritide. Several other potential therapies such as growth factors [42], erythropoeitin [51], and free- radical scavengers [20, 23] are also being investigated in animal models from which AKI pathophysiologic mechanisms were originally delineated.

6.6   Outcome of AKI

Children requiring acute dialysis for AKI have high mortality rates. Depending on the AKI definition used and the population studied, mortality ranges up to 70% [12, 31, 54, 56]. A recent multicenter study of children receiving CRRT revealed that patients with nonrenal organ disease or multiple organ system dysfunction syndrome (MODS) have a higher mortality rate (>50%) compared to other diagnoses (<30%) [56]. Because pediatric MODS tends to occur early in the PICU course [47], death also often occurs in these patients within the first week of MODS diagnosis. Infants demonstrate even higher mortality rates when compared with older children [56, 62].

Little data exist to describe the long-term outcome of children with PICU-acquired AKI. Two-thirds of patients who had hospital acquired AKI in a tertiary health care center had complete recovery of their renal dysfunction by hospital discharge, whereas 30% had improved renal function but some element of chronic kidney disease, and 5% required ongoing renal replacement therapy at discharge [31]. In a 3–5 year follow-up study of patients who suffered from AKI during PICU admission, patient survival was 80%, although 60% of patients had some renal abnormality at follow-up (decreased GFR, hypertension, micro albuminuria, or hematuria) [6]. Premature neonates with perinatal AKI had higher SCR levels and were more likely to have proteinuria at 1 year follow-up compared with premature neonates without perinatal AKI [1]. Overall, hospital mortality of patients with AKI is related to the level of illness severity. In those who survive significant AKI, there appears to be a definite risk of long-term renal dysfunction including impaired GFR.

6.7   Summary and Future Directions

Understanding the pathophysiology, risk factors, and management of AKI is essential for the clinician in the PICU. Critically ill children rarely have one cause of AKI. They tend to be medically complex patients with multiple organ dysfunction. Early recognition of AKI and timely interventions aimed at preventing further renal injury and limiting complications are crucial to promote both renal and nonrenal recovery. AKI can no longer be considered a hospital-acquired condition that eventually resolves in survivors, but is now recognized to impact long-term renal function including the potential for future chronic kidney disease. Ongoing research should help elucidate more accurate diagnostic methods such as biomarkers to detect AKI and lead to therapeutic strategies to prevent acute injury, minimize renal damage, and promote recovery.

References

1. Abitbol CL, Bauer CR, Montane B, et al. (2003) Long-term follow-up of extremely low birth weight infants with neonatal renal failure. Pediatr Nephrol 18: 887–893
2. Abosaif NY, Tolba YA, Heap M, et al. (2005) The outcome of acute renal failure in the intensive care unit according to RIFLE: Model application, sensitivity, and predictability. Am J Kidney Dis 46: 1038–1048
3. Akcan-Arikan A, Zappitelli M, Loftis LL, et al. (2007) Modified RIFLE criteria in critically ill children with acute kidney injury. Kidney Int 71: 1028–1035
4. Andreoli S (2004) Clinical evaluation and management. In: Avner E, Harmon W, Niaudet P (eds) Pediatric Nephrology, 5th edn. Lippincott Williams and Wilkins, Philadelphia, PA
5. Andreoli SP (2002) Acute renal failure. Curr Opin Pediatr 14: 183–188
6. Askenazi DJ, Feig DI, Graham NM, et al. (2006) 3–5 Year longitudinal follow-up of pediatric patients after acute renal failure. Kidney Int 69: 184–189
7. Bailey D, Phan V, Litalien C, et al. (2007) Risk factors of acute renal failure in critically ill children: A prospective descriptive epidemiological study. Pediatr Crit Care Med 8: 29–35
8. Beaver TM, Winterstein AG, Shuster JJ, et al. (2006) Effectiveness of nesiritide on dialysis or all-cause mortality in patients undergoing cardiothoracic surgery. Clin Cardiol 29: 18–24
9. Bellomo R, Ronco C, Kellum JA, et al. (2004) Acute renal failure – Definition, outcome measures, animal models, fluid therapy and information technology needs: the Second International Consensus Conference of the Acute Dialysis Quality Initiative (ADQI) Group. Crit Care 8: R204–R212
10. Benfield MR, Bunchman TE (2004) Management of acute renal failure. In: Avner ED, Haron WE, Niaudet P (eds) Pediatric Nephrology, 5 edn. Lippincott, Williams & Wilkins Philadelphia
11. Bonventre JV, Zuk A (2004) Ischemic acute renal failure: an inflammatory disease? Kidney Int 66: 480–485
12. Bunchman TE, McBryde KD, Mottes TE, et al. (2001) Pediatric acute renal failure: outcome by modality and disease. Pediatr Nephrol 16: 1067–1071
13. Burns KE, Chu MW, Novick RJ, et al. (2005) Perioperative N-acetylcysteine to prevent renal dysfunction in high-risk patients undergoing cabg surgery: a randomized controlled trial. Jama 294: 342–350
14. Chan KL, Ip P, Chiu CS, et al. (2003) Peritoneal dialysis after surgery for congenital heart disease in infants and young children. Ann Thorac Surg 76: 1443–1449
15. Chertow GM BE, Honour M, Bonventre JV, Bates DW (2005) Acute kidney injury, mortality, length of stay, and costs in hospitalized patients. JASN 16: 3365–3370
16. Chesney RW, Jones DP, Chapter 52. Nephrotoxins. In: Avner ED, Haron WE, Niaudet P (2004) Pediatric Nephrology 5 edn. Lippincott Williams and Wilkins, Philadelphia, PA
17. Costello JM, Backer CL, Checchia PA, et al. (2005) Effect of cardiopulmonary bypass and surgical intervention on the natriuretic hormone system in children. J Thorac Cardiovasc Surg 130: 822–829
18. Costello JM, Goodman DM, Green TP (2006) A review of the natriuretic hormone system's diagnostic and therapeutic potential in critically ill children. Pediatr Crit Care Med 7: 308–318
19. Costello JM, Thiagarajan RR, Dionne RE, et al. (2006) Initial experience with fenoldopam after cardiac surgery in neonates with an insufficient response to conventional diuretics. Pediatr Crit Care Med 7: 28–33
20. de Vries B, Walter SJ, von Bonsdorff L, et al. (2004) Reduction of circulating redox-active iron by apotransferrin protects against renal ischemia-reperfusion injury. Transplantation 77: 669–675
21. Deray G (2002) Amphotericin B nephrotoxicity. J Antimicrob Chemother 49 Suppl 1: 37–41
22. Devarajan P (2005) Cellular and molecular derangements in acute tubular necrosis. Curr Opin Pediatr 17: 193–199
23. Doi K, Suzuki Y, Nakao A, et al. (2004) Radical scavenger edaravone developed for clinical use ameliorates ischemia/reperfusion injury in rat kidney. Kidney Int 65: 1714–1723
24. Farias JA, Frutos-Vivar F, Casado Flores J, et al. (2006) [Factors associated with the prognosis of mechanically ventilated infants and children. An international study]. Med Intensiva 30: 425–431
25. Fleming F, Bohn D, Edwards H, et al. (1995) Renal replacement therapy after repair of congenital heart disease in children. A comparison of hemofiltration and peritoneal dialysis. J Thorac Cardiovasc Surg 109: 322–331
26. Foland JA, Fortenberry JD, Warshaw BL, et al. (2004) Fluid overload before continuous hemofiltration and survival in critically ill children: a retrospective analysis. Crit Care Med 32: 1771–1776
27. Friedewald JJ, Rabb H (2004) Inflammatory cells in ischemic acute renal failure. Kidney Int 66: 486–491
28. Gallego N, Perez-Caballero C, Gallego A, et al. (2001) Prognosis of patients with acute renal failure without cardiopathy. Arch Dis Child 84: 258–260
29. Goldstein SL, Somers MJ, Baum MA, et al. (2005) Pediatric patients with multi-organ dysfunction syndrome receiving continuous renal replacement therapy. Kidney Int 67: 653–658
30. Hoste EA, Clermont G, Kersten A, et al. (2006) RIFLE criteria for acute kidney injury are associated with hospital mortality in critically ill patients: A cohort analysis. Crit Care 10: R73

31. Hui-Stickle S, Brewer ED, Goldstein SL (2005) Pediatric ARF epidemiology at a tertiary care center from 1999 to 2001. Am J Kidney Dis 45: 96–101
32. Kaushal GP, Basnakian AG, Shah SV (2004) Apoptotic pathways in ischemic acute renal failure. Kidney Int 66: 500–506
33. Kist-van Holthe JE, Goedvolk CA, Brand R, et al. (2002) Prospective study of renal insufficiency after bone marrow transplantation. Pediatr Nephrol 17: 1032–1037
34. Kuitunen A, Vento A, Suojaranta-Ylinen R, et al. (2006) Acute renal failure after cardiac surgery: Evaluation of the RIFLE classification. Ann Thorac Surg 81: 542–546
35. Lameire N, Van Biesen W, Vanholder R (2005) Acute renal failure. Lancet 365: 417–430
36. Lassnigg A, Donner E, Grubhofer G, et al. (2000) Lack of renoprotective effects of dopamine and furosemide during cardiac surgery. J Am Soc Nephrol 11: 97–104
37. Lopes JA, Jorge S, Neves FC, et al. (2006) An assessment of the rifle criteria for acute renal failure in severely burned patients. Nephrol Dial Transplant 22: 285
38. Loza R, Estremadoyro L, Loza C, et al. (2006) Factors associated with mortality in acute renal failure (ARF) in children. Pediatr Nephrol 21: 106–109
39. Medina Villanueva A, Lopez-Herce Cid J, Lopez Fernandez Y, et al. (2004) [Acute renal failure in critically-ill children. A preliminary study]. Ann Pediatr 61: 509–514
40. Michael M, Kuehnle I, Goldstein SL (2004) Fluid overload and acute renal failure in pediatric stem cell transplant patients. Pediatr Nephrol 19: 91–95
41. Mishra J, Dent C, Tarabishi R, et al. (2005) Neutrophil gelatinase-associated lipocalin (NGAL) as a biomarker for acute renal injury after cardiac surgery. Lancet 365: 1231–1238
42. Nishida M, Hamaoka K (2006) How does G-CSF act on the kidney during acute tubular injury? Nephron Exp Nephrol 104: e123–e128
43. Olowu WA, Adelusola KA (2004) Pediatric acute renal failure in southwestern Nigeria. Kidney Int 66: 1541–1548
44. Piper SN, Kumle B, Maleck WH, et al. (2003) Diltiazem may preserve renal tubular integrity after cardiac surgery. Can J Anaesth 50: 285–292
45. Price J, Mott A, Dickerson H, et al. (2007) Worsening renal function in children hospitalized with acute decompensated heart failure: Evidence for a pediatric cardiorenal syndrome? Ped Crit Care Med (accepted)
46. Price PM, Megyesi J, Saf Irstein RL (2004) Cell cycle regulation: Repair and regeneration in acute renal failure. Kidney Int 66: 509–514
47. Proulx F, Gauthier M, Nadeau D, et al. (1994) Timing and predictors of death in pediatric patients with multiple organ system failure. Crit Care Med 22: 1025–1031
48. Schmidt-Ott KM, Mori K, Kalandadze A, et al. (2006) Neutrophil gelatinase-associated lipocalin-mediated iron traffic in kidney epithelia. Curr Opin Nephrol Hypertens 15: 442–449
49. Schrier RW, Wang W (2004) Acute renal failure and sepsis. N Engl J Med 351: 159–169
50. Schwartz GJ, Haycock GB, Edelmann CM, Jr, et al. (1976) A simple estimate of glomerular filtration rate in children derived from body length and plasma creatinine. Pediatrics 58: 259–263
51. Sharples EJ, Yaqoob MM (2006) Erythropoietin and acute renal failure. Semin Nephrol 26: 325–331
52. Shilliday IR, Quinn KJ, Allison ME (1997) Loop diuretics in the management of acute renal failure: A prospective, double-blind, placebo-controlled, randomized study. Nephrol Dial Transplant 12: 2592–2596
53. Siegel JN, Van Why SK, Devarajan P (2004) Pathogenesis of acute renal failure. In: Avner ED, Harmon WE, Niaudet P (eds) Pediatric Nephrology, 5 edn. Lippincott Williams and Wilkins, Philadelphia, PA
54. Skippen PW, Krahn GE (2005) Acute renal failure in children undergoing cardiopulmonary bypass. Crit Care Resusc 7: 286–291
55. Sorof JM, Stromberg D, Brewer ED, et al. (1999) Early initiation of peritoneal dialysis after surgical repair of congenital heart disease. Pediatr Nephrol 13: 641–645
56. Symons JM, Chua A, Somers MJ, et al. (2007) Demographic characteristics of pediatric continuous renal replacement therapy: A report of the prospective pediatric continuous renal replacement therapy registry. CJASN 2: 732–738
57. Taber SS, Mueller BA (2006) Drug-associated renal dysfunction. Crit Care Clin 22: 357–374, viii
58. Uchino S, Doig GS, Bellomo R, et al. (2004) Diuretics and mortality in acute renal failure. Crit Care Med 32: 1669–1677
59. Uchino S, Bellomo R, Goldsmith D, et al. (2006) An assessment of the RIFLE criteria for acute renal failure in hospitalized patients. Crit Care Med 34: 1913–1917
60. Vachvanichsanong P, Dissaneewate P, Lim A, et al. (2006) Childhood acute renal failure: 22-Year experience in a university hospital in southern Thailand. Pediatrics 118: e786–e791
61. Van Why SK, Friedman AL, Wei LJ, et al. (1991) Renal insufficiency after bone marrow transplantation in children. Bone Marrow Transplant 7: 383–388
62. Williams DM, Sreedhar SS, Mickell JJ, et al. (2002) Acute kidney failure: A pediatric experience over 20 years. Arch Pediatr Adolesc Med 156: 893–900

7

Pharmacotherapy in the Critically Ill Child with Acute Kidney Injury

M.T. Bigham, T.K. Hutson, and D.S. Wheeler

Contents

Core Messages

› Several commonly used medications in the pediatric intensive care unit (PICU) are potentially toxic to the kidney.
› The kidney plays a major role in determining the absorption, distribution, metabolism, and elimination of a multitude of medications that are commonly used in the PICU. As such, dosing of these medications needs to be adjusted in critically ill children with acute kidney injury.
› Renal replacement therapy can affect the drug levels of commonly used medications in the PICU.

Case Vignette

A 13-month-old male with a history of short-gut syndrome and TPN-dependent cholestasis presents to the PICU with septic shock. He is treated aggressively with fluid resuscitation, broad-spectrum antibiotics (vancomycin, gentamicin, and cefotaxime), tracheal intubation and mechanical ventilatory support, and administration of continuous infusions of epinephrine ($0.3 \mu g \, kg^{-1} \, min^{-1}$) and dopamine ($12 \mu g \, kg^{-1} \, min^{-1}$). His cardiorespiratory and hemodynamic status stabilizes over the subsequent 48 h, though he develops oliguria progressing to anuria despite administration of diuretics. Laboratory evaluation reveals a coincident rise in blood urea nitrogen (BUN) to 95 mg dL^{-1} and serum creatinine to 2.3 g dL^{-1}. His antibiotics are dosed appropriately for his deteriorating kidney function based upon drug-monitoring studies. Because of fluid overload, impaired clearance, and modest hemodynamic instability, he is started on continuous

S.G. Kiessling et al. (eds) *Pediatric Nephrology in the ICU.*
© Springer-Verlag Berlin Heidelberg 2009

veno-venous hemofiltration (CVVH) for renal replacement therapy (RRT). Adjustments in vancomycin and gentamicin dose and intervals are required, as well as consideration of CVVH flow rates, ultrafiltration volumes, circuit anticoagulation, and replacement fluid composition.

7.1 Introduction

Acute kidney injury (AKI), formerly known as acute renal failure, continues to represent a very common and potentially devastating problem in critically ill children and adults [14, 45, 78, 105, 108]. AKI affects between 5 and 50% of critically ill children and adults in reported series [6, 18, 26, 45, 117, 118]. In the vast majority of these patients, AKI is caused by the underlying disease process itself (e.g., sepsis, shock, etc.) and is just one of many affected organ systems in the multiple organ dysfunction syndrome (MODS). However, recent studies suggest that the kidney plays more than just the role of innocent bystander. Instead, the physiologic consequences of AKI (Table 7.1) appear to contribute to a chain of events that culminate in the development of MODS [22, 44]. To this end, recent studies suggest that AKI itself may be an independent risk factor for mortality in both critically ill children [1, 6, 83] and adults [4, 23, 61, 73]. Finally, the kidney plays a major role in deter-

Table 7.1 Physiologic consequences of acute kidney injury

Volume overload
Congestive heart failure
Intra-abdominal hypertension (secondary to ascites and retroperitoneal tissue edema)
Altered lung mechanics (secondary to pulmonary edema, pleural effusions)
Electrolyte and acid–base disturbances
Hyponatremia
Hyperkalemia
Metabolic acidosis (accumulation of organic anions and unmeasured anions)
Uremia
Altered immunity (CRISIS = critical illness stress-induced immunosuppression)
Decreased erythropoietin production (*anemia of critical illness*)
Poor wound healing
Altered pharmacokinetics

mining the absorption, distribution, metabolism, and elimination of a multitude of medications that are commonly used in the pediatric intensive care unit (PICU). A clear understanding of the altered pharmacokinetics of these drugs in critically ill children with AKI is of paramountcy.

Much of what we know about pharmacology in children assumes general health. However, in the critically ill child the physiologic interplay of fluid balance related to blood pressure and capillary leak, glomerular and tubular filtration related to renal insufficiency, and even drug metabolism and disposition becomes upset. To understand the central role that the kidney plays in physiologic and pharmacologic processes in the critically ill child, we must first delineate the pharmacologic terminology. Pharmacology has been described as the science of chemical agents, including their composition, uses and effects, and their interaction with biologic systems. Pharmacology largely depends on the interplay of two entities, namely pharmacokinetics and pharmacodynamics. The former describes the study of the absorption, distribution, metabolism, and elimination of drugs, while the latter focuses on the effects of drugs on the organs and tissues. The emerging field of pharmacogenomics describes the genetic variability in biotransformation of a given medication based on the enzyme activity of specific drug-metabolizing enzymes [82]. Clinical pharmacology, or pharmacotherapy, describes the targeted use of drugs to treat disease. The task of understanding these important pharmacologic and pharmacotherapeutic concepts in critically ill children with renal insufficiency lies in understanding fluid balance and assessment of renal function, and ultimately the unique properties of specific drugs commonly used in the PICU setting. In this chapter, we will therefore briefly review the nephrotoxicity of some of the pharmacologic agents that are commonly used in the PICU. We will briefly discuss the effect of AKI and RRT on absorption, distribution, metabolism, and elimination of drugs. Finally, we will also review the several agents that have been used to prevent and treat AKI in the clinical setting.

7.2 Drug-Associated Kidney Injury

Palliative or corrective surgery requiring cardiopulmonary bypass for congenital heart disease is the most common cause of AKI in critically ill children, while sepsis is generally the second most common cause of

AKI in most reported series [6, 45, 51, 98, 118]. The impact of drug therapy on AKI is well recognized, but difficult to define. A recent review of the most frequently used medications in the intensive care units (PICU, cardiac ICU, and neonatal ICU) at C.S. Mott Children's Hospital at the University of Michigan showed that more than 25% of these medications were potentially toxic to the kidney. Moreover, these nephrotoxic medications accounted for nearly 40% of all the medication orders in these units over a 1-year period [104]. Therefore, many of the pharmacologic agents used in the PICU have the potential to at least contribute, and in some causes directly cause, AKI. We will concentrate on only a few, major classes of agents.

7.2.1   Nonsteroidal Anti-Inflammatory Drugs (NSAIDs)

NSAIDs (aspirin, ibuprofen, indomethacin, naproxen, ketorolac) were some of the most commonly prescribed medications in the aforementioned study performed at the University of Michigan [104]. This particular class of medications is frequently used for management of fever [89] and postoperative pain [39, 63] in the PICU. A recent prospective, multicenter study suggested that aspirin significantly lowers the risk of shunt thrombosis and subsequent death following surgical placement of a systemic-to-pulmonary artery shunt in children with single-ventricle physiology [62]. Finally, ibuprofen and indomethacin are used in the medical management of preterm neonates with a patent ductus arteriosus [113]. While generally safe and well tolerated in previously healthy children, the nephrotoxic potential of NSAIDs is compounded in critically ill children with preexisting kidney dysfunction, dehydration, sepsis, shock, or congestive heart failure. The body's normal compensatory response during these states results in increased sympathetic tone, activation of the renin–angiotensin–aldosterone axis, and release of vasopressin, all of which act to maintain adequate renal blood flow. However, maintenance of renal blood flow is also dependent upon the local conversion of arachidonic acid to vasodilatory prostaglandins by the two enzymes, cyclooxygenase (COX)-1 and COX-2. Increased production of prostaglandin (PG) D_2, PGE_2, and PGI_2 counteracts the vasoconstrictive effects of norepinephrine, angiotensin II, and vasopressin. NSAIDs disturb this homeostatic balance, leading to intense renal vasoconstriction, a decrease in renal blood flow, a rapid decline in glomerular filtration, and subsequent AKI [104, 116]. At the extreme,

this decrease in renal blood flow may rarely lead to papillary necrosis [54, 55, 90]. Finally, NSAIDs have been associated with acute interstitial nephritis (AIN), a relatively reversible form of AKI characterized by fever, rash, eosinophilia, and eosinophiluria [7]. The nephrotoxic potential of NSAIDs appears to be both dose- and duration-dependent. Aspirin is generally the least nephrotoxic, while indomethacin is the most likely NSAID to cause AKI. AKI secondary to the use of NSAIDs is generally reversible with supportive care and discontinuation of the NSAID.

7.2.2   Radiographic Contrast Dye

Radiographic contrast agents are generally safe and well tolerated in previously healthy children. Conditions commonly encountered in the PICU, including preexisting kidney dysfunction, dehydration, hypotension, sepsis, and congestive heart failure significantly increase the risk of AKI following administration of radiographic contrast. Radiographic contrast nephropathy is the third most common cause of hospital-acquired AKI in most adult series, though unfortunately comparable data in the pediatric population is not currently available [42]. The pathophysiology of radiographic contrast nephropathy is undoubtedly multifactorial, though evidence suggests that contrast agents induce renal vasoconstriction [43, 104], possibly through endothelin-1 [19, 36] or inhibition of locally produced nitric oxide [17, 43]. Radiocontrast is also directly toxic to the renal tubular epithelium [17]. Several evidence-based recommendations for the prevention of radiographic contrast nephropathy exist [8, 58, 96]. Fluid volume loading and avoiding other nephrotoxic drugs prior to the administration of radiographic contrast are particularly important. Hydration with sodium bicarbonate (154 meq L^{-1}) was superior to that of sodium chloride (154 meq L^{-1}) in a recently published, prospective, single-center, randomized trial [72]. Lower osmolality contrast agents are less nephrotoxic than high osmolality contrast agents and are generally preferred in high-risk patients [8, 43, 58, 104]. The administration of N-acetylcysteine (NAC) may be effective in the prevention of radiographic contrast nephropathy, though the evidence is such that routine administration of NAC is not currently recommended for all patients [8, 43, 58, 104]. Finally, prophylactic hemodialysis or hemofiltration may be effective in preventing AKI following contrast administration [66], though further studies are needed.

7.2.3 Vasopressors

Vasopressors are commonly used to restore blood pressure and tissue perfusion in critically ill children with shock, regardless of etiology. When compared with adults, children have a relatively high systemic vascular resistance (SVR) and vasoactive capacity, such that hypotension is a relatively late sign of shock (Fig. 7.1). For example, Ceneviva et al. [20] categorized 50 children with fluid-refractory shock according to hemodynamic state (based upon hemodynamic measurements performed with a pulmonary artery catheter) into one of three possible cardiovascular derangements (1) hyperdynamic, so-called *warm shock* state characterized by high cardiac output (>5.5 L min^{-1} m^{-2} BSA) and peripheral vasodilation (SVR < 800 dynes s cm^{-5}), (2) a hypodynamic state characterized primarily by myocardial depression (cardiac output < 3.3 L min^{-1} m^{-2} BSA), or (3) a hypodynamic, *cold shock* state characterized by low cardiac output and peripheral vasoconstriction (SVR > 1,200 dynes s cm^{-5}). In contrast to adults in whom the early stages of septic shock are characterized by a high cardiac output and peripheral vasodilation (warm shock), most of these children were in a hypodynamic state characterized by low cardiac output and peripheral vasoconstriction (cold shock) and required the addition of vasodilators to decrease SVR, increase cardiac index, and improve peripheral perfusion [20]. These findings have been subsequently corroborated in multiple studies [34, 71, 81, 84, 85, 87]. These results suggest that vasopressors such as high-dose epinephrine (>0.3 µg kg^{-1} min^{-1}) or

norepinephrine may worsen the cold shock state that is characteristic of pediatric septic shock. To the same extent, vasopressors in this scenario may actually worsen perfusion of the kidney and other organs, leading to worsening of AKI and ultimately, MODS.

Historically, so-called *renal-dose* dopamine (3–5 µg kg^{-1} min^{-1}) was used in critically ill children on vasopressors, to preserve perfusion to the kidney during the shock state. At these low doses, dopamine acts via the dopaminergic receptor to increase renal blood flow. While several large studies consistently showed that renal-dose dopamine increased glomerular filtration, natriuresis, and diuresis, there was no effect on either the incidence of AKI or outcome [47]. Dopamine, even at these low doses, is not completely without risk. Dopamine decreases prolactin secretion, which may contribute to the critical illness stress-induced immunosuppression (CRISIS) syndrome [33, 119]. In addition, dopamine administration may be associated with increased mortality when used in critically ill adults with shock [88]. Finally, at least one study suggested that renal-dose dopamine actually worsened renal blood flow in patients with preexisting AKI [60]. For all of these reasons, the practice of renal-dose dopamine has been largely abandoned.

7.2.4 Antibiotics

There are several antibiotics that have been associated with AKI in both children and adults. For example, the penicillins, cephalosporins, sulfonamides, fluoroquinolones, and vancomycin have all been associated with AIN [32, 80, 104]. Other medications have been linked with AIN as well, and AIN may be the primary etiology in up to 15% of hospitalized adults with AKI [74]. AIN is believed to represent a cell-mediated, hypersensitivity reaction and should be considered in the differential diagnosis of AKI in previously healthy children. Kidney function usually returns to normal after discontinuing the offending agent.

Acyclovir is cleared by the kidney through glomerular filtration and tubular secretion. The majority of the drug is excreted in the urine unchanged and may precipitate in the distal tubule, leading to crystal precipitation and obstruction of tubular flow [46, 104]. The risk of AKI following acyclovir administration appears to be dose-dependent, and the risk may be compounded in the presence of fluid restriction or dehydration [10, 110]. Kidney function generally returns to normal following cessation of the drug, though RRT may be required until that time [104].

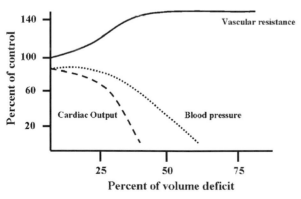

Fig. 7.1 The cardiovascular response to volume depletion in children. Tachycardia and increased systemic vascular resistance (SVR) initially maintain adequate cardiac output in the face of dramatic fluid losses (e.g., hemorrhage) during the so-called *compensated* phase of shock. Further fluid losses lead to a decrease in cardiac output, though blood pressure may be maintained until the late phases of *uncompensated* shock

The nephrotoxicity of amphotericin B is well recognized (*amphoterrible*). Several studies report rates of AKI as high as 65% for patients on amphotericin B [27, 38]. Amphotericin B induces renal vasoconstriction to reduce renal blood flow and GFR, leading to AKI. Amphotericin B is also directly toxic to the distal tubular epithelium [104]. The latter effect results in hypokalemia and the other electrolyte derangements commonly associated with this drug (namely, hyponatremia and hypomagnesemia). The risk of AKI is compounded in critically ill children with preexisting kidney dysfunction, concomitant administration of other nephrotoxic drugs, sepsis, congestive heart failure, shock, or dehydration [38]. The lipid-based formulations of amphotericin B are less nephrotoxic, and several antifungal agents with significantly less nephrotoxicity are currently available, including fluconazole, itraconazole, voriconazole, and caspofungin [104]. Sodium and volume loading prior to administration of the drug may also minimize nephrotoxicity.

The aminoglycosides are the last major class of antibiotics commonly used in the PICU that are frequently associated with AKI. These antibiotics are cleared by the kidney and excreted in the urine and are thought to be directly toxic to the renal tubular epithelium. Again, the risk of AKI is compounded in critically ill children with preexisting kidney dysfunction, concomitant administration of other nephrotoxic drugs, sepsis, congestive heart failure, shock, or dehydration. Administration of higher doses at longer dosing intervals may lessen the risk of AKI [43, 104].

7.3   Drug Disposition and Metabolism in AKI and RRT

7.3.1   Assessment of the Glomerular Filtration Rate (GFR) in Critically Ill Children

Recent studies have revealed that AKI may be an independent risk factor for mortality in both critically ill children [1, 6, 83] and adults [4, 23, 61, 73], reinforcing the need for earlier detection of renal injury to allow for prompt intervention and potential reversal of AKI. Evaluation and assessment of the GFR is but one facet in the overall management of patients with AKI. The GFR is the most commonly used and widely recognized parameter to monitor kidney function in the clinical setting. In addition, adjustments in both the dose and dosing interval of drugs cleared by the kidney are frequently necessary in patients with AKI, which depend upon the GFR to reduce the risks of drug accumulation and toxicity.

Clearance techniques for GFR assessment involve measurement of either intrinsic or intravenously administered substances that are freely filtered by the glomerulus. The premise behind all clearance techniques is the equation:

$$C_x = U_x \times V/P_x,$$

where C_x = clearance of x, U_x = urine concentration of x, V = urine flow rate (in mL min^{-1}), and P_x = plasma concentration of x. Thus, if a freely filtered substance is neither absorbed nor secreted, its plasma and urine concentrations measured after a set dose in a set period of time can be used to determine clearance. The gold standard for definitive measurement of GFR is inulin [86], though the inulin clearance technique is cumbersome in that it requires a continuous intravenous infusion of inulin followed by urine collections at timed intervals. Simplified modifications in the inulin clearance technique involving bolus dosing of inulin rather than continuous infusion or measurement of serum inulin with pharmacokinetic calculations that yield inulin clearance have been used. However, most experts feel that the inulin clearance technique is not practical for use in the critical care setting. Other clinically applicable clearance tools include isotope clearance studies such as chromium-labeled ethylenediamine tetraacetic acid (^{51}Cr-EDTA), ^{99m}Tc-diethylenetriaminepentaacetic acid (DTPA), ^{99m}Tc-mercaptoacetyltriglycine (MAG3), ^{125}I-iothalamate, and iodoth-alamate [37].

Creatinine clearance is the most frequently used method for estimation of GFR in the critical care setting. Unfortunately, there are several limitations to using creatinine clearance as a surrogate for GFR in this population as well. First, creatinine is an unreliable and insensitive indicator during early, acute changes in kidney function, as serum creatinine concentrations typically do not change until approximately 50% of kidney function has already been lost [76]. Second, the serum creatinine does not accurately reflect kidney function until a steady state has been reached, which may require several days following an acute insult [76]. Finally, as kidney function deteriorates further, a greater fraction of creatinine is secreted by the renal tubules, and creatinine clearance will then typically overestimate GFR.

In children, creatinine clearance is calculated using the Schwartz formula [93–95] and is normalized to body surface area in order to allow for comparison with published standards:

$$CrCl \ (mL \ min^{-1} per \ 1.73 \ m^2) = k \times length \ (cm)/serum \ creatinine \ (mg \ dL^{-1})$$

The constant, k varies with age. For patients with age less than 2 years, $k = 0.45$, if between 2 and less than 13 years, $k = 0.55$, and if age is 13 and less than 20 years, $k = 0.7$ for male and 0.55 for female. Cystatin C, a 13-kD nonglycosylated basic protein that is freely filtered by the glomerulus has been investigated as an alterative means to calculate clearance. The age and sex variability described earlier seems to be minimal in cystatin C measurements. Though evidence exists both in favor and against the use of cystatin C measurements as a favorable alternative to creatinine clearance equations, particularly at higher levels of GFR, it is not clear whether cystatin C measurements offer improvement in estimating GFR [101].

7.3.2 Drug Dosing in AKI

The physiologic derangements that characterize critical illness can significantly affect the pharmacokinetics and pharmacodynamics of drugs that are commonly used in the PICU [13, 56]. These effects are compounded further in the presence of AKI. AKI can adversely affect both the volume of distribution and clearance of medications, which can either increase the toxicity or decrease the efficacy of any one particular medication, depending on context. For example, critically ill children with volume overload secondary to AKI will have a higher volume of distribution for many medications (e.g., aminoglycosides, vancomycin) and thus may require a higher dose to achieve the desired therapeutic range. Changes in serum albumin frequently have untoward consequences on the relative amount of free and unbound medication in the blood. Some of the most commonly used medications in the PICU and how they are affected by AKI are described briefly in the following sections.

7.3.2.1 Antibacterials

Antibiotics are one of the most commonly administered classes of medications in the PICU. The goal for antimicrobial therapy relies on reaching adequate active drug concentrations that result in bacterial killing while avoiding drug-induced toxicity. Most antibiotics are eliminated by the kidneys, and the presence of AKI

will necessitate dosing adjustments with careful monitoring of serum drug concentrations (when available). Penicillins and cephalosporins usually do not require adjustment until the patient's GFR is ≤ 30 mL min^{-1} per 1.73 m^2. However, there are reports of neurotoxicity and seizures associated with cephalosporin therapy in patients with renal impairment, so care must be taken to adjust doses and monitor patients accordingly [21, 68]. The aminoglycosides are all cleared by the kidney and their dosage must be adjusted in patients with AKI. As discussed earlier, since the bactericidal activity of these medications is concentration-dependent, the goal is to have a high peak and a lower trough level to help minimize nephrotoxicity [64]. To achieve this, patients with AKI require longer dosing intervals to allow adequate time for drug clearance while still reaching a therapeutic peak level. These patients may also have variable volumes of distribution, requiring dosage increase to achieve the desired peak level. Several dosage guidelines have been published that can serve as a guide to initial therapy with these agents, but individual dosage adjustment based on clinical pharmacokinetic monitoring will provide the most accurate dosing to optimize therapy and minimize toxicity [25]. Dosing guidelines have been published to aid in adjusting vancomycin in patients with AKI as well, but again the guidelines are designed as initial dosing ranges with individualized therapy determined based on drug levels and the patient's unique pharmacokinetic parameters [25]. Care must be taken in patients with end-stage renal disease, however, due to falsely high vancomycin serum concentrations related to cross-reactivity of a vancomycin pseudometabolite [99]. Other antibacterials such as nafcillin, clindamycin, and linezolid are not renally eliminated and thus do not require adjustment in dosing [16]. However, patients with AKI who are receiving linezolid may have an associated increased incidence of thrombocytopenia. Imipenem-cilastatin should be used cautiously in patients with AKI, as it is more likely to cause convulsions, especially if these patients also have other risk factors for seizures [77].

7.3.2.2 Antivirals

Acyclovir is the most commonly used antiviral agent in the PICU. As discussed earlier, acyclovir has been associated with the development of transient increases in BUN and serum creatinine caused by crystal nephropathy and acute tubular necrosis. The dose of acyclovir should be adjusted in children with AKI or in children who are at risk for AKI. Adequate hydration is of paramountcy. Other commonly used antiviral agents (ganciclovir, cidofovir, foscarnet) also require dosage adjustments in patients with AKI.

7.3.2.3 Antifungals

We have already discussed the adverse effects of amphotericin B on kidney function. Whenever feasible, alternative antifungal agents should be used in lieu of amphotericin B. Voriconazole is a relatively new antifungal agent used increasingly more often in critically ill children with fungal infections, particularly aspergillosis. It is available in both oral and intravenous dosage forms. Oral voriconazole does not require dosage adjustments in patients with AKI. The intravenous formulation, however, is not recommended in patients with a GFR < 50 mL min^{-1} per 1.73 m^2 due to the accumulation of the vehicle sulfobutyl ether beta-cyclodextrin sodium. This carrier compound has been associated with proximal renal tubule vacuole formation in experimental rat models. We feel that oral voriconazole should be used in critically ill children with impaired GFR whenever voriconazole therapy is necessary.

7.3.2.4 Gastrointestinal Protective Agents

Agents commonly used in the PICU for gastric mucosal protection include the histamine (H_2) antagonists (e.g., ranitidine, famotidine), proton-pump inhibitors (e.g., omeprazole, lansoprazole, pantoprazole), and sucralfate. Thrombocytopenia has been rarely reported in patients with AKI receiving therapy with histamine antagonists. Dosages should be adjusted according to recommended guidelines and patients should have their platelet counts monitored closely while on this therapy. The proton-pump inhibitors do not require any dosage adjustments in patients with AKI. Sucralfate, a topical protectant, contains aluminum, which is effective for stress ulcer prophylaxis. In patients with normal renal function, the amount of aluminum received from the usual dose is eliminated effectively by the kidneys. However, in patients with AKI, the aluminum can accumulate and result in toxicity. Thus, it is recommended to use sucralfate cautiously if at all in patients with AKI. If long-term sucralfate therapy is required, aluminum levels should be monitored [41, 106].

7.3.2.5 Anticonvulsants

Most of the anticonvulsants do not require dosage adjustments in patients with AKI, as most of these agents are metabolized by the liver. The primary exception is the commonly used anticonvulsant, phenytoin. Though phenytoin is metabolized in the liver, dosing adjustments must be considered in patients with AKI due to the high degree of protein binding of phenytoin to albumin (~90–95% bound). This binding is often altered in patients with AKI due to a decreased serum albumin or accumulation of other drug metabolites that compete with phenytoin for the albumin binding sites [3]. Only the unbound form of phenytoin is active, thus impaired protein binding will result in higher levels of unbound drug. Increased unbound drug could result in phenytoin toxicity. In such patients, monitoring of unbound (free) drug levels is recommended for dosing accuracy. Fosphenytoin is a prodrug of phenytoin that is metabolized to phenytoin, phosphate, and formaldehyde. The advantage of fosphenytoin over phenytoin is that fosphenytoin can be administered more quickly with relatively few adverse hemodynamic effects. Most of the side effects seen with fosphenytoin are related to the parent drug phenytoin; however, one case report exists describing acute hyperphosphatemia in a patient with renal impairment who received 1,000 mg of fosphenytoin [69]. Care should be taken when administering fosphenytoin to patients with AKI, and serum phosphate levels should be closely monitored. Levetiracetam is the other anticonvulsant that has guidelines for dosage adjustment in patients with renal failure. Total body clearance of levetiracetam is decreased by up to 70% in patients with severe AKI.

7.3.3 Drug Dosing in RRT

As discussed in the preceding section, the dose of drugs that are cleared primarily by the kidney must be adjusted in critically ill children with impaired kidney function. However, once RRT is initiated, these same drugs may in fact be cleared by dialysis or hemofiltration, potentially resulting in clinically significant underdosing and lack of therapeutic effect. Unfortunately, the literature on the pharmacokinetics of specific drugs during RRT is rather limited, and the majority of these pharmacokinetic studies is limited to adults. There are few pediatric studies detailing the effects of RRT on drug disposition and clearance. However, a basic understanding of drug pharmacokinetics during RRT is absolutely essential to the care of critically ill children in the PICU, and several excellent reviews on this topic are available [12, 48, 57, 91].

Drug disposition and clearance during RRT requires an understanding of basic pharmacokinetic principles, such as protein binding, clearance, and volume of distribution (Box 7.1), all of which determine the peak concentration (C_{max}), trough concentration (C_{min}), half-life ($T_{1/2}$), and area under the plasma concentration vs. time curve (AUC). Only the unbound fraction of a drug is available for removal by RRT; therefore, drugs that are highly bound to plasma proteins are not efficiently removed by RRT. To a similar extent, drugs with a large volume of distribution (generally >0.7 L kg^{-1}) are not efficiently removed by RRT, as less of the drug is available for hemofiltration or dialysis. Drugs that are highly lipid soluble will accumulate in adipose tissues and therefore exhibit two and three compartment kinetics. The extent of drug removal by RRT will then depend upon the extent to which the drug is transferred between the plasma and these tissue compartments. Some drugs are eliminated by interactions with the hemofiltration membrane, through adsorption to the membrane itself, or via interactions between the negatively charged proteins along the membrane.

Box 7.1

Simplified pharmacokinetic equations

Volume of Distribution (V_d): $V_d = \dfrac{D}{\Delta C}$

V_d in L kg^{-1}, ΔC is peak minus trough concentration in mg L^{-1}, and D is dose in mg kg^{-1}.

Plasma Clearance (Cl$_p$): $Cl_p = V_d \times K_d$

Cl$_p$ in L kg^{-1} h^{-1}, V_d in L kg^{-1}, and K_d is the elimination rate constant in first hour.

Elimination Half-Life
$(t_{1/2})$: $t_{1/2} = t_{\frac{1}{2}} = \dfrac{0.693 V_d}{Cl_p}$ or $t_{\frac{1}{2}} \dfrac{0.693}{K_d}$

$t_{1/2}$ in h, Cl$_p$ in L kg^{-1} h^{-1}, V_d in L kg^{-1}, and K_d.

Elimination Rate Constant (K_d): $t_{1/2} = \dfrac{\text{Ln (C1} \div \text{C2)}}{T1 - T2}$

K_d in first hour, $C1$ is concentration at time 1 ($T1$) in mg L^{-1}, $C2$ is concentration at time 2 ($T2$) in mg L^{-1}, and Ln is the natural log.

Loading Dose (D_l): $D_l = C_d \times V_d$

D_l in mg kg^{-1}, C_d is desired plasma concentration in mg L^{-1}, and V_d

---

Most drugs have a molecular weight less than 500 Da (vancomycin is one notable exception, with a molecular weight of approximately 1,400 Da) and pass freely through the membrane. However, only that portion of the drug that is not bound to protein will pass through the membrane via either diffusion or convection. If a drug has significant protein binding, no relevant clearance by RRT can be expected, and hence, no dosage adjustment for RRT is necessary. The free, unbound fraction of drugs that are freely filtered through the membrane is generally calculated by the following:

Free fraction = (1 − protein bound fraction).

The capacity of a drug to pass through the membrane by convection (i.e., during hemofiltration) is determined by the sieving coefficient (S):

$$S = C_f / C_p,$$

where C_f is the concentration of the drug in the ultrafiltrate and C_p is the concentration of the drug in plasma. The primary determinant of S for most drugs with molecular weight less than 500 Da is the drug's protein binding, so that:

$$S = (1 - \text{protein bound fraction}).$$

The extent to which a particular drug is cleared during hemofiltration depends upon whether hemofiltration is performed with the use of predilution replacement fluids or postdilution replacement fluids. With postdilution, clearance equals the rate of ultrafiltration and may be calculated as follows:

$$Cl = S \times Q_f,$$

where Q_f is the ultrafiltration rate and S is the sieving coefficient, discussed earlier. Conversely, with predilution, clearance will be less than in postdilution, as the blood passing through the membrane is diluted. The concentration of the drug in the plasma passing through the membrane is less than the actual concentration of the drug in the plasma. Clearance during predilution is therefore calculated as follows:

$$Cl = S \times Q_f \times Q_b / (Q_b + Q_r),$$

where Q_b is the blood flow and Q_r is the predilution fluid replacement rate.

The extent to which a particular drug is eliminated during hemodialysis depends on the molecular weight of the drug. Clearance during hemodialysis occurs via diffusion – dialysate and blood are separated by the semipermeable dialysis membrane. As the rate of diffusion is inversely proportional to the molecular weight, drugs with lower molecular weights will diffuse across the membrane faster compared with drugs with higher molecular weights. However, the dialysate flow rate also is important to consider. Low dialysate flow rates fail to maintain a higher concentration gradient across the dialysis membrane, and in this scenario, the molecular weight of the drug is not as important. Conversely, with high dialysate flow rates, there is a higher concentration gradient maintained, and hence, smaller molecules will diffuse much faster. Other factors, such as the degree of protein binding, membrane pore size and thickness, and the surface area available for diffusion also play a role in determining the clearance. The extent to which a drug is cleared by hemodialysis can be determined by the following equation:

$$Cl = S_d \times Q_d \times K_d,$$

where S_d is the dialysate saturation (derived by dividing the drug concentration in the dialysate outflow by the drug concentration in the plasma), Q_d is the dialysate flow rate, and K_d is a diffusive mass transfer coefficient that depends upon the molecular weight and electrical charge of the drug.

Finally, when hemofiltration is combined with hemodialysis (continuous hemodiafiltration), drug clearance occurs via both convection and diffusion. Drug clearance can be approximated by the sum of the clearance by hemofiltration and the clearance by hemodialysis (using the earlier equations).

Dosing adjustments in critically ill children on RRT will therefore depend upon many factors. In some cases, there is some residual kidney function, so that drug clearance by the kidney must be taken into consideration. The fractional drug clearance via RRT is calculated as follows:

$$FC_{RRT} = Cl_{RRT} / (Cl_{RRT} + Cl_{liver} + Cl_{kidney}).$$

Clearance by the liver, kidney, or RRT is clinically important if its contribution to total body drug clearance exceeds 25%. Therefore, clearance via RRT is not important if Cl_{RRT} is less than 25% (due to either significant protein binding, large V_D, low Q_f, or low dialysate flow rates), clearance in the liver exceeds 25%, or clearance by residual kidney function exceeds 25%.

While there are several different proposed methods to adjust drug dosing in critically ill children on RRT

[12, 48, 91, 114], some important generalizations can be made. First, administration of a loading dose based upon the desired target plasma concentration and V_D is usually safe. The maintenance dose of the drug is adjusted for the estimated GFR. The maintenance dose is increased if the clearance by RRT is greater than 25%. Close monitoring of drug levels is important, especially for drugs with a narrow therapeutic index. Finally, whether the dosing interval or maintenance dose for antibiotics is adjusted depends upon the pharmacodynamic properties of the antibiotic in question. For example, the efficacy of aminoglycoside antibiotics depends upon a high peak concentration. A longer dosing interval with a higher maintenance dose may be appropriate in this circumstance, as aminoglycosides are readily cleared by RRT. In contrast, the efficacy of beta-lactam antibiotics depends upon the time the plasma drug concentration is above the MIC. Frequent administration of a lower drug dose is preferred in this circumstance.

7.4   Renal Protection and Prevention of AKI

7.4.1   Fluid Management

Currently, effective treatments to prevent AKI are lacking [50, 53], and management is largely directed toward reversing the underlying cause and providing supportive care. Supportive care in PICU has traditionally included optimizing nutrition and fluid status, avoiding potentially nephrotoxic medications, and maintaining cardiorespiratory stability with the use of vasoactive medications and mechanical ventilatory support. Fluid balance in critically ill children who are at risk for or are developing AKI is of absolute paramountcy. Volume overload appears to be a consistent and important marker of increased morbidity and mortality in the PICU [9, 35, 92, 107]. Volume overload is directly associated with significant derangements in cardiovascular and respiratory function. Therefore, once AKI has been recognized, the daily fluid intake should be adjusted to equal the daily output. Output includes both insensible losses, estimated to be 500 mL m^{-2} day^{-1}, as well as urine output. Insensible losses should be replaced with 5% dextrose, while urinary losses should be replaced with intravenous fluid matching the urinary electrolyte profile. As discussed in previous chapter of this textbook, electrolyte and acid–base homeostasis also require meticulous management.

7.4.2 Diuretics

Diuretics are frequently used in the PICU for the management of volume overload. Historically, diuretics have been used in critically ill patients in an attempt to *jump start* the kidneys and reestablish adequate urine output in the setting of oliguria [11, 103]. For example, Anderson et al. reported a reduction in mortality from 50 to 26% in critically ill adults with oliguria and AKI with the use of high-dose diuretic therapy [2]. Unfortunately, several investigators have been unable to replicate these findings [11, 103, 115]. A systematic review found that diuretics alone could not prevent AKI in critically ill patients [49]. More importantly, the Project to Improve Care on Acute Renal Disease (PICARD) study group that reported the results of a large cohort study involving over 500 critically ill patients from 1989 to 1995 suggested that the use of diuretics to convert oliguric to nonoliguric AKI was associated with a significant increase in the risk of death or nonrecovery of renal function (odds ratio: 1.77; 95% confidence interval: 1.14–2.76) [70]. A more recent cohort study involving over 50 centers in more than 20 countries and over 1,700 patients showed that while diuretics were not associated with increased mortality, there was no appreciable benefit either [109]. Therefore, while the use of diuretics does not alter the natural history of AKI, they can potentially simplify fluid, electrolyte, and nutritional management.

7.4.3 Fenoldopam

As discussed in the preceding section, there is no evidence to support the routine use of so-called *renal-dose* dopamine for the prevention or management of AKI [47, 49, 50, 60, 115]. Recently, however, there has been growing interest in the selective dopaminergic-1 receptor agonist, fenoldopam. Similar to renal-dose dopamine, fenoldopam has been shown to improve renal blood flow and decrease serum creatinine [50, 115]. More interesting, a recently published meta-analysis of 16 randomized studies involving over 1,200 critically ill adults showed that fenoldopam consistently and significantly reduced the risk for AKI [59]. While there is still insufficient experience with the use of fenoldopam in critically ill children [102], a recent retrospective review suggested that fenoldopam may improve urine output in critically ill neonates following cardiopulmonary bypass [24].

7.4.4 *N*-acetylcysteine

While the administration of NAC may be effective in the prevention of radiographic contrast nephropathy (see preceding discussion and Chap. 21), there is currently no evidence that routine administration of NAC prevents AKI in critically ill patients [11, 40, 50, 53, 115]. There are several potential reasons to be optimistic, however, as the reasons for the failure of these trials may be related more to the lack of early recognition and intervention than to the efficacy of the drug itself. Animal models have taught us that while AKI can be effectively prevented and/or treated by several maneuvers, there is an extremely narrow *window of opportunity* to accomplish this, and treatment must be instituted very early after the initiating insult [100]. Unfortunately, the lack of early biomarkers of renal injury in humans has hitherto crippled our ability to launch these potentially effective therapies in a timely manner. Not surprisingly, clinical studies to date examining a variety of promising interventions have been uniformly unsuccessful, primarily because the treatments were initiated based on elevation of serum creatinine, a late and unreliable measure of kidney function in AKI [14, 29, 31, 78, 79, 100, 105]. The recent identification of several promising biomarkers of early AKI [28] offers a reason to be optimistic for the potential of drugs such as NAC to prevent AKI in critically ill patients.

7.5 Pharmacology of Diuretics

As stated in the preceding paragraphs, diuretics are among the most frequently used medications in the PICU. Therefore, a thorough understanding of the pharmacology of these medications is warranted. The interested reader is referred to several excellent recent reviews for additional information [5, 15, 30, 67, 112]. The most commonly used diuretics are listed in Table 7.2.

7.5.1 Carbonic Anhydrase Inhibitors

Acetazolamide is a derivative of the sulfonamide antibiotic, sulfanilamide – sulfanilamide was frequently noted to cause a diuresis and metabolic acidosis as a side effect, which was subsequently attributed to inhibition of the enzyme, carbonic anhydrase [15]. The diuretic effects of acetazolamide first require secretion into the proximal tubular lumen by the OAT1 and OAT3 organic acid transporters [112]. Carbonic

Table 7.2 Diuretic quick reference

Diuretic	Dose	Dosing interval	Site of action	Mechanism of action
Furosemide	Oral: 1–2 mg kg^{-1} dose^{-1}	Oral: every 6–8 h	Ascending loop of Henle and distal renal tubule	Inhibits reabsorption of sodium and chloride, interfering with the chloride-binding cotransport system
	I.V.: 1–2 mg kg^{-1} dose^{-1}	I.V.: every 6–12 h		
Bumetanide	Oral, I.V.: 0.015–0.1 mg kg^{-1} dose^{-1}	Oral, I.V.: every 6–24 h	Ascending loop of Henle and proximal renal tubule	Inhibits reabsorption of sodium and chloride, interfering with the chloride-binding cotransport system
Ethacrynic acid	Oral: 1 mg kg^{-1} dose^{-1}	Oral: once daily	Ascending loop of Henle and distal renal tubule	Inhibits reabsorption of sodium and chloride, interfering with the chloride-binding cotransport system
	I.V.: 1 mg kg^{-1} dose^{-1}	I.V.: every 8–12 h[a]		
Acetazolamide	Oral, I.V.: 5 mg kg^{-1} dose^{-1}	Oral, I.V.: 1–3 times per day	Proximal tubular lumen	Competitive, reversible inhibition of the enzyme carbonic anhydrase; increased renal excretion of sodium, potassium, bicarbonate, and water
Metolazone	Oral: 0.1–0.2 mg kg^{-1} day^{-1}	Oral: every 12–24 h	Cortical diluting site and proximal convoluted tubules	Inhibits sodium reabsorption
Mannitol	I.V.: 0.25^{-1} g kg^{-1}	I.V.: every 4–6 h	Proximal tubule and thick ascending loop of Henle	Increases the osmotic pressure of glomerular filtrate
Spironolactone	Oral: 0.5–2 mg kg^{-1} dose^{-1}	Oral: every 6–12 h	Distal tubules	Aldosterone antagonist; decreased potassium secretion and decreased sodium and chloride reabsorption
Amiloride	Oral: 0.2–625 mg kg^{-1} dose^{-1}	Oral: every 12–24 h	Distal tubules	Directly inhibit sodium reabsorption through the sodium channels
Chlorothiazide[b]	Oral: 10 mg kg^{-1} dose^{-1}	Oral: every 12 h	Distal tubules	Inhibit the thiazide-sensitive Na$^+$/Cl$^-$ cotransporter; decreasing reabsorption of sodium
	I.V.: 2–4 mg kg^{-1} dose^{-1}	I.V.: every 8–24 h		
Hydrochloro-thiazide	Oral: 1–1.5 mg kg^{-1} dose^{-1}	Oral: every 12 h	Distal tubules	Inhibit the thiazide-sensitive Na$^+$/Cl$^-$ cotransporter; decreasing reabsorption of sodium

[a] Repeat dosing is not usually recommended
[b] Effectively administered 30–60 min prior to loop diuretics

anhydrase facilitates virtually all of the bicarbonate that is filtered by the glomerulus. By inhibiting carbonic anhydrase, acetazolamide results in decreased reabsorption of sodium and bicarbonate, resulting in reduced water reabsorption. However, most of the sodium is reabsorbed at the thick ascending loop of Henle, thereby accounting for the relatively weak diuretic effect of this class of medications. Increased delivery of sodium to the distal tubule leads to increased potassium loss. The two most common side effects of acetazolamide are therefore metabolic acidosis and hypokalemia. Acetazolamide is occasionally used in patients with hypochloremic metabolic alkalosis secondary to diuretic use (i.e., loop diuretics) [75].

7.5.2 Osmotic Diuretics

Mannitol is freely filtered by the glomerulus and is not reabsorbed, and its osmotic effect prevents reabsorption of sodium (and hence, water) at the proximal tubule and thick ascending loop of Henle. The onset of action is rapid, and the drug is eliminated by the kidney relatively quickly. Mannitol is rarely used as a diuretic in the clinical setting, and there is no evidence to support the practice of mannitol administration to patients with AKI in an attempt to *flush* the kidneys [15, 50, 115].

7.5.3 Loop Diuretics

The loop diuretics are the most potent diuretics in clinical use today. They require transport into the proximal tubular lumen by the organic anion transporters, OAT1 and OAT2 [112]. Here, the loop diuretics inhibit carbonic anhydrase, but their main site of action is the $Na^+/K^+/2Cl^-$ transporter in the thick ascending loop of Henle. They bind to the chloride binding site of the transporter to inhibit virtually all of the sodium reabsorption (20–30% of all sodium reabsorption in the nephron) that occurs in the loop of Henle [15, 30, 112]. Blockade of the $N^+/K^+/2Cl^-$ transporter also decreases potassium secretion and chloride reabsorption – the result is a decrease in the luminal-positive transepithelial potential difference, which thereby inhibits paracellular reabsorption of sodium, calcium, and magnesium. Increased sodium delivery to the distal tubule causes a compensatory increase in sodium reabsorption, which leads to increased potassium secretion. The most common side effects of this class of diuretics are therefore hypocalcemia, hypomagnesemia, and hypokalemia. It is also important to note that larger doses of the

loop diuretics must be administered in patients with AKI to assure adequate drug delivery to the proximal tubule. Traditionally, loop diuretics have been administered orally or intravenously via intermittent dosing. The trade name for furosemide, in fact, derives from the fact that the diuretic effects of furosemide lasted approximately 6 h (*last six*). Alternatively, continuous intravenous infusions of furosemide have been used in critically ill children to achieve a more predictable urine output with decreased urinary losses of sodium and chloride, decreased total drug requirements, and less hemodynamic instability [52, 65, 97, 111]. Additionally, continuous dosing permits more gentle fluid shifts, allowing diuresis in the critically ill patient who may be at risk for hemodynamic instability.

7.5.4 Thiazide Diuretics

Thiazide diuretics also require transport into the proximal tubular lumen by OAT1 and OAT3 [112]. This class of diuretics also blocks carbonic anhydrase at the proximal tubule, prior to delivery to the distal tubule where they exert most of their effects. The thiazide diuretics inhibit the thiazide-sensitive Na^+/Cl^- cotransporter, thereby decreasing reabsorption of sodium, potassium, and chloride. There is no significant change in the luminal-positive transepithelial difference, and therefore thiazides do not result in calcium or magnesium wasting in the urine. While thiazides are generally ineffective in patients with low GFR (GFR < 30 mL min^{-1} per $1.73 m^2$), coadministration of thiazides will increase the efficacy of the loop diuretics [15, 30, 112]. Blockade of sodium reabsorption in the distal tubule by the thiazides will decrease the compensatory increase in sodium reabsorption in the distal tubule that commonly occurs with administration of the loop diuretics. Metolazone is unique among the thiazides, in its ability to inhibit reabsorption of sodium in the proximal tubule in addition to the distal tubule effects. By blocking proximal tubular reabsorption of sodium and perpetuating substrate delivery to the loop of Henle, metolazone further enhances loop diuretic effects [30].

7.5.5 Potassium-Sparing Diuretics

Potassium sparing diuretics (amiloride, triamterene) are secreted into the proximal tubular lumen by the organic cation transporter, OCT2. These diuretics directly inhibit sodium reabsorption through the sodium channels in the distal tubule, which also leads to decreased potassium secretion and chloride reabsorption. Spironolactone is also included in this category, but unlike all of the other diuretics, spironolactone does not have to reach the tubular lumen to exert its effects. Rather, spironolactone is an aldosterone antagonist, and by blocking the mineralocorticoid receptor, causes decreased potassium secretion and decreased sodium and chloride reabsorption [15, 112].

Take-Home Pearls

> AKI often causes alterations in the patient's elimination of medications, drug distribution, and metabolites.
> NSAID effects are compounded in critically ill children potentially leading to AKI via renal vasoconstriction, a decrease in renal blood flow, and a rapid decline in glomerular filtration.
> Inulin clearance is the gold standard for measurement of GFR, though creatinine clearance calculated using the Schwartz formula is a most frequently used estimate of GFR in children.
> During hemodialysis, the most efficient removal occurs of medications with a molecular weight of less than 500 Da, less than 90% protein binding, and small volumes of distribution.
> Volume overload associated with AKI appears to be a consistent and important marker of increased morbidity and mortality in the PICU.
> Renal-dose dopamine does not affect either the incidence of AKI or outcome, though fenoldopam may provide renal protection via dopamingergic-1 receptor agonism.
> Loop diuretics are the most potent diuretics in use, though they often require higher doses in AKI for delivery of the drug to the proximal tubule.

References

1. Akcan-Arikan A, Zappitelli M, Loftis LL et al. (2007) Modified RIFLE criteria in critically ill children with acute kidney injury. Kidney Int 71:1028–1035
2. Anderson RJ, Linas SL, Berns AS et al. (1977) Nonoliguric acute renal failure. N Engl J Med 296:1134–1138
3. Aweeka FT, Gottwald MD, Gambertoglio JG et al. (1999) Pharmacokinetics of fosphenytoin in patients with hepatic or renal disease. Epilepsia 40(6):777–782
4. Bagshaw SM, Mortis G, Doig CJ et al. (2006) One-year mortality assessment in critically ill patients by severity of kidney dysfunction: A population-based assessment. Am J Kidney Dis 48:402–409
5. Bagshaw SM, Delaney A, Haase M (2007) Loop diuretics in the management of acute renal failure: A systematic review and meta-analysis. Crit Care Resusc 9:60–68
6. Bailey D, Phan V, Litalien C et al. (2007) Risk factors of acute renal failure in critically ill children: A prospective descriptive epidemiological study. Pediatr Crit Care Med 8:29–35
7. Becker-Cohen R, Frishberg Y (2001) Severe reversible renal failure due to naproxen-associated acute interstitial nephritis. Eur J Pediatr 160:293–295
8. Benko A, Fraser-Hill M, Magner P (2007) Canadian Association of Radiologists: Consensus guidelines for the prevention of contrast-induced nephropathy. Can Assoc Radiol J 58:79–87
9. Benoit G, Phan V, Duval M (2007) Fluid balance of pediatric hematopoietic stem cell transplant recipients and intensive care unit admission. Pediatr Nephrol 22:441–447
10. Bianchetti MG, Roduit C, Oetliker OH (1991) Acyclovir-induced renal failure: Course and risk factors. Pediatr Nephrol 5:238–239
11. Block CA, Manning HL (2002) Prevention of acute renal failure in the critically ill. Am J Respir Crit Care Med 165(3):320–324
12. Bohler J, Donauer J, Keller F (1999) Pharmacokinetic principles during continuous renal replacement therapy: Drugs and dosage. Kidney Int 56 Suppl 72:S24–S28
13. Boucher BA, Wood GC, Swanson JM (2006) Pharmacokinetic changes in critical illness. Crit Care Clin 22:255–271
14. Brady H, Singer G (1995) Acute renal failure. Lancet 346:1533–1540
15. Brater DC (2000) Pharmacology of diuretics. Am J Med Sci 319:38–50
16. Brier ME, Stalker DJ, Aronoff GR et al. (2003) Pharmacokinetics of linezolid in subjects with renal dysfunction. Antimicrob Agents Chemother 47(9):2775–2780
17. Briquori C, Tavano D, Colombo A (2003) Contrast agent-associated nephrotoxicity. Prog Cardiovasc Dis 45:493–503
18. Brivet FG, Kleinknecht DJ, Loirat P et al. (1996) Acute renal failure in intensive care units – Causes, outcome, and prognostic factors of hospital mortality: A prospective, multicenter study French Study Group on Acute Renal Failure. Crit Care Med 24:192–198
19. Cantley LG, Spokes K, Clark B et al. (1993) Role of endothelin and prostaglandins in radiocontrast-induced renal artery constriction. Kidney Int 44:1217–1223
20. Ceneviva G, Paschall JA, Maffei F et al. (1998) Hemodynamic support in fluid refractory pediatric septic shock. Pediatrics 102:e19
21. Chatellier D, Jourdain M, Mangalaboyi J (2002) Cefepime-induced neurotoxicity: An underestimated complication of antibiotherapy in patients with acute renal failure. Intensive Care Med 28(2):214–217
22. Chien C-C, King LS, Rabb H (2004) Mechanisms underlying combined acute renal failure and acute lung injury in the intensive care unit. Contrib Nephrol 144:53–62
23. Clermont G, Acker CG, Angus DC et al. (2002) Renal failure in the ICU: Comparison of the impact of acute renal failure and end-stage renal disease on ICU outcomes. Kidney Int 62:986–996
24. Costello JM, Thiagarajan RR, Dionne RE et al. (2006) Initial experience with fenoldopam after cardiac surgery in neonates with an insufficient response to conventional diuretics. Pediatr Crit Care Med 7:28–33

25. Daschner M (2005) Drug dosage in children with reduced renal function. Pediatr Nephrol 20(12):1675–1686

26. de Mendonca A, Vincent JL, Suter PM et al. (2000) Acute renal failure in the ICU: Risk factors and outcome evaluated by the SOFA score. Intensive Care Med 26:915–921

27. Deray G (2002) Amphotericin B nephrotoxicity. J Antimicrob Chemother 49 Suppl 1:37–41

28. Devarajan P (2007) Emerging biomarkers of acute kidney injury. Contrib Nephrol 156:203–212

29. DuBose TDJ, Warnock DG, Mehta RL et al. (1997) Acute renal failure in the 21st century: Recommendations for management and outcomes assessment. Am J Kidney Dis 29:793–799

30. Eades SK, Christensen ML (1998) The clinical pharmacology of loop diuretics in the pediatric patient. Pediatr Nephrol 12:603–616

31. Edelstein CL, Ling H, Schrier R (1997) The nature of renal cell injury. Kidney Int 51:1341–1351

32. Ellis D, Fried WA, Yunis EJ et al. (1981) Acute interstitial nephritis in children: A report of 13 cases and review of the literature. Pediatrics 67:862–870

33. Felmet KA, Hall MW, Clark RSB et al. (2005) Prolonged lymphopenia, lymphoid depletion, and hypoprolactinemia in children with nosocomial sepsis and multiple organ failure. J Immunol 174:3765–3772

34. Feltes TF, Pignatelli R, Kleinart S et al. (1994) Quantitated left ventricular systolic mechanics in children with septic shock utilizing noninvasive wall-stress analysis. Crit Care Med 22:1647–1658

35. Foland JA, Fortenberry JD, Warshaw BL et al. (2004) Fluid overload before continuous hemofiltration and survival in critically ill children: A retrospective analysis. Crit Care Med 32:1771–1776

36. Fujisaki K, Kubo M, Masuda K et al. (2003) Infusion of radiocontrast agents induces exaggerated release of urinary endothelin in patients with impaired renal function. Clin Exp Nephrol 7:279–283

37. Gaspari F, Perico N, Remuzzi G (1997) Measurement of glomerular filtration rate. Kidney Int 63:S151–S154

38. Goldman RD, Koren G (2004) Amphotericin B nephrotoxicity in children. J Pediatr Hematol Oncol 26:421–426

39. Gupta A, Daggett C, Drant S (2004) Prospective randomized trial of ketorolac after congenital heart surgery. J Cardiothorac Vasc Anesth 18:454–457

40. Haase M, Haase-Fielitz A, Bagshaw SM (2007) Phase II, randomized, controlled trial of high-dose N-acetylcysteine in high-risk cardiac surgery patients. Crit Care Med 35:1324–1331

41. Hemstreet BA (2001) Use of sucralfate in renal failure. Ann Pharmacother 35(3):360–364

42. Hirsch R, Dent C, Pfriem H et al. (2007) NGAL is an early predictive biomarker of contrast-induced nephropathy in children. Pediatr Nephrol 22:2089–2095

43. Hock R, Anderson RJ (1995) Prevention of drug-induced nephrotoxicity in the intensive care unit. J Crit Care 10:33–43

44. Hoste EAJ, De Waele JJ (2005) Physiologic consequences of acute renal failure on the critically ill. Crit Care Clin 21:251–260

45. Hui-Stickle S, Brewer ED, Goldstein SL (2005) Pediatric ARF epidemiology at a tertiary care center from 1999 to 2001. Am J Kidney Dis 45:96–101

46. Izzedine H, Launay-Vacher V, Deray G (2005) Antiviral drug-induced nephrotoxicity. Am J Kidney Dis 45:804–817

47. Jones D, Bellomo R (2005) Renal-dose dopamine: From hypothesis to paradigm to dogma to myth and, finally, superstition? J Intensive Care Med 20:199–211

48. Joy MS, Matzke GR, Armstrong DK et al. (1998) A primer on continuous renal replacement therapy for critically ill patients. Ann Pharmacother 32:362–375

49. Kellum JA (1997) The use of diuretics and dopamine in acute renal failure: A systematic review of the evidence. Crit Care 1:53–59

50. Kellum JA, Leblanc M, Gibney RT et al. (2005) Primary prevention of acute renal failure in the critically ill. Curr Opin Crit Care 11:537–541

51. Kist-van Holthe tot Echten JE, Goedvolk CA, Doornaar MB et al. (2001) Acute renal insufficiency and renal replacement therapy after pediatric cardiopulmonary bypass surgery. Pediatr Cardiol 22:321–326

52. Klinge JM, Scharf J, Hofbeck M (1997) Intermittent administration of furosemide versus continuous infusion in the postoperative management of children following open heart surgery. Intensive Care Med 23:693–697

53. Komisarof JA, Gilkey GM, Peters DM (2007) N-acetylcysteine for patients with prolonged hypotension as prophylaxis for acute renal failure (NEPHRON). Crit Care Med 35:435–441

54. Kovacevic L, Bernstein J, Valentini RP et al. (2003) Renal papillary necrosis induced by naproxen. Pediatr Nephrol 18:826–829

55. Krause I, Cleper R, Eisenstein B et al. (2005) Acute renal failure, associated with non-steroidal anti-inflammatory drugs in healthy children. Pediatr Nephrol 20:1295–1298

56. Krishnan V, Murray P (2003) Pharmacologic issues in the critically ill. Clin Chest Med 24:671–688

57. Kuang D, Verbine A, Ronco C (2007) Pharmacokinetics and antimicrobial dosing adjustment in critically ill patients during continuous renal replacement therapy. Clin Nephrol 67:267–284

58. Lameier NH (2006) Contrast-induced nephropathy – Preven-tion and risk reduction. Nephrol Dial Transplant 21:11–23

59. Landoni G, Biondi-Zoccai GG, Tumlin JA (2007) Beneficial impact of fenoldopam in critically ill patients with or at risk for acute renal failure: A meta-analysis of randomized clinical trials. Am J Kidney Dis 49:56–68

60. Lauschke A, Teichgraber UK, Frei U et al. (2006) 'Low-dose' dopamine worsens renal perfusion in patients with acute renal failure. Kidney Int 69:1669–1674

61. Levy EM, Viscoli CM, Horwitz RI (1996) The effect of acute renal failure on mortality. A cohort analysis. JAMA 275:1489–1494

62. Li JS, Yow E, Berezny KY et al. (2007) Clinical outcomes of palliative surgery including a systemic-to-pulmonary artery shunt in infants with cyanotic congenital heart disease: Does aspirin make a difference? Circulation 116:293–297

63. Lieh-Lai MW, Kauffman RE, Uly HG (1999) A randomized comparison of ketorolac tromethamine and morphine for postoperative analgesia in critically ill children. Crit Care Med 27:2786–2791

64. Livornese LL, Jr, Slavin D, Gilbert B (2004) Use of antibacterial agents in renal failure. Infectious disease. Clin North Am 18(3):551–579, viii–ix

65. Luciani GB, Nichani S, Chang AC (1997) Continuous versus intermittent furosemide infusion in critically ill infants after open heart operation. Ann Thorac Surg 64:1133–1139

66. Marenzi G, Marana I, Lauri G et al. (2003) The prevention of radiocontrast agent-induced nephropathy by hemofiltration. N Engl J Med 349:1333–1340

67. Martin SJ, Danziger LH (1994) Continuous infusion of loop diuretics in the critically ill: A review of the literature. Crit Care Med 22:1323–1329

68. Martinez-Rodriguez JE, Barriga FJ, Santamaria J (2001) Nonconvulsive status epilepticus associated with cephalosporins in patients with renal failure. Am J Med 111(2): 115–119

69. McBryde KD, Wilcox J, Kher KK (2005) Hyperphosphatemia due to fosphenytoin in a pediatric ESRD patient. Pediatr Nephrol 20(8):1182–1185

70. Mehta RL, Pascual MT, Soroko S (2002) Diuretics, mortality, and nonrecovery of renal function in acute renal failure. JAMA 288:2547–2553

71. Mercier J-C, Beaufils F, Hartmann J-F et al. (1988) Hemodynamic patterns of meningococcal shock in children. Crit Care Med 16:27–33

72. Merten GJ, Burgess WP, Gray LV et al. (2004) Prevention of contrast-induced nephropathy with sodium bicarbonate: A randomized controlled trial. JAMA 291:2328–2334

73. Metnitz PG, Krenn CG, Steltzer H et al. (2002) Effect of acute renal failure requiring renal replacement therapy on outcome in critically ill patients. Crit Care Med 30:2051–2058

74. Michel DM, Kelly CJ (1998) Acute interstitial nephritis. J Am Soc Nephrol 9:506–515

75. Moffett BS, Moffett TI, Dickerson HA (2007) Acetazolamide therapy for hypochloremic metabolic alkalosis in pediatric patients with heart disease. Am J Ther 14:331–335

76. Moran SM, Myers BD (1985) Course of acute renal failure studied by a model of creatinine kinetics. Kidney Int 27:928–937

77. Mouton JW, Touzw DJ, Horrevorts AM et al. (2000) Comparative pharmacokinetics of the carbapenems: Clinical implications. Clin Pharmacokinet 39(3): 185–201

78. Nolan CR, Anderson RJ (1998) Hospital-acquired acute renal failure. J Am Soc Nephrol 9:710–718

79. Paller MS (1998) Acute renal failure: Controversies, clinical trials, and future directions. Semin Nephrol 18:482–489

80. Papachristou F, Printza N, Farmaki E (2006) Antibiotics-induced acute interstitial nephritis in six children. Urol Int 76:348–352

81. Parr GV, Blackstone EH, Kirklin JW (1975) Cardiac performance and mortality early after intracardiac surgery in infants and young children. Circulation 51:867–874

82. Perazella MA, Parikh C (2005) Pharmacology. Am J Kidney Dis 46:1129–1139

83. Plotz FB, Hulst HE, Twist JW et al. (2005) Effect of acute renal failure on outcome in children with severe septic shock. Pediatr Nephrol 20:1177–1181

84. Pollack MM, Fields AI, Ruttiman UE (1984) Sequential cardiopulmonary variables of infants and children in septic shock. Crit Care Med 12:554–559

85. Pollack MM, Fields AI, Ruttiman UE (1985) Distributions of cardiopulmonary variables in pediatric survivors and nonsurvivors of septic shock. Crit Care Med 13:454–459

86. Rahn KH, Heidenreich S, Bruckner D (1999) How to assess glomerular function and damage in humans. J Hypertens 17(3):309–317

87. Reynolds EM, Ryan DP, Sheridan RL et al. (1995) Left ventricular failure complicating severe pediatric burn injuries. J Pediatr Surg 30:264–270

88. Sakr Y, Reinhart K, Vincent JL et al. (2006) Does dopamine administration in shock influence outcome? Results of the Sepsis Occurrence in Acutely Ill Patients (SOAP) Study. Crit Care 34:589–597

89. Sarrell EM, Wielunsky E, Cohen HA (2006) Antipyretic treatment in young children with fever: Acetaminophen, ibuprofen, or both alternating in a randomized, double-blind study. Arch Pediatr Adolesc Med 160:197–202

90. Schaller S, Kaplan BS (1998) Acute nonoliguric renal failure in children associated with nonsteroidal antiinflammatory agents. Pediatr Emerg Care 14:416–418

91. Schetz M (2007) Drug dosing in continuous renal replacement therapy: General rules. Curr Opin Crit Care 13:645–651

92. Schroeder VA, DiSessa TG, Douglas WI (2004) Postoperative fluid balance influences the need for antihypertensive therapy following coarctation repair. Pediatr Crit Care Med 5:539–541

93. Schwartz GJ, Feld LG, Langford DJ (1984) A simple estimate of glomerular filtration rate in full-term infants during the first year of life. J Pediatr 104(6):849–854

94. Schwartz GJ, Gauthier B (1985) A simple estimate of glomerular filtration rate in adolescent boys. J Pediatr 106(3):522–526

95. Schwartz GJ, Haycock GB, Edelmann CM, Jr, et al. (1976) A simple estimate of glomerular filtration rate in children derived from body length and plasma creatinine. Pediatrics 58(2):259–263

96. Schweiger MJ, Chambers CE, Davidson CJ et al. (2007) Prevention of contrast induced nephopathy: Recommendations for the high risk patient undergoing cardiovascular procedures. Catheter Cardiovasc Interv 69:135–140

97. Singh NC, Kissoon N, al Mofada S (1992) Comparison of continuous versus intermittent furosemide administration in postoperative pediatric cardiac patients. Crit Care Med 20:17–21

98. Skippen PW, Krahn GE (2005) Acute renal failure in children undergoing cardiopulmonary bypass. Crit Care Resusc 7:286–291

99. Smith PF, Morse GD (1999) Accuracy of measured vancomycin serum concentrations in patients with end-stage renal disease. Ann Pharmacother 33(12):1329–1335

100. Star RA (1998) Treatment of acute renal failure. Kidney Int 54:1817–1831

101. Stevens LA, Coresh J, Greene T et al. (2006) Assessing kidney function – Measured and estimated glomerular filtration rate. N Engl J Med 354:2473–2483

102. Strauser LM, Pruitt RD, Tobias JD (1999) Initial experience with fenoldopam in children. Am J Ther 6:283–289

103. Subramanian S, Ziedalski TM (2005) Oliguria, volume overload, Na+ balance, and diuretics. Crit Care Clin 21:291–303

104. Taber SS, Mueller BA (2006) Drug-associated renal dysfunction. Crit Care Clin 22:357–374

105. Thadhani R, Bonventre JV (1996) Acute renal failure. N Engl J Med 334:1448–1460

106. Thorburn K, Samuel M, Smith EA et al. (2001) Aluminum accumulation in critically ill children on sucralfate therapy. Pediatr Crit Care Med 2(3):247–249

107. Tomaske M, Bosk A, Eyrich M et al. (2003) Risks of mortality in children admitted to the paediatric intensive care unit after haematopoietic stem cell transplantation. Br J Haematol 121:886–891

108. Uchino S (2006) The epidemiology of acute renal failure in the world. Curr Opin Crit Care 12:538–543

109. Uchino S, Doig GS, Bellomo R et al. (2004) Diuretics and mortality in acute renal failure. Crit Care Med 32:1669–1677

110. Vachvanichsanong P, Patamasucon P, Malagon M et al. (1995) Acute renal failure in a child associated with acyclovir. Pediatr Nephrol 9:346–347

111. van der Vorst MM, Ruys-Dudok van Heel I, Kist-van Holthe JE (2001) Continuous intravenous furosemide in haemodynamically unstable children after cardiac surgery. Intensive Care Med 27:711–715

112. van der Vorst MMJ, Kist JE, van der Heijden AJ (2006) Diuretics in pediatrics: Current knowledge and future prospects. Pediatr Drugs 8:245–264

113. Van Overmeire B, Smets K, Lecoutere D (2007) A comparison of ibuprofen and indomethacin for closure of patent ductus arteriosus. N Engl J Med 343:674–681

114. Veltri MA, Neu AM, Fivush BA (2004) Drug dosing during intermittent hemodialysis and continuous renal replacement therapy: Special considerations in pediatric patients. Pediatr Drugs 6:45–65

115. Venkataraman R, Kellum JA (2007) Prevention of acute renal failure. Chest 131:300–308

116. Whelton A (1999) Nephrotoxicity of nonsteroidal anti-inflammatory drugs: Physiologic foundations and clinical implications. Am J Med 106:13S–24S

117. Wilkins RG, Faragher EB (1983) Acute renal failure in an intensive care unit: Incidence, prediction and outcome. Anaesthesia 38:628–634

118. Williams DM, Sreedhar SS, Mickell JS, et al. (2002) Acute kidney failure: A pediatric experience over 20 years. Arch Pediatr Adolesc Med 156:893–900

119. Zellweger R, Wichmann MW, Ayala A (1996) A novel and safe immunomodulating hormone for the treatment of immunodepression following severe hemorrhage. J Surg Res 63:53–58

Renal Replacement Therapy in the ICU

8

K.E. Luckritz and J.M. Symons

Contents

Case Vignette

A 9-year-old boy who underwent mismatched unrelated donor stem cell transplant for acute lymphocytic leukemia, complicated by graft-vs.-host disease treated with steroids, cyclosporine, and tacrolimus, develops

S.G. Kiessling et al. (eds) *Pediatric Nephrology in the ICU.*
© Springer-Verlag Berlin Heidelberg 2009

> **Core Messages**
>
> › Physical principles of dialysis
> › Renal replacement modalities
>   – Peritoneal dialysis
>   – Hemodialysis
>   – Continuous renal replacement therapies (CRRT)
> › General techniques for renal replacement in the ICU
> › Comparison of renal replacement modalities
> › Outcomes of renal replacement therapy

bacteremia and sepsis. He is transferred to the pediatric intensive care unit where he receives volume resuscitation, intubation, and mechanical ventilation. At the time of intubation, bloody secretions come up from the endotracheal tube, suggesting alveolar hemorrhage. He becomes hypotensive and requires support with vasopressor infusion. The critical care team consults the nephrology service that recommends CRRT for volume and metabolic control, using citrate regional anticoagulation to avoid systemic heparinization. Hemodynamic instability limits fluid removal; for the first 72 h of CRRT, the patient achieves even fluid balance and does not become more fluid overloaded. With improving blood pressure and discontinuation of vasopressors, the net ultrafiltration rate is increased and the child has a negative fluid balance over the next week, returning him to his appropriate volume status. CRRT continues to maintain metabolic status and neutral fluid balance while the patient receives parenteral nutrition and other intravenous medications. After 14 days of mechanical ventilation, the patient's respiratory status recovers and he is extubated. The critical care team is able to adjust his regimen such that full daily nutrition and medications are provided in a volume less than 1,000 mL, which permits transition to intermittent hemodialysis. Over the next few weeks, urine output begins to increase and renal function improves. Intermittent hemodialysis is discontinued when the patient can maintain fluid and metabolic balance on his own.

8.1 Introduction/History

The indications for renal replacement therapy in the pediatric intensive care unit vary and, with advances in care, children may now be supported through the initial phases of a critical illness to the point where renal dysfunction complicates ongoing care. Modalities of dialysis used in the ICU setting include intermittent hemodialysis, peritoneal dialysis, and CRRT. The modality utilized in each child depends on clinical circumstances and local resources. To date, no randomized trials have been performed in pediatric patients investigating indications or outcomes of the various modalities of renal replacement therapy.

8.2 Principles of Dialysis

All dialysis systems operate by leveraging physical principles that govern molecular movement between solutions separated by a semipermeable membrane. A brief review of these properties is provided later and greater detail can be found in texts devoted to dialysis methods [9, 37].

8.2.1 Diffusion

Diffusion is defined as "the random movement of molecules or ions or small particles in solution or sus-

pension under the influence of Brownian (thermal) motion toward a uniform distribution throughout the available volume [32]." As illustrated in Fig. 8.1a, two solutions, separated by a semipermeable membrane, will eventually reach equilibrium as solutes randomly move across the membrane from the more concentrated solution A to the less concentrated solution B. Solutes in higher concentration in solution B will flow in the reverse. Eventually this traffic across the membrane will be equal in both directions and the two solutions will be in equilibrium. Smaller molecules will tend to diffuse more easily than larger molecules.

8.2.2 Convection

Convection refers to the movement of molecules across a semipermeable membrane due to a pressure gradient, rather than a concentration gradient as described in diffusion. This phenomenon can be imagined by a piston pushing down on one of the two solutions described earlier (Fig. 8.1b). The positive pressure *pushes* molecules small enough to pass through the membrane pores to the other side. Since convection does not depend on the random movement and energy of individual particles to cause molecular transit, small and larger molecules tend to pass across the membrane with equal efficiency, up to the size limit of the membrane pores. Convective movement of particles can be achieved through positive pressure as described earlier or through application of negative pressure to *pull* molecules across the semipermeable membrane.

8.2.3 Ultrafiltration

Ultrafiltration refers to the movement of water molecules across a semipermeable membrane under the

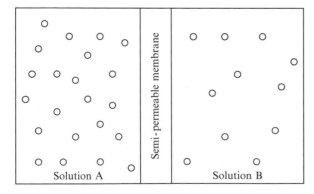

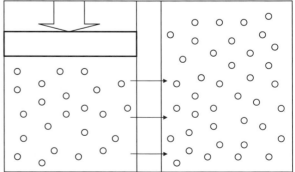

Fig. 8.1 **a** *Diffusion*: solution A has a greater concentration of solute than solution B. With the random movement of molecules across the membrane, the two solutions will reach equilibrium.

b *Convection*: hydrostatic pressure forces molecules across the semipermeable membrane effects of pressure. The physical principles are the same as convection. Particles dissolved in solution will also traverse the semipermeable membrane with the water flux, although solute movement or so-called solute drag will be limited again by the pore size of the membrane.

8.3   Modalities: Peritoneal Dialysis

Peritoneal dialysis (PD) utilizes the peritoneal membrane as the filter for dialysis. PD requires a surgically implanted catheter to access the abdominal compartment. A dialysate solution is placed into the abdomen; it dwells for a period of time and is later drained, effectively removing wastes and fluid that have been filtered by the peritoneal membrane. In PD, molecular mass transfer is mostly by diffusion or concentration differences between the peritoneal vascular space and the dialysate. Ultrafiltration occurs through osmotic pressure generated by osmotically active particles in the dialysate, usually dextrose, and there is some concomitant convective solute transfer in the fluid removed by ultrafiltration.

8.3.1   Advantages/Disadvantages

Benefits of PD for pediatric patients include the relative ease with which it can be performed, limiting the need for specialized equipment or specially trained personnel [12]. PD requires no extracorporeal perfusion and therefore no vascular access, relying instead on the peritoneal membrane as an innate filter. Electrolyte and fluid shifts are more gradual with PD as compared with other modalities such as intermittent hemodialysis; for this reason, PD may be preferred with critically ill pediatric patients in whom there is concern about cardiovascular stability [12, 31]. PD also avoids the risks of systemic anticoagulation required for modalities that employ extracorporeal perfusion.

Despite these benefits of PD, some clinical situations are better treated with hemodialysis. These include acute intoxications, hyperkalemia, severe metabolic imbalances, or profound fluid overload where the gradual shifts of PD may not provide a rapid enough response to preclude significant morbidity or mortality. Extensive abdominal surgery may be a contraindication for PD but patients should be evaluated individually in consultation with the surgeon. Eagle–Barrett (*prune belly*) syndrome and the presence of a ventriculoperitoneal shunt are not considered contraindications [12].

8.3.2   Access

PD requires the placement of a catheter providing access to the abdominal compartment. In the acute situation, a temporary catheter can be placed. This is usually done by blind percutaneous technique making perforation of internal organs a risk. Temporary PD catheters have also been associated with a higher risk of leak and malfunction [7]. A recent study found, however, that the Cook Mac-Loc Multipurpose Drainage catheter [Cook Inc., Bloomington, IN] for acute PD had no greater rate of complications than the traditional surgically placed Tenckhoff catheter [1].

A *permanent* catheter, such as the Tenckhoff style, is used for chronic maintenance PD and can also be employed for acute PD. Permanent catheter placement requires abdominal surgery to tunnel the catheter, ensuring proper catheter placement and limiting the risk of intra-abdominal perforation. Although PD catheters placed for chronic dialysis use are generally allowed to heal for days to weeks prior to first use [26], in the acute setting the catheter can be used immediately. Usually, low fill volumes should be used and care should be taken to monitor for evidence of wound dehiscence or leaking of fluid.

With initial catheter placement, heparin can be added to the dialysate to avoid fibrin deposition and subsequent catheter malfunction. The systemic absorption of heparin is felt to be minimal [13] thus reducing the risk of systemic anticoagulation. The heparin can be mixed directly into the dialysate and is typically started at 500 units L^{-1} of fluid. This is continued for 48 h or until the fluid is no longer bloody [31].

8.3.3   Technique/Prescription

8.3.3.1   Dialysate

Peritoneal dialysis solutions come in a variety of commercially available mixtures with varying concentrations of key electrolytes and dextrose. Dextrose generates an osmotic pressure within the dialysate to cause ultrafiltration of water across the peritoneal membrane. With ultrafiltration, there will also be some convective clearance of molecules small enough to traverse the peritoneal membrane. Some dextrose will be metabolized in the peritoneum, so prolonged dialysate dwells may decrease fluid removal ability as well as provide caloric supplements. In the USA, commercially available dextrose concentrations currently include 1.5, 2.5, and 4.25%. Slightly different concentrations are available in other regions. Icodextrin, a nonabsorbable glucose polymer used instead of dextrose, is also available as an osmotic agent for fluid removal in commercially available dialysate in some countries. It is more appropriate if longer dwells are necessary [31], and thus it may have a limited role in the acute ICU setting.

Currently lactate is the buffer used in peritoneal dialysate solutions available in the USA. Absorbed lactate is converted to bicarbonate by the liver. In the setting of hepatic dysfunction, such lactate may contribute to a metabolic acidosis.

Commercial dialysate solutions may provide a choice of calcium level but the remaining components tend to be fixed. Commercial dialysate is potassium-free but potassium may be added by pharmacy if potassium losses are excessive. Rare clinical situations may require the use of custom-made peritoneal dialysate prepared through the local pharmacy but extreme care must be taken with quality control measures in place to prevent inadvertent errors and potentially disastrous clinical consequences.

8.3.3.2 Volume

Therapy is usually initiated at low fill volumes of 10–20 mL kg^{-1} and gradually increased to a long-term goal of 40–50 mL kg^{-1} [16, 31]. Care must be taken to follow for discomfort and signs of leaking or hernias as the volumes are increased [16].

8.3.3.3 Dwell Times

Since the membrane properties of peritoneal dialysis are fixed, it is the dialysate flow rate that will determine clearance. This can be adjusted by volumes (which may be limited in the critically ill period) or the number of exchanges performed in a 24-h period (e.g., dwell times) [29].

Initially, shorter dwell times up to 1 h are recommended [31], but in smaller children and neonates the dwell times may be as short as 15–30 min. Dwell times should be adjusted for the individual patient's ultrafiltration and clearance needs and subsequent response to therapy. Since the critically ill patient is often not ambulatory, PD in the intensive care unit is often provided around the clock to maximize therapy.

The patient can receive PD through manual exchanges of solution or through the use of an automated cycling system. Automated PD using a cycler device can simplify care for bedside staff. The cycler is programmed to fill and drain the patient's abdomen at the prescribed volumes and intervals. For small pediatric patients, the desired prescription may be outside the limits of the

cycler's capabilities. Under such circumstances manual exchanges of fluid must be performed. With either method, the system must be kept closed and careful sterile technique must be employed to limit the chances of infection [31].

8.3.4 Complications

Constipation or bladder distension may obstruct fluid flow through the PD catheter, and stool softeners or bladder drainage may be indicated. Malposition or kinking of the catheter may also limit flow and may require surgical intervention. This is often easily identified with an abdominal X-ray.

Other possible causes of catheter obstruction include fibrin deposition within or covering the catheter or the presence of omentum actually obstructing the pores of the catheter. It is for these reasons that heparin is typically added in the initial dialysate dwells, and a partial omentectomy may be performed at the time of surgical catheter placement, although this is generally reserved for chronic catheter placement. Tissue-type plasminogen activator (tPA) is an effective fibrinolytic that has been successfully used in peritoneal dialysis catheters that remain obstructed despite heparinization and attempts at flushing [30]. Catheter leak or abdominal wall hernia may occur as a result of increased abdominal pressure. Such complications may require reduction of fill volumes or surgical intervention to better secure the catheter.

Peritonitis is a significant complication of peritoneal dialysis, and monitoring for signs of infection must be ongoing in any critically ill patient with a catheter in place. Chronic ambulatory patients with peritonitis may complain of fever or abdominal pain as a presenting symptom. In a critically ill or sedated patient, signs may be as subtle as a rise in acute phase reactants or changes in cardiovascular status. Obvious signs such as fever or cloudy peritoneal effluent require prompt evaluation. Regardless of presenting symptoms, if peritoneal infection is suspected, a sample of the peritoneal effluent should be sent for cell count and gram stain and, if appropriate, bacterial and fungal culture. In patients undergoing PD, peritonitis should be suspected if the white cell count in a sample of recently infused dialysate exceeds 100 cells mm^{-3} with more than 50% neutrophils [35]. Empiric antibiotic therapy may need to be instituted immediately with coverage for both Gram-positive and Gram-negative organisms while awaiting culture results. Intraperitoneal antibiotics are used for the ambulatory patient and can also be employed for the acute patient. Other antibiotic coverages should be customized by patient status. Specific consensus recommendations for peritonitis therapy have been developed and may help in guiding local practice [35].

8.4 Modalities: Hemodialysis

For the purposes of this text, hemodialysis will refer to the generic modality of dialysis utilizing a pumped extracorporeal circuit to move blood past an artificial membrane (dialyzer or hemofilter). A review of properties shared by intermittent hemodialysis and continuous therapies is provided followed by modality-specific descriptions. Advantages and disadvantages will be addressed individually for each modality.

The extracorporeal dialysis circuit is best described by dividing it into a blood circuit and a dialysate circuit. These two circuits interact via the filter (dialyzer) where fluid and solute exchange occurs across an artificial membrane. Blood flow rates, dialysate rates, and types of dialysate will vary with the modality chosen.

8.4.1 Access

Most acute hemodialysis is performed through a hemodialysis catheter. A multilumen catheter placed in the femoral position can usually provide sufficient blood flow for effective emergent therapy. Alternative locations include the jugular and subclavian positions, although the subclavian position is discouraged due to risk of venous stenosis and potential complication for future chronic dialysis access. Temporary catheters can be placed at the bedside by the Seldinger technique, or a tunneled catheter can be placed if long-term therapy is indicated.

To maximize blood flow, the largest gauge catheter that can be placed safely is ideal. Catheter size is often limited by the patient's vessel size. Ideally, a dual-lumen catheter should be placed to allow continuous flow through the dialyzer. If a triple-lumen hemodialysis catheter is available in an appropriate size for the patient, this may be desired if limited vascular access is a concern. In the event that a single-lumen catheter is the largest able to be placed safely, two catheters can be placed to provide continuous flow. If this is not feasible, some dialysis machines can perform single-needle dialysis. This involves the rapid alternation of flow and has similar efficacy [34]. Its use is often limited by

available technology. With the commercial availability of very small diameter multilumen dialysis catheters, use of single-lumen catheters or single-needle dialysis should be extremely rare.

If a chronic dialysis patient presents for critical care support, permanent vascular access for hemodialysis may already be in place. Existing tunneled catheters, mature arteriovenous fistulas, or hemodialysis grafts may be used in this setting. In the ICU, use of any permanent dialysis access should be discussed with the patient's nephrologists and, outside of an acute resuscitation with no other vascular access, should be restricted to dialysis access.

8.4.2 Anticoagulation

Heparin is the most commonly used anticoagulant. Heparin provides systemic anticoagulation and complications from bleeding can occur. A loading dose of $2,000 \, u \, m^{-2}$ body surface area (BSA) may be given at the start of dialysis with a continuous infusion of $400 \, u \, m^{-2} h^{-1}$ for the remainder of the session ($0–50 \, u \, kg^{-1}$ bolus with $0–30 \, u \, kg^{-1} h^{-1}$ maintenance) [31]. Activated partial thromboplastin time (aPTT) or activated clotting time (ACT) can be used to monitor therapy and guide heparin infusion. Goal ACT is $120–180 \, s$ and the aPTT should be 1.2–1.5 times the baseline. Goal levels should be confirmed by the testing modality and equipment used by your facility. Suboptimal anticoagulation of the system can result in insufficient dialysis, clotting of the filter, and blood loss.

When heparin is contraindicated, such as in patients with high risk for bleeding or heparin-induced thrombocytopenia (HIT), other therapies are available. With intermittent hemodialysis, systemic anticoagulation may be omitted and the filter can be flushed frequently with small bolus infusions of saline. In this case, active monitoring of the filter pressures and visual inspection of the filters may allow saline flushes as necessary to prevent clotting. It is important to recognize that each time saline is flushed, time is lost dialyzing and fluid added to the patient's ultrafiltration goal. While this technique may permit successful intermittent hemodialysis sessions lasting only a few hours, continuous therapies performed without anticoagulation tend to have greatly reduced circuit life, and some equipment for CRRT are closed systems precluding access to the filter to allow flushes [4].

Citrate is a commonly used alternative to heparin in continuous therapy and can also be used in intermittent hemodialysis. Its main advantage is the ability to regionally anticoagulate the circuit rather than systemically anticoagulate the patient. More details can be found in the continuous therapy section. Danaparoid and lepirudin are two other anticoagulation alternatives that have been used in dialysis patients with HIT [23, 24]. Prostaglandin E1 and low-molecular-weight heparin [27] have also been successfully used as anticoagulants in continuous hemofiltration [18].

8.4.3 Dialyzers

Most current dialysis filters employ a hollow fiber system in which blood flows through a series of fibers secured together at each end of the dialyzer cartridge with dialysate flowing in a countercurrent direction around the fibers (Fig. 8.2).

Several membrane properties affect dialysis efficiency, often reported as clearance for a particular molecule. These properties include pore size, pore density, and membrane thickness. Dialyzers come in varying sizes depending on the number of filters in each cartridge. Further details on hemodialyzer design can be found in dialysis reference texts [9].

The total available surface area of the dialyzer will often be considered when choosing a dialyzer. The surface area of the dialyzer should approximate the surface area of the patient [31], although some clinical situations may warrant the use of larger dialyzers. The total extracorporeal blood volume should also be determined including necessary tubing and the volume of the dialyzer itself. In the event that the extracorporeal blood volume exceeds 10–15% of the patient's total blood volume, a blood prime is recommended [16]. Depending on the patient's hemodynamic stability, even in circumstances where extracorporeal volume is <10% of estimated blood volume, lines may need to be primed with isotonic saline or albumin.

Two types of membranes are currently in use; cellulose based and synthetic. Because of their decreased antigenicity, synthetic membranes are preferred. Choice of dialyzer type and size is best made in consultation with clinicians familiar with local resources.

Dialyzers made with the synthetic AN69 membrane deserve special mention for their risk of an entity termed bradykinin release syndrome (BRS). This syndrome presents as a sudden sepsis-like or anaphylactic episode with hypotension, tachycardia, vasodilation, and even death [3]. Some devices for CRRT are designed to work only with the AN69 membrane; see section on CRRT for more details. Maneuvers to avoid this reaction have

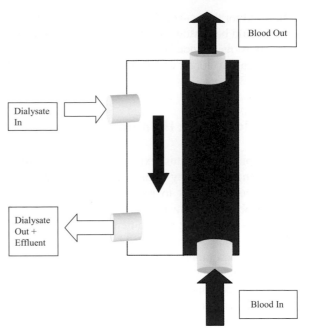

Fig. 8.2 Schematic of counter current flow of dialysate past blood in dialysis filter

been developed and need to be considered in any circuit employing this membrane [3, 17, 25].

8.4.4 Intermittent Hemodialysis

8.4.4.1 Advantages/Disadvantages

When a patient is hemodynamically stable and can tolerate relatively rapid fluid and electrolyte shifts, intermittent hemodialysis has many advantages. The efficiency of mass transfer in intermittent hemodialysis makes it an ideal modality in toxic poisonings, severe electrolyte imbalance, metabolic abnormalities, and acute fluid overload. Hemodialysis also offers the opportunity to perform ultrafiltration without solute removal, as well as allowing titration of the dialysate that may be desired in metabolic derangements such as hypernatremia. Other advantages include an intermittent schedule allowing the patient to be disconnected from the device, whether for further testing, procedures, or for therapeutic mobilization and limited periods of necessary anticoagulation [12].

In a patient who cannot tolerate rapid fluid removal or positive fluid balance in the interdialytic period, or in whom fluid restriction is not feasible, a continuous renal replacement modality may be more appropriate. In the event that equipment for continuous hemofiltration is not available, some hemodialysis machines permit slow extended dialysis sessions, variously termed slow low-efficiency dialysis or slow extended dialysis (SLED). In these modalities, the slower flow rates and less efficient dialysis are compensated for by extended duration of dialysis, allowing for achievement of both adequate solute clearance and ultrafiltration [2, 20].

8.4.4.2 Prescription

There are multiple components to the hemodialysis prescription. Choice and adjustment depends on the clinical situation and available equipment. Special considerations are necessary when performing hemodialysis in a pediatric patient.

Dialyzer: As noted earlier, the dialyzer membrane can be cellulose-based or fully synthetic. Both can function well in the critical care setting. Although a larger dialyzer will permit greater mass transfer per unit time, solute clearance that occurs too rapidly may be problematic in certain clinical settings. The size of the dialyzer is generally not a factor impacting ultrafiltration volumes in critically ill children who usually do not tolerate rapid volume shifts. Dialyzer size may also be limited by the required extracorporeal blood volume, which may exceed a safe volume for the small pediatric patient. Total extracorporeal volume can be reduced by choosing a low-volume tubing set, but if extracorporeal volume remains excessive, blood priming of the extracorporeal circuit may be necessary [16].

Tubing set: Several companies make low-volume tubing sets that may be useful with small children since they can help to limit extracorporeal blood volume. When unable to reduce volume sufficiently, blood prime may be used.

Circuit prime: As discussed earlier, in small children large-volume circuits may require priming with blood to prevent cardiovascular collapse at the time of hemodialysis initiation. The circuit is filled with the priming fluid and then attached to the patient, allowing the priming fluid to enter the circulation. At many pediatric institutions, it is the practice to prime the extracorporeal circuit with a mix of packed red blood cells and 5% albumin when the extracorporeal volume exceeds 10% of the patient's blood volume. Blood prime might also be employed for a patient with severe anemia or profound hypotension. Other patients with concerns regarding hemodynamic instability with initiation of hemodialysis tolerate circuit primes of 5% albumin alone or 0.9% sodium chloride (normal saline). For the very stable or volume overloaded patient, one may initiate hemodialysis with a *self-prime*; no priming fluid would enter the patient in this setting.

Blood flow rate (Q_B): Q_B is often dependent on the adequacy of vascular access. A rough estimate for target flow rate is 6–$8\,mL\,kg^{-1}\,min^{-1}$ up to adult flow rates of 300–$400\,mL\,min^{-1}$ [31]. Inadequate blood flow prevents adequate dialysis and, as such, needs to be addressed promptly. If access is by catheter, which is often the case in children in the ICU with acute renal dysfunction, catheter replacement may need to be considered.

Dialysate flow rate (Q_D): In intermittent hemodialysis, dialysate flow rate is generally kept at least 1.5 times the blood flow rate to insure diffusional gradients. Standard dialysate flow rate is $500\,mL\,min^{-1}$ with many modern dialysis machines allowing flow rates up to $800\,mL\,min^{-1}$ if indicated.

Dialysate composition: Dialysate composition should be altered based on the patient's current electrolyte status. Modern machines for intermittent hemodialysis mix dialysate online from concentrates using a sophisticated proportioning system. The user can vary final concentrations of sodium, calcium, potassium, and bicarbonate according to the clinical situation.

Anticoagulation: Heparin is the most commonly used anticoagulant for intermittent hemodialysis [4], although intermittent hemodialysis sessions for the critically ill patient can at times be performed successfully without anticoagulation or with alternative anticoagulation as detailed earlier in this chapter.

Ultrafiltration plan: Fluid removal is often a key goal of the hemodialysis session. Since the critically ill patient may tolerate rapid ultrafiltration poorly, careful consideration must be given to ultrafiltration rate, total fluid removal goals, and the need for supportive measures during the hemodialysis session such as the use of vasoactive medications to support blood pressure. For those patients who do not tolerate the more rapid ultrafiltration that occurs with intermittent hemodialysis, CRRT with slower continuous ultrafiltration may provide an alternative.

SLED is a modality that has been used as an alternative to continuous therapy. It involves significantly extended hemodialysis sessions with decreased flows that reduce the efficiency but is compensated for by the extended session length [2, 20].

8.4.4.3 Complications

Although serious complications from hemodialysis are infrequent, such sequelae can be severe and should be watched for diligently. With any form of hemodialysis, there is a significant volume of extracorporeal blood. While measures are taken to minimize the volume, with the rapid blood flows necessary, any break in the system can result in rapid blood loss or even exsanguination. Just as bleeding is a risk with hemodialysis, clotting of the circuit or catheter can result in loss of the blood volume of the circuit.

Similar to peritoneal dialysis, infection is a concern in any patient with an indwelling foreign body. The catheter exit site needs monitoring for signs of infection, and appropriate cultures and consideration of empiric antibiotic therapy should follow fever or other signs of infection.

Disequilibrium syndrome secondary to rapid osmolar shifts is a potential complication of hemodialysis, especially when initiating dialysis in a patient with significant uremia and related increased serum osmolarity. Without appropriate monitoring and management, disequilibrium syndrome can result in cerebral edema leading to mental status changes and even seizures. Manipulation of the dialysis prescription can limit risk. In the significantly uremic patient starting dialysis, the decrease in blood urea nitrogen should be kept to less than a 30% decrease in the first session, with gradual increases in ensuing dialysis treatment goals to maintenance levels [9]. Some clinicians also argue that longer sessions (2–3 h) with less rapid clearance may be equally effective [31].

8.4.5 Continuous Renal Replacement Therapy

CRRT was first reported by Kramer in 1977 [19]. In 1986, Ronco published a case series of four critically ill infants treated with CRRT [28]. As the techniques and equipment have improved, this modality is becoming more popular in pediatric ICUs [36].

8.4.5.1 Advantages/Disadvantages

One of the key benefits of CRRT is the gradual rate of solute and fluid removal. This makes it an ideal modality in patients with hemodynamic instability [12, 15]. Similar to hemodialysis, continuous therapy allows adjustment of the dialysate, which may be advantageous in states of metabolic derangement. The gradual nature of continuous therapy also may decrease osmolar shifts, thus reducing the risk of disequilibrium syndrome.

8.4.5.2 Technique

Free-flow arteriovenous techniques for CRRT have largely been abandoned in favor of pumped venovenous methods. These systems yield more consistent blood flow and minimize the risk of bleeding from an arterial access. The generic term CRRT is used to describe all modalities, whether based on convection, diffusion, or a combination of the two (see previous sections on physiology). For specifics on how the modalities differ, please refer to Table 8.1.

8.4.5.3 Prescription

Many aspects of the CRRT prescription are similar to that for intermittent hemodialysis. Specific differences will be highlighted later.

Hemofilter: While fundamentally similar, choices for CRRT hemofilter may be limited more than those for a dialyzer for intermittent hemodialysis. Some CRRT devices require the use of a proprietary hemofilter; others permit the use of any brand.

Tubing set: Depending on the manufacturer, the tubing set may be chosen separately from the hemofilter or may be an integrated part of the filter set. Total extracorporeal volume must be considered as noted earlier for intermittent hemodialysis.

Table 8.1 Continuous renal replacement therapy modalities

CRRT modality	Type of infused fluids		Form of molecular transfer	
	Dialysate	Replacement fluid	Diffusion	Convection
SCUF				Minimal
CVVH		●		●
CVVHD	●		●	
CVVHDF	●	●	●	●

SCUF slow continuous ultrafiltration, *CVVH* continuous veno-venous hemofiltration, *CVVHD* continuous veno-venous hemodialysis, *CVVHDF* continuous veno-venous hemodiafiltration

Circuit prime: Priming considerations for CRRT are similar as for intermittent hemodialysis. Blood priming seems to increase the risk for the BRS when using the AN-69 membrane (see section on complications later) [3].

Blood flow rate (Q_B): Initial targets for blood flow rate can be similar to targets for intermittent hemodialysis 5–10 mL min^{-1} kg^{-1} [31], adjusted for the vascular access. Some devices have maximum blood flows that are much lower than the rates possible on intermittent hemodialysis machines. Since dialysate or replacement fluid flow rates are much slower in CRRT than dialysate flow in intermittent hemodialysis, solute clearance is less dependent on blood flow and there is little advantage to high blood flow rates for most children undergoing CRRT.

Infused fluids for CRRT (dialysate and replacement fluids): CRRT procedures may employ dialysate, replacement fluids, or both. A variety of commercially prepared premixed solutions from several manufacturers are available for use as dialysate in the USA. These come in sterile bags for use with the CRRT device. Each manufacturer offers a range of electrolyte concentrations to address varied clinical situations. The prescribers should be familiar with their electrolyte composition. The solution utilized will depend on the metabolic status of the patient.

Replacement fluids are used to compensate for volume lost with high levels of convective clearance. Commercially prepared replacement fluids have also recently become available in the USA. These options have been available in Europe for many years. Simpler solutions such as normal saline and lactated Ringers may also be used as replacement fluids; consideration must be given to the biochemical status of the patient. Solutions prepared by local pharmacy permit custom-made electrolyte content but may be more costly and have a higher risk of preparation errors.

Total infused fluid rate (dialysate plus replacement fluid) depends on the clinical goals of the procedure. One common approach in pediatric centers uses dialysate or replacement fluid flow rates of 2,000 mL hr^{-1} per 1.73 m^2 [6, 21]. If both diffusion and convection are desired, the fluid can be divided between dialysate and replacement fluid, for instance, 75% dialysate and 25% replacement fluid as a starting point. The patient's volume and electrolyte status must be monitored closely and the CRRT prescription adjusted as indicated. Higher fluid rates increase mass transfer. Similarly, adjusting the proportion of dialysate and replacement fluid will alter the relative contribution of diffusion and convection to overall mass transfer.

Anticoagulation: Unique to CRRT is the need for continuous anticoagulation. Similar to intermittent hemodialysis, heparin infusion adjusted to a target ACT or aPTT can be used. In the event that continuous systemic anticoagulation with heparin is contraindicated, citrate is a commonly used alternative. Citrate infused into the extracorporeal circuit chelates calcium and prevents clotting, serving as a regional anticoagulant. With citrate use, calcium must be replaced to the patient to avoid systemic hypocalcemia. Several protocols have been developed for the use of citrate anticoagulation in CRRT [6, 8, 10].

Ultrafiltration plan: CRRT offers an opportunity for slow ultrafiltration that may be better tolerated by the critically ill patient. The continuous nature of treatment allows ultrafiltration goals to be divided across an entire 24-h period and may be much more successful than rapid ultrafiltration in intermittent hemodialysis. Ultrafiltration rate can be adjusted to remove daily input and also to achieve net fluid loss in the volume-overloaded patient. In children undergoing CRRT, there is less concern regarding fluid restriction and clinicians can, for instance, maximize parenteral nutrition.

8.4.5.4   Complications

The complications with CRRT are similar to those of intermittent hemodialysis although there are several additional concerns. As mentioned previously, the use of replacement fluids can influence the patient's electrolyte and acid/base status, especially if there is significant ongoing ultrafiltration. The electrolyte content of the ultrafiltrate should parallel plasma electrolyte concentration. Use of the AN-69 membrane has been associated with BRS [3]. BRS is characterized by tachycardia, hypotension, vasodilation, and potential death. The symptoms occur within minutes of the contact of blood with the membrane and symptoms will resolve with discontinuation of therapy and removal of the membrane. Bradykinin release results from blood contact with the negatively charged hemofilter made from the AN-69 material. Acidosis exacerbates the reaction [3]. Interventions to limit the likelihood of BRS include avoiding use of blood prime, pH correction of the patient prior to CRRT initiation, blood bypass [3] and recirculation systems [17, 25], and use of membranes other than AN-69.

Unique complications of acid/base status may occur with citrate anticoagulation. Unmetabolized citrate may act as a weak acid, but fully metabolized citrate yields bicarbonate and may cause alkalosis. If citrate infusion exceeds metabolism, then citrate overload, sometimes known as *citrate lock*, can occur. This will result in systemic total hypercalcemia due to ongoing calcium infusion but systemic ionized hypocalcemia. Correction requires a decrease in citrate delivery, an increase in citrate removal, or both. Citrate infusion can be held for approximately 30 min and then resumed at a slower rate, or increased solute clearance can be achieved by augmenting replacement fluid rates and dialysate rates, or these interventions can be combined [22]. Close monitoring is warranted.

8.5 RRT Outcomes

Randomized studies comparing outcomes of dialysis modalities for critically ill children are lacking. Some retrospective studies may be limited by provider bias; for instance, patients assigned to CRRT rather than intermittent hemodialysis are more likely to be hemodynamically unstable with a risk for higher mortality. Others suggest that the need for vasopressors or the underlying disease process is the better predictor of mortality [5]. These explanations may account for the findings by Bunchman et al. of survival rates of 40% for CRRT, 49% for peritoneal dialysis, and 81% for hemodialysis in children undergoing dialysis in the ICU [5].

Timing of initiation of renal replacement therapy may influence outcome. Several studies found that the early initiation of CRRT and prevention of significant fluid overload (<10%) has improved patient outcome [11, 14, 15]. A recent review of pediatric CRRT with data drawn from a registry of pediatric centers showed better overall outcomes than previously reported; this may suggest an improvement in CRRT techniques and overall application of this technology in the care of the critically ill patient [33].

8.6 Conclusion

Renal replacement techniques are an important adjunct to the successful care of critically ill children. Renal support during periods of acute kidney injury or multisystem organ dysfunction can bridge the patient through the period of critical illness, preventing further complications from volume overload and metabolic imbalance, permitting the delivery of necessary medications and nutrition, and leading to better patient outcomes. Ongoing refinement of renal replacement

techniques, coupled with careful coordination between nephrology and critical care services, will help to improve these outcomes further.

Take-Home Pearls

> Dialysis utilizes the physical properties of convection and diffusion to transfer molecules from the blood.
> Peritoneal dialysis uses the peritoneum as an intrinsic dialysis membrane and provides a slower more gradual correction of metabolic abnormalities.
> Peritoneal dialysis has the advantages of simplicity and no need for systemic anticoagulation.
> Hemodialysis employs an extracorporeal blood circuit and an artificial dialysis membrane that can rapidly and efficiently transfer molecules from the patient.
> Intermittent hemodialysis requires a level of cardiovascular stability for the rapid fluid and electrolyte shifts. Slower techniques such as CRRT and SLED may be more successful in the unstable patient.
> Choice of dialysis modality and prescription must be tailored to the individual patient and clinical situation.
> Successful therapy requires coordination between critical care and dialysis teams.

References

1. Auron A, Warady BA, Simon S, et al. (2007) Use of the multipurpose drainage catheter for the provision of acute peritoneal dialysis in infants and children. American Journal of Kidney Diseases 49(5):650–655
2. Berbece AN, Richardson RMA (2006) Sustained low-efficiency dialysis in the ICU: Cost, anticoagulation, and solute removal. Kidney International 70:963–968
3. Brophy PD, Mottes TA, Kudelka TL, et al. (2001) AN-69 membrane reactions are pH-dependent and preventable. American Journal of Kidney Diseases 38(1):173–178
4. Brophy PD, Somers MJG, Baum MA, et al. (2005) Multicentre evaluation of anticoagulation in patients receiving continuous renal replacement therapy (CRRT). Nephrology Dialysis Transplantation 20:1416–1421
5. Bunchman TE, McBryde KD, Mottes TE, et al. (2001) Pediatric acute renal failure: Outcome by modality and disease. Pediatric Nephrology 16:1067–1071
6. Bunchman TE, Maxvold NJ, Barnett J, et al. (2002) Pediatric hemofiltration: Normocarb dialysate solution with citrate anticoagulation. Pediatric Nephrology 17:150–154
7. Chadha V, Warady BA, Blowey DL, et al. (2000) Tenckhoff catheters prove superior to cook catheters in pediatric acute peritoneal dialysis. American Journal of Kidney Diseases 35(6):1111–1116
8. Chadha V, Garg U, Warady BA, Alon US (2002) Citrate clearance in children receiving continuous venovenous renal replacement therapy. Pediatric Nephrology 17:819–824

9. Daugirdas JT, Blake PG, Ing TS (2001) Handbook of Dialysis, 3rd edn. Lippincott Williams & Wilkins, Philadelphia, PA

10. Elhanan N, Skippen P, Nuthall G, et al. (2004) Citrate anticoagulation in pediatric venovenous hemofiltration. Pediatric Nephrology 19:208–212

11. Foland JA, Fortenberry JD, Warshaw BL, et al. (2004) Fluid overload before continuous hemofiltration and survival in critically ill children: A retrospective analysis. Pediatric Critical Care 32(8):1171–1176

12. Flynn JT (2002) Choice of dialysis modality for management of pediatric acute renal failure. Pediatric Nephrology 17:61–69

13. Furman KI, Gomperts ED, Hockley J (1978) Activity of intraperitoneal heparin during peritoneal dialysis. Clinical Nephrology 9(1):15–18

14. Gillespie RS, Seidel K, Symons JM (2004) Effect of fluid overload and dose of replacement fluid on survival in hemofiltration. Pediatric Nephrology 19:1394–1399

15. Goldstein SL, Currier H, Graf JM, et al. (2001) Outcome in children receiving continuous venovenous hemofiltration. Pediatrics 107:1309–1312

16. Goldstein SL (2003) Overview of pediatric renal replacement therapy in acute renal failure. Artificial Organs 27(9):781–785

17. Hackbarth RM, Eding D, Gianoli Smith C, et al. (2005) Zero balance ultrafiltration (Z-BUF) in blood-primed CRRT circuits achieves electrolyte and acid–base homeostasis prior to patient connection. Pediatric Nephrology 20:1328–1333

18. Kozek-Langenecker SA, Kettner SC, Oismueller C, et al. (1998) Anticoagulation with prostaglandin E1 and unfractionated heparin during continuous venovenous hemofiltration. Critical Care Medicine 26(7):1208–1212

19. Kramer P, Wigger W, Rieger J, et al. (1977) Arteriovenous haemofiltration: A new and simple method for treatment of over-hydrated patients resistant to diuretics. Klin Wochenschr 55:1121–1122

20. Marshall MR, Golper TA, Shaver MJ, et al. (2001) Sustained low-efficiency dialysis for critically ill patients requiring renal replacement therapy. Kidney International 60:777–785

21. Maxvold NJ, Smoyer WE, Custer JR, Bunchman TE (2000) Amino acid loss and nitrogen balance in critically ill children with acute renal failure: A prospective comparison between classic hemofiltration and hemofiltration with dialysis. Critical Care Medicine 28(4):1161–1165

22. Maxvold NJ, Bunchman TE (2003) Renal failure and renal replacement therapy. Critical Care Clinics 19:563–575

23. Neuhaus TJ, Goetschel P, Schmugge M, Leumann E (2000) Heparin-induced thrombocytopenia type II on hemodialysis: Switch to danaparoid. Pediatric Nephrology 14:713–716

24. Nowak G, Bucha E, Brauns I, Czerwinski R (1997) Anticoagulation with r-hirudin in regular haemodialysis with heparin-induced thrombocytopenia (HIT II). The first long-term application of r-hirudin in a haemodialysis patient. Wien Klin Wochenschr 109(10):354–355

25. Pasko DA, Mottes TA, Mueller BA (2003) Pre-dialysis of blood prime continuous hemodialysis normalizes pH and electrolytes. Pediatric Nephrology 18:1177–1183

26. Rahim KA, Seidel K, McDonald RA (2004) Risk Factors for catheter-related complications in peritoneal dialysis. Pediatric Nephrology 19:1021–1028

27. Reeves JH, Cumming AR, Gallagher L, et al. (1999) A controlled trial of low-molecular weight heparin (dalteparin) versus unfractionated heparin as anticoagulant during continuous venovenous hemodialysis with filtration. Critical Care Medicine 27(10):2224–2228

28. Ronco C, Brendolan A, Bragantini L, et al. (1986) Treatment of acute renal failure in newborns by continuous arteriovenous hemofiltration. Kidney International 29:908–915

29. Ronco C, Brendolan A, LaGreca GL (1998) The peritoneal dialysis system. Nephrology Dialysis and Transplantation 13(S6):94–99

30. Shea M, Hmiel SP, Beck AM (2001) Use of tissue plasminogen activator for thrombolysis in occluded peritoneal dialysis catheters in children. Advances in Peritoneal Dialysis 17:249–252

31. Strazdins V, Watson AR, Harvey B (2004) Renal replacement therapy for acute renal failure in children: European Guidelines. Pediatric Nephrology 19:199–207

32. Stedman's (1994) Medical Dictionary, 27th edn. Lippincott Williams & Wilkins, Philadelphia, PA

33. Symons JM, Chua AN, Somers MJG, et al. (2007) Demographic characteristics of pediatric CRRT: A report of the prospective pediatric continuous renal replacement therapy (ppCRRT) registry. Clinical Journal of the American Society of Nephrology 2:732–738

34. Trakarnvanich T, Chirananthavat T, Ariyakulnimit S, et al. (2006) The efficacy of single-needle versus double-needle hemodialysis in chronic renal failure. Journal of the Medical Association of Thailand 89(S2):196–206

35. Warady BA, Schaefer F, Holloway M, et al. (2000) Consensus guidelines for the treatment of peritonitis in pediatric patients receiving peritoneal dialysis. Peritoneal Dialysis International 20:610–624

36. Warady BA, Bunchman TE (2000) Dialysis therapy for children with acute renal failure: Survey results. Pediatric Nephrology 15:11–13

37. Warady BA, Schaefer FS, Fine RN, Alexander SR (eds) (2004) Pediatric Dialysis. Kluwer Academic, Dordrecht

Nutrition for the Critically Ill Pediatric Patient with Renal Dysfunction

9

N.M. Rodig

Contents

Case Vignette

Λ 3-year-old previously healthy girl presents for assessment of fever, cough, increased respiratory effort, and lethargy. Her parents report that she has had decreased intake of solid nutrition for approximately 5 days and decreased liquid intake for 3 days. Her urine output had decreased, and her parents are unsure when she voided last. Upon arrival, she is ill appearing, poorly responsive, and has tachypnea. Urgent assessment reveals temperature of 39.5°C, pulse of 150, blood pressure of 65/30, shallow respirations with respiratory rate of 44, and oxygen saturation of 88% on room air. Her extremities are warm, though her peripheral pulses are weak. A chest radiograph reveals left lobar pneumonia with associated large effusion. Arterial blood gas assessment demonstrates respiratory acidosis. She is intubated, receives a 20 mL kg^{-1} intravenous bolus of 0.9 NaCl, and initial doses of broad-spectrum antibiotics. She

Core Messages

> ❱ During critical illness, total energy expenditure will be increased proportionate to the severity of the underlying illness. The aim of nutritional support is to blunt the negative nitrogen balance that may accompany a hypermetabolic or catabolic state.

> ❱ Careful assessment of energy requirements in critically ill children with acute kidney injury (AKI) is essential to optimize the nutritional plan. Inadequate nutritional support will result in poor protein retention and excessive support may predispose to metabolic derangements and fluid excess.

> ❱ In addition to the increased protein catabolism associated with critical illness, patients supported with dialysis will have additional nitrogen losses. These losses should be accounted for when protein intake is prescribed.

> ❱ Water-soluble vitamins will be removed with dialysis and should be supplemented accordingly to avoid deficits.

> ❱ If nutritional support is indicated due to inadequate oral intake, enteral nutrition is the preferred method of support. If volume restriction is necessary, feeds can be fortified to increase energy density. To optimize digestibility, similar proportions of fat, protein, and carbohydrate as the base formula should be provided.

is admitted to the intensive care unit for further care of pneumonia complicated by respiratory failure and sepsis. Serum laboratory studies return and are notable for white blood count of 25,000 cells μL^{-1} with a left shift, hematocrit of 31%, and platelet count of 660,000 cells μL^{-1}. Electrolytes are notable for serum potassium of 6.2 meq L^{-1} and serum bicarbonate of 12 meq L^{-1}. Her BUN and serum creatinine are elevated at 90 and 3.5 mg dL^{-1}, respectively. Because of continued poor perfusion, further volume resuscitation is provided. Volume resuscitation is not sufficient, however, and she requires dopamine and epinephrine continuous infusions to maintain hemodynamic integrity. She initially passes a small amount of urine, but then becomes anuric. Plans to initiate continuous venovenous hemodialysis are made. Given her hemodynamic instability, she is not provided with enteral nutrition but total parenteral nutrition is initiated.

9.1 Introduction

The prevalence of malnutrition among critically ill patients has remained relatively constant over the past two decades [29, 51], and preexisting or hospital-acquired malnutrition has been identified as a contributing factor resulting in the poor outcome of severe acute kidney injury (AKI) [23]. There is consensus that nutritional support improves anthropometric outcomes as assessed by body weight and mid-arm muscle mass. However, controversy persists as to whether nutritional support improves clinical outcomes, such as length of stay and mortality [33, 34]. During serious illness, the aim of nutritional support is to blunt the negative nitrogen balance, though this trend cannot be entirely prevented. During the recovery phase, anabolism exceeds catabolism, and nutrition serves to replenish stores and maintain positive nitrogen balance. As significant renal dysfunction results in impairment of nitrogenous waste excretion and altered regulation of water, electrolyte, and acid–base homeostasis, the provision of optimal nutrition may be challenged. The following chapter will outline principles for the nutritional management of critically ill children with disturbances in renal function. The nutritional care of children with severe AKI will be emphasized. When indicated, specific considerations for children with chronic kidney disease (CKD) will be discussed. As the clinical manifestations of both acute and chronic renal failure are varied, the need for individualized nutritional prescription is emphasized throughout.

9.2 Energy Metabolism and Requirements

Careful assessment of energy requirement in children with AKI is essential to optimize nutritional support. Inadequate caloric provision will result in poor protein retention, and excessive nutrition increases the risk for metabolic derangements and fluid excess. Assessment

of total energy requirements should consider resting energy expenditure, energy needed for physical activity, and diet- induced thermogenesis. In patients with AKI not associated with critical illness, energy expenditure has been shown to be comparable to its expenditure as measured by indirect calorimetry in healthy subjects [59]. Adult patients with sepsis or severe trauma develop an increase in energy expenditure, and the increase is proportionate to the severity of the underlying process [12, 49]. In addition, critically ill adults with sepsis and systemic inflammatory response syndrome (SIRS) were found to have increased oxygen consumption and resting energy expenditure when compared with patients with SIRS unrelated to sepsis [45]. This hypermetabolic response apparent in adults has not been a consistent finding in critically ill pediatric patients [16, 25]. Though data are limited, renal failure itself does not appear to increase overall energy requirements. A study of critically ill adults compared the energy expenditure of those who required dialysis for severe renal dysfunction to those who required only supportive measures for normal or moderately impaired renal function. The average measured hypermetabolism was 28% for those who required dialysis and 42% for those who did not. It was proposed that AKI reduced energy demand secondary to diminished renal metabolic activity [63].

Knowledge of a child's total energy expenditure is essential to optimize nutritional support. Basal metabolic rate is the largest component of total energy expenditure, though energy is also utilized for growth, activity, and the thermic effect of food. Determining the energy requirement of a critically ill patient may be challenging as potential stress factors such as fever and sepsis will increase metabolic demand. Additionally, hospitalized patients will often have altered activity levels, blunted or absent growth, and reduced enteral intake of food. Indirect calorimetry accurately measures resting energy expenditure and allows nutrition to be tailored to the needs of the individual. A comprehensive review of the principles and methodology of indirect calorimetry was recently published [27]. Though indirect calorimetry is the preferred method when available, measurement requires equipment and trained staff. When assessment by indirect calorimetry is not possible, resting energy expenditure can be estimated by one of the equations to calculate basal metabolic rate. Commonly used equations include the Harris–Benedict equation for adults and Schofield equations for children [60]; the reader is referred elsewhere for further details regarding the use of these predictive equations

[21]. Numerous studies evaluating the accuracy of such predictive equations relative to measured resting energy expenditure have, however, demonstrated considerable error in both children and adults [9, 25, 67, 69].

A general recommendation for critically ill adult patients with AKI is to tailor energy intake to the individual, aiming not to exceed 130% of the patient's resting energy expenditure [18, 19, 40, 59]. Pediatric-specific data or practice guidelines for energy requirements in AKI are lacking. A group of critically ill pediatric patients on continuous renal replacement therapy (CRRT) was provided total calories of 20–30% above their resting energy expenditures based on indirect calorimetry, including 1.5 g kg^{-1} day^{-1} of protein [41]. Despite this nutritional support, positive nitrogen balance was often not met. For practical purposes, it is reasonable to start at the recommended dietary caloric intake for an aged matched healthy child and adjust as indicated based on indirect calorimetry or results of predictive calculations.

Modification of nutritional support should be made to account for calories provided by any dextrose-containing intravenous fluids or dextrose-containing dialysate solutions. During acute peritoneal dialysis, passive uptake of dextrose from the dextrose-rich dialysate may augment significantly total energy provision. Grodstein et al. studied the amount of energy derived from dialysate in a group of adult patients undergoing chronic continuous ambulatory peritoneal dialysis (CAPD) and developed an equation to predict daily glucose absorption. The quantity of glucose absorbed per liter of dialysate (y) varied with the concentration of glucose in the dialysate (x), ($y = 11.3x - 10.9$, $r = 0.96$) [26]. Though this formula can be utilized to assess glucose absorption during CAPD, dwell time is not included as an independent variable. Dwell times during acute peritoneal dialysis are generally shorter, and this may render the estimation inaccurate. Actual measurement of glucose absorption during acute peritoneal dialysis was performed in nine adult patients and compared with the result calculated by the Grodstein formula [50]. The calculated method overestimated glucose absorption when using 4.25% dialysate and underestimated glucose absorption when using 1.5% dialysate. The authors of this study recommended the use of a percentage estimate of 40–50% of glucose in dialysate to account for additional calories provided during acute peritoneal dialysis.

As there is lack of evidence to suggest that children with kidney dysfunction have increased total caloric needs, recommended energy intake for children with CKD and children on maintenance dialysis has been based on data acquired in healthy children without kidney dysfunction. Should a child with CKD become critically ill, energy expenditure will be increased proportionately to the severity of the underlying illness. As for children on acute peritoneal dialysis, peritoneal absorption of dialysate glucose should be considered when calculating energy intake. When children on CAPD were studied, glucose absorption accounted for approximately 7–10 kcal kg^{-1} day^{-1} [55].

Dextrose is the major source of calories provided by parenteral nutrition, and hyperglycemia may be an unintended consequence. Hyperglycemia is not an uncommon finding during critical illness and has been associated with increased mortality and adverse outcome [22, 64]. Acute renal injury may increase the risk for hyperglycemia due both to accelerated hepatic gluconeogensis and insulin resistance. AKI is a state of increased protein catabolism, and increased hepatic gluconeogenesis results from conversion of amino acids released during protein degradation [14]. The kidney plays a direct role in glucose homeostasis, which is regulated by insulin [66]. During acute renal injury, insulin resistance may be more likely given the loss of the kidney as a major target organ for insulin action. Critically ill patients with AKI have demonstrated insulin resistance as evidenced by higher blood glucose and insulin concentrations [6]. The consequences of insulin resistance and hyperglycemia have been shown to be significant. In a retrospective study, hyperglycemia was found to be independently associated with mortality in a group of 152 critically ill children [64]. A prospective, randomized study of more than 1,500 adults in a surgical intensive care unit was undertaken to determine if intensive insulin therapy would improve prognosis when compared with conventional therapy. By employing a strategy of strict glycemic control and maintaining blood glucose levels between 80 and 110 mg dL^{-1}, the morbidity and mortality among these ICU patients fell significantly [68]. Well-designed studies determining the effect of insulin therapy on the outcome of critically ill children are needed [70].

9.3 Protein Metabolism and Requirements

AKI is a state of increased catabolism, the extent of which parallels the severity of the underlying illness. During metabolic stress, counterregulatory hormones and cytokines are produced with subsequent release of glucose, fatty acids, and amino acids from the body stores. The catabolism of skeletal muscle allows for the generation of glucose, which is the preferred substrate for the brain, red blood cells, and renal medulla. This stress response is an effective short-term adaptation, though a prolonged response is maladaptive and will lead to reduction of lean body mass. Clinically, significant negative protein balance may be characterized by skeletal muscle wasting, weight loss, and immune dysfunction.

The protein catabolic rate of critically ill adults with AKI has been reported to be $1.4–1.8\,g\,kg^{-1}\,day^{-1}$ [11, 18, 37]. Virtually all nitrogen arising from amino acids liberated during protein degradation is converted to urea, and the extent of protein catabolism may be assessed by calculating the urea nitrogen appearance (UNA). While on dialysis, the UNA is the sum of the urea in the dialysis ultrafiltrate, urine, and the change in the body nitrogen pool. UNA was studied in a group of critically ill children with anuric AKI maintained on CRRT and was greater than $180\,mg\,kg^{-1}\,day^{-1}$ [35]. This compares with a mean UNA of approximately $100\,mg\,kg^{-1}\,day^{-1}$ in well children on chronic peritoneal dialysis [43]. Increased protein catabolic rate was confirmed in a subsequent report of critically ill pediatric patients on CRRT [41]. The mean UNA while on continuous venovenous hemofiltration (CVVH) and continuous venovenous hemodiafiltration (CVVHD) were 291 and $245\,mg\,kg^{-1}\,day^{-1}$, respectively. Nitrogen balance, defined as the difference between nitrogen intake and UNA, was often negative despite the provision of $1.5\,g\,kg^{-1}\,day^{-1}$ of protein.

In addition to increased protein catabolism associated with critical illness, patients supported with dialysis have additional nitrogen losses. During an intermittent hemodialysis session, amino acids and small peptides are lost to filtration across the dialysis membrane [30, 31], and these losses will be continuous if a CRRT dialysis modality is employed. CVVH provides clearance solely by convection, whereas clearance by CVVHD is primarily diffusive. The previously mentioned pediatric study compared amino acid losses between CVVH and CVVHD [41]. With the exception of glutamic acid, individual free amino acid clearances were greater on CVVH than on CVVHD, though there was no significant difference in daily losses over the 48-h period of the study. Amino acid losses by dialysis clearance represented 12 and 11% of daily protein intake on CVVH and CVVHD, respectively.

Peritoneal dialysis can result in significant protein losses through the dialysis effluent, and the degree of loss varies inversely with body surface area. When peritoneal protein loss was studied in children supported with chronic peritoneal dialysis, protein loss was highest in infants ($277 \pm 22\,mg\,kg^{-1}\,day^{-1}$) and lowest in children who weighed greater than $50\,kg$ ($91 \pm 15\,mg\,kg^{-1}\,day^{-1}$) [52].

Few studies have attempted to define protein or amino acid requirements in adult patients with AKI, and similar pediatric data are nonexistent. A child with uncomplicated AKI who is not critically ill should be provided protein based on the amount recommended for age and adjusted as clinically indicated. Protein requirements in critically ill pediatric patients will be increased, though data specific to AKI are lacking. Protein should be provided based on recommendations for critically ill children and adjusted for individual needs [3]. While protein intake is increased, electrolytes, acid–base balance, and uremia should be assessed daily. Patients supported with dialysis will have additional nitrogen loss, and protein provision should be adjusted accordingly. The American Society for Parenteral and Enteral Nutrition (ASPEN) has put forth recommendations for protein intake and estimated losses for children undergoing dialysis for AKI (Table 9.1) [4]. Estimated protein losses from dialysis, particularly from PD, vary widely and data is limited. Few studies are available that allow estimation of optimal protein to energy ratio in critically ill children, though standard maintenance diets typically provide a ratio of nonprotein energy (kcal) to nitrogen (g) between 150 and 250:1 [15].

9.4 Micronutrient Requirements

Trace element requirements in AKI are not clearly defined, and most recommendations are derived from data in patients with chronic renal failure. Many of the findings regarding trace element metabolism in AKI may reflect the effect of the acute phase response and not necessarily reflect specific effects induced by AKI. As trace elements have small molecular weights and critical illness results in altered protein binding, hemodialysis will likely alter trace element homeostasis. When studied using in vitro methods, trace elements including selenium, chromium, copper, and zinc were cleared during CVVH [46], with convective fluid rates significantly affecting clearance. When trace element losses were studied in actual patients on CRRT, however, the results were variable [7, 65, 71]. The variability likely stemmed from differences in patient population, CRRT method, and assays utilized. A recent study of trace element removal during CRRT confirmed

Table 9.1 Recommended protein intake and estimated protein losses during dialysis therapy for acute renal failure

Age (weight range)	RDI	Estimated PD losses	Estimated HD losses	Estimated CRRT losses	Daily protein intake goal
Infant (≤10 kg)	1.6–2.2	2.0–4.0	0.5–1.0	2.0–3.0	2.0–6.0
Small child (>10 and ≤25 kg)	1.0–1.2	2.0–3.0	0.5–1.0	2.0–3.0	1.0–3.0
Older child (>25 and ≤40 kg)	0.8–1.2	1.0–2.0	0.5–1.0	2.0–3.0	1.0–3.0
Adolescent (>40 kg)	0.8–1.0	1.0–2.0	0.5–1.0	2.0–3.0	1.0–3.0

Adapted from [4]
Values are expressed as grams of protein kg^{-1} day^{-1}. *RDI* recommended dietary intake for normal children, *PD* peritoneal dialysis, *HD* hemodialysis, *CRRT* continuous renal replacement therapy

Table 9.2 Recommendations for oral water-soluble vitamin supplementation in acute kidney injury and composition of pediatric and adult parenteral vitamin preparations

Supplement	ASPEN recommendation	ASPEN enteral dose	M.V.I. pediatric for infusion	M.V.I. adult for infusion
Thiamine	Recommended	0.2–1 mg day^{-1}	1.2 mg	6 mg
Riboflavin	Recommended	0.3–1 mg day^{-1}	1.4 mg	3.6 mg
Pyridoxine	Recommended	6.25–50 mg day^{-1}	1 mg	6 mg
Folate	Recommended	0.4–1 mg day^{-1}	140 μg	600 μg
Vitamin B12	Recommended	0.5–2.5 μg day^{-1}	1 μg	5 μg
Vitamin C	Caution	≤60 mg day^{-1}	80 mg	200 μg

Adapted from [4]

removal of chromium, copper, manganese, selenium, and zinc in ten adult patients [13]. As selenium is a cofactor for antioxidant enzymes, impaired defense against antioxidant stress may be of concern. However, the standard trace element supplementation provided in parenteral nutrition to these patients exceeded their losses during CRRT. Nonetheless, further studies are needed to clarify micronutrient requirements in AKI. Until these data are available, patients on parenteral nutrition should be provided standard supplements of trace elements.

Water-soluble vitamins will be removed with dialysis. Therefore, when assessing the need for vitamin supplementation in children with AKI, the effect of dialysis should be considered. For children on chronic dialysis, clear guidelines for supplementation are provided [1]. Recommended intake of thiamin (B_1), riboflavin (B_2), pyridoxine (B_6), vitamin B_{12}, and folic acid should achieve 100% of the daily reference intake (DRI) for age. If the patient with AKI is supported with dialysis, additional water-soluble vitamins should be provided to avoid deficiencies. The recommendations for oral vitamin supplementation during AKI provided by the ASPEN guidelines and composition of pediatric and adult parenteral multivitamin preparations are listed in Table 9.2 [4]. If enteral nutrition is an option, infants and small children may be given liquid or chewable multivitamin preparations and additional folic acid dosed for age. Older children and adults may be provided B complex vitamins containing folic acid, such as Nephrocaps (Fleming & Company). Vitamin C should not be supplemented beyond the DRI. Vitamin C is metabolized to oxalate, which can accumulate in patients with CKD. Oxalate accumulation in AKI has not been adequately studied. Fat-soluble vitamins are not removed during dialysis and may accumulate, though little data pertinent to AKI are available. With the exception of Vitamin K, deficiencies of other fat-soluble vitamins during AKI have been reported [20] and further studies are needed. ASPEN guidelines recommend supplementation of fat-soluble vitamins if the duration of AKI is expected to be limited (i.e., <2 weeks), with dosing not to exceed the DRI.

9.5 Electrolyte Considerations

With significant deterioration in renal function, there is increased risk for electrolyte abnormalities. Common disorders include hyperkalemia, hyperphosphatemia, and hypocalcemia. Extensive discussion of electrolyte physiology in the setting of acute disturbances of renal function is beyond the scope of this chapter. A limited discussion is provided to serve as a basis for nutritional planning.

Given the potential for increased risk of life-threatening arrythmias, hyperkalemia is a dreaded consequence of AKI. Potassium is the most abundant intracellular cation with less than 2% of total body potassium present in the extracellular fluid. As potassium is primarily excreted by glomerular filtration and tubular secretion, decreased renal function and renal tubular damage will predispose to hyperkalemia. In addition to decreased excretion, movement of potassium from the intracellular space to the extracellular space may further aggravate potassium homeostasis. Acidosis, enhanced cell turnover, and hemolysis all increase extracellular potassium concentration. If transfusion of red blood cell products is necessary, attempts to secure relatively fresh packed red blood cells should be made or washing the product should be considered. When 52 units of packed red blood cells transfused in a pediatric intensive care unit were assessed, approximately 30% had a potassium concentration >25 mmol L^{-1} [47]. Another study reported mean potassium concentrations of ~37–40 mmol L^{-1} when assessed in units as old as 30 days [5]. If AKI is evolving, nutritional sources of potassium should be limited or withheld until acceptable potassium homeostasis is assured. Potassium provision should then be based on serial assessment of serum levels. If dialysis is initiated, potassium clearance should be anticipated if the dialysate contains little or no potassium. If clinically appropriate, potassium salts can be added to the dialysate at concentrations of 1–3 meq L^{-1} to avoid hypokalemia but necessitates close monitoring of serum potassium levels.

Similar to hyperkalemia, hyperphosphatemia is a common electrolyte disturbance in oliguric or anuric renal failure. Serum phosphorus occurs in two forms, organic and inorganic. The inorganic fraction is the principal circulating form and routinely assayed for clinical use. When glomerular filtration rate (GFR) is within the normal range and tubular function is intact, approximately 80–90% of serum inorganic phosphorus is filtered, and typically more than 80% of filtered phosphorus is reabsorbed. In AKI, hyperphosphatemia may result and may in turn lead to hypocalcemia due to precipitation of calcium–phosphorus salts.

Treatment of hyperphosphatemia includes restricting phosphorus intake and intitating oral phosphorus binders if enteral feeds are provided. In children who require phosphorus restriction, intake of milk, milk products, eggs, nuts, dried beans, peanut butter, whole grains, chocolate, and other high-phosphorus containing foods should be limited. Options for phosphorus binders include calcium-based preparations (calcium acetate, calcium carbonate), noncalcium and nonmetal-based (sevelamer hydrochloride, lanthanum carbonate) binders, and aluminum-based binders (aluminum hydroxide).

First-line enteral binding therapy for hyperphosphatemia in children is often a calcium-based binder, which may provide added benefit if hypocalcemia is present but may also predispose to hypercalcemia if large doses are needed. Sevelamer hydrochloride has been shown to be effective and safe in children and may be associated with less hypercalcemia [38, 48, 57]. The other noncalcium and nonmetal-based binder lanthanum carbonate has not been adequately studied in children and is generally not used in pediatric patients. Aluminum-containing binders are very effective and were once the mainstay of phosphate binding in children. If their use is expected to be prolonged, however, especially in the setting of CKD, these binders are now avoided due to the potential for aluminum retention, neurotoxicity, and osteodystrophy [56, 61, 62]. The only phosphate binders readily available in liquid or powdered form are calcium carbonate and aluminum hydroxide, limiting the options for small children and infants. Methods to prepare a sevelamer hydrochloride oral suspension have also recently been published [42].

9.6 Route of Nutrition

When it is evident that oral intake of nutrition is inadequate or projected to remain suboptimal, nutritional support should be provided. If allowable, enteral nutrition is the preferred method of support for the critically ill patient. Proposed benefits of enteral nutrition include intestinal trophism, reducing bacterial translocation, stimulation of the immune system, and cost effectiveness [2, 17, 32, 39]. Early initiation of enteral feeds was shown to reduce complications from sepsis in adult surgical patients when compared with patients receiving parenteral nutrition [44] and was also well tolerated in critically ill pediatric patients [10]. A specific benefit of enteral feeds is the potential for providing concentrated nutrition in a smaller volume. This is of particular advantage to those patients with oliguric renal failure or evolving or existing volume excess. Nasogastric feeds were well tolerated when provided carefully to an adult population with AKI and did not result in significant increase in major gastrointestinal complications [24]. To decrease the risk of aspiration and improve tolerance of feeds when gastric emptying is delayed, transpyloric feeds should be considered. In a cadre of critically ill children including pediatric patients with AKI, continuous transpyloric feeds were overall effective and well tolerated, although associated with increased gastrointestinal sequelae including abdominal distension and excessive gastric residuals [36, 58].

If enteral feeds are initiated, both standard formulas and formulas appropriate for decreased renal function are available. Table 9.3 lists a selection of formulas appropriate for infants, children, and adults. For infants, Good Start Supreme (Nestle Clinical Nutrition) has lower phosphorus content when compared with other standard cow's milk formula. Similac PM 60/40 (Ross Products) is designed for infants with impaired renal function and has overall lower mineral content. The calcium content of PM 60/40 is lower than that of standard infant formulas, however, and calcium supplementation may be necessary. Suplena (Ross Products) and Nepro (Ross Products) are available for children and adults and are designed for patients with reduced renal function and on dialysis, respectively. Both provide $1.8 \, \text{kcal mL}^{-1}$. Feeds should be initiated with hypo- or standard caloric formula at low rates of $0.5-1 \, \text{mL kg}^{-1} \, \text{h}^{-1}$ with gradual increase to normal caloric delivery for age over 36–48 h as tolerated. Gastric residual volumes and abdominal exams should be monitored closely with each advancement [58].

If volume restriction is indicated, the rate of formula delivery should be increased to the target volume and then gradually fortified using modular components to meet nutritional needs (Table 9.4) [53]. Both breast milk and commercial formulas may be fortified, though it is generally not advisable to increase the energy density of formula by concentration alone due to increased sodium, potassium, phosphorus, and overall renal solute load. Caloric density may be increased gradually in $2-4 \, \text{kcal oz}^{-1}$ increments, and

Table 9.3 Nutrient content of selected infant, pediatric, and adult formulas

Formula (manufacturer)	Energy (kcal mL^{-1})	Protein (g L^{-1})	Fat (g L^{-1})	Carb (g L^{-1})	Na/K (mg L^{-1})	Ca/P (mg L^{-1})	mOsm kg^{-1} H$_2$O
Infant formulas							
Enfamil LIPIL Mead Johnson	0.67	14.2	35.8	73.7	182/730	527/290	270
Good Start Supreme Nestle Clinical Nutrition	0.67	14.7	34.2	75	181/724	449/255	280
Similac PM 60/40 (Ross Products)	0.67	15	37.9	69	162/541	379/189	280
Pediatric and adult formulas							
Pediasure (Ross Products)	1	30	38	131	380/1310	972/845	480
Suplena (Ross Products)	1.8	45	96	205	785/1120	1055/700	600
Nepro (Ross Products)	1.8	81	96	167	1060/1060	1060/700	585

Information based on manufacturer's literature as of 2008 and is subject to change. For the most current nutrient content, please see product labels. Data are from manufacturers: Mead Johnson (Evansville, IN 47721), Nestle Clinical Nutrition (Deerfield, IL 60015), Ross Products (Abbott Laboratories, Columbus, OH 43215)

Carb carbohydrate, *Na* sodium, *K* postassium, *Ca* calcium, *P* phosporus

Table 9.4 Nutrient content of selected modular products

Modular product (manufacturer)	Energy (kcal)	Protein (g)	Fat (g)	Carb (g)	Na (mg)	K (mg)	P (mg)
Carbohydrate (per 100 g)							
Moducal (Mead Johnson)	375	0	0	95	70	5	trace
Polycose (Ross Products)	380	0	0	95	110	10	12
Fat (per 100 mL)							
Canola oil	813	0	92	0	0	0	0
Microlipid (Mead Johnson)	449	0	51	0	0	0	0
Carbohydrate and fat (per 100 g)							
Duocal (SHS International)	492	0	73	22	≤20	≤5	≤5
Protein (per 100 g)							
Beneprotein (Resource)	357	86	0	0	214	500	286

Adapted from [53]

For the most current nutrient content, please see product labels

Carb carbohydrate, *Na* sodium, *K* potassium, *P* phosphorus

the tempo of fortification will depend on individual tolerance. In children with CKD, caloric density up to $60 \, \text{kcal oz}^{-1}$ has been used to achieve intended goals [72]. To optimize digestibility, similar proportions of fat, protein, and carbohydrate as in the base formula should be provided. If the patient is on CRRT, amino acid and small peptide losses may challenge the ability to supply adequate protein enterally. If indicated, intravenous administration of 10% amino acids can be provided to achieve desired goals.

Though enteral feeds are preferred, they may not be tolerated in critically ill patients. The underlying illness and need for vasoactive medications may compromise gastrointestinal perfusion and function. An additional concern in the setting of chronic or acute renal failure is the potential detrimental effect of uremia on gastrointestinal motility, though this has been studied primarily in patients on chronic dialysis [8, 28, 54]. Contraindications to enteral feeds include intestinal obstruction, severe or protracted ileus, gastrointestinal ischemia, and hemodynamic instability. If enteral feeds are not possible or cannot provide the intended nutritional support, parenteral nutrition (PN) combined with enteral support or total parenteral nutrition

alone may be necessary. An adequate discussion of parenteral nutrition is beyond the scope of this chapter and is detailed elsewhere [15]. Modification of PN should be performed based on anticipated amino acid losses and dextrose absorption from dialysis therapies if applicable. Electrolyte composition should be guided by regular assessment of the patient's laboratory studies.

9.7 Conclusion

Optimal nutritional management of critically ill children is challenging and becomes more complex should there be an acute or chronic disturbance in renal function. The provision of both adequate and appropriate nutrition support should be viewed as a critical element in the therapeutic effort. To achieve this end, repeated evaluations of renal function, metabolic balance, volume status, and energy expenditure should be made to guide adjustment of any nutritional care plan. If available, the assessment and counseling provided by a renal dietician is a valuable resource in formulating and implementing a successful nutrition plan.

Take Home Pearls

> The aim of nutritional support during AKI associated with critical illness is to blunt the tendency towards negative nitrogen balance.

> AKI is a state of increased catabolism, the extent of which parallels the severity of the underlying illness.

> In addition to an increased protein catabolic rate, patients supported with dialysis will have additional nitrogen losses.

> Calories provided by dextrose-containing intravenous fluids and dialysate should be considered when planning nutritional support.

> Water-soluble vitamins will be removed with dialysis and should be supplemented to avoid deficiencies.

References

1. (2000) Clinical practice guidelines for nutrition in chronic renal failure. K/DOQI, National Kidney Foundation. Am J Kidney Dis 35:S1–S140

2. (2002) Guidelines for the use of parenteral and enteral nutrition in adult and pediatric patients. JPEN J Parenter Enteral Nutr 26:1SA–138SA

3. (2004) Nutrition of children who are critically ill. In: Kleinman R (ed) Pediatric nutrition handbook. American Academy of Pediatrics, Elk Grove Village, IL, p 643–652

4. Abitbol CL, Rossique M, Rios M (2005) Nutritional support of the pediatric pateint with acute renal failure. In: American Society of Parenteral and Enteral Nutrition (ed) The ASPEN nutrition support practice manual. American Society of Parenteral and Enteral Nutrition, Silver Spring, MD, p 287–295

5. Bansal I, Calhoun BW, Joseph C, et al. (2007) A comparative study of reducing the extracellular potassium concentration in red blood cells by washing and by reduction of additive solution. Transfusion 47:248–250

6. Basi S, Pupim LB, Simmons EM, et al. (2005) Insulin resistance in critically ill patients with acute renal failure. Am J Physiol Renal Physiol 289:F259–F264

7. Berger MM, Shenkin A, Revelly JP, et al. (2004) Copper, selenium, zinc, and thiamine balances during continuous venovenous hemodiafiltration in critically ill patients. Am J Clin Nutr 80:410–416

8. Bird NJ, Streather CP, O'Doherty MJ, et al. (1994) Gastric emptying in patients with chronic renal failure on continuous ambulatory peritoneal dialysis. Nephrol Dial Transplant 9:287–290

9. Boullata J, Williams J, Cottrell F, et al. (2007) Accurate determination of energy needs in hospitalized patients. J Am Diet Assoc 107:393–401

10. Chellis MJ, Sanders SV, Webster H, et al. (1996) Early enteral feeding in the pediatric intensive care unit. JPEN J Parenter Enteral Nutr 20:71–73

11. Chima CS, Meyer L, Hummell AC, et al. (1993) Protein catabolic rate in patients with acute renal failure on continuous arteriovenous hemofiltration and total parenteral nutrition. J Am Soc Nephrol 3:1516–1521

12. Chiolero R, Revelly JP, Tappy L (1997) Energy metabolism in sepsis and injury. Nutrition 13:45S–51S

13. Churchwell MD, Pasko DA, Btaiche IF, et al. (2007) Trace element removal during in vitro and in vivo continuous haemodialysis. Nephrol Dial Transplant 22:2970–2977

14. Cianciaruso B, Bellizzi V, Napoli R, et al. (1991) Hepatic uptake and release of glucose, lactate, and amino acids in acutely uremic dogs. Metabolism 40:261–269

15. Collier S, Gura K, Richardson D, et al. (2005) Parenteral nutrition. In: Hendricks KM, Duggan C (eds) Manual of pediatric nutrition. BC Decker, Hamilton

16. Coss-Bu JA, Klish WJ, Walding D, et al. (2001) Energy metabolism, nitrogen balance, and substrate utilization in critically ill children. Am J Clin Nutr 74:664–669

17. de Lucas C, Moreno M, Lopez-Herce J, et al. (2000) Transpyloric enteral nutrition reduces the complication rate and cost in the critically ill child. J Pediatr Gastroenterol Nutr 30:175–180

18. Druml W (2001) Nutritional management of acute renal failure. Am J Kidney Dis 37:S89–S94

19. Druml W (2005) Nutritional management of acute renal failure. J Ren Nutr 15:63–70

20. Druml W, Schwarzenhofer M, Apsner R, et al. (1998) Fat-soluble vitamins in patients with acute renal failure. Miner Electrolyte Metab 24:220–226

21. Duggan C (2005) Nutritional assessment in sick or hospitalized children. In: Hendricks KM, Duggan C (eds) Manual of pediatric nutrition. BC Decker, Hamilton, p 239–251

22. Falciglia M (2007) Causes and consequences of hyperglycemia in critical illness. Curr Opin Clin Nutr Metab Care 10:498–503

23. Fiaccadori E, Lombardi M, Leonardi S, et al. (1999) Prevalence and clinical outcome associated with preexisting malnutrition in acute renal failure: A prospective cohort study. J Am Soc Nephrol 10:581–593

24. Fiaccadori E, Maggiore U, Giacosa R, et al. (2004) Enteral nutrition in patients with acute renal failure. Kidney Int 65:999–1008

25. Framson CM, LeLeiko NS, Dallal GE, et al. (2007) Energy expenditure in critically ill children. Pediatr Crit Care Med 8:264–267

26. Grodstein GP, Blumenkrantz MJ, Kopple JD, et al. (1981) Glucose absorption during continuous ambulatory peritoneal dialysis. Kidney Int 19:564–567

27. Haugen HA, Chan LN, Li F (2007) Indirect calorimetry: A practical guide for clinicians. Nutr Clin Pract 22: 377–388

28. Hubalewska A, Stompor T, Placzkiewicz E, et al. (2004) Evaluation of gastric emptying in patients with chronic renal failure on continuous ambulatory peritoneal dialysis using 99mTc-solid meal. Nucl Med Rev Cent East Eur 7:27–30

29. Hulst J, Joosten K, Zimmermann L, et al. (2004) Malnutrition in critically ill children: From admission to 6 months after discharge. Clin Nutr 23:223–232

30. Hynote ED, McCamish MA, Depner TA, et al. (1995) Amino acid losses during hemodialysis: Effects of high-solute flux and parenteral nutrition in acute renal failure. JPEN J Parenter Enteral Nutr 19:15–21

31. Ikizler TA, Flakoll PJ, Parker RA, et al. (1994) Amino acid and albumin losses during hemodialysis. Kidney Int 46:830–837

32. Jolliet P, Pichard C, Biolo G, et al. (1998) Enteral nutrition in intensive care patients: A practical approach. Working Group on Nutrition and Metabolism, ESICM. European Society of Intensive Care Medicine. Intensive Care Med 24:848–859

33. Koretz RL (2007) Do data support nutrition support? Part I: Intravenous nutrition. J Am Diet Assoc 107:988–996; quiz 998

34. Koretz RL (2007) Do data support nutrition support? Part II. Enteral artificial nutrition. J Am Diet Assoc 107:1374–1380

35. Kuttnig M, Zobel G, Ring E, et al. (1991) Nitrogen and amino acid balance during total parenteral nutrition and continuous arteriovenous hemofiltration in critically ill anuric children. Child Nephrol Urol 11:74–78

36. Lopez-Herce J, Sanchez C, Carrillo A, et al. (2006) Transpyloric enteral nutrition in the critically ill child with renal failure. Intensive Care Med 32:1599–1605

37. Macias WL, Alaka KJ, Murphy MH, et al. (1996) Impact of the nutritional regimen on protein catabolism and nitrogen balance in patients with acute renal failure. JPEN J Parenter Enteral Nutr 20:56–62

38. Mahdavi H, Kuizon BD, Gales B, et al. (2003) Sevelamer hydrochloride: An effective phosphate binder in dialyzed children. Pediatr Nephrol 18:1260–1264

39. Major K, Lefor AT, Wilson M (2002) Route of nutrition support. Nutrition 18:445–446

40. Marin A, Hardy G (2001) Practical implications of nutritional support during continuous renal replacement therapy. Curr Opin Clin Nutr Metab Care 4:219–225

41. Maxvold NJ, Smoyer WE, Custer JR, et al. (2000) Amino acid loss and nitrogen balance in critically ill children with acute renal failure: A prospective comparison between classic hemofiltration and hemofiltration with dialysis. Crit Care Med 28:1161–1165

42. McElhiney LF (2007) Sevelamer suspension in children with end stage renal disease. Int J Pharm Compound 11:20–24

43. Mendley SR, Majkowski NL (2000) Urea and nitrogen excretion in pediatric peritoneal dialysis patients. Kidney Int 58:2564–2570

44. Moore FA, Feliciano DV, Andrassy RJ, et al. (1992) Early enteral feeding, compared with parenteral, reduces postoperative septic complications. The results of a meta-analysis. Ann Surg 216:172–183

45. Moriyama S, Okamoto K, Tabira Y, et al. (1999) Evaluation of oxygen consumption and resting energy expenditure in critically ill patients with systemic inflammatory response syndrome. Crit Care Med 27:2133–2136

46. Nakamura AT, Btaiche IF, Pasko DA, et al. (2004) In vitro clearance of trace elements via continuous renal replacement therapy. J Ren Nutr 14:214–219

47. Parshuram CS, Joffe AR (2003) Prospective study of potassium-associated acute transfusion events in pediatric intensive care. Pediatr Crit Care Med 4:65–68

48. Pieper AK, Haffner D, Hoppe B, et al. (2006) A randomized crossover trial comparing sevelamer with calcium acetate in children with CKD. Am J Kidney Dis 47:625–635

49. Plank LD, Hill GL (2000) Sequential metabolic changes following induction of systemic inflammatory response in patients with severe sepsis or major blunt trauma. World J Surg 24:630–638

50. Podel J, Hodelin-Wetzel R, Saha DC, et al. (2000) Glucose absorption in acute peritoneal dialysis. J Ren Nutr 10:93–97

51. Pollack MM, Wiley JS, Kanter R, et al. (1982) Malnutrition in critically ill infants and children. JPEN J Parenter Enteral Nutr 6:20–24

52. Quan A, Baum M (1996) Protein losses in children on continuous cycler peritoneal dialysis. Pediatr Nephrol 10:728–731

53. Rock J, Secker DJ (2004) Nutrition management of chronic kidney disease in the pediatric patient. In: Byham-Gray L, Wiesen K (eds) A clinical guide to nutrition care in kidney disease. American Dietetic Association, Chicago, p 127–149

54. Ruley EJ, Bock GH, Kerzner B, et al. (1989) Feeding disorders and gastroesophageal reflux in infants with chronic renal failure. Pediatr Nephrol 3:424–429

55. Salusky IB, Fine RN, Nelson P, et al. (1983) Nutritional status of children undergoing continuous ambulatory peritoneal dialysis. Am J Clin Nutr 38:599–611

56. Salusky IB, Foley J, Nelson P, et al. (1991) Aluminum accumulation during treatment with aluminum hydroxide and dialysis in children and young adults with chronic renal disease. N Engl J Med 324:527–531

57. Salusky IB, Goodman WG, Sahney S, et al. (2005) Sevelamer controls parathyroid hormone-induced bone disease as efficiently as calcium carbonate without increasing serum calcium levels during therapy with active vitamin D sterols. J Am Soc Nephrol 16:2501–2508

58. Sanchez C, Lopez-Herce J, Carrillo A, et al. (2007) Early transpyloric enteral nutrition in critically ill children. Nutrition 23:16–22

59. Schneeweiss B, Graninger W, Stockenhuber F, et al. (1990) Energy metabolism in acute and chronic renal failure. Am J Clin Nutr 52:596–601

60. Schofield WN (1985) Predicting basal metabolic rate, new standards and review of previous work. Hum Nutr Clin Nutr 39 Suppl 1:5–41

61. Sedman AB, Miller NL, Warady BA, et al. (1984) Aluminum loading in children with chronic renal failure. Kidney Int 26:201–204

62. Sedman AB, Wilkening GN, Warady BA, et al. (1984) Encephalopathy in childhood secondary to aluminum toxicity. J Pediatr 105:836–838

63. Soop M, Forsberg E, Thorne A, et al. (1989) Energy expenditure in postoperative multiple organ failure with acute renal failure. Clin Nephrol 31:139–145

64. Srinivasan V, Spinella PC, Drott HR, et al. (2004) Association of timing, duration, and intensity of hyperglycemia with intensive care unit mortality in critically ill children. Pediatr Crit Care Med 5:329–336

65. Story DA, Ronco C, Bellomo R (1999) Trace element and vitamin concentrations and losses in critically ill patients treated with continuous venovenous hemofiltration. Crit Care Med 27:220–223

66. Stumvoll M, Chintalapudi U, Perriello G, et al. (1995) Uptake and release of glucose by the human kidney.

Postabsorptive rates and responses to epinephrine. J Clin Invest 96:2528–2533

67. Suman OE, Mlcak RP, Chinkes DL, et al. (2006) Resting energy expenditure in severely burned children: Analysis of agreement between indirect calorimetry and prediction equations using the Bland-Altman method. Burns 32:335–342

68. van den Berghe G, Wouters P, Weekers F, et al. (2001) Intensive insulin therapy in the critically ill patients. N Engl J Med 345:1359–1367

69. Vazquez Martinez JL, Martinez-Romillo PD, Diez Sebastian J, et al. (2004) Predicted versus measured energy expenditure by continuous, online indirect calorimetry in ventilated, critically ill children during the early postinjury period. Pediatr Crit Care Med 5:19–27

70. Verbruggen SC, Joosten KF, Castillo L, et al. (2007) Insulin therapy in the pediatric intensive care unit. Clin Nutr 26:677–690

71. Wooley JA, Btaiche IF, Good KL (2005) Metabolic and nutritional aspects of acute renal failure in critically ill patients requiring continuous renal replacement therapy. Nutr Clin Pract 20:176–191

72. Yiu V, Harmon WE, Spinozzi N, et al. (1996) High-calorie nutrition for infants with chronic renal disease. J Ren Nutr 6:203–206

Tools for the Diagnosis of Renal Disease

10

K. Mistry and J.T. Herrin

Contents

S.G. Kiessling et al. (eds) *Pediatric Nephrology in the ICU.*
© Springer-Verlag Berlin Heidelberg 2009

Core Messages

> › Kidney function abnormalities are associated with increased morbidity and mortality in critically ill ICU patients.
> › Even modest increases in serum creatinine of 0.3–0.4 mg dL^{-1} lead to a 70% greater risk of death compared with patients without an increase.
> › Physiologic changes that occur during illness may affect solute and water handling as well as renal function. These changes can easily be assessed using a combination of readily available clinical and laboratory data or what can be considered *diagnostic tools*.
> › These tools can be used to do the following:
> – Determine the appropriateness of the renal response for a particular clinical circumstance.
> – Make or confirm a diagnosis.
> – Guide and monitor therapy.

10.1 Introduction

Abnormalities in body chemistry, urine flow, and renal function are relatively common occurrences in hospitalized patients. Critically ill patients who present with or develop acute renal failure have persistently poorer outcomes and higher mortality rates than patients without renal failure [8, 11]. Even modest increases in serum creatinine of 0.3–0.4 mg dL^{-1} in adult patients lead to a 70% greater risk of death compared with patients without an increase [10, 36, 42]. Mortality is even higher in the subgroup of patients who require renal replacement therapy [8, 11, 65]. This increased morbidity and mortality cannot be explained solely by the loss of renal function, but likely reflects the impact of deranged regulatory responses in multiorgan failure. Often isolated renal failure in previously healthy children such as may occur with drug toxicity or even in milder forms of hemolytic uremic syndrome does not require admission to the ICU, but can be safely managed on the regular medical unit. Nonetheless, the loss of GFR places these children at risk for further clinical morbidity and underscores the importance of careful attention to ongoing fluid, electrolyte, and biochemical balance.

Similarly, the pathophysiology of multiple disease processes that afflict ICU patients often interferes with normal renal and endocrine function, necessitating adjustments to drug dosing and fluid administration to prevent electrolyte or acid–base imbalance. This chapter focuses on the diagnostic approach to a range of renal and biochemical abnormalities that may prompt renal consultation in the ICU. Our goal is to provide the clinician with objective scientific measures or tools, which can be reliably used to make a diagnosis and guide therapy.

While some definitive tests may take days or weeks to obtain results, these tools will allow prompt recognition of the nature of the renal response or abnormality, using readily available serum and urinary parameters, with results that are available within hours. This approach enables timely institution of appropriate interventions and the means to effectively monitor the response to these interventions, for instance, the use of the transtubular potassium gradient (TTKG) in hyperkalemia and its response to a therapeutic trial of fludrocortisone (Florinef) or acetazolamide (see Sect. 10.3.5).

Investigational tools supplement the clinical findings. While some provide anatomic information, e.g., renal ultrasound, others provide a snapshot of the physiologic or pathologic responses to various conditions. Examples include urine sodium (UNa) and urine chloride (UCl) as indicators of volume status, and fractional excretion of sodium (FE_{Na}) as an indicator of the tubular response to volume depletion vs. tubular injury, thus permitting its use for differentiating between causes of renal failure [26, 42].

All investigations require careful interpretation, and results need to be put in perspective by a clinician cognizant of the patient's clinical status when the data were obtained. As such, awareness of the limitations of each of the tools is of paramount importance in the interpretation of the results.

10.2 Available Tools

10.2.1 Clinical History and Physical Examination

It is helpful to approach any clinical problem in a stepwise fashion, using objective supportive data whenever possible to build a clear and logical picture of how homeostatic mechanisms have been perturbed. We must emphasize the importance of obtaining the complete history upon presentation to the ICU. This will provide strong clues to the etiology of presenting renal and electrolyte abnormalities. For example, a history of fluid loss by diarrhea or vomiting associated with poor intake, difficulty in replacing losses, or decreasing urine output should alert one to the likelihood of prerenal acute renal failure.

Ingestion of nephrotoxic agents is of particular interest as they may result in renal failure, electrolyte and acid–base abnormalities, acute tubular necrosis, or interstitial nephritis, an effect potentiated by dehydration. Predisposing existing medical conditions, chronic medications, and knowledge about preexisting kidney disease will assist in determining the nature of the underlying renal abnormality and predicting outcome.

Meticulous physical examination will provide additional clues. Fever, state of hydration (reflected as poor tissue turgor in dehydration, or edema in fluid overload), heart rate, blood pressure, need for ventilatory support, cardiac abnormalities, abdominal pathology, and neurologic state are important in discerning the nature of the biochemical and renal abnormalities within the context of the patient's general condition.

Clinical history and physical examination with special emphasis on weight *change*, careful evaluation of mass balance (calculated from consideration of input and output), chemical composition of intravenous fluid, enteral feeds, urine, and stool, and measured losses from drains provide the basis for initial ICU renal recommendations [17]. Consideration of changes produced by both ongoing therapy (for instance, water retention with positive pressure respiration vs. evaporative fluid loss from phototherapy and use of radiant warmers) and changes in body temperature (increased insensible losses with fevers) is necessary to fully assess adequacy of fluid and solute input or losses that may otherwise remain unappreciated [27, 38, 39].

One must differentiate total body water (TBW) status from effective circulating blood volume. Effective circulating volume, that portion of the body water actually perfusing the tissues and accomplishing homeostasis, can be clinically assessed for adequacy by measuring and following changes in blood pressure, heart rate, and central venous pressure (if indicated or available) and by gauging peripheral perfusion by capillary refill. In instances when, despite TBW overload, the effective circulating blood volume is reduced, for example, in patients with capillary leak syndromes postoperatively or with sepsis, or in poor cardiac output states, an increase in both hematocrit and total protein occurs concurrently, reflecting continuing or increasing intravascular depletion.

Bladder catheterization provides valuable information about urine flow rate. At the same time, urine samples can be obtained for biochemical, microscopic, and microbiological analysis. Urine flow rate is sensitive to changes in circulating blood volume, but does not always predict renal function, as evidenced in nonoliguric renal failure. Arbitrary targets for urine output as a marker of adequacy of renal function are often promulgated in the ICU but are of limited clinical utility. Rather, attention to the patient's ongoing volume balance by comparing total input vs. total output and interpreting this in light of the specific clinical circumstances at that point in time is more likely to allow proper clinical interpretation of the adequacy of urine output.

10.2.2 Direct Chemical Measurements

Serum electrolytes, blood urea nitrogen (BUN), creatinine [41], osmolality (P_{Osm}), calcium, phosphorus, albumin, total protein, and hematocrit: These laboratory parameters are followed serially in most ICU patients, and their values allow assessment of the general pattern of response to a clinical condition and its therapy. They may also be indicative of overall adequacy of circulation (for instance, alteration in usual BUN/Cr ratio and parallel changes in hematocrit and total protein suggestive of intravascular volume fluctuations, with an increase with dehydration or a fall with rehydration or fluid overload).

Changes in serum calcium during intensive care treatments demonstrate distinct response patterns for survivors vs. nonsurvivors. The magnitude of increase in the serum calcium after fluid resuscitation is a marker correlating with the patient's ability to withstand physiologic stress, especially after major trauma. Uncorrected calcium provides a better guide to calcium replacement therapy in trauma patients than albumin-adjusted calcium [66].

Certain serum patterns of chemistries can also provide clues as to underlying etiology, for example, (1) the combination of hyponatremia and hyperkalemia with/without hypercalcemia, and minimal change in BUN and creatinine suggests adrenal insufficiency, (2) hypercalcemia and hypophosphatemia with mild elevation in BUN and creatinine suggest primary hyperparathyroidism, while (3) hypocalcemia, hyper-

phosphatemia, and elevated BUN and creatinine suggest secondary hyperparathyroidism.

Urinary sodium (UNa), potassium (UK), chloride (UCl), pH, osmolality (U_{Osm}), urinary urea nitrogen (UUN), glucose, calcium (UCa), phosphorus, and magnesium: Low UNa (<20 mmol L^{-1}) and high urinary osmolality (>500 mOsm kg^{-1}) suggest volume depletion and are the most common urinary assessments for volume. Evaluation of both UNa and UCl concentrations may be necessary to evaluate volume status. Although UNa concentration usually correlates well with volume status, apparent variation may occur in the presence of restricted tubular sodium reabsorption, for example, in renal tubular acidosis (RTA) or significant systemic alkalosis where sodium diuresis needs to occur with bicarbonate loss to maintain electroneutrality. Under these circumstances, the UNa concentration and FE_{Na} will not reflect sodium or intravascular volume status, while UCl concentration will still mirror the changes in circulating volume.

Biochemical excretion patterns in the urine can also provide clues as to the site of tubular abnormality or damage (proximal vs. distal). Fanconi syndrome characterizes generalized proximal tubular dysfunction, resulting in phosphaturia (determined by a low tubular reabsorption of phosphate (TRP)), glucosuria (on dipstick), aminoaciduria, and normal anion gap hyperchloremic metabolic acidosis.

Determination of the electrolyte composition of measured fluid losses may be necessary as a guide to replacement therapy to prevent or treat electrolyte abnormalities, especially if the volume loss is high or renal function is abnormal.

Serum organic acids (lactic acid, pyruvic acid), serum ammonia levels, and urinary amino and organic acid screening is helpful in differentiation of potential metabolic abnormalities, particularly in the neonatal period. Examples include aminoacidopathies such as maple syrup urine disease, tyrosinemia, urea cycle abnormalities and galactosemia, and organic acidopathies such as congenital lactic acidosis and isovaleric acidemia.

10.2.3 Twenty-Four Hour Urinary Excretion

10.2.3.1 Glomerular Filtration Rate (GFR) Estimation

In clinical practice, GFR in children is generally estimated based on the serum creatinine and the child's age and length using the Schwartz formula. In rare circumstances, a 24-h urine collection for creatinine clearance may provide a useful estimation of GFR, for instance, in individuals with exceptional dietary intake (vegan diet or ingestion of creatine supplements), or in the presence of abnormal muscle mass because of amputation, malnutrition, muscle-wasting disease, spinal injury, or myelodysplasia [29, 45]. It is extremely important to be sure to discard the first bladder urine at time zero, measure the time accurately, and obtain the total urine volume for optimal results. A serum creatinine must be obtained during the collection interval.

As renal function declines, increased tubular secretion of creatinine results in overestimation of GFR by this method [54]. For estimation of GFR under these circumstances, it is wise to perform both a creatinine and urea clearance and average the results.

In the ICU setting, rapid and wide variations in GFR follow changing circulation patterns, electrolyte surfeits or deficits, and renal injury, making frequent estimations or measurements over shorter time intervals necessary to allow for medication dosage adjustments. Again, most estimation is done with serum creatinine values and the Schwartz formula. If a bladder catheter is in place, however, a rapid assessment can be done using urine collection periods as short as 15–60 min for measurement of creatinine and urea clearance. Averaging 2–3 sequential collections and using a single midpoint serum creatinine measurement can attain increase in accuracy.

In the assessment of nutritional status, 24-h excretion of sodium, potassium, protein, urea nitrogen, and calcium is necessary to assess changes, particularly if there are significant variations in urinary volume or where balance studies are necessary. The need for such measurements in the ICU setting is rare, however, and careful attention to fluctuations in biochemistries in light of on-going fluid and electrolyte therapy and underlying renal function will generally be adequate.

10.2.4   Derived Values

These values, calculated from direct chemical measurements allow a more sensitive index of renal tubular function and integrity with which to compare *expected values* in response to an observed stimulus. There are no absolute normal values and there is a wide range in *normal* expected responses depending on dietary intake, fluid balance, and intercurrent medications. It is best to compare values obtained in any patient with expected values under similar clinical circumstances.

Derived values commonly used as tools and expected results are outlined in Table 10.1 and include the following:

10.2.4.1   *Fractional Excretion of Sodium*

This measures sodium excreted in the urine as a percentage of sodium filtered at the glomerulus. It may be used in assessment of either volume status or tubular function in renal failure. In infancy, FE_{Na} varies with gestational age: 28-week gestation 12–15%, 32 weeks 10%, and 36 weeks or later 2–5% [35, 39, 56, 62].

Values for FE_{Na} are higher in obstructive uropathy and other states of solute diuresis, e.g., loop diuretic usage, which increases sodium excretion and hence FE_{Na}. Under these circumstances, FE_{Na} cannot be used reliably to interpret volume status. Otherwise, a $FE_{Na} < 1\%$ generally suggests volume depletion or sodium avidity. In the setting of acute kidney injury, a $FE_{Na} < 1\%$ also points toward maintained integrity of tubular reabsorption and prerenal azotemia other than intrinsic renal failure.

10.2.4.2   *Fractional Excretion of Urea (FE_{Urea})*

Like FE_{Na}, this can also be used in the assessment of volume status or tubular function in renal failure. FE_{Urea} has the advantage of being less influenced by volume expansion and diuretic therapy, which are common events in the ICU, and is thus helpful in the evaluation of oliguric states when FE_{Na} cannot be reliably interpreted [9, 14, 43]. A $FE_{Urea} < 40\%$ is generally considered indicative of volume depletion.

10.2.4.3   *Urinary Osmolality to Plasma Osmolality Ratio (U_{Osm}/P_{Osm})*

This may be used as a surrogate for clearance of free water (C_{H2O}) and tubular reabsorption of water (TC_{H2O}). It allows for evaluation of solute excretion and urinary concentrating ability. U_{Osm}/P_{Osm} is also helpful in distinguishing between the various causes of acute renal failure (Table 10.2).

10.2.4.4   *Transtubular Potassium Gradient (TTKG)*

By providing a ratio of tubular fluid potassium to plasma potassium corrected for water reabsorption, this tool provides an indication of adequacy of tubular handling of potassium and the driving force for its excretion in the distal tubule. TTKG is an estimate of potassium excretion under the influence of

Table 10.1   Description of calculations and interpretation of data

Function	What to measure	Formula	Expected value	Interpretation
FE_{Na}	Na and creatinine in plasma and urine	$[(U_{Na}/P_{Na}) \times (P_{Cr} \times U_{Cr})] \times 100$	<1% in oliguria	Dependent on urine flow and Na balance Varies with age
FE_{Urea}	Urea and creatinine in plasma and urine	$[(UUN/BUN) \times (P_{Cr} \times U_{Cr})] \times 100$	40%	Low with decreased circulation High in renal damage Surrogate for FE_{Na} when FE_{Na} cannot be reliably interpreted, e.g., fluid or diuretic administration
U_{osm}/P_{osm}	Urine and plasma osmolality	U_{osm}/P_{osm}	If $P_{osm} > 290$: > 2.5; if $P_{osm} < 275$: < 1	Surrogate for free water clearance (C_{H2O})
TTKG	Urine and plasma osmolality	$[U_K/P_K] \times [P_{osm}/U_{osm}]$	Hypokalemia <5	Adjusts K for water reabsorption beyond the terminal collecting tubule
	Urine and plasma potassium		Hyperkalemia >10	TTKG cannot be reliably interpreted if (1) UNa is <30 mmol L^{-1} and (2) urine is hypotonic
FE_K	Urine and plasma potassium and creatinine	$[(U_K/P_K) \times (P_{Cr} \times U_{Cr})] \times 100$	Use nomograms [5]	Varies with GFR. Can be used when TTKG cannot be used
UK/UNa	Urine Na and K	U_K/U_{Na}	>1 suggestive of aldosterone activity	Gives an indication of aldosterone effect
TRP	Plasma and urine phosphorus and creatinine	$(1 - FE_{phos}) \times 100$	>85%	60–85% in hyperparathyroidism <60% implies tubular leak, e.g., Fanconi syndrome, familial Vit D resistant rickets
Random urine calcium/ creatinine (UCa/UCr)	Urine calcium and creatinine	Urine calcium (mg dL^{-1})/urine creatinine (mg dL^{-1})	Age [49] <7 months: <0.86 7–18 months: <0.60 19 months to 6 years: <0.42 >6 years: <0.2	Varies with calcium intake Higher postprandial Higher in infants
Random urine protein/ creatinine (UProt/UCr)	Urine protein and creatinine	Urine protein (mg dL^{-1})/urine creatinine (mg dL^{-1})	Age [25] <6 months: <0.70 6–12 months: <0.55 1–2 years: 0.4 2–3 years: 0.3 >3 years: 0.2	Approximates urinary protein excretion in grams per day Infants have higher values
Serum anion gap	Serum Na, Cl, HCO_3	$Na - (Cl + HCO_3)$	8–16 mmol L^{-1}	When high, this is caused by unmeasured anions, e.g., ketoacids, lactic acid Normal AG is due to hyperchloremia, due to renal or GI bicarbonate loss

(continued)

Table 10.1 (continued)

Function	What to measure	Formula	Expected value	Interpretation
Urine anion gap	Urine Na, K, Cl	If U pH < 6.1: $UNa + UK - UCl$	± 10 Adult $UNH_4 = -0.8$ $(UAG) + 82$ meq day^{-1}	Approximately 2 meq kg^{-1} acid production for infant; 1 meq kg^{-1} for adult
U_{osm} gap	Urine osmolality, Na, K, UUN, glucose	Measured $U_{osm} -$ $[(2(U_{Na} + U_K)$ $+ (UUN/2.8) +$ $(glucose/18)]$	100–160 mOsm L^{-1}	Used in calculation of NH$_4$ excretion NH$_4$ excretion $= 0.5(U_{Osm}$ gap)

aldosterone and tubular electromotive force (EMF). When urine is hypotonic, or UNa concentration is very low (<30 mmol L^{-1}), TTKG is inaccurate. In general, in hyperkalemic states TTKG should be high (>10) and in hypokalemic states it should be low (<5).

10.2.4.5   Fractional Excretion of Potassium (FE$_K$)

When TTKG cannot be reliably interpreted, FE$_K$ is helpful in the assessment of potassium excretion and aldosterone activity [5, 6, 26]. FE$_K$ corrects urine potassium for the ratio of creatinine in urine and plasma, thus adjusting for reabsorption of water along the whole nephron. Changes in GFR influence FE$_K$; hence, normal values need correction for simultaneous GFR. Although nomograms are available, it is cumbersome to have to balance FE$_K$ for GFR and this is used infrequently [5] unless urine is hypotonic or a low UNa concentration renders TTKG inaccurate.

10.2.4.6   Urinary Potassium/Sodium Ratio

When this ratio is greater than 1.1–1.2 it suggests the presence of aldosterone and resulting kaliuresis. It may be used as a rough guide to aldosterone activity if the urine osmolality is low, precluding the use of TTKG.

10.2.4.7   Tubular Reabsorption of Phosphate (TRP)

TRP may be helpful in assessing a low serum phosphorus concentration suggesting tubular damage, decreased intrinsic tubular reabsorptive capacity, or hyperparathyroidism. This measurement can be helpful in patients taking drugs that have the potential for producing Fanconi syndrome, for example, valproic acid, where the development of hypophosphatemia could be dangerous and consideration of alternative anticonvulsants warranted.

10.2.4.8   Spot or Random Urinary Calcium to Creatinine Ratio (UCa/UCr)

This will vary with dietary calcium loading. It may be necessary to monitor in patients on long-term continuous enteral feedings to prevent nephrocalcinosis, renal calculi, or cholelithiasis. Hypercalciuria is a particular problem in the face of prolonged loop diuretic usage.

Random UCa/UCr ratios vary with age (see Table 10.1) [49] and dietary calcium intake. Ultimately, a 24-h urine collection for calcium, creatinine, and volume provides the most accurate measure of excretion, normal being less than 4 mg kg^{-1} day^{-1}. However, this is rarely necessary in the ICU setting.

10.2.4.9   Spot or Random Urinary Protein to Creatinine Ratio (UProt/UCr)

This may be used as a surrogate for 24-h urine protein excretion to assist in monitoring of glomerular damage. There is good evidence that this correlates well with 24-h protein excretion [29, 31]. Proteinuria must be quantitated and, if significantly elevated, followed for resolution or persistence. Persistent proteinuria is prognostically important in most renal diseases. Variations in degree of proteinuria may occur following pressor therapy, sympathomimetic stimulation, and albumin infusion, and thus may be seen transiently in the ICU patient.

10.2.4.10   Serum Anion Gap (SAG)

This is helpful in determining the cause of metabolic acidosis and differentiating organic acidemia (unmeasured anions) from hyperchloremic metabolic acidosis. See Sect. 10.3.4.1 later.

10.2.4.11   Urinary Anion Gap (UAG) or Urinary Net Charge

This may be used as a surrogate for urinary ammonium and therefore, hydrogen ion excretion. Provided the

Table 10.2 Differential features of acute renal failure

	Prerenal	Renal	Postrenal	Nonoliguric
Urine volume	Decreased	Decreased, normal, or increased	Decreased	Variable
Urinary sediment	Usually normal, there may be some granular or hyaline casts	Evidence of glomerular (dysmorphic red blood cells, red cell casts, granular casts) or tubular injury (red blood cells, epithelial cells, granular and epithelial cell casts)	Usually normal. May have scant granular or hyaline casts. May have eumorphic red blood cells if nephrolithiasis	Usually normal. Occasional tubular epithelial cells
Serum BUN: creatinine ratio	>20:1	<20:1	<20:1	<20:1
Urine sodium (mmol L^{-1})	<20	>40	15–40+	<20
Serum sodium (mmol L^{-1})	Decreased/normal/ increased	Mildly decreased	Variable	Variable
FE_{Na} (%)	<1	>2	>2	1–2
FE_{Urea} (%)	<40	>40	>40	20–40
U_{osm} (mOsm L^{-1})	>350–500	<or about 300	<or about 300	<300
Urine specific gravity	1.020–1.030	1.010–1.015	1.010–1.015	1.008–1.010
U_{osm}/P_{osm}	>1	<1.1	1.1–1.2	<1.1
Renal ultrasound	Normal	Echogenic kidneys, decreased corticomedullary differentiation but otherwise normal	Hydronephrosis, hydroureter, possibly obstructing stone visible, variable bladder size	Normal or mild increase in echogenicity
Nuclear renal scan	Early uptake	Early uptake	Delayed uptake	Early uptake
	Delayed excretion	Delayed or absent excretion	Delayed excretion	Decreased concentration
			Decreased concentration	

urine pH is less than 6.2, a negative UAG is suggestive of the presence of ammonium. It may be used to differentiate between gastrointestinal and renal bicarbonate losses as a cause of metabolic acidosis (see Sect. 10.3.4.2).

10.2.4.12   Urinary Osmolar Gap

This is a useful surrogate for urinary ammonia concentration and can be applied even when urine pH is elevated above 6.2 (showing that some bicarbonate or another unmeasured anion is present in the urine), rendering calculation of urinary ammonium concentration from a UAG invalid.

10.2.4.13   Strong Ion Difference (SID)

May be used to provide similar data as the SAG [13, 15] but is less widely used in practice because of complexities in calculation (see Sect. 10.3.4.2).

10.2.4.14 Plasma Ratios of BUN and Creatinine

This may be helpful in assessment of renal failure (Table 10.2) [55].

10.2.5 Estimating GFR

Estimates of GFR are the best overall indices of the level of kidney function (Table 10.3). It is best to estimate GFR in children and adolescents from predictive equations that take into account the serum creatinine concentration together with the patient's height and gender. Measurement of creatinine clearance using a timed (usually 24 h) sample does not improve the estimate of GFR over predictive equations [16, 29]. However, under certain circumstances, for instance in individuals with exceptional dietary intake (vegetarian or vegan diet, ingestion of creatine supplements) or those with an abnormal muscle mass as a result of amputation, malnutrition, or muscle wasting disease, a timed collection may be more accurate (see Sect. 10.2.3.1).

10.2.6 Urinalysis with Sediment Analysis

When there is renal dysfunction or variation in usual urine output or color, the biochemical and micro-scopic analysis of urine is a rapid and valuable way to determine the etiology and magnitude of these changes [28].

10.2.6.1 Abnormal Urine Color and Hematuria

Sediment analysis is particularly helpful in the evaluation of hematuria. A red or brown urine color together with urine dipstick positive for heme (peroxi-dase-like activity) suggests either frank hematuria or free heme pigment as occurs in hemoglobinuria and myoglobinuria. These entities can be differentiated by microscopic examination of the urinary sediment. The absence of red blood cells on microscopy suggests that the positive heme test on dipstick is due to hemoglob-inuria or myoglobinuria, while the presence of a significant number of red blood cells confirms hematuria.

Free hemoglobin produces a clear *cranberry* colored urine while myoglobin more commonly produces a brownish and slightly opaque appearance to the urine. Measurement of the respective heme pigment in the urine also helps differentiate between these entities. It may take several days, however, before these results are available, so suggestive history and indirect measures of muscle damage (creatine kinase) or hemolysis (falling hemoglobin, reticulocytosis, low haptoglobin, elevated

Table 10.3 Derived values for estimates of GFR

Formula [Reference]	When to use	Calculation	Notes
Schwartz [51]	Children under 70 kg and age < 18 years	C_{Cr} (mL min^{-1} per 1.73 m^2) = k × height (cm)/serum creatinine (mg dL^{-1})	k is dependent on age
			Low birth weight infant: 0.33
			<12 months: 0.45
			>12 months and <14 years: 0.55
			Adolescent boys: 0.7
Counahan-Barratt [16]		C_{Cr} (mL min^{-1} per 1.73 m^2) = 0.43 × height (cm)/serum creatinine (mg dL^{-1})	
Cockcroft-Gault [12]	Age 20 years and older	[(140 − age (years) × weight (kg))/[72 × serum creatinine (mg dL^{-1})]	Multiply result × 0.85 if female
MDRD[a] [37]	Age > 18 years	eGFR (mL min^{-1} per 1.73 m^2) = 186 × (0.742 if female) × (1.212 if black) × serum creatinine (mg dL^{-1})$^{-1.154}$ × age (years)$^{-0.203}$	

[a] Modification of diet in renal disease study

indirect bilirubin, and positive Coombs test) can serve to differentiate between the two more rapidly.

Myoglobin, a small protein (16,700 Da), is readily filtered, whereas the larger hemoglobin (approximately 68,000 Da) is not well filtered unless it dissociates into smaller dimers. Acutely, simply examining a sample of the patient's serum can differentiate between the two conditions: the plasma will be red in hemoglobinuria, but clear in myoglobinuria.

Red or brown urine that is negative by dipstick suggests the presence of nonheme-containing pigment, most often derived from food coloring or drugs such as pyridium or rifampin.

Urinary sediment revealing the presence of *dysmorphic and small red blood cells* associated with cellular casts is suggestive of glomerular etiology, while normal sized *eumorphic red blood cells* without casts imply lower tract bleeding from trauma such as placement of transurethral catheters, hypercalciuria, cystic disease, calculi, or cystitis.

10.2.6.2   Pyuria

Polymorphonuclear leucocytes in the urine imply inflammation from infection or interstitial nephritis. Leukocytes may also be seen in glomerulonephritis with associated inflammation. Although urinary tract infection must be considered in the differential of pyuria, pertinent current clinical signs and symptoms as well as past renal history must be taken into account before a presumptive diagnosis of urinary infection is made before culture results are known.

10.2.6.3   Casts

The pattern of casts and cells in the sediment is helpful in the differentiation of renal failure types (Table 10.2). For instance, hematuria with *muddy brown casts*, granular casts, waxy casts, and epithelial casts is indicative of tubular damage and suggests acute tubular necrosis. Muddy brown casts may also be present in the sediment with minimal or absent hematuria on dipstick, and thus could be missed if the urine is sent for routine laboratory analysis where sediment analysis may often not be performed if the dipstick is negative [64].

10.2.7   Renal Biopsy

When there are features suggestive of a significant glomerular lesion, or rapidly progressive loss of renal function that warrants immediate therapy to slow or halt progression, a diagnostic percutaneous renal biopsy will aid in guiding therapy. This procedure carries an added

risk in ICU patients who often have coagulopathies. Furthermore, technical limitations may arise when positioning for the procedure in a critically ill patient who may be intubated with multiple intravenous lines. Judicious use of plasma or clotting factors or DDAVP, adequate sedation or anesthesia, and careful control of the airway must all be coordinated. Preliminary treatment with steroids, cyclophosphamide, or plasmapheresis may be necessary in rapidly progressive glomerulonephritis or potential Goodpasture's syndrome while awaiting the results of a full diagnostic evaluation. In rare patients, the clinical circumstances may preclude immediate biopsy, but in most circumstances the risk–benefit analysis will favor the information obtained by biopsy.

10.2.8   Tools for Anatomical Assessment

Studies aimed at making an anatomic diagnosis include urinalysis, radiologic imaging, and even histologic and immunohistologic examination of renal tissue obtained at biopsy. While some imaging studies provide static anatomic data, others provide a more dynamic evaluation of relative kidney function [4].

Renal and bladder ultrasound is a noninvasive and portable study. In the ICU, ultrasound is a valuable tool to evaluate general anatomy and exclude abnormality such as hydronephrosis, hydroureter, or other obstruction. Ultrasound precludes the necessity for radioopaque contrast media with its potential for allergic reaction and nephrotoxicity to which critically ill ICU patients are particularly vulnerable [40].

Renal ultrasound provides specific information about kidney size, parenchymal echogenicity, presence or absence of urinary outflow tract dilation, and the state of the bladder. Renal ultrasound can also detect the presence of calcifications, calculi, mass or cystic lesions [4]. Although its sensitivity is limited in detecting calculi less than 5 mm, such small stones are less likely to require emergent intervention since they tend to be nonobstructing [22].

Doppler studies evaluate arterial and venous renal blood flow, and can aid in the diagnosis of arterial or venous thrombosis. Measured arterial resistive indices may also be high in renal allograft rejection.

Other imaging studies such as CT, MR, and angiography can be used to further evaluate renal and vascular anatomy but these studies are infrequently indicated in the ICU patient except in those undergoing trauma evaluation. These studies carry the significant added risk of contrast toxicity, particularly in patients with functional renal impairment or inadequate renal perfusion. A cystogram or urethrogram may be necessary to assess potential bladder or urethral trauma but is rarely otherwise indicated in the ICU patient.

Isotope studies are helpful in evaluation of perfusion. MAG3, DMSA, and Tc[99] labeled DPTA or EDTA scans provide information about the differential kidney function and the contribution of each kidney to total GFR. Furthermore, the excretion phase of a MAG3 scan, with or without furosemide, assesses the adequacy of drainage. These scans also provide evidence of anatomic or functional obstruction as the cause of delayed allograft function in the early posttransplant period.

Measurement of GFR using labeled iothalamate or iohexol provides the *gold standard* for assessment of renal function. These studies are rarely indicated in ICU patients, however, especially since serum creatinine can be used to estimate creatinine clearance in most clinical circumstances (Table 10.3).

10.3 Practical Scenarios: Using the Tools

Using patterns of serum and urine chemistries can help determine whether the renal response to a clinical stress is appropriate or expected. The following clinical scenarios are presented to examine the physiology of *expected* urinary response patterns and to indicate the basis for selection of appropriate tools. Table 10.4 lists the tools that may be helpful in the evaluation of various clinical scenarios. Optimal assessment requires intact renal and endocrine (adrenal, pituitary, and thyroid) function and no recent fluid bolus or diuretic administration. Clearly this is rare in the ICU, and consideration of the clinical scenario and comparison of the observed and expected responses will be necessary.

10.3.1 Change in Renal Physiology Secondary to Circulatory Change

The expected response to hypovolemia is decreasing urine volume (oliguria) with low UNa concentration (usually <20 mmol L^{-1}) and increased U_{Osm} (>500 mOsm kg^{-1}). If the response in oliguria is a higher than expected UNa concentration or decreased U_{Osm}, this pattern suggests tubular damage and further investigation and treatment for renal failure can be instituted. FE$_{Urea}$ may be helpful (see Sect. 10.2.4.2),

particularly if urine sample is not obtained before a fluid bolus or diuretic therapy [9, 14, 43].

10.3.2 Assessment of Effective Circulating Blood Volume in Hyponatremic Metabolic Alkalosis

Metabolic alkalosis may follow primary or secondary hyperaldosteronism. Low intravascular volume leads to secondary hyperaldosteronism, stimulating the physiological changes leading to reabsorption of sodium, chloride, and water. Low UNa and UCl concentration and decrease in urine output reflect this. The changes in UNa and UCl usually occur in parallel if the effective blood volume is contracted.

If there is a chloride deficit in the setting of sodium depletion or sodium avidity, however, reabsorption of bicarbonate becomes necessary to allow for electroneutrality in the face of continued sodium reabsorption [34]. When urine sodium is excreted with bicarbonate for electroneutrality, then UNa no longer reflects volume status. *Both* UNa and UCl concentrations are thus required for evaluation [34]. Treatment consists of sufficient fluid to replete sodium, potassium, and chloride.

In mineralocorticoid excess where circulatory volume is normal or increased, in salt-losing tubulopathies such as Bartter and Gitelman syndromes [50], or in renal dysplasia with intrinsic tubular dysfunction, UCl concentration may be elevated or normal. UCl will not be a good measure of volume, and BUN/creatinine ratio may be used to assess volume status along with other measures such as parallel changes in hematocrit and total protein.

In primary mineralocorticoid abnormalities, weight will generally remain stable and edema is rare, but blood pressure is often elevated. In secondary hyperaldosteronism, volume and weight change more closely parallel one another. In cases of hypovolemia, review of other clinical factors such as diuretic overuse or other drug exposure may figure in the development of alkalosis.

Initial laboratory assessment should include concurrent serum and urine chemistries including sodium, potassium, chloride, urea nitrogen, creatinine, osmolality, calcium, and magnesium (see Tables 10.4 and 10.5) to determine response to tubular damage. Both calcium and magnesium wasting occur in the presence of lesions of the loop of Henle, while magnesium wasting alone occurs in Gitelman syndrome accompanied by extremely low urinary calcium excretion.

Table 10.4   Expected changes from nephron damage

Nephron segment	Effective exchange	Effect of lesion at site
Glomerulus	Ultrafiltrate	Decreased GFR
		Low tubular fluid delivery distally
Proximal convoluted tubule	Na and Cl reabsorption	Na diuresis
	HCO_3^- reabsorption	Excretion of HCO_3^-, K, glucose, amino acids, Phosphate and uric acid
	K reabsorption	
	Glucose reabsorption	
	Amino acids reabsorption	
	Phosphate reabsorption	
	Organic acids and uric acid reabsorption	
Loop of Henle (thick ascending limb)	Na, K, Cl reabsorption	Na, Cl, K wasting
	Ca, Mg reabsorption	Ca, Mg wasting
		Low U_{Osm} max
Distal convoluted tubule	Na, Cl reabsorption/ excretion (regulated)	Na, Cl wasting
	K secretion/absorption (regulated)	K wasting
	Ca reabsorption	Mg wasting
		Low Ca
		U_{Osm} max retained
Cortical collecting duct	Na, Cl reabsorption	Na, Cl wasting
	Free water reabsorption under influence of ADH	No effect on Ca, Mg
		Low K excretion
		Low TTKG
Medullary collecting duct	Cl reabsorption paracellular	Na, Cl retention
	Ca, Mg (paracellular)	Dilute urine – diabetes insipidus
	Free water reabsorption under influence of ADH	Na, Cl wasting
	Na, Cl reabsorption (late)	No Ca, Mg wasting

With occult electrolyte losses, comparison of UNa and UCl can assist in making a diagnosis. In the acute phase, vomiting leads to a high UNa and low UCl as there are obligate urinary losses of sodium with bicarbonate in the face of evolving alkalosis. With ongoing volume depletion, however, urinary sodium will eventually fall with increased proximal reabsorption of filtered sodium. Laxative abuse usually leads to low UNa and high UCl. Recent diuretic abuse leads to high UNa and UCl, but chronically, with volume contraction and chloride depletion, UNa and UCl will be low. Continuing high UNa and UCl losses in the presence of contracted extracellular fluid volume suggest a tubulopathy, for example, Bartter or Gitelman syndromes [26].

10.3.3 Assessment of Acute Renal Failure (ARF)

In the ICU, renal consultation is often called for acute kidney injury with oliguria and rising levels of BUN and creatinine. The etiology of acute kidney injury

Table 10.5 Helpful tools for various clinical scenarios

Clinical Scenario	Clinical tools	Biochemical tools
1. Determination of effective circulating blood volume	Sequential weights	UNa, UCl, UUN, U_{Osm}
	Urine output	FE_{Na}, FE_{Urea}
	Blood pressure	U_{Osm}/P_{Osm}
	Heart rate	UUN, BUN
	Peripheral perfusion	$U_{Creatinine}$, $P_{Creatinine}$
	Central venous pressure	Hematocrit, total protein
2. Oligoanuria	Sequential weights	UNa, UCl, UUN, U_{Osm}
	Urine output	FE_{Na}, FE_{Urea}
	Blood pressure	U_{Osm}/P_{Osm}
	Heart rate	UUN, BUN
	Peripheral perfusion	$U_{Creatinine}$, $P_{Creatinine}$
	Central venous pressure	
3. Dysnatremia	Sequential weights	UNa, U_{Osm}
	Urine output	FENa
	Central venous pressure	U_{Osm}/P_{Osm}
		Serum Na, Cl, uric acid
4. Dyskalemia	Blood pressure	TTKG
		FE_K
		Renin, aldosterone, cortisol
		Serum electrolytes, bicarbonate
		UNa, U_{Osm}
5. Disturbance in osmolality:	Sequential weights	Free water clearance (C_{H2O})
SIADH vs. cerebral salt wasting	Urine output	Urine and plasma sodium and osmolality
Diabetes insipidus vs. solute diuresis	Urine volume	Plasma uric acid
6. Acid–base disturbances	Blood pressure	Arterial/venous pH, pCO_2 and HCO_3
	Heart rate	Serum anion gap if normal serum albumin
	Peripheral perfusion	Adjusted serum anion gap if hypoalbuminemia present
	Respiratory rate	Urine anion gap
	Losses from drains/fistulae	Osmolar gap
7. Miscellaneous	Urine output	Urine Ca/creatinine ratio
Calcium/phosphorus metabolism		Serum Ca, phosphorus, PTH, 25 vitamin D, 1.25 vitamin D
Fanconi syndrome		Proximal tubular function: amino aciduria, TRP, glycosuria
		Serum uric acid, calcium, phosphorus, creatinine

(*continued*)

Table 10.5 (continued)

Clinical Scenario	Clinical tools	Biochemical tools
8. Magnesium		Proximal tubular function: amino aciduria, TRP, glycosuria
		Serum uric acid, calcium, phosphorus, creatinine
9. Tumor lysis syndrome	Urine output	Serum uric acid, calcium, phosphorus, creatinine
	Sequential weights	TRP, TTKG
	Blood pressure	

is often made based on comparison of normal renal tubular function with an abnormal response from damaged tubules. Chemical assessment includes UNa, urine creatinine, UUN, U_{Osm}, FE_{Na}, FE_{Urea}, and U_{Osm}/P_{Osm} [55].

Acute renal failure represents a recent abrupt decline in GFR, as measured indirectly by a rise in serum creatinine. Renal failure may occur with sustained urine output and thus be nonoliguric, or may occur with oliguria or complete anuria.

The causes of acute kidney injury are traditionally divided into three broad categories: prerenal, intrinsic renal, and postrenal. History and laboratory parameters help to differentiate between these categories and will point the clinician toward effective therapy.

10.3.3.1   Prerenal Renal Failure

Here, the underlying reason for rise in serum BUN and creatinine is due to reduced renal perfusion or an increase in catabolism. The cause for hypoperfusion may be actual volume depletion, as occurs in severe blood loss from trauma or surgical complication, dehydration from gastrointestinal illness, renal losses from polyuria or diuretics, capillary leak syndromes with sepsis or malignancy, or hypoalbuminemia and subsequent fluid loss from the intravascular to interstitial compartment due to reduced capillary oncotic pressure. Alternatively, there may be a state of *perceived volume depletion* such as may occur in low cardiac output states, hepatorenal syndrome, or renal artery stenosis where a smaller decrease in intravascular volume leads to an exaggerated decrease in renal perfusion secondary to an activated rennin–angiotensin system [1].

Renal hypoperfusion, irrespective of cause, generally leads to an appropriate renal tubular response with sodium, chloride, and water retention, and resultant

oliguria. UNa concentration will be low, usually less than $20\,\mathrm{mmol}\,L^{-1}$ on a random sample and U_{Osm} high. As well, appropriate reduction in free water clearance results in U_{Osm}/P_{Osm} ratio of >1. In hypoperfusion, the salt and water avidity and increased ADH activity result in decreased tubular filtrate flow and an increased reabsorption of urea both proximally and distally. As a result, there is a disproportionate rise in urea compared with creatinine (serum BUN: creatinine >20:1).

Therapy for prerenal renal failure involves measures to improve renal perfusion to reverse the physiologic response that has caused renal dysfunction. Maneuvers may involve rehydration or transfusions to restore circulating blood volume, management of renal artery stenosis, or therapy to improve cardiac output. Patient weight and urine output compared with fluid intake must be monitored closely, especially while giving intravenous fluids for volume repletion. Prolonged or severe dehydration may lead to acute tubular necrosis that will not respond to hydration alone, and overzealous fluid administration, particularly in the presence of such tubular dysfunction, may lead to clinically significant volume imbalance manifested by edema, hypertension, or pulmonary edema.

10.3.3.2   Intrinsic (Parenchymal) Renal Failure

Intrinsic renal failure may arise from a number of causes. Many patients with critical illness have been exposed to nephrotoxins and initial clinical assessment should include a history of drug exposure. These include (1) toxic agents such as antibiotics, particularly synthetic penicillins, cephalosporins, amphotericin B, or proton pump blockers, (2) arteriolar vasoconstrictor agents such as calcineurin inhibitors and radiocontrast agents, or (3) drugs that increase the susceptibility to renal failure such as non steroidal anti-inflammatory drugs and angiotensin-converting enzyme inhibitors or angiotensin receptor blockers [1]. Additionally, factors impacting volume status such as adequacy of circulation, sepsis with vascular leak, and weight changes should be reviewed. It is important to define whether acute renal dysfunction has followed a single insult (expect early recovery), a more prolonged insult (prolonged recovery), or whether the episode follows a complication during recovery from a prior episode of ARF (when recovery is usually delayed and often incomplete). The injury due to acute interstitial nephritis or nephrotoxic medications may result in tubulointerstitial damage and swelling, leading to water and sodium retention, and inflammation with pyuria, often eosinophilouria or white cell casts.

When the abnormality is a decrease in intrinsic renal function due to a glomerulonephritis, then glomerulotubular imbalance and decreased urine flow lead to increased proximal reabsorption of sodium and water. Stimulation of the renin–angiotensin system results in increased urinary specific gravity or U_{Osm}, low UNa, and TBW and sodium retention frequently manifested by edema.

By comparison, in acute tubular necrosis, the damaged nephron is unable to handle solutes and water appropriately, and intratubular cellular debris and cast formation lead to increased intratubular pressure, decreased glomerular filtration, and increased tubular fluid reabsorption.

Since most of these processes result in an inability to handle solutes and water appropriately, particular attention to monitoring the patient's fluid balance and serum chemistries is warranted. Certain forms of glomerular injury such as lupus nephritis and rapidly progressive glomerulonephritis such as ANCA-associated disease and Goodpasture's syndrome may require specific therapy. Other disorders will likely recover spontaneously with time with supportive management including avoidance or discontinuation of toxic agents and restoration of circulation.

10.3.3.3 Postrenal Acute Renal Failure

This form of acute renal failure is usually due to obstruction of the urinary tract. Prompt recognition by appropriate imaging (renal and bladder ultrasound, MAG3 scan) will allow for timely intervention for relief of the obstruction and improvement in kidney drainage and function. Following relief of an obstruction, a diuresis may ensue and attention must be paid to overall solute and water loss to prevent clinical compromise.

10.3.4 Assessment of Acid–Base Balance

The assessment of acid–base balance in the ICU differs from that in the general ward setting in that complex mixed disturbances are more common, and interference with compensation occurs more commonly because of change in respiratory and renal function. It becomes necessary to consider both traditional measures of acid–base balance such as pH and blood gases, *and* electrolyte pattern, serum anion gap (SAG), and P_{Osm}, to avoid overlooking an underlying *occult* disorder in the presence of a mixed acid–base disorder.

SAG, adjusted SAG, base excess, buffer base, and SID represent attempts to (1) adjust the anionic contribution of plasma proteins and phosphate ion in acid–base balance, (2) compensate for the complex changes seen with fever, which increases hydrogen ion generation, (3) reflect changes in plasma osmolality, (4) pCO_2, and (5) electrolyte balance. These complex interactions make any single assessment of acid–base homeostasis unlikely to provide a complete picture of acid–base balance [53].

Multiple tools are available that attempt to integrate gas exchange, changes in the anion contribution of albumin on pH, and osmolar changes. As outlined later, each of the tools described has advantages in examination of a portion of the acid–base spectrum, but also has limitations.

As with many clinical assessments, the history and physical findings are important first steps. Clinical history needs to examine (1) elements associated with volume control, for example, sepsis, nausea, vomiting, ongoing losses from drains and fistulae, the potential for *third-space* sequestration; (2) water and solute balance including composition of feeds, increased losses with fever and polyuria, or decreased losses in antidiuretic states (SIADH); and (3) the presence of renal or respiratory disease. Physical examination notes the state of hydration, weight gain or loss, pulse and respiratory rate, and pattern of respiration (Kussmal respiration).

Assessment of serum electrolytes and serum bicarbonate will allow calculation of the SAG, while pH and blood gases will assist in determining respiratory vs. metabolic components. Urine pH and urine chemistries will allow calculation of UAG (net charge) and, if the urine pH exceeds 6.2, calculation of the urine osmolar gap to estimate urine ammonium and, therefore, hydrogen ion excretion. These tools will assist in differentiating between renal and gastrointestinal (extrarenal) bicarbonate losses. UCa and TRP measurement may be necessary in patients with a chronic metabolic acidosis when use of phosphate bone buffer stores limits pH changes.

10.3.4.1   *Blood Gases*

Arterial gases are only required if pO_2 is a critical variable, otherwise venous gases suffice. The Henderson–Hasselbach equation attributes variation in plasma pH to modifications in plasma bicarbonate or pCO_2 and categorizes acid–base disturbances into four primary disturbances based on pCO_2 and bicarbonate concentration: (1) respiratory acidosis (increased pCO_2), (2) respiratory alkalosis (decreased pCO_2), (3) metabolic acidosis (decreased extracellular base excess), and (4) metabolic alkalosis (increased extracellular base excess). Regulation of the pCO_2/bicarbonate buffer pair fixes the hydrogen ion concentration and determines the ratio of other body buffer pairs [46]. The pCO_2/HCO_3 pair is unique in being an open system with CO_2 elimination by respiration and potential regeneration of bicarbonate by the kidney.

Since pCO_2 and HCO_3 are dependent variables and their calculation does not consider the effect of albumin as an anion, consideration of pCO_2 and HCO_3 alone may lead to misrepresentation of complex acid–base imbalances. In mixed acid–base disturbances, the diagnosis rests on comparison of the pCO_2 or HCO_3 with *expected* compensatory changes for that acid–base aberration.

The serum bicarbonate concentration or total CO_2 content can be used as a screen of metabolic vs. respiratory acid–base disturbance. Remember that disturbances in hydrogen ion result in change in electrolyte composition due to transcellular shifts to maintain electroneutrality, but changes in electrolyte composition are not always associated with change in hydrogen ion concentration.

SAG reflects the contribution of unmeasured anions, largely albumin and phosphate, on total anion/cation balance [20]. Metabolic acidosis can be classified according to whether the anion gap is increased above its normal range of 8–12 [20]. In the former situation, unmeasured anions lead to apparent excess in cation (measured as sodium). The presence of an increased anion gap suggests that the acidosis is the likely result of lactic acidosis, diabetic or alcoholic ketoacidosis, uremia, or toxin ingestion (methanol, ethylene glycol, aspirin, paraldehyde). On the other hand, hyperchloremic metabolic acidosis results in a normal anion gap (nonanion gap acidosis) where an increase in chloride concentration parallels decrease in serum bicarbonate. This is most commonly associated with bicarbonate losses from the GI tract or kidney.

Concurrent calculation of the anion gap with blood gases can suggest a mixed acid–base disorder and has the potential to detect a *hidden* acidosis in approximately 30% of cases where SAG is not adjusted for change in albumin. The SAG works best clinically when the serum total protein, albumin, and phosphate concentrations are approximately normal.

Another limitation to the use of SAG in the ICU rests with differences in techniques used for electrolyte measurements [20, 53]. The laboratory measurement by indirect electrolyte assay, as used in most standard clinical chemistry departments, and direct electrode methods, commonly used in ICU/anesthesia laboratories can show significant differences in sodium and chloride concentrations. Sodium measurements by indirect methods are usually higher than those by direct electrode method, whereas chloride measurements by indirect methods tend to be lower. Furthermore, these changes increase in magnitude as plasma albumin concentration decreases [63]. These factors result in an inaccurate calculated SAG in patients with hypoalbuminemia (critically ill patients, nephrotic and cirrhotic patients) and, under these circumstances, an adjusted SAG may be more helpful.

10.3.4.2   *Adjusted SAG*

Hypoalbuminemia lowers the expected SAG and thereby can mask an anion gap metabolic acidosis, especially if clinicians do not appreciate that in hypoalbuminemia an anion gap that falls in the normal range may denote a metabolic acidosis. Since significant hypoalbuminemia is common in critically ill patients in the ICU, the SAG should be corrected for change in albumin concentration and pH effect [47, 60]. This value is called an *adjusted SAG* and may be calculated according to the following equations [21]:

If albumin is measured in grams per liter (international units):

Adjusted SAG = observed SAG + 0.25 [normal serum albumin − measured serum albumin].

If American standard units for albumin in grams per deciliter are used

Adjusted SAG = observed SAG + 2.5 [normal serum albumin − measured serum albumin].

UAG or net charge gives an idea of hydrogen ion generation as ammonium, or potential anion loss [6]. Gastrointestinal bicarbonate loss results in a negative UAG, while renal bicarbonate loss is associated with a positive UAG. Thus in a normal anion gap metabolic acidosis, UAG can suggest the site of generation of the acidosis.

Base excess (BE) and buffer base (BB) are measured from the Siggaard Anderson nomogram for pH and gas measurement [2, 3, 57–59]. BE is a measure of change in strong acid or strong base needed to restore serum pH to normal at normal pCO_2, and is numerically the difference between BB measured and BB at normal pH/PCO_2, thus representing a measure of non-respiratory acid–base status. BE and pCO_2 can completely characterize acid–base disorders assuming that nonbicarbonate buffers are normal [15, 59, 60].

BB = $[A^-] + [HCO_3^-]$, where A represents the negative charge on albumin and phosphate ion yielding similar information to A_{TOT} calculation (see following section). Base excess or deficit caused by unmeasured anion, or an albumin-adjusted anion gap, are good predictors of plasma lactate concentration, while acid–base variables are not.

10.3.4.3 Strong Ion Difference (SID)

Calculations in this model proposed by Stewart [15, 61] are based on the physicochemical premise of electroneutrality, where plasma pH results from the degree of plasma water dissociation. This dissociation is determined by three independent variables (1) SID, (2) the total nonvolatile weak acids in plasma (A_{TOT}), and (3) pCO_2. SID and A_{TOT} represent a measure of the metabolic components and pCO_2 the respiratory contribution.

At the bedside, both the apparent and effective SID can be calculated and used to determine the strong ion gap (SIG), which can then be used in a manner similar to anion gap [13, 15, 60]. The benefits of the SIG rest in its detection of otherwise unidentified anions in plasma whenever the serum total protein, albumin, and phosphate concentrations are markedly abnormal. SIG can be valuable in clinical settings or in research studies investigating acid–base balance and help provide an understanding of acid–base properties of administered intravenous fluids [41].

In terms of calculations:

Apparent SID (SIDa) = [Na + K] − [arterial lactate + Cl].
Effective SID (SIDe) = [Na + K] − [albumin + phosphorus + pCO_2].
SIG = SIDa − SIDe.

The SID approach categorizes eight primary acid–base disturbances: (1) respiratory acidosis (increased pCO_2), (2) respiratory alkalosis (decreased pCO_2), (3) strong ion acidosis (decreased SID), (4) strong ion alkalosis (increased SID), (5) nonvolatile buffer ion acidosis (increased A_{TOT}), (6) nonvolatile buffer ion alkalosis (decreased A_{TOT}), (7) temperature acidosis (increased body temperature), and (8) temperature alkalosis (decreased body temperature).

The measurement and calculation of SID is more complex than that of SAG. Although the compensation for more variables is appealing, practically, the increased number of measurements and complexities of calculation has hindered more widespread acceptance. This led to attempts at simplifying the formulae, providing approximations of SIDa and SIDe, or using the independent variables of SID to define the pH of body fluids since for a given value of pCO_2 the pH of body fluids is essentially determined by a difference between SID and A_{TOT}.

In practice, use of the SID better pinpoints the etiology of an acid–base abnormality than relying on bicarbonate concentration, uncorrected anion gap (S AG), and BE measurements. When *adjusted SAG* is included in the analysis, however, the SID approach did not offer any diagnostic or prognostic advantages [18]. Given the complexities of calculations with the SID and lack of clear benefit over *adjusted SAG*, we recommend using an adjusted SAG (see 10.3.4.2) rather than SID for typical bedside calculation.

10.3.4.4 Winter's Formula to Check the Degree of Compensation

When metabolic acidosis is present, Winter's formula estimates the expected compensatory decrease in pCO_2. Expected pCO_2 mmHg = (serum bicarbonate mmol/L × 1.5) + 8 [68]. The actual pCO_2 should be within 2 mmHg of the expected pCO_2 calculated by this formula. A discrepancy of > 2 mmHg implies the presence of an additional respiratory component other than compensation. For example, a patient has the following blood gas finding: pH 7.32, pCO_2 15 mmHg, and bicarbonate 8 mmol/L. With the decreased systemic pH and bicarbonate, a primary metabolic acidosis exists. To determine if the pCO_2 of 15 mmHg is an appropriate compensatory respiratory alkalosis, Winter's formula can be applied. With Winter's formula, the expected pCO_2 should be (8 × 1.5) + 8, or 20 mmHg. Since the actual pCO_2 is lower than expected at 15 mmHg, this implies an additional acid–base anomaly: a respiratory alkalosis.

10.3.5   Assessment of Dyskalemia

Aberrations in renal potassium handling are found frequently in ICU patients. The tools for evaluation of potassium imbalance are based on the expectation that, under normal circumstances, potassium intake is balanced by potassium excretion. Since most of the factors that modulate potassium balance impact excretion, evaluation of factors affecting renal excretion is most important [24].

If the estimated potassium excretion rate is not that expected for the degree of hyper- or hypokalemia, the problem can be assumed to be renal in origin. Renal dyskalemias are usually the result of either abnormal aldosterone response (alterations in secretion or change in receptor response) or result from an inability to generate the negative EMF required for potassium excretion.

To assess the nature of the problem, one must examine (1) body volume status, which influences both cortical collecting tubular flow and aldosterone secretion, (2) components of the driving force influencing potassium concentration in the urine (TTKG), and (3) relative sodium (aldosterone driven) and chloride reabsorption rate (electroneutral sodium and chloride shunting either at the ascending loop Na–K–2Cl exchanger site or in the distal and collecting tubules under the influence of WNK1 or WNK4) [23, 24, 69].

Since a net negative tubular luminal charge (EMF negative) is necessary to provide the electrogenic force for potassium excretion, either an increase in sodium reabsorption or decrease in chloride reabsorption will enhance potassium excretion. Conversely, a decrease in sodium reabsorption or increase in chloride reabsorption will limit potassium excretion.

Clinical history and physical examination should aim at defining (1) aldosterone stimulation due to decreased effective circulating blood volume (BP, pulse, state of hydration, weight change), (2) agents that change the EMF negativity, and (3) medications that decrease potassium secretion such as potassium-sparing diuretics, antibiotics, and calcineurin inhibitors, or that increase sodium delivery such as furosemide or acetazolamide.

In addition to serum potassium, sodium, and calcium to assess electrolyte influence on cell membrane function, useful diagnostic tools include UNa, UK, urinary flow rate, urine volume, U_{Osm}, P_{Osm}, TTKG, and FE_K that will allow a measure of the driving force to secrete potassium.

Tubular fluid volume delivered to the collecting duct is modified by ADH that causes reabsorption of water and urea. An estimate of the tubular fluid volume traversing the cortical collecting duct is made by dividing the final urinary concentration of sodium or potassium by U_{Osm}/P_{Osm} to correct for water reabsorption, allowing the use of TTKG as an estimate of the driving force for potassium excretion [5, 32, 48, 52, 67]. Dilute or hypotonic urine with high flow, or limited delivery of sodium distally, changes the driving force, precluding the use of TTKG. Under these circumstances, FE_K can be used to assess tubular handling of potassium. FE_K varies with GFR, reabsorption from the proximal tubule and ascending loop, and distal secretion, thereby necessitating comparison to GFR using a nomogram as previously discussed [5].

Optimally, blood and urine samples for evaluation of any dyskalemia are obtained before commencement of specific treatment to correct the imbalance. This is often challenging in the ICU setting. Remember that plasma renin and aldosterone levels will be acutely depressed for some hours by a fluid bolus. High urine flow may be produced and UNa, UK, and TTKG will also change, but to a lesser degree in response to the fluid bolus.

Hyperkalemia resulting from low potassium excretion may follow decreased sodium reabsorption or a more positive tubular EMF. Review of clinical volume status, urinary TTKG, and UNa concentration is necessary to evaluate the physiological cause, postulate etiology, and design therapy. Although changes in plasma renin and aldosterone concentrations can be diagnostic, knowledge of the conditions under which the samples were obtained is necessary for interpretation, noting the presence of volume expansion, which is likely to suppress these levels or diuretic usage that will stimulate levels. In addition, the results are rarely available rapidly enough to guide therapy.

Hyperkalemia secondary to low urinary potassium excretion may also result from (1) decreased aldosterone activity in adrenal disease (decreased production), (2) interference with receptor function (pseudohypoaldosteronism), or (3) drugs such as potassium-sparing diuretics, antibiotics (trimethoprim and pentamidine), and calcineurin inhibitors. Hypoaldosteronism leads to decreased sodium reabsorption and high UNa (even in the presence of low extracellular fluid volume) with a low TTKG, high plasma renin, and low plasma aldosterone level [67]. Therapy is fludrocortisone and sodium supplementation as necessary.

With pseudohypoaldosteronism type 1, TTKG is low but plasma renin and aldosterone levels are normal or elevated, and response to fludrocortisone is limited [67]. In the presence of potassium-sparing diuretics (spironolactone, amiloride), antibiotics (trimethoprim or pentamidine), or calcineurin inhibitors, response to fludrocortisone will be blunted as will be the ability to generate an EMF gradient. Treatment is symptomatic if it is not possible to withdraw or modify drug dose.

Increased sodium chloride reabsorption (chloride shunting or what is termed pseudohypoaldosteronism type 2 [23, 24, 69]) with change in EMF is demonstrated by a low TTKG not responsive to Florinef, low UNa, high extracellular fluid volume often with hypertension, and low plasma renin and aldosterone levels. Treatment in this group of patients is aimed at (1) increase in distal sodium delivery to produce a negative EMF with sodium bicarbonate supplementation or acetazolamide administration, and (2) therapy for life-threatening hyperkalemia with insulin and glucose, administration of beta agonists, and Kayexalate. A response to changing the EMF may be tested using TTKG pre and post therapy. Renin and aldosterone can also be assayed but TTKG can be calculated immediately [26, 32]. Thiazide administration in patients with WNK-chloride shunt abnormalities will correct both the hyperkalemia and also treat the hypertension mediated by the anomaly in sodium chloride reabsorption.

10.3.6 Approach to Dysnatremia

Although referral for dysnatremia is prompted by serum sodium values, a change in sodium implies a change in TBW in relation to total body sodium. Thus, assessment requires review of both water and sodium balance. The clinician should remember that serum sodium correlates with change in TBW, and UNa concentration correlates with changes in total body sodium.

The brain is the target organ for dysnatremia and the predominant symptoms are neurological. The generation and persistence of the water abnormalities seen in dysnatremia are, however, dependent on changes in renal function or renal free water clearance. Classification of dysnatremic states is based on body weight, volume status, and osmolar status [7, 19, 44].

Hyperosmolar hyponatremia occurs in severe hyperglycemia or after exposure to mannitol, ethanol, or methanol. Hyponatremia with normal osmolality occurs in hypoproteinemic states. Hypoosmolar hyponatremia is associated with SIADH, renal failure, or hyponatremic dehydration.

Sodium levels may be factitiously low in the presence of hyperlipidemia if sodium is measured by flame photometry methods, or in hyperosmolar states such as hyperglycemia, where intracellular water moves to the plasma. For each 100 mg dL^{-1} rise in glucose, there will be a decrease in plasma sodium of 1.2–1.4 mmol L^{-1} [19].

Assessment of dysnatremia includes evaluation of hydration status (fluid overload, edema, dehydration, body weight) [17]. Serum electrolytes may suggest a pattern of endocrine dysfunction, or demonstrate hypokalemia or hypercalcemia, which interfere with tubular response to ADH and promote a diuresis. BUN and creatinine are used as indirect measures of renal function and UNa, UK, UCa, UUN, urine creatinine, and U_{Osm} (or specific gravity) provide a measure of urinary solute excretion and allow calculation of derived values FE_{Na}, TTKG, and U_{Osm}/P_{Osm}. Hematocrit, total protein, and serum uric acid can demonstrate dilution or contraction of TBW.

10.3.6.1 Hyponatremia

Hyponatremia usually results from an increase in TBW under conditions where the kidney cannot excrete free water. To generate hypotonic urine it is necessary to provide sufficient tubular fluid to the diluting segment of the nephron's thick ascending limb and early distal tubule where reabsorption of sodium, potassium, and chloride (but not water) leads to a hypotonic tubular fluid. The presence or absence of vasopressin in the collecting tubule will determine if water reabsorption leads to concentrated or dilute urine. In the presence of vasopressin/ADH, the U_{Osm} is >300 mOsm kg^{-1} and free water clearance (C_{H2O}) becomes negative, demonstrating water reabsorption.

Since cells are freely permeable to urea, it cannot produce translocation of water. Any translocation of water results from electrolyte transmembrane exchange. This realization led to the concept of *electrolyte free water clearance* (C^e_{H2O}) to estimate translocation of water. Electrolyte free water clearance is calculated by modifying the formula for free water clearance.
Free water clearance,

$$C_{H2O} = V - C_{Osm} = V(1 - U_{Osm}/P_{Osm}).$$

Electrolyte free water clearance,

$$C^e_{H2O} = V[1 - (U_{Na} + U_K)/P_{Na}].$$

where C_{H2O} represents free water clearance, V urine volume flow per minute, C_{Osm} osmolar clearance, U_{Osm}

urine osmolality, P_{Osm} plasma osmolality, C^e_{H2O} electrolyte free water clearance, U_{Na} urinary sodium concentration, U_K urinary potassium concentration, and P_{Na} plasma sodium concentration [19].

C^e_{H2O} will be negative with water retention and positive with losses of free water. In practice, this provides a tool to assess response to therapy and can guide fluid restriction in hyper or hyponatremia. When $[U_{Na} + U_K] < P_{Na}$ there is excretion of electrolyte free water with an expected rise in serum sodium, while $[U_{Na} + U_K] > P_{Na}$ indicates electrolyte free water reabsorption that will result in a fall in serum sodium [19].

10.3.6.2 Indices Useful in Assessing Water Balance in Perioperative States

A number of factors that lead to altered water balance preoperatively, including hydration state, will alter the potential for water retention postoperatively. Urinary concentrating defects may lead to dehydration or electrolyte imbalance, while ongoing losses (e.g., in inflammatory bowel disease, malrotation, paralytic ileus with increased losses, or fluid sequestration) can exaggerate ADH response [19, 30, 33, 44].

Postoperative water balance is influenced by elevated ADH levels mediated by conditions described earlier and other factors such as pain, anxiety, response to anesthesia, circulatory changes intraoperatively, and renal water handling. Decreases in GFR and tubular solute presentation affect renal water handling. For example, diluting segment dysfunction will result from low solute presentation caused by avid proximal reabsorption due to preoperative volume deficits or unreplaced intraoperative fluid losses. Excessive water intake either by mouth or by hypotonic intravenous fluid administration results in hyponatremia. Administration of drugs such as opiates and some sedatives lead to decreased GFR and potentially increased ADH secretion, reflected as low urine volume with $U_{Osm} > P_{Osm}$ and $[U_{Na} + U_K] > P_{Na}$. Thus, measurement of these parameters will assist in discerning the etiology of dysnatremia and planning appropriate therapy.

Hyponatremia from sodium loss is less common and most often arises from GI loss of sodium. Generally, this condition is associated with volume depletion and obvious signs of dehydration early in the course. If the renal response is appropriate, UNa and UCl concentrations are low, with oliguria and an increase in U_{Osm}. Even in the setting of brain injury, cerebral salt wasting is a condition seen much less frequently than alterations in ADH secretion. With cerebral salt wasting, there are high urinary sodium levels but, unlike SIADH, there is concomitant volume depletion. As a result, the hyponatremia is due to urinary Na losses and not due to water excess. Thus, clinical history, physical exam, and consideration of changes in weight are key initial diagnostic tools. Since there is volume depletion with cerebral salt wasting, assessing other markers such as uric acid that increase with volume depletion and tubular solute avidity may be helpful, especially if there is difficulty in assessing volume state clinically.

10.3.6.3 Hypernatremia

Hypernatremia results from an increase in exchangeable sodium due to decreased TBW, either from hypotonic fluid losses when water loss exceeds sodium loss or from sodium retention.

With hypernatremia, clinical evaluation should include history, and physical examination for signs of dehydration or volume overload such as edema and hypertension. Search for sources of increased insensible water loss such as high fever, use of radiant warmers in the ICU [27, 38, 39], phototherapy for hyperbilirubinemia, or tachypnea [27]. There may be an osmotic or solute diuresis due to administration of high osmolar feeds, hypertonic saline, and bicarbonate or dietary supplements. Check for presence of a renal concentrating defect and review clinical history for factors that could impact ADH production or function such as recent cranial surgery or medications such as diuretics or lithium. Recent weight changes will provide additional clues, with the expectation of weight loss with inadequate or delayed replacement of ongoing gastrointestinal tract, fistula or drain losses.

Classification of hypernatremic states is based on the serum osmolality, weight, and volume status. Measures of volume status and renal water and solute clearance are helpful in evaluation. These include serum and urine Na, K, Ca, urea nitrogen, creatinine, as well as hematocrit, total protein, and uric acid. For finer points of differentiation, FE_{Na}, U_{Osm}/P_{Osm} as a surrogate for free water clearance and consideration of C^e_{H2O} are required. If $[U_{Na} + U_K]$ is less than P_{Na}, monitoring is necessary since the continued loss of free water is likely to lead to a further increase in serum sodium.

UNa and UCl concentration can also help in determining the inciting factor and guide therapy. In hypovolemic states such as hypernatremic dehydration, UNa is still expected to be low despite the increased serum sodium, while increase in exchangeable sodium from increased salt loading (salt poisoning) results in a significantly elevated UNa. Review of U_{Osm}/P_{Osm} compared with P_{Osm} will assist in the diagnosis of concentrating defects and potential diabetes insipidus, indicating the potential need for a trial of ADH therapy.

10.3.7 Assessment of Polyuria and Oliguria in the ICU

The stimulus for ADH secretion may be (1) osmotic, in response to an approximately 1% change in plasma osmolality through hypothalamic osmoreceptors, or (2) nonosmotic stimuli acting through the baroreceptors, stimulated by volume instability that is common in the ICU setting.

Urine volume and flow rate is dependent on water balance, solute load, presence or absence of ADH, renal tubular integrity, and delivery of water and sodium to the distal tubule. Clinical evaluation should include weight change, total fluid and solute intake by both intravenous and enteral sources, review of medications, as well as consideration of coexisting medical conditions that may impact hydration status or contribute to potential renal abnormalities.

10.3.7.1 *Tools to Examine Polyuria*

We provide an outline for the assessment of polyuric states in Fig. 10.1. U_{Osm}/P_{Osm} is a surrogate for free water clearance and as such allows examination of ADH activity. Review of solute excretion ($U_{Osm} \times V h^{-1}$) allows comparison of water diuresis ($<1 mOsm kg^{-1} h^{-1}$) vs. solute diuresis ($>1 mOsm kg^{-1} h^{-1}$). Additional helpful investigations include serum electrolytes, including serum potassium and calcium to exclude the effects of hypokalemia and hypercalcemia on ADH, BUN, and serum creatinine to provide a coarse measure of renal function, and UNa, UK, UCa, UUN, U_{Osm}, and UCr to provide data on solute load and renal concentrating and diluting ability (Fig. 10.1).

10.3.7.2 *Assessment of Antidiuretic (Oliguric) States*

In the ICU, oliguria can result from renal failure with decreased GFR and decreased urine production or from appropriate or inappropriate ADH activity. The tools required to differentiate these conditions begin with historical details of circulation, hydration, and fluid or electrolyte losses. Chemical measures provide information about renal function (BUN and creatinine) and

ADH activity and response (serum and urine osmolality). UNa, UCl, and FE_{Na} provide an idea of intravascular circulating volume and tubular function that can be used to monitor the changes following fluid administration.

Volume depletion, circulatory insufficiency, or marked ongoing water and sodium losses as in inflammatory bowel disease, fistulae, or prolonged gastric suction lead to an appropriate or sometimes exaggerated appropriate ADH response. The result is avid water reabsorption and oliguria with an elevated U_{Osm}. Correction of circulatory depletion by administration of fluid or saline leads to an increase in urine volume, decrease in U_{Osm}, and rise in UNa and UCl. BUN and creatinine may show only mild increases but an elevated BUN/creatinine ratio reflects the degree of volume depletion and ADH activity.

Inappropriate ADH activity occurs in association with certain infections such as meningitis or pneumonia; with drugs such as carbamazepine, opiates, vincristine, and cyclophosphamide; with significant pCO_2 retention; and following head trauma or surgery or any condition with significant pain and anxiety. The decrease in urine volume is usually less than in appropriate or exaggerated responses to ADH. The biochemical picture is very similar to appropriate ADH activity, with $U_{Osm} > P_{Osm}$, however, UNa and UCl concentrations are elevated rather than decreased because of natriuretic peptide activity secondary to volume expansion. Administration of water or saline is followed by a modest increase in urinary volume flow with no significant fall in U_{Osm} and a significant rise in UNa and UCl. BUN and creatinine concentrations are low initially and may fall after fluid administration. Administration of isotonic or hypotonic saline will be followed by a further decrease in serum sodium. Appropriate therapy is fluid restriction and treatment of any underlying condition promoting ADH release.

In renal failure, decreased GFR leads to decreased tubular fluid delivery to the distal nephron, possible fluid reabsorption from damaged tubules, and low water and solute delivery to the distal tubule, all contributing to oliguria and fluid retention. In this group of patients, clinical and chemical changes are consistent with those previously described in Sect. 10.3.3. Clues to the correct diagnosis include the lower U_{Osm} (isotonic or hypotonic), elevated or rising BUN and creatinine, and characteristic changes of urinary indices and the urinary sediment (Tables 10.1 and 10.2).

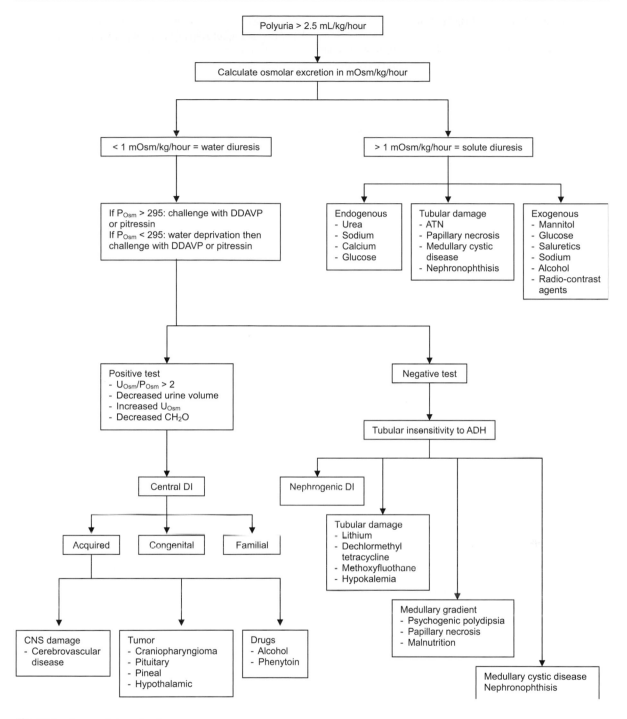

Fig. 10.1   Approach to polyuria

10.3.8 Approach to Tumor Lysis Syndrome

Tumor lysis syndrome is both an oncologic and renal metabolic emergency. It is caused by massive tumor cell death that may be spontaneous or secondary to antitumor therapy. The resultant release of intracellular potassium and phosphorus and the production of uric acid from rapid cell turnover lead to characteristic electrolyte derangements.

Hyperphosphatemia leads to secondary hypocalcemia due to precipitation of calcium phosphate in tissues. When this process occurs in the renal tubules, it can result in acute kidney injury due to tubular necrosis. Additionally, acute kidney injury may occur secondary to uricosuria and ensuing uric acid nephropathy. The risk of acute kidney injury in tumor lysis syndrome increases when there is preexisting kidney dysfunction or intravascular volume depletion.

Usually, the tools to evaluate this condition include clinical history and physical examination, as well as assessment of electrolytes, phosphorus, uric acid, calcium, BUN, and creatinine. Urinalysis with microscopic examination of the sediment may help to confirm acute tubular injury if casts are present, and calcium phosphate or uric acid crystals may also be visualized in the urine. Macroscopically, calcium phosphate crystals may appear as white urinary solute or even sludge, and uric acid crystals as orange or pink powder or sludge. In the face of oliguria with tumor lysis, renal ultrasound should be performed to determine the presence of obstructing calculi or parenchymal infiltration.

Calculation of TRP, TTKG, uric acid excretion in mg/dL^{-1} GFR ($[U_{Uric\ acid} \times P_{Creat}]/U_{Creat}$), and FE$_{Uric\ acid}$ will usually reveal an appropriate response by the kidneys to increase excretion of phosphorus, potassium, and uric acid, indicating that these metabolic abnormalities are due to an overwhelmed renal excretory capacity rather than any intrinsic renal dysfunction. These calculations are rarely required in practice since the process is usually advanced when renal consultation is initiated, and the clinical condition is generally anticipated or recognized.

Take-Home Pearls

> History and physical examination are invaluable tools in the assessment of any derangement in fluid or electrolyte status and in differentiating between expected vs. abnormal response.

> FE$_{Urea}$ is helpful even in the presence of diuretic therapy or after saline fluid bolus when interpretation of FENa may be limited.

> Several assessments are usually more helpful than single tests.
>   – FE$_{Na}$ and FE$_{Urea}$ used concurrently in oligoanuria
>   – Arterial/venous blood gases, bicarbonate, SAG and UAG in metabolic acidosis
>   – UNa, UCl, and FE$_{Na}$ in low circulating blood volume

> Tests repeated before and after a clinical maneuver are helpful in interpreting expected vs. actual response. Rather than yielding an absolute value, renal physiological testing must be corrected for expected response in the particular clinical circumstance.

References

1. Abuelo JG (2007) Normotensive ischemic acute renal failure. N Eng J Med 357:797–805
2. Astrup P, Jorgensen K, Andersen OS, et al. (1960) The acid–base metabolism. A new approach. Lancet 1:1035–1039
3. Astrup P (1963) Acid–base disorders. N Eng J Med 269:817
4. Barozzi L, Valentino M, Santoro A, et al. (2007) Renal ultrasonography in critically ill patients. Crit Care Med 35 (Suppl):S198–S205
5. Batlle DC, Arruda JAL, Kurtzman NA (1981) Hyperkalemia distal renal tubular acidosis associated with obstructive uropathy. N Eng J Med 304:373–380
6. Batlle DC, Hizon M, Cohen E, et al. (1988) The use of the urine anion gap in the diagnosis of hyperchloremic metabolic acidosis. N Eng J Med 318:594–599
7. Berl T (1976) Hypernatremia. Clinical disorders of water metabolism. Kidney Int 110:117
8. Brivet FG, Kleinknecht DJ, Loirat P, et al. (1996) Acute renal failure in intensive care units: causes, outcome, and prognostic factors of hospital mortality; a prospective, multicenter study. French Study Group on Acute Renal Failure. Crit Care Med 24(2):192–198
9. Carvounis CP, Nisar S, Guro-Razuman S (2002) Significance of the fractional excretion of urea in the differential diagnosis of acute renal failure. Kidney Int 62:2223–2229
10. Chertow GM, Burdick E, Honour M, et al. (2005) Acute kidney injury, mortality, length of stay, and costs in hospitalized patients. J Am Soc Nephrol 16:3365–3370
11. Clermont G, Acker CG, Angus DC, et al. (2002) Renal failure in the ICU: comparison of the impact of acute renal failure and end-stage renal disease on ICU outcomes. Kidney Int 62:986–996
12. Cockcroft DW, Gault MH (1976) Prediction of creatinine clearance from serum creatinine. Nephron 16:31–41
13. Constable PD (1999) Clinical assessment of acid–base status. Strong ion difference theory. Vet Clin N Am Food Anim Pract 15:447–471
14. Corey HE, Greifer I, Greenstein SM, et al. (1993) The fractional excretion of urea; a new diagnostic test for acute renal allograft rejection. Pediatr Nephrol 7:268–272

15. Corey HE (2003) Stewart and beyond: numeral goals of acid–base balance. Kidney Int 64:777–787

16. Counahan R, Chandler C, Ghazali S, et al. (1976) Estimation of glomerular filtration rate from plasma creatinine concentration in children. Arch Dis Child 51:875–878

17. Chung HM, Kluge R, Schrier RW, et al. (1987) Clinical assessment of extracellular fluid volume in hyponatremia. Am J Med 83:905–908

18. Dubin A, Menises MM, Masevicius FD, et al. (2007) Comparison of three different methods of evaluation of metabolic acid-based disorders. Crit Care Med 35:1264–1270

19. Ellison DH, Berl T (2007) The syndrome of inappropriate antidiuresis. N Eng J Med 356:2064–2072

20. Emmett M, Nairns RG (1977) Clinical use of the anion gap. Medicine 56:38–54

21. Figge J, Jabor A, Kazda A, et al. (1998) Anion gap and hypoalbuminemia. Crit Care Med 26(11):1807–1810

22. Fowler KA, Locken JA, Duchesne JH, Williamson MR (2002) US for detecting renal calculi with nonenhanced CT as a reference standard. Radiology 222:109–113

23. Gamba G (2005) Role of WNK kinases in regulating tubular salt and potassium transport and in the development of hypertension. Am J Physiol Renal Physiol 288:F245–F252

24. Giebisch G, Krapf R, Wagner C (2007) Renal and extra renal regulation of potassium. Kidney Int 72:397–410

25. Guignard J, Santos F (2004) Laboratory investigations. In: Avner ED, Harmon WE, Niaudet P (eds) Pediatric nephrology, 5th edn. Lippincott Williams and Wilkins, Philadelphia, PA, p 401

26. Halperin ML, Kamel KS (2000) Use of the composition of the urine at the bedside: emphasis on this physiologic principles to provide insights into diagnostic and therapeutic issues. In: Seldin DW, Giebish G (eds) The Kidney-physiology and pathophysiology, 3rd edn. Lippincott Williams and Wilkins, Philadelphia, PA, pp 2297–2327

27. Herrin JT, Fluid and electrolytes (1997). In: Graef JW (ed) Manual of pediatric therapeutics, 6th edn. Lippincott-Raven, Philadelphia, PA, pp 63–75

28. Herrin JT (1999) General urology. workup of hematuria and tubular disorders. In: Gonzáles ET, Bauer SB (eds) Pediatric urology practice. Lippincott-Raven, Philadelphia, PA, pp 69–78

29. Hogg RJ, Furth S, Lemley KV, et al. (2003) National kidney foundation kidney disease outcomes quality initiative clinical practice guidelines for chronic kidney disease in children and adolescents: evaluation, and classification, and stratification. Pediatrics 111:1416–1421

30. Holliday MA, Friedman AL, Segar WE, et al. (2004) Acute hospital induced hyponatremia in children: a physiologic approach. J Pediatr 145:584–587

31. Houser MT (1990) Assessment of proteinuria using random urine samples. J Pediatr 166:243–247

32. Kamel KS, Halperin ML (1998) Clinical approach to a patient with hypokalemia or hyperkalemia. Lancet 352:1206–1212

33. Kaplan SL, Feigin RD (1980) Syndrome of inappropriate antidiuretic hormone in children. Adv Pediatr 27:247–258

34. Kassirer JP, Schwartz WB (1966) The response of normal man to selective depletion of hydrochloric acid. Am J Med 40:10–18

35. Kim MS, Herrin JT (2003) Renal conditions. In: Cloherty JP, Eichenwald EC, Stark AR (eds) Manual of neonatal care, 5th edn. Lippincott Williams and Wilkins, Philadelphia, PA, pp 621–642

36. Lassnig A, Schmidlin D, Mouhieddine M, et al. (2004) Minimal changes in serum creatinine predict prognosis in patients after cardiothoracic surgery: a prospective cohort study. J Am Soc Nephrol 15:1597–1605

37. Levey AS, Greene T, Kusek JW, et al. (2000) MDRD Study Group. A simplified equation to predict glomerular filtration rate from serum creatinine. J Am Soc Nephrol 11:A0828

38. Lorenz JM (2001) Fluid and electrolyte management in the first week of life summary data chart from Polin RA, Yoder MC, Burg FD (eds) Workbook in practical neonatology, 3rd edn. WB Saunders, Philadelphia, PA

39. Lorenz JM (2002) Fluid and electrolyte therapy in the newborn infant. In: Burg FD, Ingelfinger JR, Wald ER, Pollin RA (eds) Pediatric therapeutics, 17th edn. W.B. Saunders, Philadelphia, PA, pp 29–36

40. McCullough PA, Adam A, Becker CR, et al. (2006) Risk prediction of contrast induced nephropathy. Am J Cardiol 98:26K–36K

41. Morgan TJ (2005) The meaning of acid–base abnormalities in the intensive care unit, Part 3: Effects of fluid administration. Crit Care 9:204–211

42. Murray PT, Palevsky PM (2007) Acute kidney injury. NephSAP 6:281–286

43. Musch W, Thimpoint J, Vandervelde D, et al. (1995) Combined fractional excretion of sodium and urea better predicts response to saline in hyponatremia than do the usual clinical and biochemical parameters. Am J Med 99:348–355

44. Oh MS, Carroll HJ (1992) Disorders of metabolism: hypernatremia and hyponatremia. Crit Care Med 20:94–103

45. Perrone RD, Madias NE, Levey AS (1992) Serum creatinine as an index of renal function: new insights into old concepts. Clin Chem 38:1933–1953

46. Pitts RF (1974) Renal regulation of acid–base balance. In: Physiology the kidney and body fluids, 3rd edn. Year Book Medical Publishers, Chicago, IL, p 204–205

47. Rastegar A (2007) Use of the delta anion gap/delta bicarbonate ratio in the diagnosis of mixed acid–base disorders. J Am Soc Nephrol 18:2429–2431

48. Rodriguez-Soriano J (1995) Potassium homeostasis and it's disturbances in children. Pediatr Nephrol 9:364–374

49. Sargent JD, Stukel TA, Kresel J, et al. (1993) Normal values for random urinary calcium to creatinine ratios in infancy. J Pediatr 123:393–397

50. Scheinman SJ, Guay-woodford LM, Thacker RV, et al. (1999) Genetic disorders of renal electrolyte transport. N Eng J Med 340:1177–118

51. Schwartz GJ, Haycock GB, Edelman CM, et al. (1976) A simple estimate of glomerular filtration rate in children derived from body length and plasma creatinine. Pediatrics 58:259–263

52. Schwartz G, Potassium (2004) In: Avner ED, Harmon WE, Niaudet P (eds) Pediatric nephrology, 5th edn. Lippincott Williams and Wilkins, Philadelphia, PA, pp 147–188

53. Schwartz WB, Relman A (1963) A critique of the parameters used in the evaluation of acid–base disorders. "Whole blood buffer base" and "standard bicarbonate" compared with blood pH in plasma bicarbonate concentration. N Eng J Med 268:1382–1398

54. Shemesh O, Golbetz H, Kriss JP, et al. (1985) Limitations of creatinine as a filtration marker in glomerulopathic patients. Kidney Int 28:830–838

55. Siegel NJ, Acute renal failure (1984) In: Brenner BM, Stein JH (eds) Contemporary issues in nephrology: pediatric nephrology, vol. 12. Churchill Livingstone, Edinburgh, pp 297–320

56. Siegel SR, Oh W (1976) Renal function as a marker of human fetal maturation. Acta Pediatr Scand 65:481–485

57. Siggaard-Anderson O, Engel K (1960) A new acid–base nomogram, an improved method for calculation of the relevant blood acid–base data. Scand J Clin Lab Invest 12:177–186

58. Siggaard-Andersen O (1962) The pH-log pCO2 blood acid–base nomogram revised. Scand Clin Lab Invest 14:598–604

59. Siggaard-Anderson O (1963) Blood acid–base alignment nomogram. Scales for pH, PCO2, base excess of whole blood of different hemoglobin concentrations. Plasma bicarbonate and plasma total CO2. Scand J Clin Lab Invest 15:211–217

60. Siggaard-Andersen O, Fogh-Andersen N (1995) Base excess or buffer base (strong ion difference) as a measure of non-respiratory acid–base disturbance. Acta Anesthesiol Scand Suppl 107:123–128

61. Stewart PA (1983) Modern quantitative acid–base chemistry. Can J Physiol Pharmacol 61:1444–1461

62. Stonestreet BS, Rubin L, Pollak A, et al. (1980) Renal function of low birth weight infants with hyperglycemia and glucosuria produced by glucose infusions. Pediatrics 66:561–567

63. Story DA, Morimatsu H, Bellomo R (2007) The effect of albumin concentration on plasma sodium and chloride measurements in critically ill patients. Anesth Analg 104:893–897

64. Tsai JJ, Yuen JY, Kumar VA, et al. (2005) Comparison and interpretation of urinalysis performed by a nephrologist versus a hospital based clinical laboratory. Am J Kidney Dis 46:820–829

65. Wang Y, Cui Z, Fan M (2007) Hospital acquired and community acquired acute renal failure in hospitalized Chinese: the 10-year review. Ren Fail 29:163–168

66. Ward RT, Coltin DM, Meade PC, et al. (2004) Serum levels of calcium in albumin in survivors versus non-survivors after critical injury. J Crit Care 19:54–64

67. White PC (1994) Disorders of aldosterone biosynthesis and action. N Engl J Med 331:250–258

68. Winters RW, Dell RB (1962) Clinical physiology of metabolic acidosis. Postgrad Med 31:161–168

69. Xie J, Craig L, Cobb MH, et al. (2006) Role of withno-lysine [K] kinases in the pathogenesis of Gordon's syndrome. Pediatr Nephrol 21:1231–1236

Urosepsis

11

G. Abuazza and C. Nelson

Contents

Core Messages

> ❯ The development of bacteremia from a urinary focus is called urosepsis.
> ❯ Urosepsis as a result of urinary tract infection (UTI) is commonly caused by Gram-negative bacteria.
> ❯ Early identification and treatment of urosepsis in infants and children is very crucial.
> ❯ Urosepsis can lead to systemic symptoms that may result in multiorgan failure.
> ❯ Patients with urosepsis who have systemic symptoms are best managed in the intensive care setting.
> ❯ Optimum management of urosepsis requires collaboration between several subspecialties.

Case Vignette

A 6-week-old female baby was admitted to the hospital because of fever, poor feeding, vomiting, and lethargy for 2 days. A workup revealed pyuria (WBCs = 9 per high-power field in spun urine sediment) and bacteriuria. Treatment was initiated with intravenous ampicillin and cefotaxime after septic workup was done. The urine and blood cultures grew *Escherichia coli*. The spinal fluid examination was unremarkable, and culture of the fluid showed no growth. A renal ultrasound obtained on the day after admission, when the urine culture result was reported, showed a normal left kidney and a duplicated collecting system on the right with moderate to severe hydronephrosis. Several days later a voiding cystourethrogram (VCUG) was performed, and it revealed grade IV–V vesicoureteral reflux (VUR) on the right kidney.

S.G. Kiessling et al. (eds) *Pediatric Nephrology in the ICU.*
© Springer-Verlag Berlin Heidelberg 2009

11.1 Introduction

Urosepsis is a systemic inflammatory response caused by a primary infection in the urinary system that has spread into the general vascular circulation. It is commonly used to describe the sepsis syndrome secondary to UTI. However, urosepsis patients do not always have renal involvement of their infections [39]. About 20–30% of all sepsis cases within a hospital originate from the urogenital tract. About half of them can be considered as primary sepsis due to the combination of infection and obstruction within the upper or lower urinary tract, which is due to congenital or acquired causes; however, the other half may be induced by any urologic intervention [35]. The development of urosepsis can lead to severe sepsis or septic shock, a life-threatening condition that should be treated in an intensive care unit (ICU) with continuous monitoring.

Septicemia as a result of UTI is a serious condition, even though the mortality has been reported lower compared with other causes of sepsis [54]. The UTI is the main source of hospital-acquired secondary bloodstream infection. It is the third most common nosocomial infection after primary bloodstream infections and pneumonia in the ICU [44]. UTIs are common in childhood, occurring in about 5% of febrile infants and 2% of febrile children of <5 years of age [1, 21]. In pediatric ICUs, nosocomial UTIs comprise 13% of all nosocomial infections, with a median incidence of 4.3 episodes per 1,000 catheter days [58]. Review of the literature indicates that secondary bacteremia, or urosepsis, is uncommon, except in young febrile infants and catheterized critically ill children in whom it occurs in up to 3% [42]. The actual number can be higher and varies by age. Fungal infections of the urinary tract are increasing in frequency [27], likely due to use of invasive devices that impair physical host defenses and use of broad-spectrum antimicrobial agents that eliminate commensal flora. Fungal UTIs seem to be associated with increase in morbidity and mortality, particularly in very-low-birth weight, premature infants, and immunocompromised children [23].

11.2   Risk Factors for the Development of Urosepsis

Although the urinary tract is a common source of infection in children and infants, the implications of UTIs in children and infants are different from those in adults. These differences are reflected in the bacteriology, pathogenesis, and epidemiology of UTI. Although retrograde ascending infection is probably the most common pathway, seeding from systemic and nosocomial infection is a significant pathway to infection in infants and immunocompromised children. There are three mechanisms through which the urinary tract may become infected: (1) retrograde ascent of fecal-perineal bacteria, (2) nosocomial or bacterial introduction in a medical setting through instrumentation, and (3) urinary tract involvement as part of a systemic infection [7]. The most common mechanism is retrograde ascent. The bacteria associated with retrograde ascent most often come from the host's bowel. Once entrance into the urinary outlet occurs, bacteriuria may result from pathogens possessing virulence factors allowing increased bacterial adherence to the epithelia. The second mechanism is the introduction of pathogens by way

of a foreign body or instrument. One prospective study estimated the incidence of nosocomial UTI as 0.6 cases per 1,000 patients per day, with newborns and infants affected disproportionately [26]. Finally, infants, young children, and some immunocompromised individuals may have Gram-positive bacteriuria that may be caused by urinary tract seeding from a systemic infection [7]. Intrarenal abscesses can also be caused by certain hematogenously borne pathogens, most commonly *Staphylococcus aureus, Candida* spp., and *Mycobacterium tuberculosis* [41]. Infant boys with intact foreskins have a higher risk of urosepsis and may not have specific anatomic findings. These boys should undergo renal ultrasound (US) and voiding cysto urethrogram (VCUG) to rule out obstruction and reflux [57].

Patients with structural or functional obstruction at any level of the urinary tract, such as calculi, neurogenic bladder, spinal cord injury, and other uropathies, as well as those with biomaterials or foreign bodies in the urinary tract, are at greater risk for developing urosepsis [11, 37]. Posterior urethral valves and other congenital obstructions of the urethra are particularly important clinical disorders because severe urethral obstruction results in widespread damage and dysfunction of the entire urinary tract, affecting glomerular filtration, ureteral and bladder smooth muscle function, and urinary continence. Severely affected neonates who are not recognized at birth most commonly present within a few weeks with urosepsis, dehydration, and electrolyte abnormalities [25]. Posterior urethral valves remain the single most common urologic cause for renal failure and need for subsequent renal transplantation in children. These anomalies are unique to male children. Occasionally girls with bladder outlet obstruction secondary to ureteroceles or neoplasm may present with a similar clinical picture [22, 28].

Pyelonephritis results from ascending bacteriuria from the bladder via the ureter to the renal pelvis and the renal parenchyma. This transport may be facilitated by host factors such as anatomic defects of the ureters or the kidneys, VUR, or, in patients without anatomic defects, adhesion to the ureteral mucosa. In about one-third of patients with pyelonephritis there also is bacteremia, which can result in urosepsis [17, 33].

In renal transplant patients urosepsis can occur as a result of UTIs, which may occur at any period but are most frequent shortly after transplantation because of catheterization, stenting, and aggressive immunosuppression. Other risk factors for urosepsis after renal transplant are anatomic abnormalities and neurogenic bladder. There is evidence that acute pyelonephritis in the early posttransplant period predisposes to acute rejection [29].

Although fungal infection of the urinary tract is rare among healthy children, the incidence of fungal UTI is increased in hospitalized patients. In large tertiary care neonatal ICUs, Bryant et al. [6] found the overall incidence of candiduria to be 0.5%, whereas Phillips and Karlowicz [42] reported *Candida* sp in 42% of patients with UTI. Risk factors for the development of funguria include long-term antibiotic treatment, use of urinary drainage catheters, parenteral nutrition, and immunosuppression [24]. The overwhelming majority of fungal UTIs are caused by *Candida* spp followed by *Aspergillus* spp, *Cryptococcus* spp, and *Coccidioides* spp [46]. The clinical presentation of patients with funguria ranges from an absence of symptoms to fulminant sepsis. The urinary tract is most frequently the primary entry point but also may represent the site of disseminated infection.

Neonates and infants in the first few months of life are at a higher risk for UTI, which may lead to urosepsis. This susceptibility has been attributed to an incompletely developed immune system [18]. Breastfeeding has been proposed as a means of supplementing the immature neonatal immune system via the passage of maternal IgA to the infant [30], providing the presence of lactoferrin [20], and providing the effect of antiadhesive oligosaccharides [8]. Several studies have demonstrated the protective effect of breastfeeding against UTI in the first 7 months of life [19, 30].

Another rare cause of urosepsis is ureteral injuries. Although a small extravasation of urinary contrast in the intrarenal collecting system in the setting of a renal injury can often be observed, any ureteral injury should be stented and/or repaired immediately. Delay in diagnosis or delay in therapy leads to increased complications from urinary leakage, including infected urinoma and possible urosepsis [43].

11.3   Pathogenesis of Urosepsis

The human urinary tract is a unique space, its mucosa lined with transitional cells. Unlike the gastrointestinal tract, it is usually a sterile space with an impermeable lining. UTI occurs with entrance of pathogens into the urinary tract and subsequent adherence to it. Although normal voiding with intermittent urinary outflow usually clears pathogens within the bladder, human urine has enough nutrients

(e.g., amino acids, glucose) for bacterial growth. In addition, when abnormal voiding with residual urine or bacterial adherence occurs, mechanical clearance by voiding may be inadequate, and UTI may result. Many urinary pathogens possess fimbrial or nonfimbrial adhesins (type-1 fimbriae and P fimbriae) for introital and periurethral mucosal adhesion and subsequent colonization into the urinary tract [48]. After these strains colonize host mucosal surfaces, they injure and invade host tissues, evade host defense mechanisms, and incite an injurious host inflammatory response. P fimbriae also appear to be important in the pathogenesis of bloodstream invasion from the kidney [10, 12]. A multitude of cytokines are produced in response to the presence of certain organisms or their toxins in the bloodstream. They include tumor necrosis factor (TNF)-α and interleukins (IL)-1, IL-6, and IL-8. Together, these proinflammatory mediators trigger the systemic inflammatory response syndrome (SIRS), including vasodilation, increased vascular permeability, abnormal coagulation, superoxide radical production, and granulocyte chemotaxis [13]. In urosepsis, urokinase plasminogen activator receptor production is also upregulated, which appears to play a role in the inflammatory response, particularly in the renal tubular epithelium [13, 59].

11.4   Causative Organisms of Urosepsis

In the pediatric population the etiologic agent causing UTI, as well as the propensity to invade the bloodstream and cause urosepsis, varies with age. For neonates born at term, Gram-negative bacteria comprise the predominate organisms causing urosepsis. *Escherichia coli* alone accounts for 80% of such infections in neonates and young infants with other Gram-negative organisms such as *Enterobacter, Klebsiella, Proteus, Citrobacter, Morganella, Providencia, Serratia*, and *Salmonella* species causing infection less frequently. In the hospitalized neonate or infant, additional Gram-negative pathogens such as *Pseudomonas* and *Acinetobacter* species may cause urosepsis. These organisms carry the potential risk of being multidrug-resistant, complicating antibiotic management and increasing potential morbidity and mortality. The infrequent episode of Gram-positive urosepsis in the neonate may be caused by Group B *Streptococcus, Enterococcus* or *Staphylococcus (saprophyticus* or *aureus)* species. In the context of UTI and urosepsis, premature infants represent a microbiologically distinct group of patients because in addition to the bacterial etiologies discussed earlier, these infants are at increased risk for fungal urosepsis. The majority of these infections are caused by *Candida* species [42]. Hematogenous seeding of multiple organs such as liver, spleen, eyes, brain, and endocardium, as well as fungus ball obstruction of the urinary tract are complications that may be seen in premature neonates with *Candida urosepsis* [3]. It is clear that the incidence of concomitant UTI and bacteremia decreases with increasing age. In a study of urinary tract infection in 100 infants aged 5 days to 8 months of age, sepsis was documented in 31 percent of neonates, 21 percent of infants aged 1 to 2 months, 14 percent of infants aged 2 to 3 months and 5.5 percent of infants aged greater than 3 months of age [16]. What remains unclear is the chicken-and-egg dilemma that arises when the two (urinary tract infection and bacteremia) coincide as to whether ascending UTI results in extension to the bloodstream or if the urinary tract is seeded hematogenously from the bloodstream. Regardless, gram negative organisms predominate over the occasional gram positive organism in patients with urosepsis from infancy through childhood, with the incidence of urosepsis falling off sharply after the first few months of life.

11.5 Evaluation of the Patient with Urosepsis

Sepsis is suspected in a patient with a known infection who develops systemic signs of inflammation or organ dysfunction. Similarly, a patient with otherwise unexplained signs of systemic inflammation should be evaluated for infection by history, physical examination, and further lab workup. A typical presentation includes fever (temperature > 38°C or >100.4°F) or hypothermia (temperature <36°C or <96.8°F), tachycardia, tachypnea, hypotension, oliguria (<0.5 mL kg^{-1} h^{-1}). Later, extremities become cool and pale, with peripheral cyanosis and mottling. As severe sepsis or septic shock develops, the first neurological signs may be confusion or altered mental status. Organ failure may develop, producing additional signs and symptoms specific to the organ involved, including the lungs, kidneys, liver, and nervous system. Appropriate laboratory evaluation includes urinalysis and urine culture, serial blood cultures, and cultures of other suspect body fluids, complete blood count (CBC), arterial blood gas (ABG), chest X-ray, serum electrolytes, serum lactate levels, and liver function. At the onset of septic shock, the peripheral white blood cell (WBC) count may initially decrease to <4,000 µL^{-1}, and polymorphonuclear leukocytes (PMNs) may be as low as 20% immature band forms. However, this situation usually reverses within 1–4 h of initiation of resuscitative efforts, and a significant increase in both the total WBC count to >15,000 µL^{-1} and PMNs to >80% usually occurs. A sharp decrease in platelet count to ≤50,000 µL^{-1} is often present early. Blood levels of procalcitonin and C-reactive protein are elevated in severe sepsis and may facilitate diagnosis, but these are not specific. Hyperventilation with respiratory alkalosis (low PaCO$_2$ and increased arterial pH) occurs early, in part as compensation for lactic acidemia. Serum HCO$_3$ is usually low, and serum lactate increases. As shock progresses, metabolic acidosis worsens, and serum pH decreases. Early respiratory failure leads to hypoxemia with PaO$_2$ < 70 mmHg. Blood urea nitrogen (BUN) and creatinine usually increase progressively as a result of renal insufficiency. Bilirubin and serum transaminase levels may rise, although overt hepatic failure is uncommon.

Renal ultrasonography (US) should be performed on an emergency basis in patients with septic shock caused by presumed urosepsis because if the underlying pathologic problem is obstruction of the urinary tract, patients usually do not respond adequately to supportive treatments until the obstruction is relieved by a drainage procedure. In centers that do not have special competence in US, a computed tomography (CT) with contrast may be the preferred imaging study, which allows for CT-guided abscess drainage [38]. It is very important in hospitalized patients who suddenly develop signs and symptoms of septic shock to consider the possibility of urosepsis even in the absence of urinary symptoms. This is particularly true after recent instrumentation or catheterization of the urinary tract [47].

In an infant presenting with sepsis, evaluation for a possible urinary source should be undertaken. A urine specimen obtained by catheterization or suprapubic aspiration must be obtained for culture before the institution of antibiotic therapy. If pyuria is present, urosepsis should be strongly considered. A screening renal ultrasound is an excellent means to quickly and accurately assess the urinary tract in such infants. The most common causes of urosepsis are obstructive uropathy with anatomic abnormalities or massive VUR. However, a normal renal ultrasound does not rule out VUR, and in the presence of urosepsis a VCUG is essential. This should be obtained during the acute hospital admission [52, 59].

11.6 Management of Urosepsis

The first priority in severe cases of urosepsis is the initiation of basic resuscitative measures within the first 6 h of presentation [9, 31, 45]. It is essential to establish intravenous access and to administer fluids. If the patient is in shock or fails to respond to fluids alone, vasopressors may be needed to assist in maintaining organ perfusion. The first-line vasopressors in this context are norepinephrine bitartrate or dopamine although some data suggest that norepinephrine has greater initial efficacy [32]. Because norepinephrine has little effect on cardiac output, dobutamine may be used concomitantly for inotropic support. Phenylephrine, epinephrine, and vasopressin should not be used as first-line therapies in septic shock. Low-dose dopamine is also not recommended for renal protection [2]. Additional measures may be necessary in specific circumstances as part of the initial resuscitation such as close monitoring of fluid status particularly with regard to urine output. Urine output should be at least 0.5 mL kg^{-1} h^{-1}. Patients should be monitored closely for renal insufficiency secondary to sepsis, which may require adjustment of fluid status, electrolytes, and frequent assessment of renal function as well as monitoring drug levels while using antibiotics such as aminoglycosides, or other renally excreted medications [4, 14, 15, 36, 49, 50].

In addition to basic supportive therapy, optimal management of urosepsis consists of elimination of the infectious focus or foci and initiation of appropriate empiric antimicrobial therapy. A list of commonly used parental antibiotics can be found in Table 11.1. It is important that free drainage of urine from both kidneys is established by means of a bladder catheter,

retrograde catheterization, or percutaneous nephrostomy. As soon as the necessary cultures have been taken (at least two blood cultures as well as cultures from urine and other appropriate body sites and fluids), the patient should be started on broad-spectrum IV antibiotics. The best outcome is seen when IV antibiotics are initiated within the first hour of presentation [9, 40].

11.6.1 Antimicrobial Therapy for Urosepsis

The selection of initial empiric antibiotics is based upon the most likely organisms involved, and the agents should be capable of penetrating the suspected source of infection [5]. A history of previous antibiotic therapy should always be elicited in patients with urosepsis because such treatment may have resulted in selection of resistant organisms [17, 51]. Because the predominate organisms responsible for urosepsis at all ages are Gram-negative rods, empiric therapy is necessarily aimed at these organisms. This is not to say, however, that empiric treatment decisions should be made with disregard to Gram-positive organisms, especially *Enterococcus* species. It is also important to understand that in the context of a chapter addressing empiric antimicrobial recommendations for urosepsis, it is implied that the treating clinician's impression is that the urinary tract is the source for the sepsis syndrome. The recommendations offered here are not necessarily appropriate for sepsis in general, as a number of other potential organisms not often associated with infection of the urinary tract such as *Neisseria meningitidis*, *Streptococcus pneumonia*, and *Streptococcus pyogenes* must be considered in the broader clinical context of sepsis and septic shock in children. Of course, empiric antimicrobial choices must always be modified once original blood and urine culture and susceptibility data as well as other laboratory testing results (urinalysis, cerebrospinal fluid cell counts, etc.) become available. Changes in empiric antimicrobial therapy must also be considered when a patient is failing to improve clinically within the first 24–48 h of initiation of therapy. In this setting, one must consider the possibility of alternative pathogens not affected by the chosen antimicrobial agents, or the possibility that one is dealing with a pathogen that is resistant to the antimicrobial agents that the patient is receiving. Ampicillin plus gentamicin remains a reasonable empiric combination therapy for newborns, infants, and children with urosepsis. Alternatively,

Table 11.1 Commonly used parenteral antibiotics for empiric therapy of urosepsis

Antibiotic	Dosing for normal renal function
Ampicillin	100–200 mg kg^{-1} per 24 h divided every 6 h, max 12 g per 24 h
Ceftriaxone	75 mg kg^{-1} per 24 h single daily dose, max 2 g per 24 h
Gentamicin	7.5 mg kg^{-1} per 24 h divided every 8 h, check peaks/troughs
Cefepime	100 mg kg^{-1} per 24 h divided every 12 h, max 6 g per 24 h
Cefazolin	50–100 mg kg^{-1} per 24 h divided every 8 h, max 6 g per 24 h
Cefotaxime	100–200 mg kg^{-1} per 24 h divided every 8 h, max 12 g per 24 h

an expanded spectrum cephalosporin such as cefotaxime or ceftriaxone may be appropriate in addition to or in place of gentamicin, especially when other body foci such as the meninges are documented or suspected to be infected. Many experts recommend use of an expanded spectrum cephalosporin in this setting based on the fact that 50% or more of *E. coli* are resistant to ampicillin. For patients who have been hospitalized for more than 7 days and for newborn infants born to mothers who were hospitalized for more than 7 days prior to delivery, antibiotic-resistant Gram-negative and Gram-positive pathogens must be considered. For these patients, ampicillin or vancomycin plus gentamicin plus an extended spectrum, antipseudomonal cephalosporin such as cefepime should be considered. For premature neonates, especially those hospitalized for more than 7 days and for those whose mothers were hospitalized for more than 7 days prior to delivery, empiric antibiotic considerations are the same for those as term newborns above with regard to the possibility of encountering an antibiotic-resistant pathogen. However, because these infants may commonly develop urosepsis caused by *Candida* species, additional consideration should be given to initiation of antifungal therapy with amphotericin B, especially when such infants are not showing signs of clinical improvement within 24–48 h of initiation of appropriate antibacterial therapy.

11.6.2 Antimicrobial Resistance and Urosepsis

An important issue pertinent to patients with urosepsis is the emergence of infections caused by antibiotic-resistant bacteria such as extended spectrum ß lactamase (ESBL)-producing *Enterobacteriaceae*, vancomycin-resistant *Enterococcus* (VRE), and community and health care-associated, methicillin-resistant *Staphylococcus aureus* (MRSA). Each of these may be urinary tract pathogens, and each requires special antimicrobial therapy to successfully treat. The clinician treating patients with urosepsis caused by one of these pathogens should work closely with an experienced, state-of-the-art microbiology laboratory as well as consult a specialist in infectious diseases to assist in managing these difficult and potentially life-threatening infections. Organisms producing ESBLs generally demonstrate resistance to extended spectrum cephalosporins such as cetriaxone, cefotaxime, and cefepime as well as semisynthetic penicillins such as ticarcillin and piperacillin. Although patients with urosepsis caused by ESBL-producing

bacteria may respond to antibiotics to which these bacteria appear to be resistant to in-vitro, recommended therapy for such infections usually includes the use of a carbapenem (imipenem, meropenem, ertapenem) in combination with an aminoglycoside (gentamicin, tobramycin, or amikacin). For patients with urosepsis caused by VRE, optimal therapy formerly consisted of the use of the dual peptide antibiotic, quinupristin/dalfopristin. However, due to increasing resistance to this agent and the potential for infusion-related side effects, the use of oral or intravenous linezolid has become the recommended therapy for this pathogen. Patients with urosepsis caused by MRSA may be treated with a variety of antibiotics, including vancomycin, trimethoprim-sulfamethoxazole, clindamycin, and linezolid. Newer agents that have proven efficacy in adult trials against infections caused by MRSA include daptomycin and tigecycline, but these antibiotics have not been studied sufficiently in children to recommend their use at the present time. In the near future, anti-MRSA cephalosporins such as ceftobiprole medocaril may offer new therapeutic alternatives for patients with urosepsis and other infections caused by MRSA.

Fungus balls in the collecting system may cause obstruction in children. Patients with these upper tract foci of funguria should be treated with systemic therapy that consists of amphotericin B or fluconazole. In cases of urinary tract obstruction caused by fungi, emergency percutaneous nephrostomy should be pursued in order to reestablish normal urinary tract drainage and to allow for local irrigation. Surgical removal may be necessary should the fungal balls persist [45, 55, 56].

When there is obstruction to urine flow (e.g., by a calculus or tumor), the obstruction must be relieved, either by percutaneous nephrostomy or ureteral stenting [34, 53]. Both are very effective options that may be used acutely to relieve the obstruction. When possible, removal of urinary calculi from patients who have pyelonephritis is probably best delayed until the bacterial load can be reduced and the patient stabilized with medical therapy [53]. The indications for nephrostomy tube placement include the preservation of renal function, relief of pain; and, in the most extreme circumstances, the emergent drainage of a pyocalix or pyonephrosis in a patient with urosepsis in whom retrograde ureteral stent placement is not possible or is contraindicated [53]. Renal replacement therapy should be considered in patients with urosepsis who have developed renal insufficiency and no improvement of renal function after placement of percutaneous nephrostomy tubes.

11.7 Conclusion

Early identification and treatment of urosepsis in infants and children is crucial. Urosepsis as a result of UTI is a serious condition, commonly caused by Gram-negative bacteria. Urosepsis leads to profound disruption in the normal hemodynamic status of affected patients, with deleterious effects on renal, cardiac, respiratory, and hepatic function. Such patients are best managed in the intensive care setting with IV fluids and broad-spectrum antibiotics as soon after presentation as possible. This severe and often life-threatening condition is a paradigm for the need for collaboration between various specialties because the fate of the patient often will be determined within the first hours following admission. During these critical early hours collaborative treatment involving the pediatric intensivist, nephrologist, the urologist, and the infection disease specialist is necessary to optimize patient outcomes.

Take-Home Pearls

> UTI is the third most common nosocomial infection in the ICU.

> UTI is caused mainly by retrograde ascending infection; however, seeding from systemic infection is a significant pathway in infants and immune-compromised patients.

> Urosepsis can lead to severe septic shock, which can result in a life-threatening condition that requires intensive care.

> Neonates and infants are at increased risk for developing UTI, therefore any infant or young child with an unexplained fever should be evaluated for a UTI.

> Infants with a UTI often present with nonspecific signs and symptoms, such as irritability, vomiting, diarrhea, and failure to thrive.

> Patients with obstruction or anatomic abnormalities at any level of the urinary tract are at high risk of developing urosepsis, and these patients may not present with the typical laboratory findings of pyuria and bacteriuria.

> It is important in patients with sepsis to perform urine analysis and urine culture in addition to the other septic workup even in the absence of urinary symptoms.

> In urosepsis it is very crucial to initiate treatment in the first 6 h of presentation including fluid support, stabilization of hemodynamic state with pressors if indicated, and empiric intravenous antimicrobial therapy.

> Renal ultrasound should be performed in cases of urosepsis to rule out obstruction of the urinary tract. If obstruction is the underlying cause of urosepsis, a drainage procedure is warranted to relieve the obstruction.

References

1. Bauchner H, Philipp B, Dashefsky B, et al. (1987) Prevalence of bacteriuria in febrile children. Pediatr Infect Dis J 6:239–242
2. Beale RJ, Hollenberg SM, Vincent JL, et al. (2004) Vasopressor and inotropic support in septic shock: an evidence-based review. Crit Care Med 32(11 Suppl):455–465
3. Benjamin DK, Poole C, Steinbach WJ, et al. (2003) Neonatal candidemia and end-organ damage: a critical appraisal of the literature using meta-analytic techniques. Pediatrics 112(3, Part 1):634–640
4. Bernard GR, Vincent JL, Laterre F, et al. (2001) Efficacy and safety of recombinant human activated protein C for severe sepsis. N Engl J Med 344(10):699–709
5. Bochud PY, Bonten M, Marchetti O, et al. (2004) Antimicrobial therapy for patients with severe sepsis and septic shock: an evidence-based review. Crit Care Med 32(11 Suppl):495–512
6. Bryant K, Maxfield C, Rabalais G (1999) Renal candidiasis in neonates with candiduria. Pediatr Infect Dis J 18:959–963
7. Chon HC, Lai FC, Shortliffe LD (2001) Pediatric urinary tract infections. Pediatr Clin North Am 48:1441–1459
8. Coppa G, Gabrielli O, Giorgi P, et al. (1990) Preliminary study of breastfeeding and bacterial adhesion to uroepithelial cells. Lancet 335:569–571
9. Dellinger RP, Carlet JM, Masur H, et al. (2004) Surviving sepsis: campaign guidelines for management of severe sepsis and septic shock. Crit Care Med 32(3):858–873
10. Donnenberg MS, Welch RA (1996) Virulence determinants of uropathogenic *Escherichia coli*. In: Mobley HLT, Warren JW (eds) Urinary tract infections: molecular pathogenesis and clinical management. ASM Press, Washington, DC
11. Dow G, Rao P, Harding G (2004) A prospective, randomized trial of 3 or 14 days of ciprofloxacin treatment for acute urinary tract infection in patients with spinal cord injury. Clin Infect Dis 39:658–664
12. Eisenstein BI, Jones GW (1988) The spectrum of infections and pathogenic mechanisms of *Escherichia coli*. Adv Intern Med 33:231–252
13. Florquin S, van den Berg JG, Olszyna DP, et al. (2001) Release of urokinase plasminogen activator receptor during urosepsis and endotoxemia. Kidney Int 59:2054–2061
14. Gainer JA, Yost NP (2003) Critical care infectious disease. Obstet Gynecol Clin North Am 30(4):695–709
15. Gea-Banacloche JC, Opal SM, Jorgensen J, et al. (2004) Sepsis associated with immunosuppressive medications: an evidence-based review. Crit Care Med 32(11 Suppl):578–590
16. Ginsburg CM, McCracken GH (1982) Urinary tract infections in young infants. Pediatrics 69(4):409–412
17. Goldman (2004) Urinary tract infections. In: Cecil textbook of medicine, 22nd edn. Saunders, Philadelphia, PA, Chapter 344
18. Hanson LA (1976) Esch. coli infections in childhood significance of bacterial virulence and immune defense. Arch Dis Child 51:737–742

19. Hanson LA, Korotkova M, Haversen L, et al. (2002) Breast-feeding, a complex support system for the offspring. Pediatr Int 44:347–352

20. Haversen L, Ohlsson BG, Hahn-Zoric M, et al. (2002) Lactoferrin down-regulates the LPS-induced cytokine production in monocytic cells via NF-kappa B. Cell Immunol 220:83–95

21. Hoberman A, Chao HP, Keller DM, et al. (1993) Prevalence of urinary tract infection in febrile infants. J Pediatr 123:17–23

22. Hrair-George O, Mesrobian, MD, Balcom, AH, et al. (2004) Urologic problems of the neonate. Pediatr Clin of North Am 51:4

23. Karlowicz MG (2003) Candidal renal and urinary tract infection in neonates. Semin Perinatol 27:393–400

24. Kauffman CA, Vazquez JA, Sobel JD, et al. (2000) Prospective multicenter surveillance study of funguria in hospitalized patients. The National Institute for Allergy and Infectious Diseases (NIAID) Mycoses Study Group. Clin Infect Dis 30:14–18

25. Langley JM (2005) Defining urinary tract infection in the critically ill child. Pediatr Crit Care Med 6:25–29

26. Langley JM, Hanakowski M, Leblanc JC (2001) Unique epidemiology of nosocomial urinary tract infection in children. Am J Infect Control 29(2):94–98

27. Lundstrom T, Sobel J (2001) Nosocomial candiduria. Clin Infect Dis 32:1602–1607

28. Ma JF, Dairiki Shortliffe LM (2004) Urinary tract infection in children: etiology and epidemiology. Urol Clin North Am 31(3):517–526

29. Magee CC, Milford EL (2004) Clinical aspects of renal transplantation. In: Brenner BM (ed) Brenner and Rector's – The Kidney. Saunders, Philadelphia, PA

30. Marild S, Hansson S, Jodal U, et al. (2004) Protective effect of breastfeeding against urinary tract infection. Acta Paediatr 93:164–168

31. Marshall JC, Maier RV, Jimenez M, et al. (2004) Source control in the management of severe sepsis and septic shock: an evidence-based review. Crit Care Med 32(11 Suppl):513–526

32. Martin C, Papazian L, Perrin G, et al. (1993) Norepinephrine or dopamine for the treatment of hyperdynamic septic shock? Chest 103(6):1826–1831

33. McCammon KA, McCammon CF (2006) Acute pyelonephritis. In: Rakel Conn's current therapy, 58th edn. W.B. Saunders, St. Louis, MO

34. Millberg JA, Davis DR, Steinberg KP, et al. (1983–1993) Improved survival of patients with acute respiratory distress syndrome (ARDS). JAMA 273(4):306–309

35. Naber KG (2006) Urogenital infections: the pivotal role of the urologist. Eur Urol 50:657–659

36. Naber KG, Bergman B, Bishop MC, et al. (2001) EAU guidelines for the management of urinary and male genital tract infections. Urinary Tract Infection (UTI) Working Group of the Health Care Office (HCO) of the European Association of Urology (EAU). Eur Urol 40(5):576–588

37. Nadler RB, Loeb S, Vardi I (2005) Contemporary management of urosepsis: updated critical care guidelines. Contemp Urol 17(7):35–39

38. Noble J (2001) Textbook of primary care medicine, 3rd edn. Mosby, Amsterdam, Chapter 146 (Laboratory studies and diagnostic procedures, urinary tract infections)

39. Norrby R (2004) Urinary tract infection. In: Goldman L, Bennett JC (eds) Cecil textbook of medicine, 22nd edn. WB Saunders, Philadelphia, PA

40. Paradisi F, Corti G, Mangani V (1998) Urosepsis in the critical care unit. Crit Care Clin 14(2):165–180

41. Patterson JE, Andriole VT (1987) Renal and perirenal abscesses. Infect Dis Clin North Am 1:907–926

42. Phillips JR, Karlowicz MG (1997) Prevalence of Candida species in hospital-acquired urinary tract infections in a neonatal intensive care unit. Pediatr Infect Dis J 16:190–194

43. Rakel RE, Bope ET, Conn HF (2006) Conn's current therapy. Trauma to the genitourinary tract-ureteral trauma. Elsevier Saunders, Philadelphia, PA

44. Richards MJ, Edwards JR, Culver DH, et al. (1999) Nosocomial infections in pediatric intensive care units in the United States. National Nosocomial Infections Surveillance System. Pediatrics 103:e39

45. Rivers E, Nguyen B, Havstad S, et al. (2001) Early goal-directed therapy in the treatment of severe sepsis and septic shock. N Engl J Med 345(19):1368–1377

46. Sobel JD, Vazquez JA (1999) Fungal infections of the urinary tract. World J Urol 17:410–414

47. Sussman M, Cattell WR, Jones KV (1998) Urinary tract infection. In: Cameron S, et al. (eds) Oxford textbook of clinical nephrology, 2nd edn. Oxford University Press, New York

48. Sussman M, Gally DL (1999) The biology of cystitis: host and bacterial factors. Annu Rev Med 50:149–158

49. van den Berghe G, Wouters P, Weekers F, et al. (2001) Intensive insulin therapy in the critically ill patients. N Engl J Med 345(19):1359–1367

50. Vincent JL, Gerlach H (2004) Fluid resuscitation in severe sepsis and septic shock: an evidence-based review. Crit Care Med 32(11 Suppl):451–454

51. Walsh PC, Retik AB, Vaughan ED, et al. (2002) Infections of the urinary tract. In: Cambpell's urology, 8th edn. Saunders, Philadelphia, PA

52. Walsh PC, Retik AB, Vaughan ED, et al. (2002) Perinatal urology, neonatal urologic emergencies. In: Campbell's Urology, 8th edn. Saunders, Philadelphia, PA

53. Walsh PC, Retik AB, Vaughan ED, et al. (2002) Percutanous approaches to upper urinary tract. In: Campell's urology, 8th edn. Saunders, Philadelphia, PA

54. Watson RS, Carcillo, JA (2005) Scope and epidemiology of pediatric sepsis. Ped Crit Care Med 6(3) Suppl:3–5

55. Wise GJ, Kozinn PJ, Goldberg P (1982) Amphotericin B as a urologic irrigant in the management of noninvasive candiduria. J Urol 128:82–84

56. Wise GJ, Talluri GS, Marella VK (1999) Fungal infections of the genitourinary system: manifestations, diagnosis, and treatment. Urol Clin North Am 26:701–718

57. Wiswell TE, Hachey WE (1993) Urinary tract infections and the uncircumcised state: an update. Clin Pediatr 32:130–134

58. National Nosocomial Infections Surveillance (NNIS) System Report: data summary from January 1992 through June 2003, issued August 2003. Am J Infect Control 31:481–498

59. Practice parameter. The diagnosis, treatment, and evaluation of the initial urinary tract infection in febrile infants and young children. American Academy of Pediatrics. Committee on Quality Improvement. Subcommittee on Urinary Tract Infection. Pediatrics 1999;103(4, Part 1): 843–852

12

Hypertension in the Pediatric Intensive Care Unit

A.Z. Traum and M.J.G. Somers

Contents

Case Vignette

A 14-year-old boy with end-stage renal disease secondary to obstructive uropathy on maintenance hemodialysis presents to the Emergency Department (ED). He suffered a generalized tonic–clonic seizure at home lasting 8 min and was transported by ambulance. The seizure abated without intervention. His

Core Messages

> Severe hypertension can lead to acute end-organ dysfunction in children. In the ICU, hypertension is most likely a sequela of the critical illness rather than the primary reason for ICU admission.

> The treatment and evaluation of pediatric hypertension should occur simultaneously, and renal parenchymal or vascular etiologies of high blood pressure must be considered high in the differential diagnosis.

> Multiple short-acting intravenous agents are available as continuous infusions for the rapid lowering of blood pressure and may be used emergently along with the institution of longer acting maintenance antihypertensive therapy.

blood pressure at home was 186/124 mmHg and upon arrival to the ED was 178/116. His home blood pressures had recently been more labile, although they were improved after dialysis and ultrafiltration on the day before, with ongoing counseling regarding the importance or adherence to his daily fluid restriction and his antihypertensive regimen consisting of enalapril and amlodipine.

In the ED, intravenous access is quickly achieved and he is administered hydralazine 10-mg IV. His blood pressure is unchanged and a second dose is given. In the interim, a CT scan of the head is normal. Thirty minutes later, with a blood pressure of 180/120, he has another 4-min seizure that abates without provision of antiepileptic medication.

He is transferred to the Pediatric Intensive Care Unit where a continuous infusion of sodium nitroprusside is initiated at a dose of 0.25 mcg kg^{-1} min^{-1}.

S.G. Kiessling et al. (eds) *Pediatric Nephrology in the ICU*.
© Springer-Verlag Berlin Heidelberg 2009

The infusion is titrated up to a dose of $5\,mcg\,kg^{-1}\,min^{-1}$ with eventual lowering of his blood pressure to 146/88. His chronic dialysis prescription is reviewed with focus on his presumed dry weight and ultrafiltration requirements. His maintenance oral antihypertensive regimen is reinstituted and his nitroprusside drip weaned off, with stable blood pressures in the 120/80 range documented. A referral is made to the Coping Clinic for ongoing psychosocial support and help with adherence to his medication and dietary routine.

12.1 Introduction

In children, hypertension is a relatively uncommon finding and its presence often suggests some underlying disease. Unlike in adults, where hypertension is generally deemed to be primary or essential and frequently no diagnostic evaluation ensues after diagnosis, in children primary hypertension is considered a diagnosis of exclusion. Regardless of its cause, significant elevations of blood pressure can lead to acute organ dysfunction, and the hypertensive child almost always warrants a diagnostic evaluation while treatment is ongoing. In the hospitalized child, there is the additional burden of determining if hypertension is a problem in itself or if it stems from another ongoing illness or condition. The approach to evaluating and treating hypertension is oftentimes both more directed and more urgent in the hospitalized child than in the ambulatory setting, especially in children whose acute illness has resulted in ICU admission.

Hypertension is relatively uncommon as the root cause of admission to the general pediatric ward or the pediatric ICU. Acute elevations of blood pressure are frequently categorized into hypertensive urgencies and hypertensive emergencies, the difference being the presence of actual end organ dysfunction in emergencies. In children, a hypertensive emergency most often manifests with seizures or encephalopathy, although congestive heart failure and impairment of renal function may also be seen. Thrombotic microangiopathy secondary to severe hypertension is a rarer consequence. Many children found to have severe elevations of blood pressure can be managed on the general pediatric ward. Those children with hypertensive emergencies or with symptomatic blood pressures refractory to intermittent medication dosing will often require ICU admission for continuous infusion of antihypertensive agents and close clinical monitoring.

12.2 Background

12.2.1 Blood Pressure Norms

Adult blood pressure standards are based on epidemiologic outcome measures related to chronic end-organ damage. In contrast, blood pressure standards in children are based on statistical population norms stratified by age, gender, and height percentile. The Fourth Report on the Diagnosis, Evaluation, and Treatment of High Blood Pressure in Children and Adolescents of the National High Blood Pressure Education Program (NHBPEP) [1] describes the most recent normative pediatric blood pressure data in a fashion similar to previously published standards in adults [3]. Normal blood pressure is defined as consistent blood pressure measurements less than the 90th percentile compared with blood pressure readings from a peer reference group. Prehypertension is defined as typical blood pressure ≥90th percentile but <95th percentile. Stage 1 hypertension is defined as typical blood pressure ≥95th percentile with stage 2 or severe hypertension exceeding the 99th percentile. Children with sustained blood pressure readings >30% above the 99th percentile for age, size, and gender are at particular risk of developing acute sequelae from their high blood pressure and, even if asymptomatic, blood pressure control must be immediately addressed to prevent further deterioration.

12.2.2 Auscultation vs Oscillometry

Accurate measurement of blood pressure is essential for diagnosis and for allowing ongoing management decisions. The blood pressure norms in pediatrics are based on measurement by auscultation in an upper extremity while sitting [1]. In spite of this, oscillometric measurements of blood pressure are widely used because of the ease in obtaining these readings, especially in the hospitalized child and in urgent care settings such as the ICU. Oscillometric measurements of blood pressure are typically at least 5–10 mmHg higher than those obtained by auscultation [25, 26]. As a result, any high blood pressure measurements should be confirmed with auscultation.

In the ICU setting, arterial lines may be placed to assist with monitoring of a patient's hemodynamic stability and will be an additional resource to follow blood pressures. Although blood pressures from arterial lines should, ostensibly, be superior to measurements from cuffs, technical complications such as positional line placement or microthrombus formation often cause erroneous readings, and concern regarding ongoing vascular integrity often limits the duration of an arterial catheter placement.

12.2.3 Cuff Size

Cuff size is another important factor that affects accuracy of blood pressure measurement. Generally, a cuff that is too small will overestimate blood pressure. Conversely, cuffs that are too large may underestimate blood pressure, although clinically the impact of overestimated blood pressure measurements from small cuffs is far more significant. Although there are controversies regarding the most precise method for measuring cuff size [2, 4, 19], the recommendations of NHBPEP Working Group on High Blood Pressure in Children and Adolescents should be followed as a consensus guideline [1]. This guideline delineates that the width of the cuff bladder should be at least 40% of the arm circumference measured midway between the olecranon and acromion. This measurement also tends to correlate with the bladder length covering 80–100% of the arm circumference. Appropriate sized cuffs should be available for both manual and oscillometric blood pressure measurements. In particularly obese or muscular adolescents, a thigh cuff may be necessary to cover appropriately the arm.

Blood pressure standards are based on cuff readings from upper extremities. In the normal child with no aortic or lower extremity arterial compromise, readings from the lower extremities (thighs or calves) should be higher than upper extremity blood pressures. Although lower extremity readings may provide information about blood pressure trends when compared with other lower extremity readings, these measurements should not be used to determine if a patient actually has hypertension or if medication doses need to be augmented.

12.2.4 Auscultatory Technique

As noted earlier, auscultation is the modality that has been used to create pediatric norms for blood pressure. With the child at rest, the diaphragm of the stethoscope should be placed over the brachial artery at the antecubital fossa. The right arm is used both by convention as well as to assist in the diagnosis of coarctation of the aorta, as the left subclavian artery usually comes off the aorta after a thoracic coarctation and will thus have lower blood pressure. The systolic blood pressure is the pressure noted at auscultation of the first tapping or Korotkoff sound, signifying turbulent blood flow through a previously compressed vessel. The diastolic blood pressure is the disappearance of Korotkoff sounds. In some children, the Korotkoff sounds may continue until a diastolic blood pressure of zero. Although unlikely in the presence of significant hypertension, if this occurs the diastolic blood pressure should be measured at the muffling, or fourth Korotkoff sound.

In severely ill children in the ICU, it is likely that blood pressure will be monitored by a variety of invasive and noninvasive means and, along with other clinical assessments such as peripheral perfusion, will assist in allowing the clinician to gauge the child's hemodynamic status. Regardless of the modality used, any single blood pressure measurement is less important than the trend of the blood pressures. In children with hypertensive urgencies or emergencies, or in whom blood pressures have been chronically quite elevated, it is important to make sure that any therapy aimed at decreasing blood pressure does not result in too rapid a fall from the aberrant baseline since this may trigger further CNS compromise. In these settings, the importance of being able to assess blood pressure reliably by a consistent modality cannot be overemphasized.

12.3 Diagnostic Evaluation

Most hospitalized children with identified high blood pressure have a secondary form of hypertension, although as the incidence of obesity rises so too does the incidence of primary, or essential, hypertension in all children [8, 16, 31, 33]. Although obesity and the metabolic syndrome result in measurable physiologic changes including increased vascular endothelial activity, obesity-related hypertension in children is still generally categorized as primary. Hypertension in children admitted to the ICU is rarely primary in nature and such a diagnosis would need to be predicated on a rather extensive diagnostic evaluation.

The diagnostic evaluation of a hospitalized hypertensive child should be undertaken concurrent with lowering blood pressure, most especially in the setting of hypertensive urgencies or emergencies. Unlike in outpatients or children on the general ward, the evaluation should focus on the assumption of a secondary cause until proven otherwise. Not to be underestimated, especially in the ICU setting, is the influence of pain and anxiety on increased blood pressure. All children with evidence of sustained or recurrent hypertension, especially in the face of adequate analgesia and sedation, should be evaluated for secondary hypertension. This evaluation can be done in a stepwise fashion and individualized based on findings of the history, physical exam, screening tests, and the child's clinical condition.

Children with more persistent significant elevations of blood pressure, as well as younger children with hypertension, are more likely to have definable causes of their hypertension. Aside from pain and anxiety, the most common cause of secondary hypertension in hospitalized children is renal parenchymal disease [24, 30], and the diagnostic evaluation should emphasize this etiology. An algorithm for the diagnostic evaluation of hypertension in the hospitalized child is provided in Fig. 12.1.

12.3.1 History

In the hypertensive child in the ICU, although the initial focus will be on patient stabilization and initial treatment of any life-threatening hypertension, eventually the clinician will want to begin a diagnostic evaluation with a careful patient history. The history should focus on disorders or conditions that predispose to hypertension and, in the hospitalized patient, should begin with the history of present illness leading to the child's admission and the hospital course following admission, especially the child's renal function, volume status, and medications. For instance, in the postoperative child who is otherwise healthy and heretofore had normal blood pressures, pain or anxiety may play a role in hypertension as can agitation from rapid weaning of sedation after prolonged intubation or other procedures. Similarly, in the child hospitalized with severe reactive airway disease, frequent administration of beta-agonists may be problematic. In the absence of such an obvious precipitating factor to the child's hypertension, a comprehensive medical history is crucial and should begin with the child's perinatal history. Prematurity itself is a risk factor for hypertension later in life [1, 14, 30]. Interventions in the neonatal period, such as placement of umbilical catheters, or periods of hypotension or diminished effective volume, may lead to renal hypoperfusion and subsequent renal scarring. Upper urinary tract infections, and especially repeated episodes of pyelonephritis in the first few years of life, may predispose to renal parenchymal scars that lead to renin-mediated hypertension. These infections may have

been undiagnosed and any past history of unexplained recurrent febrile illnesses should be elicited [38].

Glomerulonephritis often presents with a nephritic syndrome with edema, hematuria, and hypertension and may be isolated to a primary renal condition or associated with systemic inflammatory disorders such as systemic lupus erythematosus. Relevant historical features should focus on joint symptoms, edema, rashes, and unexplained fevers. Recent systemic infections may also lead to postinfectious glomerulonephritis and may be associated with gross hematuria.

The family history should focus on relatives with early-onset hypertension as well as inherited disease that affect the kidneys such as any polycystic kidney disease complex, tuberous sclerosis, and neurofibromatosis. A strong family history of cardiovascular disease such as coronary artery disease, stroke, and hyperlipidemia suggests a similar risk in the hypertensive child.

Certain medications are known to cause hypertension, such as oral contraceptives, corticosteroids, stimulants used for attention deficit disorder, decongestants, and the calcineurin inhibitors cyclosporine and tacrolimus that are often the mainstay of immunosuppression in solid organ transplant patients. Recreational drugs with stimulant effects such as cocaine, nicotine, and ephedra may also raise blood pressure, as can withdrawal from the effects of CNS depressants such as ethanol or narcotic analgesics.

The review of systems should evaluate for symptoms such as headaches, chest pain, visual changes, or mental status changes as these may be related to severe hypertension or CNS end-organ damage. Moreover, symptoms such as headaches and sleep disturbances are often associated with hypertension and may improve with normalization of blood pressure [6]. Sweating, palpitations, and flushing are associated with states of catecholamine excess such as that accompanies a pheochromocytoma.

12.3.2 Physical Exam

Height, weight, and body mass index should be measured to assess for poor growth or to document an overweight state or frank obesity. As outlined earlier, the accurate measurement of blood pressure is an essential part of the physical assessment of the child with suspected or confirmed hypertension. In children with an unclear etiology to their hypertension, blood pressure should be measured in all four extremities. The blood pressure in the lower extremities is typically

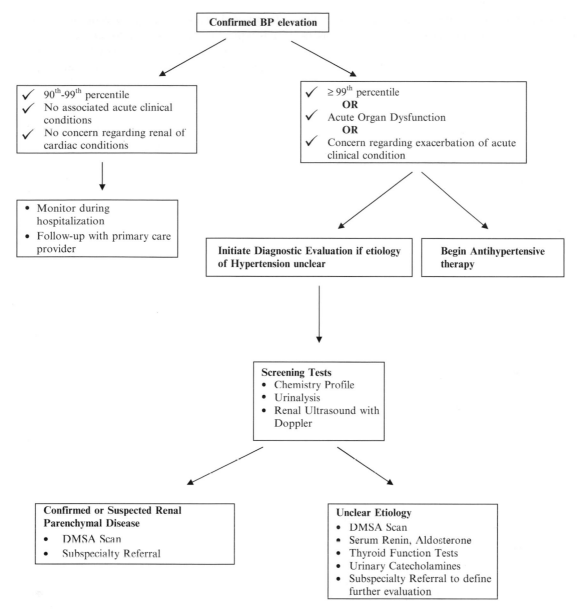

Fig. 12.1   Algorithm for the evaluation and management of the hospitalized child with hypertension

10–20 mmHg higher than in the right arm and may even be higher. Blood pressure in the lower extremities that is not higher than measurements in the upper extremity is suggestive of a coarctation or other narrowing of the aorta and is often associated with diminished femoral pulses.

The physical exam should include attention to signs of end-organ damage from hypertension. Previous studies have shown that children presenting with hyper-

tension even at younger ages often show evidence of end-organ damage, such as left ventricular hypertrophy, arteriolar narrowing and hyperreactivity, and structural and functional measures of endothelial dysfunction such as elevated carotid intimal medial thickness and impaired flow mediated dilation after occlusion of the brachial artery [15, 17, 18, 20, 21, 23, 32, 37]. Thus, the physical exam should also include fundoscopic, cardiovascular, pulmonary, and neurologic exams. The abdomen should be auscultated for abdominal bruits that, although uncommon, can accompany renovascular hypertension.

The physical exam should seek to uncover any evidence of a systemic disease that may explain the elevated blood pressure. Similarly, several genetic syndromes have elevated blood pressure often related to renovascular anomalies and they have characteristic physical findings. These include neurofibromatosis (café-au-lait spots, axillary freckling, Lisch nodules), tuberous sclerosis (ash leaf macules, adenoma sebaceum, subungual fibromas, retinal hamartomas), Turner syndrome (short stature, shield chest, upturned mouth, webbed neck), and Williams syndrome (overfriendly personality, cognitive impairment, prominent ears).

12.3.3 Laboratory and Radiologic Evaluation

Often, in the ICU setting, the first emphasis may not be on precise assignment of an etiology to the child's hypertension. As the medical condition stabilizes, ongoing successful management will necessitate a systematic review of pertinent features of the history and physical exam as well as judicious use of laboratory and imaging studies. A urinalysis should be performed on a freshly voided urine sample and, if the dipstick is positive for blood or protein, should include microscopy to look for casts or other formed elements. Screening blood tests should include blood urea nitrogen (BUN), creatinine, and electrolytes to evaluate renal function and screen for states of mineralocorticoid excess that may lead to hypokalemia and alkalosis. The uric acid level is commonly elevated in children with primary hypertension [9, 10] and may be helpful in the absence of an identified secondary cause, although significant hyperuricemia may be seen in the ICU in children with dehydration, significant cell turnover or lysis, or with renal insufficiency.

Other studies should be sent based on findings in the history or physical exam. For example, tachycardia in the absence of pain or agitation suggests hyperthyroidism or high-catecholamine states and should trigger blood thyroid function tests and urinary catecholamine quantification. A history concerning for urinary tract infections with unexplained fevers or positive urine cultures should precipitate a DMSA nuclear scan to determine the presence of cortical scars.

Plasma renin activity and aldosterone levels are helpful only if their results are unequivocally low or high. They are most useful when a diagnosis of mineralocorticoid excess is suspected as plasma renin activity is typically suppressed. Aldosterone levels may be low or high, depending on the specific etiology of the mineralocorticoid excess. As these studies are typically sent out to reference laboratories, their values are not helpful in the acute management of hypertension. Additionally, these studies may be secondarily elevated by vasodilators and, if possible, should be sent with the initial screening studies, prior to use of potent vasodilatory antihypertensives.

All children with hypertension should have a renal ultrasound performed. An ultrasound provides information about differential renal size, hydronephrosis, echotexture, and cystic change and, thus, is a good screening test for many forms of kidney disease. Subtle renal scarring may not be seen on ultrasound, but a size discrepancy between kidneys of >1 cm in length is uncommon and may reflect scarring in the smaller kidney. A DMSA renal scan is a more sensitive way to diagnose renal scars and should be considered if renal scarring needs to be confirmed or is highly suspected.

Doppler assessment of renal vessels measure changes in flow rates and, if abnormal, may suggest the presence of renovascular hypertension. A normal Doppler study does not, however, rule out renal artery stenosis, especially stenosis in smaller segmental arteries not appreciated well by Doppler. More precise renovascular imaging such as MR or CT angiography may be useful in some patients, although formal renal arteriography is often necessary to appreciate smaller segmental stenoses and allows for concomitant angioplasty.

Echocardiography is necessary in any child with concern for a structural cardiac lesion causing hypertension. Additionally, echocardiography may be useful as a very sensitive tool to measure cardiac changes such as left ventricular hypertrophy that accompanies sustained hypertension as an end-organ effect [18, 20, 32]. In some hospitalized patients with hypertension, a careful ophthalmologic exam may also give information as to the chronicity of the child's hypertensive state.

12.4 Treatment

12.4.1 Acute Management

In the child with sustained blood pressures exceeding the 99th percentile, diagnostic evaluation and therapy need to be very carefully considered. The tempo and urgency

Table 12.1 Medications for pediatric hypertensive urgency or emergency

Drug	Mechanism	Dose	Onset	Duration
Hydralazine	Arteriolar dilator	IV: 0.1–0.4 mg kg^{-1} to max dose of 20 mg	5–15 min	3–8 h
Labetalol	α/β Blocker	Initial IV bolus: 0.25 mg kg^{-1}; repeat q 15 min at increasing doses up to 1.0 mg kg^{-1} until effective or total dose of 4 mg kg^{-1}. Maintenance IV drip: 1–3 mg kg^{-1} h^{-1}	5 min	2–6 h
Nitroprusside	Venodilator and arteriolar dilator	IV: start at 0.5 μg kg^{-1} min^{-1}	1–2 min	3–5 min
Nifedipine	Ca Chan blocker	PO: 0.25–0.5 mg kg^{-1}	10–20 min	3–6 h
Nicardipine	Ca Chan blocker	IV: 0.5–5 μg kg^{-1} min^{-1}	10 min	2–6 h
Esmolol	β-Blocker	Loading dose of 500 μg kg^{-1} over 2 min. Maintenance IV drip: 50–250 μg kg^{-1} min^{-1}	Seconds	10–20 min
Enalaprilat	ACE inhibitor	IV: 5–10 μg kg^{-1} dose^{-1} q8–24 h	0.5–4 h	6 h
Furosemide	Loop diuretic	IV: Intermittent: 0.5–2 mg kg^{-1} dose^{-1} q6–24 h. Continuous: 0.1–0.5 mg kg^{-1} min^{-1}	2–5 min	2 h

See text for details of use

of the intervention is again guided on an individual basis by the child's clinical presentation and course.

Severe hypertension with actual acute end-organ dysfunction or the concern of impending end-organ dysfunction should be treated with short-acting intravenous antihypertensive medications. The medications most commonly used in a hypertensive crisis are outlined in Table 12.1. The blood pressure should be lowered by 20–30% in the first 2–3 h. Once the blood pressure is in a range that is not acutely dangerous for the patient, the blood pressure should be lowered more gradually to at least the 95th percentile reference blood pressure over the next several days or even longer.

Hypertension in the ICU can be effectively managed with continuous infusions of agents that can be carefully titrated to achieve target blood pressure goals. The choice of agent should focus on the presumed underlying mechanism of the hypertension as well as local custom and clinician's familiarity with specific agents. Intravenous hydralazine and nitroprusside were for years the mainstay of parenteral antihypertensive therapy in the pediatric ICU but medications initially introduced for care of adults have now gained more widespread use in children, with a number of studies leading to FDA approval for specific efficacy and safety labeling for several antihypertensive agents in children.

As the blood pressure is controlled, oral therapy needs to be initiated to allow a transition off drips or infused medications. In children hospitalized in the ICU for hypertension, this transition needs to be coordinated carefully and is best accomplished in a monitored unit.

12.4.1.1 Nitroprusside

Sodium nitroprusside is a powerful arteriolar and venous dilator. For decades, its rapid onset of action with short half life has made it a first-line option for continuous antihypertensive infusion. Nitroprusside acts as a donor of nitric oxide, which mediates its potent vasodilatory characteristics. Its use is limited, however, by toxicity of its metabolites. Nitroprusside is converted by tissue sulfhydryl groups to cyanide, and this cyanide is then converted to thiocyanate in the liver. Patients with liver disease or reduced renal function should have cyanide levels followed. More specifically, thiocyanate levels should be monitored in patients on nitroprusside for more than 72 h or in patients with renal insufficiency and a GFR < 60 mL per min per 1.73 m^2. Thiocyanate toxicity manifests primarily as neurotoxicity, and includes psychosis, blurred vision, confusion, weakness, tinnitus, and seizures. An early sign of cyanide toxicity includes metabolic acidosis, while other signs of toxicity include tachycardia, pink skin, decreased pulse, decreased reflexes, altered consciousness or even coma, almond smell on breath, methemoglobinemia, and dilated pupils.

Additionally, nitroprusside may increase intracranial pressure (ICP). In the ICU setting where there may be children with both increased ICP and hypertension, this possible sequela needs to be considered when individualizing therapy for relevant patients.

12.4.1.2   Adrenergic Blockers: Labetalol and Esmolol

Labetalol may be used both via continuous infusion and intermittent IV dosing. It is the only drug that is both an alpha- and beta-blocker. Some consider its alpha-blockade more pronounced in the IV form. Its dosing is independent of renal function and thus may be safely used in renal insufficiency. It may also be effective in the treatment of hypertension related to pheochromocytoma. Furthermore, its function as both a continuous and intermittent agent makes it a good bridge off a continuous drip when stability of blood pressure is achieved. It should be used judiciously in children with asthma as it may precipitate bronchospasm.

Esmolol is a selective beta-blocker used as a continuous infusion in children primarily in the setting of cardiac disease. Like labetalol, its use may be contraindicated in certain children with asthma. Its toxicities include bradycardia and congestive heart failure.

12.4.1.3   Nicardipine

Nicardipine is a dihydropyridine calcium channel blocker of the same class as nifedipine and amlodipine. While generally less familiar as an anti hypertensive agent for hypertensive urgencies or emergencies, it has been used safely in children with hypertensive crises. In spite of earlier concerns of cardiovascular collapse in young infants from calcium channel blockers, nicardipine has been used safely in both preterm and term neonates and, in three studies involving neonates, no adverse events were reported [13, 22, 36]. Nicardipine has also been used safely in older children for the acute management of hypertension [11, 35, 36]. Moreover, nicardipine was found as effective as nitroprusside in adult cohorts. Given its safety profile, this drug will likely find increased use in the pediatric ICU in the coming years. Use of nicardipine also allows transition over to a long-acting oral calcium channel blocker such as amlodipine or extended release nifedipine.

12.4.1.4   Fenoldopam

Fenoldopam is in a unique class of dopamine D1 receptor agonists. The pediatric experience with fenoldopam is most extensive in children after cardiopulmonary bypass surgery for congenital cardiac disease. In one study, while lowering blood pressure, fenoldopam also promoted diuresis in neonates who were fluid overloaded after cardiac surgery in spite of therapy with conventional diuretics [5]. Its toxicities are relatively limited but include reflex tachycardia and tachyphylaxis within days of its onset. This agent will likely find greater use given its therapeutic profile, especially in children with hypertension who may also benefit from increased renal perfusion. Its cost and limited clinician familiarity with its use may impact its widespread acceptance as first-line therapy for hypertensive emergencies.

12.4.1.5   Other Agents

Although a continuous infusion is often ideal for careful titration of blood pressure in the ICU setting, there may be situations where dosing intermittently with other agents may be appropriate or effective.

Hydralazine is a commonly used vasodilator with rapid onset that often can be titrated to achieve good blood pressure control. It is generally well tolerated and can be given in a non-ICU setting.

Nifedipine is another short-acting agent and has the advantage of oral administration. Its use in adults is rare due to reports of myocardial infarction related to its use [27]. The use of short-acting nifedipine in children has been found to be very widespread among clinicians treating children with hypertension, and although a higher incidence of adverse events was seen in patients with preexisting CNS disease [7], it is considered a safe general therapy. The sublingual route is suboptimal compared with oral ingestion of an intact capsule. Sublingual administration requires aspiration of liquid from within the gelcap and subsequent dose estimation; moreover, absorption after sublingual provision is erratic.

Enalaprilat is the IV form of the angiotensin converting enzyme (ACE) inhibitor enalapril. Its use is appropriate for those scenarios where renin-mediated hypertension is a concern. Enalaprilat, like its prodrug enalapril, is longer acting than many other IV antihypertensives and is dosed every 8–24 h in infants and children [41]. Its use for hypertension in neonates or in children with cystic kidney disease, congenital urologic malformations, or clinical conditions where afterload reduction is indicated makes enalaprilat a unique choice that addresses specific mechanisms of hypertension. It should be used with caution in renovascular disease as renal perfusion is renin-dependent in those settings. Careful attention to potassium and creatinine should also be given, as these levels may be adversely affected with ACE inhibitors, as discussed further later.

Diuretics are frequently used in adults with hypertension. Their use in children is more focused, especially in the ICU. Loop diuretics (furosemide, bumetanide) are the most potent diuretics in clinical use, blocking 25% of tubular sodium reabsorption at the thick ascending limb of the loop of Henle. Thiazides (hydrochlorothiazide, chlorothiazide, metolazone) are less potent but are often used for chronic diuretic monotherapy or as an adjunctive medication with a loop diuretic. Metolazone may be particularly effective in the setting of renal insufficiency, heart failure, or refractory nephrotic syndrome. Many of the diuretic agents have IV forms that are used most commonly in the ICU to treat volume overload when oral diuretics cannot be utilized or have been ineffective. Additionally, because of the compensatory sodium retention that follows long-term vasodilator and calcium channel blocker use, diuretics can mitigate this volume expansion. Thiazides may serve a similar adjunctive function for loop diuretics, as increased sodium reabsorption more distal to the thick ascending limb can blunt the natiuresis and water loss expected with loop diuretics [29]. Finally, aside from its intermittent dosing, furosemide or bumetanide can be administered as a continuous infusion for refractory volume overload.

12.4.2 Long-Acting Medications

As blood pressure is controlled by intravenous medication, it is important to initiate oral antihypertensives to allow transition off continuous infusions and transfer out of the ICU onto the ward. Table 12.2 reviews the drugs used most often for pediatric antihypertensive therapy. The choice of antihypertensive agent should address the presumed underlying pathophysiology of the blood pressure perturbation. For instance, children with fluid overload related to glomerulonephritis should be treated with diuretics and vasodilators. Hyperreninemic hypertension due to renal parenchymal scarring should be treated with ACE inhibitors or angiotensin receptor blockers (ARBs). Generally, one medication is initiated and its dose escalated until maximal dosing has been reached at which point an additional agent is started and dose is adjusted as needed. The use of the fewest medications is optimal clinically to maximize adherence and minimize drug sequelae. Once blood pressure is normalized, medications should be maintained to allow ongoing blood pressure control and not held because of *good* blood pressures unless

there is symptomatic hypotension. Goal blood pressure with chronic therapy should be no higher than the 95th percentile for reference group. In other words, therapy should be escalated or augmented until at least high normal blood pressure readings are obtained consistently. Depending on particular clinical circumstance, some children may benefit from even lower chronic blood pressure readings.

The dihydropyridine calcium channel blockers nifedipine and amlodipine are now among the most common agents used for pediatric hypertension since these agents are generally well tolerated and need no specific laboratory parameters followed during therapy. At higher doses, they may cause headache and reflex tachycardia. The salt retention that may occur with prolonged use may lead to tachyphylaxis, and the addition of low-dose diuretic augments the antihypertensive effect. Rare patients develop extremity edema that may also respond to diuretics. Extended-release nifedipine is formulated as a capsule that must be swallowed intact and may be difficult for younger children to swallow. Amlodipine has been studied in specific pediatric trials [12, 28, 34] and is approved for use in children over 6 years of age. Although formulated to be swallowed as a whole tablet, amlodipine may be crushed and there is extensive clinical use with compounded suspensions.

ACE inhibitors have also found widespread use in pediatrics, related both to their antihypertensive action as well as their renoprotective effect in patients with proteinuria and chronic kidney disease. Many of the agents in this class have been studied in children, and enalapril, fosinopril, lisinopril, and benazepril all have specific pediatric labeling for hypertension [39, 40]. These drugs are especially effective in patients with hyperreninemic hypertension due to renal parenchymal scarring. In patients with a suspicion of renal artery stenosis, tenuous renal perfusion, or in whom the etiology of the hypertension is unclear, ACE inhibitors should be used with caution, as they may precipitate acute renal failure in patients with bilateral renal artery stenosis or with borderline or diminished effective intravascular volume. By decreasing GFR, ACE inhibitors may also cause elevations of serum creatinine and potassium, and these biochemical parameters should be followed in children taking these drugs. ACE inhibitors should generally be avoided as first-line therapy in patients with acute renal failure in whom alterations of glomerular hemodynamics may impede recovery. These medications may also lead to anemia via bone marrow suppression and a CBC should be

Table 12.2 Long-acting oral antihypertensive agents in children

Medication	Initial dose (mg kg^{-1} day^{-1})	Maximal dose (mg kg^{-1} day^{-1})	Dosing frequency
Calcium blocker			
Nifedipine	0.25	3	XL or SR forms bid
Amlodipine	0.1	0.4	qd – bid
ACE inhibitor			
Captopril (neonate)	0.03–0.15	2	bid – tid
Captopril (child)	1.5	6	bid – tid
Enalapril	0.15	Up to 40 mg total per day	qd – bid
Diuretic			
Hydrochlorothiazide	1	2–3	qd – bid
Furosemide	0.5–1.0	10	qd – bid
Adrenergic agent			
Atenolol (β blocker)	0.5	2–3	qd – bid
Propranolol (β blocker)	1	6–8	Bid
Labetalol (α/β blocker)	1	3	Bid
Vasodilator			
Hydralazine	0.5	10	tid – qid
Minoxodil	0.1–0.2	1	qd – bid

checked periodically, especially if the patient is on any other myelosuppressive medications. Although cough is reported frequently in adults on ACE inhibitors, this is seen less often in children unless higher doses are used. Finally, this class is teratogenic and postmenarchal girls taking these medications should be counseled about abstinence or contraception.

As a result of specific pediatric studies, two ARBs (irbesartan, losartan) are approved for use in children over 6 years of age. With respect to biochemical changes and teratogenicity, these agents have a side effect profile similar to ACE inhibitors, although the effect on potassium may not be as dramatic as for ACE inhibitors.

Beta-blockers are widely used in adults for primary hypertension, due to their ability to decrease mortality after cardiovascular events and for some children with specific cardiac anomalies they will also be prescribed as first-line therapy. Beta blockers may cause exercise intolerance due to their effect on heart rate, can contribute to depression in some individuals, and may be problematic with asthma or diabetes. They may, nonetheless, play a role in antihypertensive therapy even in children with normal baseline cardiac status, for instance, in individuals already on vasodilator therapy but with tachycardia and suboptimal blood pressure control or in

hypertensive children with migraines who may benefit from headache prophylaxis.

Diuretic therapy is increasingly recommended as the mainstay of antihypertensive therapy in adult patients. In the hospitalized hypertensive child, diuretics are used primarily in glomerulonephritis where volume overload is a concern, or as an adjunct to vasodilators as secondary salt and water retention may develop as noted earlier. As chronic therapy in the ambulatory setting, diuretics may also be beneficial, again generally as an adjunctive medication; however, their prescription may be problematic in children without free access to lavatories or who are embarrassed or reluctant to use school restroom facilities.

12.5 Conclusion

While hypertension is an uncommon reason for pediatric ICU admission, especially in the setting of a hypertensive urgency or emergency where acute organ dysfunction is present, prompt management and evaluation is essential. As most causes of severe hypertension are related to kidney disease, the evaluation should focus on these etiologies. Early consultation with a pediatric nephrologist will facilitate the evaluation, focus laboratory investigation and imaging, and optimize pharmaceutical interventions. The evaluation of acute hypertension should be simultaneous with its treatment. The choice of antihypertensive agent should reflect the putative etiology of the hypertension. In addition to mainstays of antihypertensive therapy in the pediatric ICU such as nitroprusside and labetalol, there are a growing number of other medications available for continuous or intermittent infusion or oral provision. As no single continuous infusion drug has been shown to be superior, the choice of agent should be based on the mechanism of action and the experience of the center, with transition to oral therapy as soon as feasible to facilitate long-term care. Therapy should utilize the fewest medications with sequential maximization of dosing prior to initiation of an additional agent. Goal blood pressure readings should be less than the 90th to 95th percentile for age, size, and gender.

Take Home Pearls

> Hypertension in children and adolescents is assumed to be secondary and should trigger a diagnostic evaluation.
> Treatment of severe hypertension should be simultaneous with the diagnostic evaluation.
> Multiple intravenous agents are available as continuous and intermittent infusions for the rapid lowering of blood pressure in children.
> Once blood pressure is controlled with an intravenous agent, patients should be transitioned to oral medication or a similar class.

References

1. National High Blood Pressure Education Program Working Group on High Blood Pressure in Children and Adolescents. (2004) The fourth report on the diagnosis, evaluation, and treatment of high blood pressure in children and adolescents. Pediatrics 114:555–76
2. Arafat M, Mattoo TK (1999) Measurement of blood pressure in children: recommendations and perceptions on cuff selection. Pediatrics 104:e30
3. Chobanian AV, Bakris GL, Black HR, et al. (2003) The Seventh Report of the Joint National Committee on Prevention, Detection, Evaluation, and Treatment of High Blood Pressure: the JNC 7 report. JAMA 289:2560–72
4. Clark JA, Lieh-Lai MW, Sarnaik A, et al. (2002) Discrepancies between direct and indirect blood pressure measurements using various recommendations for arm cuff selection. Pediatrics 110:920–3
5. Costello JM, Thiagarajan RR, Dionne RE, et al. (2006) Initial experience with fenoldopam after cardiac surgery

in neonates with an insufficient response to conventional diuretics. Pediatr Crit Care Med 7:28–33
6. Croix B, Feig DI (2006) Childhood hypertension is not a silent disease. Pediatr Nephrol 21:527–32
7. Egger DW, Deming DD, Hamada N, et al. (2002) Evaluation of the safety of short-acting nifedipine in children with hypertension. Pediatr Nephrol 17:35–40
8. Falkner B, Gidding SS, Ramirez-Garnica G, et al. (2006) The relationship of body mass index and blood pressure in primary care pediatric patients. J Pediatr 148:195–200
9. Feig DI, Johnson RJ (2003) Hyperuricemia in childhood primary hypertension. Hypertension 42:247–52
10. Feig DI, Nakagawa T, Karumanchi SA, et al. (2004) Hypothesis: uric acid, nephron number, and the pathogenesis of essential hypertension. Kidney Int 66:281–7
11. Flynn JT, Mottes TA, Brophy PD, et al. (2001) Intravenous nicardipine for treatment of severe hypertension in children. J Pediatr 139:38–43
12. Flynn JT, Newburger JW, Daniels SR, et al. (2004) A randomized, placebo-controlled trial of amlodipine in children with hypertension. J Pediatr 145:353–9
13. Gouyon JB, Geneste B, Semama DS, et al. (1997) Intravenous nicardipine in hypertensive preterm infants. Arch Dis Child Fetal Neonatal Ed 76:F126–F127
14. Huxley RR, Shiell AW, Law CM (2000) The role of size at birth and postnatal catch-up growth in determining systolic blood pressure: a systematic review of the literature. J Hypertens 18:815–31
15. Im JA, Lee JW, Shim JY, et al. (2007) Association between brachial-ankle pulse wave velocity and cardiovascular risk factors in healthy adolescents. J Pediatr 150:247–51
16. Jago R, Harrell JS, McMurray RG, et al. (2006) Prevalence of abnormal lipid and blood pressure values among an ethnically diverse population of eighth-grade adolescents and screening implications. Pediatrics 117:2065–73
17. Lande MB, Carson NL, Roy J, et al. (2006) Effects of childhood primary hypertension on carotid intima media thickness: a matched controlled study. Hypertension 48:40–4
18. Litwin M, Niemirska A, Sladowska J, et al. (2006) Left ventricular hypertrophy and arterial wall thickening in children with essential hypertension. Pediatr Nephrol 21:811–19
19. Mattoo TK (2002) Arm cuff in the measurement of blood pressure. Am J Hypertens 15:67S–68S
20. McNiece KL, Gupta-Malhotra M, Samuels J, et al. (2007) Left ventricular hypertrophy in hypertensive adolescents: analysis of risk by 2004 National High Blood Pressure Education Program Working Group staging criteria. Hypertension 50:392–5
21. Meyer AA, Kundt G, Steiner M, et al. (2006) Impaired flow-mediated vasodilation, carotid artery intima-media thickening, and elevated endothelial plasma markers in obese children: the impact of cardiovascular risk factors. Pediatrics 117:1560–7
22. Milou C, Debuche-Benouachkou V, Semama DS, et al. (2000) Intravenous nicardipine as a first-line antihypertensive drug in neonates. Intensive Care Med 26:956–8
23. Mitchell P, Cheung N, de Haseth K, et al. (2007) Blood pressure and retinal arteriolar narrowing in children. Hypertension 49:1156–62

24. Pappadis SL, Somers MJ (2003) Hypertension in adolescents: a review of diagnosis and management. Curr Opin Pediatr 15:370–8

25. Park MK, Menard SW, Yuan C (2001) Comparison of auscultatory and oscillometric blood pressures. Arch Pediatr Adolesc Med 155:50–3

26. Podoll A, Grenier M, Croix B, et al. (2007) Inaccuracy in pediatric outpatient blood pressure measurement. Pediatrics 119:e538–e543

27. Psaty BM, Heckbert SR, Koepsell TD, et al. (1995) The risk of myocardial infarction associated with antihypertensive drug therapies. JAMA 274:620–5

28. Rogan JW, Lyszkiewicz DA, Blowey D, et al. (2000) A randomized prospective crossover trial of amlodipine in pediatric hypertension. Pediatr Nephrol 14:1083–7

29. Scheinman SJ, Guay-Woodford LM, Thakker RV, et al. (1999) Genetic disorders of renal electrolyte transport. N Engl J Med 340:1177–87

30. Sinaiko AR (1996) Hypertension in children. N Engl J Med 335:1968–73

31. Sorof J, Daniels S (2002) Obesity hypertension in children: a problem of epidemic proportions. Hypertension 40:441–7

32. Sorof JM, Cardwell G, Franco K, et al. (2002) Ambulatory blood pressure and left ventricular mass index in hypertensive children. Hypertension 39:903–8

33. Sorof JM, Lai D, Turner J, et al. (2004) Overweight, ethnicity, and the prevalence of hypertension in school-aged children. Pediatrics 113:475–82

34. Tallian KB, Nahata MC, Turman MA, et al. (1999) Efficacy of amlodipine in pediatric patients with hypertension. Pediatr Nephrol 13:304–10

35. Tenney F, Sakarcan A (2000) Nicardipine is a safe and effective agent in pediatric hypertensive emergencies. Am J Kidney Dis 35:E20

36. Treluyer JM, Hubert P, Jouvet P, et al. (1993) Intravenous nicardipine in hypertensive children. Eur J Pediatr 152:712–14

37. Urbina EM, Kieltkya L, Tsai J, et al. (2005) Impact of multiple cardiovascular risk factors on brachial artery distensibility in young adults: the Bogalusa Heart Study. Am J Hypertens 18:767–71

38. Van Der Voort JH, Edwards AG, Roberts R, et al. (2002) Unexplained extra visits to general practitioners before the diagnosis of first urinary tract infection: a case-control study. Arch Dis Child 87:530–2

39. Wells T, Rippley R, Hogg R, et al. (2001) The pharmacokinetics of enalapril in children and infants with hypertension. J Clin Pharmacol 41:1064–74

40. Wells TG (1999) Trials of antihypertensive therapies in children. Blood Press Monit 4:189–92

41. Wells TG, Bunchman TE, Kearns GL (1990) Treatment of neonatal hypertension with enalaprilat. J Pediatr 117:664–7

Acute Glomerulonephritis

13

J. Dötsch

Contents

Core Messages

> ❯ Glomerulonephritis is infrequently the cause of an ICU admission but children with significant glomerulonephritis may develop severe fluid and electrolyte perturbations or acute kidney injury requiring urgent dialysis therapy necessitating intensive care.

> ❯ The evaluation of acute glomerulonephritis is directed at both discerning an etiology and determining if there is rapid deterioration in renal function.

> ❯ Any glomerulonephritis with rapid accompanying loss of renal function needs an extensive immediate evaluation including consideration of diagnostic renal biopsy.

> ❯ The therapy for acute glomerulonephritis varies according to the underlying etiology. In cases of a rapidly progressive glomerulonephritis with loss of renal function, aggressive therapies including plasmapheresis, steroid pulses, and cytotoxic agents may be useful.

Case Vignette

A 12 year old girl presents with fever and hemoptysis. She was well until 4 months ago when she developed an upper respiratory infection that seemed to linger with persistent cough and sinus discomfort. She has been treated with several courses of oral antibiotics without improvement. She has also developed progressive fatigue and has frequently been unable to go to school or participate in her dance class. One week ago she developed fever to 39°C with night sweats.

A PPD was placed by her pediatrician and showed negative. Diagnostic evaluation included anemia on a CBC, negative sinus radiograph, a 3 cm area of nodular opacity in the left upper lung on chest radiograph, normal serum BUN and creatinine, and a urinalysis with 2+ protein and 3+ blood with red blood cell casts. Physical examination is noteworthy for a blood pressure of 132/86, mild pallor, irritated nasal mucosa, and diminished breath sounds at the left apex. Further diagnostic studies including complement levels, anti-nuclear antibodies, anti- glomerular basement membrane antibodies, and anti-neutrophil cytoplasm antibody (ANCA) serologies are obtained. Indirect immunofluorescence testing for ANCA is positive and anti-proteinase 3 ELISA titer is high. A diagnosis of Wegener's Granulomatosis is confirmed after the

S.G. Kiessling et al. (eds) *Pediatric Nephrology in the ICU.*
© Springer-Verlag Berlin Heidelberg 2009

patient undergoes biopsies of her kidneys and lungs. Renal biopsy reveals occasional glomeruli with cresentic changes. She receives three days of pulse solumedrol intravenously as well as an intravenous pulse of cyclophosphamide.

13.1 Introduction

Acute glomerulonephritis (GN) per se rarely is an actual indication for admission of a child or adolescent to the intensive care unit. Several complications of the illness may, however, lead to the need for critical care management, including:

1. Referral of the patient to the ICU for urgent hemodialysis, hemofiltration, or peritoneal dialysis
2. Admission of a patient with a complication from GN or GN therapy, for instance severe hypertension or infection in a child receiving immunosuppressive medications
3. Management of a patient with severe multisystem disease including GN from systemic lupus erythematosus (SLE), Goodpasture's syndrome, and Wegener's granulomatosis

As a consequence, the ICU specialist should

1. Recognize GN and organize the initial diagnostic evaluation
2. Know the course and prognosis of different forms of acute GN
3. Know the potentially underlying systemic diseases
4. Anticipate complications of acute GN in the intensive care setting
5. Know the mainstays of treatment and their complications

The major focus of this chapter will be on rapidly progressive GN (RPGN), also termed crescentic GN for its histologic appearance on renal biopsy. Despite being rare in presentation, its potential devastating clinical course and its propensity to cause severe acute kidney injury make it a form of GN likely to be encountered in the pediatric IUC.

13.2 Causes and Classification of Acute GN

According to the WHO classification of glomerulopathies [6], the most frequently encountered forms of acute GN will either be found in a group of primary glomerulopathies or in glomerulopathies secondary to systemic disease. Among children, the most common cause of acute GN is a primary post-infectious process from a preceding bacterial or viral infection. Found in the group of systemic diseases with GN are conditions such as Henoch–Schönlein purpura (HSP), SLE-nephritis, Goodpasture's syndrome, or anti-glomerular basement membrane (anti-GBM) disease. Found in the third WHO group are vascular diseases with renal complications such as the anti-neutrophil cytoplasm antibody (ANCA) positive vasculitides including polyarteris nodosa and Wegener's granulomatosis.

13.2.1 Causes of Rapidly Progressive or Crescentic GN

The causes of a rapidly progressive GN (RPGN) or crescentic GN vary substantially in reports from different medical centers and countries. While RPGN refers to the clinical course with a decrease in effective GFR occurring over a relatively compressed time frame, crescentic GN refers to the actual biopsy findings. Since RPGN may not always be easily distinguished from the acute exacerbation of a heretofore undiagnosed glomerulopathy, biopsy may indicate chronic diseases as well.

Information on four larger series of children and adolescents with an RPGN with at least 50% crescentic glomeruli on renal biopsy have been published. In European studies with data on 41 children from France [19] and Great Britain [13], HSP was by far the most common cause of crescentic GN in up to a third of children. RPGN from vasculitis (about 15%), poststreptococcal GN (about 10%), and anti-GBM disease (about 5%) followed in frequency. An RPGN from IgA-nephropathy or SLE was rare, and non-specific mesangioproliferative changes were common in almost a quarter of affected children.

These findings are in contrast to data from other parts of the world. In 50 American children with RPGN, 26% had non-specific immune complex disease, 18% had SLE, 14% idiopathic GN and 12% post-streptococcal GN [24]. Interestingly, RPGN related to HSP was rare (6%).

In 43 Indian children and adolescents with crescentic GN, 60% of renal biopsies were classified idiopathic and 26% post-streptococcal GN [25].

A very rare cause of RPGN in any series is a complement consuming nephritis associated with a chronic infection such as subacute bacterial endocarditis, an infected permanent central venous line, or an infected ventriculo-peritoneal or ventriculo-atrial shunt. In the context of medically complex pediatric patients in the ICU, however, this form of nephritis should be included if applicable in broad initial differential diagnoses.

13.3 Diagnosis of Acute GN

The diagnosis of an acute GN necessitates differentiation from a chronic renal disorder with similar symptoms and signs. Most important in the ICU setting is anticipation of any rapidly progressive course that may complicate patient management or impact patient morbidity or mortality. A proposed scheme of diagnostic evaluation in acute GN is shown in Fig. 13.1.

13.3.1 Clinical Presentation (Table 13.1)

The classical clinical symptoms of acute GN are hematuria, often with one or more episodes of macroscopic

hematuria, sterile pyuria, and proteinuria. Oliguria, edema, hypertension, functional renal impairment, and anemia are seen to a variable degree.

13.3.1.1 RPGN: Epidemiology and Clinical Presentation

As discussed above, in the pediatric ICU, RPGN is without doubt the most important form of GN encountered. The exact incidence of an RPGN in children with any type of GN is unknown. In adults, 2–5% of all patients diagnosed with GN show crescentic lesions on renal biopsy [20]. Approximately half of children with a predominately crescentic GN have a rapidly progressive course [17].

In contrast to uncomplicated acute GN, the most important clinical hallmark of an RPGN is renal impairment. Oliguria, hypertension, edema, and anemia are more common than in uncomplicated acute GN, but

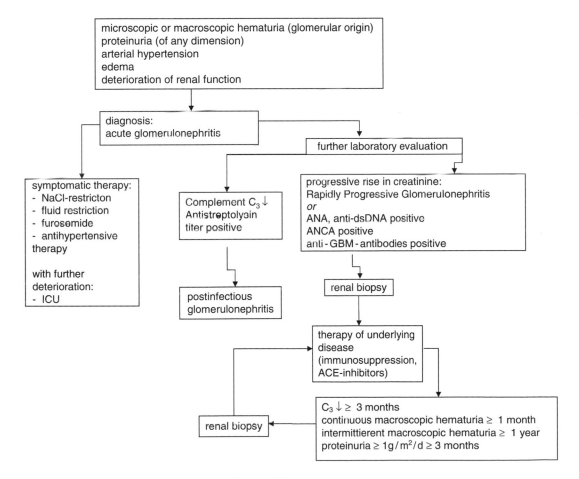

Fig. 13.1 Algorithm for the clinical management of acute GN

Table 13.1 Causes of GN and risk of a rapidly progressive course in childhood and adolescence. GN: GN, RPGN: rapidly progressive GN, CRF: chronic renal failure

GN	Age	Incidence	Risk of RPGN	Overall prognosis
Postinfectious GN	Childhood (especially 4–12 years)	Common	Low	<2% chronic kidney disease [23]
Henoch–Schönlein purpura GN	Childhood	Relatively common; in 20–60% of cases of HSP	Low	Up to 20% chronic kidney disease [28]
IgA-nephropathy	All ages, especially >10 years old	Relatively common (up to 1% of entire population)	Low	Up to 25% ESRD after 20 years in adults [8]
SLE-nephritis	Adolescents	2/1,000,000 Higher in Afro-American and Asian population	Moderate	10–20% ESRD after 10 years [5]
Polyarteritis nodosa	All age groups	Very rare	High	Mortality in adults from 10% to 45% [12]
Wegener's granulomatosis	Adolescents	Very rare	High	CRF 50% [1]
Goodpasture's syndrome	Adolescents	Very rare	High	ESRD and mortality high [3]
Shunt nephritis	All age groups	Very rare	Moderate	Reversible with appropriate treatment

are not always present [9]. The clinical spectrum of crescentic RPGN is shown in Table 13.2.

The onset of disease may be acute, or insidious and have pre-existed for a considerable time period. If the patient presents with renal failure and normocytic anemia, it may not always be easy to discriminate between acute and chronic renal failure. Signs of renal osteopathy and serious perturbations in the calcium-phosphorus-PTH axis would indicate a more chronic course. Under certain circumstances, only renal biopsy may lead to a clear diagnosis.

Extrarenal clinical symptoms of systemic disease associated with RPGN or crescentic GN may aid in the diagnosis (Table 13.3). For instance, HSP has classical dermal lesions on the lower legs and buttocks; SLE may, apart from the characteristic facial rash, present with other skin lesions and arthritis; Goodpasture's syndrome may present with pulmonary hemorrhage and Wegener's granulomatosis with epistaxis or sinopulmonary disease. The extrarenal findings in these diseases may actually precede any renal impairment or an episode of GN by up to several years [3].

Table 13.2 Clinical presentation of children and adolescents with RPGN [7,9,13,19,24,25]

Clinical presentation	Frequency (%)
Acute kidney injury	100
Microscopic hematuria	100
Macroscopic hematuria	50–90
Proteinuria	70–100
Nephrotic syndrome	up to 50
Oliguria	5–100
Edema	15–90
Anemia	up to 70
Hypertension	15–85

13.3.2 Diagnostic Evaluation

The diagnosis of acute GN is usually made by clinical evaluation and laboratory examinations. In the case of a rapidly progressive course, renal biopsy may be necessary. After symptoms such as brown urine, oliguria, or swelling are reported, ongoing clinical examination should look for findings suggesting volume imbalance such as exacerbating edema and hypertension. The urine volume as well as the patient's daily weight should be determined.

Table 13. 3 Extrarenal symptoms, clinical signs, and laboratory findings associated with acute GN

Underlying disease	Clincal sign	Characteristic laboratory findings
Postinfectious GN	History of streptococcal infection (2–6 weeks before) or preceding history of other recent infection; arthritis	Complement C3↓, Antistreptolysin Titer↑
IgA nephropathy	Acute (viral) infection precipitates gross hematuria	
Henoch–Schönlein purpura	Purpura of lower legs and buttocks, arthritis, abdominal pain	
Systemic lupus erythematosus	Facial rash, arthritis, fever, fatigue, pallor (anemia), infections (leukopenia) central nervous symptoms	Complement C3 and C4↓, anemia, leukopenia, ANA and anti-double-stranded DNA antibodies
Goodpasture's syndrome	Pulmonary hemorrhage, dyspnea	Anti GBM antibodies
Polyarteritis nodosa	Arthritis, polymorphic skin rashes (purpura, skin necrosis, nodules) neurological symptoms, gastrointestinal symptoms	pANCA elevated
Wegener's granulomatosis	Epistaxis, pulmonary hemorrhage	cANCA elevated
Shunt nephritis	Fever, ventriculo-peritoneal shunt, permanent central venous line or port	Complement C3↓, CRP↑

Laboratory examination will include urinalysis looking for positive heme and protein on dipstick and dysmorphic urinary erythrocytes and red cell casts on microscopic review. Blood chemistries including electrolytes, urea nitrogen, and creatinine help determine whether alterations of renal function or solute handling have already taken place. As a clue to underlying systemic or inflammatory disease, a CBC, C-reactive protein, erythrocyte sedimentation rate, C3 and C4 complement levels, anti-streptolysin titers, anti-nuclear antibodies, anti-double-stranded DNA-antibodies, cANCA or pANCA serologies, and anti-GBM antibodies may need to be ordered. If nephritis linked to a chronic systemic bacterial infection is suspected, blood cultures are indicated.

To assess for systemic pulmonary disease or to assess further volume overload, chest radiographs may be indicated. Specific alterations in cardiac function may best be appreciated by echocardiography. Evaluation is best done sequentially and, if there is a rapidly progressive course and no defined diagnosis, renal biopsy must not be delayed.

13.3.3   Differential Diagnosis

An acute GN has to be differentiated from a number of other entities with shared presenting characteristics:

Chronic glomerulopathies such as IgA nephropathy, membranoproliferative GN, focal segmental glomeru-losclerosis, and Alport's syndrome may be difficult to differentiate, especially if there is an acute exacerbation. Signs of chronic renal failure such as short stature, anemia, acidosis, hypocalcemia, hyperphosphatemia, and hyperparathyroidism may point to a chronic glomerular disease with pre-existing renal insufficiency. Positive family history and sensory hearing loss may indicate Alport's syndrome. Frequently, only renal biopsy establishes the etiology of a chronic disorder.

Hemolytic-uremic syndrome is occasionally a difficult diagnosis, especially if thrombocytopenia and anemia are only mild or attributed to another cause. A history of bloody diarrhea, with ensuing hematuria, schistocytes in the peripheral blood smear, and an elevation of LDH in serum will usually help to arrive at the diagnosis of typical or D+ HUS. In D− HUS or cases not related to a diarrheal prodrome, a thrombotic microangiopathy should still be a cardinal feature; various genetic, infectious, or drug-related etiologies have been described.

Acute interstitial nephritis due to infections or drugs such as penicillins and cephalosporins may present with proteinuria, microscopic hematuria, and acute kidney injury. As opposed to the proteinuria accompanying a glomerular lesion, with heavy urinary losses of albumin and potentially, immunoglobulin G, the proteinuria of interstitial nephritis is tubular in etiology and usually presents with the loss of low molecular mass proteins (α1-microglobulin or β2-

microglobulin). In addition, increased urinary losses of sodium, potassium, phophate, and glucose may be present from tubular dysfunction.

Isolated hematuria is usually easy to differentiate from acute GN since proteinuria is absent and kidney function and blood pressure is normal.

Acute urinary tract infection may sometimes mimic acute GN, in particular if macroscopic hematuria is present from cystitis. In lower tract urinary infection, the urinary erythrocytes are of non-glomerular origin and heavy proteinuria is generally not present.

13.3.4 Renal Biopsy

With advances in technical equipment and using ultrasound guidance, renal biopsies can be performed with few complications even in very small children. Although rare in experienced hands, hemorrhage, infection, arterio-venous fistula formation, and even organ loss are all reported sequelae.

Renal biopsy is indicated in any GN with progressive loss of renal function raising a suspicion of RPGN, with renal involvement in suspected systemic disease such as SLE or Goodpasture's syndrome, and in cases of GN with a nephrotic course, persisting macroscopic hematuria, or long term persistence of heavy proteinuria ($>1 \, \mathrm{g \, m^{-2} \, d^{-1}}$).

Biopsy samples should be sent for light microscopic review as well as immunofluorescence study and electron microscopy. With light microscopy, glomerular crescents can be appreciated. Although the number of crescents is somewhat predictive of the extent of disease, it may not necessarily predict the outcome of disease. In fact, a clinical RPGN can be seen with as few as 10% of glomeruli demonstrating crescents [10, 21]. A further histological feature that may be very important for the prognosis of the acute GN is the nature of the crescents. Three types are described: cellular crescents, implying recent proliferation of epithelial and inflammatory cells; fibrous crescents where all proliferating cells have been replaced by collagen indicating an advanced chronic state of disease that may no longer be remediable; and an intermediate type, so called fibrocellular crescents where there may be a mix of reversible and irreversible changes [13].

Immunohistochemical staining is an important diagnostic tool. The underlying renal disease that might be discovered by immunohistochemistry may be by far more important for the prognosis of the disease since directed therapy may induce a disease remission and allow tissue healing. Anti-glomerular basement membrane staining, for instance, may help to arrive at the diagnosis of Goodpasture's syndrome [3]. Positive IgA-staining helps to identify IgA-nephropathy [10], and the so-called "full-house" immunochemical pattern of positive staining for IgM, IgG, C3, and C1 is very suggestive of SLE. Assessment of renal vessels in the biopsy helps to exclude thrombotic microangiopathy from the differential diagnosis, and may also help to arrive at the diagnosis of GN in polyarteritis nodosa.

13.4 Complications of Acute GN Seen in the Pediatric ICU

The complications seen in acute GN may either be due to an alteration of renal function, with the consequence of volume overload and electrolyte imbalances, or due to the involvement of other organs by an underlying systemic disease (Table 13.4).

Fluid overload in the course of acute GN is quite common. Several factors add to this problem: evolving or established oligo-anuria due to functional renal impairment, iatrogenic overinfusion of crystalloids, and activation of the renin–angiotensin–aldosterone system (RAAS) on the glomerular level resulting in sodium and water retention.

As a consequence, patients often become hypertensive, which may even be further exacerbated by ongoing angiotensin II activation or further fluid provision. If hypertension is not well controlled, in any acute GN there is the risk of a hypertensive urgency or emergency potentially leading to end organ damage. Hypertension may also potentiate cardiac failure and, as a consequence, pulmonary edema may necessitate or complicate mechanical ventilation of the patient.

Electrolyte imbalance is another common complication of acute GN with renal dysfunction in the ICU. Hyperkalemia, caused by decreasing renal excretion of potassium and metabolic acidosis leading to a shift of potassium from the intracellular to extracellular space, may lead to cardiac arrhythmias. Hyponatremia from volume overload or decreased free water clearance and hypocalcemia from renal dysfunction or acid–base anomalies may also predispose to clinically relevant complications such as seizures.

In the patient with GN from systemic disease, other organ systems may be affected. Alterations of consciousness or seizures can accompany SLE or vasculitis; lung failure following pulmonary hemorrhage may be seen in Goodpasture's syndrome and in

Table 13.4 Potential complications of acute GN (seen in the pediatric ICU or leading to referral to the ICU)

Clinical characteristic	Complication
Deterioration of renal function	Therapy-refractory hypertension
	Cardiac failure (hypertension, cardiac arrythmia)
	Electrolyte derangements (hyperkalemia, acidosis, hyponatremia, hypocalcemia, hyperphosphatemia)
	Seizures (often mediated by hypertension or electrolyte disturbance)
Complications of underlying disease	Pulmonary hemorrhage (Goodpasture's syndrome, Wegener's granulomatosis)
	Seizures, cerebritis, cerebral edema (SLE, HSP, polyarteritis nodosa)
	Multi-organ function failure (SLE, generalized vasculitis)

Wegener's granulomatosis; multiorgan failure with a sepsis-like appearance is a rare manifestation of SLE.

13.5 Treatment of Acute GN

Treatment of acute GN is tailored along three lines:

1. Symptomatic therapy for fluid or electrolyte issues arising from renal dysfunction
2. Therapy based on treating any underlying disease state
3. Therapy based on addressing specific degrees of disease severity

In general, there are very little evidence-based data available on the treatment of acute GN or RPGN in children or adults, and clinical consensus generally guides management. The lack of such specific data underscores the importance of multicenter intervention studies.

13.5.1 Symptomatic Treatment

13.5.1.1 Mild or No Functional Renal Impairment

Symptomatic treatment depends on the degree of functional renal impairment. In patients with little if any change in baseline GFR, salt and fluid restriction should be considered in view of the activated RAAS. Depending on any evolving pattern, hypertension needs to be treated if it is sustained, and aggressive therapy implemented if there is any risk of hypertensive urgency. Activity level should be guided by the patient's overall clinical status, energy level, and stamina. There is no therapeutic utility to severe restrictions in activity such as bed rest and, in fact, in patients whose acute GN is also complicated by nephrosis, there may be thrombotic complications from prolonged inactivity.

13.5.1.2 Severely Impaired Renal Function, Rapidly Progressive GN

In the intensive care unit setting, oligo-anuria will be the most important therapeutic challenge since critically ill patients often require a large daily fluid volume for necessary medications, nutrition, or to maintain hemodynamic stability. Apart from judicious fluid provision and sodium restriction in the context of a highly activated RAAS, further treatment depends on the specific clinical complications. With oliguria, furosemide or other loop diuretics may be beneficial. In the setting of reduced GFR, doses as high as $2\,mg\,kg^{-1}$ body weight may need to be tried and, if increased urine flow results, repeated doses at regular intervals or diuretic drips may help to blunt volume overload, although there is little utility in maintaining the use of a diuretic if there is no significant response [4]. Continuous infusion and intermittent dosing of furosemide do not appear to have different efficacy [15].

If fluid overload leads to therapy-refractory hypertension, cardiac failure, or respiratory compromise, hemodialysis or hemofiltration are urgently indicated. Until dialysis is initiated, cardiac afterload needs to be reduced since, in the context of the high activity of the RAAS, angiotenin II-induced vasoconstriction adds to the effect of volume overload. Vasodilators such as nifedipine or hydralazine or nitroprusside may be beneficial. In certain ICU settings when fluid removal and solute clearance can proceed more slowly or where there are clinical or anatomic contraindications to hemodialysis, peritoneal dialysis may be considered.

In the case of *hyperkalemia*, the use of furosemide to encourage a kaliuresis would be an initial measure as long as the patient is not anuric. Since hyperkalemia is increased by concomitant acidosis, sodium bicarbonate infusion can be considered (1–2 mmol kg^{-1} i.v. over 15–30 min). A hypokalemic effect from shift of potassium intracellularly should be evident after approximately 15–30 min. The combined use of glucose and insulin may also promote intracellular potassium shift. The dose of glucose is 0.5 g kg^{-1} body weight and insulin 0.1 units kg^{-1} body weight, infused over 30 min with clinical effects in 30–120 min. Inhaled beta agonists such as nebulized albuterol may also cause a potassium shift intracellularly. Provision of the ion exchange resin sodium polysterene sulfonate either orally or rectally at a dose of 1 g kg^{-1} generally leads to a fall in the serum potassium by approximately 1 mEq L^{-1}. Unlike the aforementioned interventions, this maneuver actually removes potassium from the body in stools rather than merely shifting it transiently intracellularly. In case of overt cardiac arrhythmia, the first intervention should be infusion of calcium gluconate (10%) in a dose of 0.5–1 ml kg^{-1} body weight over 5–15 min to stabilize the myocardium [2]. Following calcium infusion, use of other maneuvers as outlined above can help stabilize the patient until dialysis can be initiated emergently.

Hyponatremia is usually a result of fluid overload in acute GN. Fluid restriction or ultrafiltration is usually corrective. If the serum sodium concentration drops below 120 mEq L^{-1} and the child becomes symptomatic, provision of 3% saline is indicated to raise the serum sodium by about 5 mEq L^{-1} over 2–3 h and reduce the risk of seizures. The correction of any chronic hyponatremia has to be performed slowly, often over a period of several days, to avoid the risk of central pontine myelinolysis [2].

13.5.2　Treatment of the Underlying Disease

13.5.2.1　Treatment of Mild GN

Mild forms of acute GN are usually not seen in the intensive care unit or may not be the primary indication for ICU admission. Frequent causes of a mild GN include an uncomplicated post-infectious GN or HSP associated GN. After the diagnosis is made on a combination of history, clinical findings, and laboratory assessment, treatment of the underlying renal disease is usually not necessary. The situation changes if progressive renal deterioration raises the spectre of RPGN or if the acute GN becomes chronic as indicated by persisting heavy proteinuria and hematuria (Fig. 13.1).

13.5.2.2　Treatment of Rapidly Progressive GN (Table 13.5)

With suspected RPGN, renal biopsy is indicated and treatment should commence as early as possible. A delay in treatment, or a treatment not aggressive enough, may adversely affect the chance of optimal renal recovery.

In fact, in the approximately 160 children and adolescents reported in the four studies of RPGN previously described [13,19,24,25], each series found an incidence of approximately 50% end-stage renal failure, with chronic renal impairment seen in 25%, and normal renal function regained in only 25%. In general, an RPGN with the need for dialysis support, and acutely and widespread crescentic lesions in the renal biopsy, points towards a guarded prognosis.

Because of the high risk of end-stage renal failure with RPGN, aggressive therapy is recommended [14]. Data on specific immunosuppressive therapy for RPGN in children is very scarce. In the light of poor prognosis, however, aggressive immunosuppressive therapy should be considered.

Initial treatment options and common adverse effects of therapy are shown in Table 13.5. Treatments frequently used are some combination of plasma exchange, cyclophosphamide, and methylprednisolone pulse therapy.

One disease with relative agreement on the mode of treatment is Goodpasture's syndrome or anti-GBM disease with pulmonary hemorrhage [16]. Therapy usually consists of therapeutic plasma exchange, steroids, and cyclophosphamide. Similar treatment strategies are advocated for ANCA mediated nephritides with a pauci-immune GN [27]. In SLE with significant renal disease and clinical compromise, high dose methylprednisolone pulses followed by intravenous cyclophosphamide and oral prednisone are indicated [18]. In some children with SLE refractory to this approach, the CD-20-antibody rituximab has been used with success [2]. In polyarteritis nodosa mediated RPGN, apart from therapeutic plasma exchange, corticosteroids and cyclophosphamide, a TNF-antagonist has recently been used with some efficacy [11].

There is still considerable argument on how aggressively cases of severe HSP nephritis or IgA-nephropathy, with a large number of cellular crescents on biopsy, should be treated. With concern regarding poor prognosis in a large number of patients with such crescentic disease, some advocate aggressive therapy including pulse steroids and cylophosphamide, but others do not embrace an aggressive therapy [10].

Table 13.5 Therapy in RPGN in childhood and common adverse effects [modified from [26]]

Induction therapy[a]	Methylprednisolone (3–4 pulses given daily or alternate days for total dose 900–1,800 mg m^{-2})	Hypertension, glucose intolerance, osteoporosis
	Cyclophosphamide (oral: 2–3-mg kg^{-1} d^{-1} over 3 months; IV: 6 pulses of 500–1,000 mg m^{-2} every 4 weeks)	Hemorrhagic cystitis, infertility, leukopenia, anemia, thrombocytopenia
	Plasma exchange (up to ten exchanges in 3 weeks)	Adverse effects of extracorporeal circuit (hemorrhage, hypotension, thrombocytopenia, hypocalcemia), allergic reaction, infection, immunosuppression
Maintenance therapy	Prednisone, starting at 2 mg kg^{-1} d^{-1} with slow tapering dose over months	Cushingnoid habitus, cataracts, osteoporosis, hypertension
	Mycophenolate mofetil, 1.2 g m^{-2} d^{-1} divided into two or three daily doses	Leukopenia, anemia, diarrhea, teratogenic
	Azathioprine, 2 mg kg^{-1} d^{-1}	Leukopenia, anemia, hepatitis
	Rarely used: Cyclosporine A, Methotrexate	
Rescue therapy	Humanized monoclonal antibodies such as rituximab (anti-CD20) or infliximab (anti TNF)	Not fully known, allergic reactions

[a] All immunosuppressant drugs have the potential of leading to more severe infections and a potentially increased risk of malignancy

In contradistinction to diseases treated with aggressive immunomodulation, in post-infectious GN with initial renal functional compromise immunosuppressive treatment is usually not advocated since no advantage to such therapy has been found [22,23].

13.6 Conclusions

Acute GN necessitating pediatric ICU care is a rare entity that intensivists will most likely encounter in the form of an RPGN requiring urgent dialysis. Prognosis of an acute GN varies according to etiology and depends on whether an element of rapidly progressive dysfunction exists. Because a delay in treatment may affect eventual renal outcome adversely, diagnosis should be made as soon as possible, including renal biopsy when necessary. In most cases of RPGN with concern for irreversible renal damage, a multi-agent immunosuppressive regimen is instituted, despite the lack of evidence-based data in children and adolescents supporting this approach.

References

1. Akikusa JD, Schneider R, Harvey EA, Hebert D, Thorner PS, Laxer RM, Silverman ED (2007) Clinical features and outcome of pediatric Wegener's granulomatosis. Arthritis Rheum 25;57:837–844

2. Andreoli SP (1999) Management of acute renal failure. In: Barratt TM, Avner ED, Harmon WE (eds) Pediatric Nephrology. Baltimore: Lippincott Williams & Wilkins

3. Benz K, Amann K, Dittrich K, Hugo C, Schnur K, Dötsch J (2007) Patient with antibody-negative relapse of Goodpasture syndrome. Clin Nephrol 67:240–244

4. Brater DC (1998) Diuretic therapy. N Engl J Med 339:387–395

5. Cameron JS (1994) Lupus nephritis in childhood and adolescence. Pediatr Nephrol 8:230–249

6. Churg J, Bernstein J, Glassock RJ (1995) Renal disease: Classification and atlas of glomerular diseases. Igaku-Shoin, New York, Tokyo

7. Cunningham RJ, Gilfoil M, Cavallo T, et al (1980) Rapidly progressive GN in children: a report of thirteen cases and a review of the literature. Pediatr Res 14:128–132

8. D'Amico G (1987) The commonest GN in the world: IgA nephropathy. QJ Med 245:709–727

9. Dillon MJ (2005) Crescentic GN. In: Avener ED, Harmon WE, Niaudet P (eds) Pediatric Nephrology. Baltimore: Lippincott Williams & Wilkins

10. Dittrich K (2007) Cyclophosphamide pulse-therapy in children and adolescents with severe IgA-nephropathy (review)

11. Feinstein J, Arroyo R (2005) Successful treatment of childhood onset refractory polyarteritis nodosa with tumor necrosis factor alpha blockade. J Clin Rheumatol 11:219–222

12. Guillevin L (1999) Treatment of classic polyarteritis nodosa in 1999. Nephrol Dial Transplant 14:2077–2079

13. Jardim HMPF, Leake J, Risdon RA, et al (1992) Crescentic GN in children. Pediatr Nephrol 6:231–235

14. Jindal KK (1999) Management of idiopathic crescentic and diffuse proliferative GN: evidence-based recommendations. Kidney Int 70 (Suppl):33–40

15. Klinge J (2001) Intermittent administration of furosemide or continuous infusion in critically ill infants and children: does it make a difference? Intensive Care Med 27:623–624

16. Levy JB, Turner AN, Rees AJ, Pusey CD (2001) Long-term outcome of anti-glomerular basement membrane antibody disease treated with plasma exchange and immunosuppression. Ann Intern Med 5;134:1033–1042

17. Miller MN, Baumal R, Poucell S, et al (1984) Incidence and prognostic importance of glomeruloar crescents in renal disease of childhood. Am J Nephrol 4:244–247

18. Niaudet P, Levy M (1983) Glomerulonéphritis à croissants diffuse. In: Royer P, Habib R, Mathieu H, Broyer M (eds). Néphrologie Pédiatrique, 3rd ed. Paris: Flammarion, pp 381–394

19. Niaudet P (2000) Treatment of lupus nephritis in children. Pediatr Nephrol 14:158–166

20. Rees AJ, Cameron JS (1998) Crescentic GN. In: Davison AM, Cameron JS, Grünfeld J-P, et al (eds) Oxford Textbook of Clinical Nephrology, 2nd ed. Oxford, UK: Oxford University Press, pp 625–646

21. Robson AM, Rose GM, Cole BR, et al (1981) The treatment of severe glomerulopathies in children with methyl prednisolone pulses. Proceedings of Eighth International Congress of Nephrology, Athens. Basel: Karger, pp 305–311

22. Roy S, Morphy WM, Arant BS (1981) Poststreptococcal crescentic glomerulonepehritis in children: comparison of quintuple therapy versus supportive care. J Pediatr 98:403–410

23. Sulyok E (2005) Acute proliferative GN. In: Avener ED, Harmon WE, Niaudet P (eds) Pediatric Nephrology. Lippincott Williams & Wilkins, Baltimore

24. SPNSG (Southwest Pediatric Nephrology Study Group) (1985) A clinico-pathological study of crescentic GN in 50 children. Kidney Int 27:450–458

25. Srivastava RN, Moudgil A, Bagga A, et al (1992) Crescentic GN in children: a review of 43 cases. Am J Nephrol 12:155–161

26. Willems M, Haddad E, Niaudet P, Kone-Paut I, Bensman A, Cochat P, Deschenes G, Fakhouri F, Leblanc T, Llanas B, Loirat C, Pillet P, Ranchin B, Salomon R, Ulinski T, Bader-Meunier B (2006) French Pediatric-Onset SLE Study Group. Rituximab therapy for childhood-onset systemic lupus erythematodus. J Pediatr 148:623–627

27. Wright E, Dillon MJ, Tullus K (2007) Childhood vasculitis and plasma exchange. Eur J Pediatr 166:145–151

28. Wyatt RJ, Hogg RJ (2001) Evidence-based assessment of treatment options for children with IgA nephropathies. Pediatr Nephrol 16:156–167

Acute Interstitial Nephritis

14

V.R. Dharnidharka, C.E. Araya, and D.D. Henry

Contents

Case Vignette

A previously healthy 12-year-old girl was admitted to hospital for treatment with intravenous oxacillin for a progressive cellulitis on the left leg. On the third day of treatment, though the cellulitis had shown some improvement, she developed fatigue, some joint pain, and a morbiliform generalized skin rash. Urine output and blood pressure remained normal, but laboratory tests showed microscopic hematuria and an elevated serum creatinine of $2.1\,\text{mg dL}^{-1}$ in the context of otherwise normal urinalysis, blood chemistry panel, and blood counts.

S.G. Kiessling et al. (eds) *Pediatric Nephrology in the ICU.*
© Springer-Verlag Berlin Heidelberg 2009

> **Core Messages**
>
> ❭ Acute interstitial nephritis (AIN) is a term usually reserved for an allergic inflammation of the kidney, with characteristic eosinophilic infiltrates in the renal interstitium.
> ❭ AIN should be suspected in all cases of unexplained renal failure in the intensive care setting, where the incidence of this condition is much higher than in other settings.
> ❭ Common causes include drug-induced, certain infections or autoimmune processes. Withdrawal of the offending agent, if possible, and supportive therapy are the mainstays of management.

14.1 Definition

AIN, unlike many other medical conditions, is aptly named and the term accurately describes the cardinal features: an acute inflammatory process affecting the tubule and interstitial segments of the nephron/kidney. Though the etiology of the inflammation is not explicitly stated in the term AIN, this term is typically limited to immune-mediated hypersensitivity or allergic reactions. AIN in its purest sense could also be a component of acute bacterial pyelonephritis or acute transplant rejection. However, in these cases, the predominant immune cell infiltrating the kidney is either the neutrophil or lymphocyte. In allergic AIN, the predominant immune cell seen in the interstitium is the eosinophil, one of the pathologic hallmarks of allergic injury.

14.2 Incidence and Epidemiology

AIN was first described as far back as 1898 by Councilman in an autopsy series of patients who died from scarlet fever or diphtheria [7]. The kidneys of these patients had sterile interstitial exudates and he coined the term AIN. In some texts, the longer term ATIN or acute tubulointerstitial nephritis is used and is analogous to AIN.

AIN is quite rare in the general population, even among the spectrum of kidney diseases. In Finnish army recruits who had hematuria or proteinuria, the incidence of AIN was only 2 cases among 171 biopsies, or 1.1% [24]. In pediatric patients, the reports of AIN are limited to small case series [22, 23] or case reports [10, 25, 31], so the exact incidence in the general population is not known. The incidence is presumed to be similar to that in young adults.

However, the incidence of AIN rises dramatically when considering only those patients with acute renal failure, as would be the case in an intensive care setting. In such situations, the incidence of AIN on kidney biopsy ranges between 15 and 27% in adults [9, 19] and 7% in children [12].

Several excellent reviews, both recent and prior, discuss AIN in adults [2, 16, 19] and in children [1, 13] in detail.

14.3   What Are the Causes of AIN?

The etiologies of AIN can be multiple and fall into three broad categories. Drug-induced associations, as listed in Table 14.1, are the most common and are thought to be due to allergic reactions to components or antigens within the drug. Infections form the next most common group, but the proportion of AIN cases that are attributable to infections has been on the decline due to widespread antibiotic use. This drop in incidence represents a somewhat paradoxical situation since antibiotics are among the chief culprits among drug-induced AIN cases. TINU syndrome (tubulointerstitial nephritis with uveitis) is a condition of AIN with ocular involvement (see later). Autoimmune diseases such as SLE, Sjogren's syndrome, or cryoglobulinemia can involve the kidney as AIN. TINU syndrome may also be autoimmune in etiology. The classification of etiologies is not mutually exclusive, as all three groups share a common autoimmune mechanism of injury to the kidney. The antigens may be intrarenal (such as basement membrane proteins or Tamm–Horsfall protein) or extrarenal (such as immune complexes) in origin [28, 29].

Michel and Kelly have provided an elegant diagrammatic representation of the immune mechanisms involved in AIN, adapted in Fig. 14.1 [19]. While cell-mediated immunity seems to play a major role, antibody-mediated injury may also occur. Antigen-specific activation leads to several downstream mechanisms also being activated.

14.3.1   TINU Syndrome

Dobrin et al. first described TINU in 1975 [7, 24]. Since its discovery no specific risk factors for TINU have been identified but mycoplasma or chlamydia infection may be implicated. TINU occurs more commonly in children and adolescent females but has been described in all age groups and ethnicity [7, 24]. There is a 2:1 female to male predominance of this syndrome. It can develop prior to, in conjunction with, or after AIN has been identified [9]. Clinical manifestations include the features of AIN plus the ocular symptoms of red eye, eye pain, or photophobia [7]. Examination reveals a uveitis that can be unilateral or bilateral and can be anterior or posterior [24]. Uveitis is also associated with polyarteritis nodosum, Behcet's syndrome, systemic lupus nephritis, Wegener's granulomatosis, and Sjogren's syndrome as well as multiple infectious etiologies. TINU-associated AIN may take longer to resolve than other etiologies of AIN [15].

14.3.2   Infection

Numerous infections have been associated with AIN, ranging from direct parenchymal involvement (i.e., acute pyelonephritis) to immunologically mediated AIN. These infections include but are not limited to staphylococci, streptococci, legionella, cytomegalovirus, Epstein–Barr virus, and human immunodeficency virus [7, 9] as well as salmonella [19] and strongyloides [12]. In kidney transplants, infections that are associated with predominant interstitial inflammation include polyoma virus [22] and adenovirus infection [23].

14.3.3   Systemic Disorders

Several local and systemic disorders have been implicated as the underlying cause of AIN. These include, but are not limited to, sarcoidosis, systemic

Table 14.1   Medications associated with acute interstitial nephritis

Antibiotics	Levofloxacin	Foscarnet	Piroxicam	Anticonvulsants	Famotidine
Ampicillin	Lincomycin	Indinavir	Pirprofen	Carbamazepine	Fenofibrate
Amoxacillin	Methicillin	Interferon	Rofecoxib	Diazepam	Gold salts
Aztreonam	Mezclocillin	NSAIDs	Sulfasalazine	Phenobarbital	Griseofulvin
Carbenicillin	Minocycline	Alclofenac	Sulindac	Phenytoin	Interleukin-2
Cefaclor	Moxifloxacin	Azapropazone	Suprofen	Valproate sodium	Lamotrigine
Cefamandole	Nafcillin	Aspirin	Tolemetin	Others	Lanzoprazole
Cefazolin	Nitrofurantoin	Benoxaprofen	Zomepirac	Allopurinol	Nicergoline
Cefixitin	Norfloxacin	Celecoxib	Analgesics	Alpha-methyldopa	Omeprazole
Cefotaxime	Oxacillin	Diclofenac	Aminopyrine	Amlodipine	Pantoprazole
Cefotetan	Penicillin	Diflunisal	Antipyrine	Azathioprine	Phenindione
Cephalexin	Piperacillin	Fenbufen	Antrafenine	Bethanidine	Phenothiazine
Cephaloridine	Piromidic acid	Fenclofenac	Clometacin	Bismuth salts	Phentermine
Cephalotin	Polymyxin acid	Fenoprofen	Floctafenin	Captopril	Phenylpropa-nolamine
Cephapirin	Quinine	Flubiprofen	Glafenine	Carbimazole	Probenecid
Cephradine	Rifampin	Ibuprofen	Metamizol	Chlorpro-pamide	Propranolol
Ciprofloxacin	Spiramycine	Indomethacin	Noramido-pyrine	Cyclosporine	Propylthiouracil
Cloxacillin	Sulfonamides	Ketoprofen	Diuretics	Cimetidine	Rabeprazole
Colistin	Teicoplanin	Mefenamic acid	Chlorthalidone	Clofibrate	Ranitidine
Erythromycin	Tetracycline	Meloxicam	Ethacrynic acid	Clozapine	Streptokinase
Ethambutol	TMP/SMX	Mesalazine	Furosemide	Cyamethazine	Sulphinpyrazone
Flurithromycin	Vancomycin	Naproxen	Hydrochloro-thiazide	Cytosine	Warfarin
Gentamicin	Antivirals	Niflumic acid	Indapamide	D-penicillamine	Zopiclone
Isoniazid	Acyclovir	Phenazone	Tienilic acid	Diltiazem	
Latamoxef	Atanavir	Phenylbu-tazone	Triamterene	Esomeprazole	

Compiled from several sources

lupus erythematosus, Sjogren's synderme, Wegener's granulomatosus, and malignancy. Sarcoidosis is associated with a granulomatous AIN but hypercalcemia and hypercalciuria remain the underlying cause of renal dysfunction [10, 25, 31]. In autoimmune disorders the interstitial nephritis is usually chronic and renal function is representative of the degree of the underlying glomerulopathy [10].

14.4   What Are the Clinical Features and Presentations?

The typical presentation of AIN was primarily described in the context of methicillin-induced AIN. It consisted of an abrupt onset of renal dysfunction in the presence of fever, skin rash, arthralgias, and

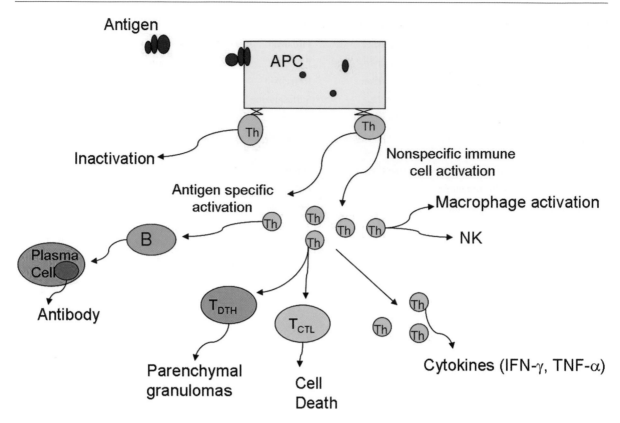

Fig. 14.1 Diagram of mechanisms underlying immune injury in acute interstitial nephritis (AIN). *APC* antigen presenting cell, *Th* T helper cell, T_{CTL} cytotoxic T lymphocyte, T_{DTH} delayed type hypersensitivity T cell, *NK* natural killer cell (adapted from [19])

eosinophilia/eosinophiluria. However, many other factors have been implicated as a cause of AIN and it is now recognized that the clinical characteristics of this condition are much more diverse. With a change in etiologies away from penicillins to other drugs, the classic triad of fever, rash, and arthralgias is now seen in only about 10% of cases [2]. Hence, AIN should be considered in any patient with unexplained acute renal failure even if there is no concomitant fever, skin rash, or eosinophilia/eosinophiluria [19]. Confirmation of the diagnosis can be challenging in hospitalized patients who develop a progressive deterioration of renal function of unclear etiology, especially in the intensive care setting, if the patient is receiving multiple medications, is septic, and is hemodynamically unstable.

The onset of AIN can be variable. It may occur rapidly, within 1 day of initiating treatment, or may develop after taking a medication for months to years. However, in drug-associated AIN most patients develop symptoms within 3 weeks of starting the causative drug. The main presenting symptom is olig-

uria, occurring in about half of the patients [5]. Other nonspecific symptoms including anorexia, nausea, vomiting, and abdominal pain may be present. Flank pain may occur as a result of renal capsular distention. The degree of renal involvement is unpredictable and can range from mild azotemia to oliguric renal failure requiring dialysis. Proteinuria is typically mild (less than 1 g day^{-1}). However, severe proteinuria and nephrotic syndrome have been reported particularly in NSAID-associated AIN, but has also been observed with the antibiotics rifampin, ampicillin, and amoxicillin [6, 8, 21, 27, 32]. In this condition, extrarenal manifestations such as fever or rash and eosinophilia/eosinophiluria are usually absent, but hypertension is more common.

Renal tubular injury is the hallmark of AIN, and dysfunction of specific nephron segments may reveal characteristic clinical and biochemical abnormalities [34]. Proximal tubular damage may lead to Fanconi syndrome. Lesions involving the loop of Henle can result in sodium and water wasting with associated polyuria and polydipsia. Distal tubular lesions may lead to renal tubular acidosis, whereas nephrogenic diabetes insipidus due to impaired water reabsorption is seen with injuries to the collecting tubules.

14.5   What Is the Pathological Picture?

On histologic examination, the characteristic abnormalities in AIN are the presence of edema and inflammatory cell infiltrates within the interstitium, as shown in Fig. 14.2 [19]. The inflammatory lesions are typically located deep in the cortex at the level of the corticomedullary junction, but can be diffuse in the most severe cases. These infiltrates principally comprise T lymphocytes and monocytes. Variable numbers of eosinophils, plasma cells, neutrophils, and basophils may also be observed. Eosinophils are more commonly noted in drug-induced AIN. However, in some cases, eosinophils have been absent from these inflammatory lesions.

Infiltrating lymphocytes in the peritubular region or across the tubular basement membrane (TBM) may also be observed. This resulting tubulitis may be difficult to distinguish from acute tubular necrosis. Tubular epithelial cell damage is variable, and necrosis can be observed in the more severe cases. The renal tubules are dilated and the lumens may contain desquamated cells.

Granulomatous inflammation of the tubulointerstitium is rare, occurring in 0.5–5.9% of AIN cases [3, 20]. Interstitial granuloma formation may be seen in drug-induced AIN, related to infections, sarcoidosis, Sjogren's syndrome, and Wegener's granulomatosis. These granulomas are nonnecrotic and contain epithelioid macrophages and multinucleated giant cells.

Classically, in AIN the glomeruli and blood vessels are uninvolved. However, there have been reports, most commonly in NSAID-associated AIN, describing a combination of AIN with lesions similar to minimal change disease [6]. Glomeruli appear to be normal by light microscopy, with foot process fusion observed by electron microscopy.

Immunofluorescence and electron microscopy findings of the kidney in AIN are typically negative. However, granular deposition of IgG, C3, and C1q along the TBM and Bowman's capsular basement membrane with electron-dense deposits within the TBM has been observed [33]. Intense and diffuse linear IgG staining along the TBM are encountered when antibodies are directed against membrane antigens (such as in anti-TBM disease). Antigens may be lodged into the interstitium from the circulation and may comprise infectious agents and drug metabolites bound to the membrane [18].

Currently, the majority of patients with AIN are not subjected to a renal biopsy and the decision to perform the procedure is not always straightforward. However, a percutaneous renal biopsy should be considered in patients in whom the diagnosis is unclear, patients who fail to improve after discontinuation of the possible precipitating drug, or when immunosuppressive therapy is considered.

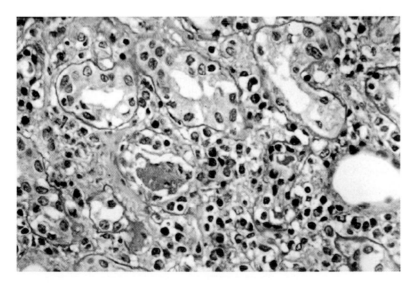

Fig. 14.2   Acute tubulointerstitial nephritis. Interstitial mononuclear cells with focal infiltration of tubular epithelium (PAS stain) (courtesy of Dr. William Clapp, University of Florida)

14.6 How Does One Make the Diagnosis?

There is no single clinical or laboratory test to diagnose AIN. Therefore, renal biopsy remains the gold standard. AIN should be suspected in patients with classic features or unexplained renal failure [16, 19, 29]. The different laboratory test results discussed later are summarized in Table 14.2.

The urinary findings in AIN vary depending on the etiology. Microscopic or gross hematuria, sterile pyuria, and white blood cell casts are common. However, red blood cell casts are usually not seen [16, 19, 29]. The degree of proteinuria will vary with AIN but is typically less than 1 g per 24 h unless the glomerulus is involved [16, 19, 29]. This is not true for nonsteroidal anti-inflammatory drugs (NSAID)-induced AIN, which can be associated with nephrotic range proteinuria and hypersensitivity symptoms. Urine eosinophilia (>1% of white blood cells being eosinophils) will reinforce the diagnosis of AIN but has been shown to have a low sensitivity of 40–67%, low positive predictive value of 50%, and moderate specificity of 72% [30]. Eosinophils are best identified with Wright's or Hanzel's stain with the latter being more sensitive. Eosinophiluria is also seen in cystitis, prostatitis, pyelonephritis, and rapidly progressive glomerulonephritis.

Other biochemical findings such as anemia, electrolyte abnormalities associated with Fanconi's syndrome, or other tubular dysfunctions and elevated hepatic function test will vary depending on the underlying etiology, acuteness of the disease, and extent of the renal insufficiency.

14.7 What Is the Differential Diagnosis?

1. Urinary obstruction
2. Vasomotor renal insufficiency
3. Acute tubular necrosis
4. Drug-induced nephropathy
5. Other causes of glomerulopathy
6. Immune-mediated systemic diseases with renal involvement
7. Vasculitis
8. Malignancy

14.8 What Are Current Treatment Concepts?

The mainstay of therapy is still supportive care, particularly for the comorbid conditions associated with acute renal failure. Fever and rash, if present,

Table 14.2 Laboratory test findings in AIN

Laboratory Evaluation	Findings	Application
Urinalysis	Proteinuria	Variable degrees <1 g per 24 h except if associated with NSAIDs
	Sterile pyuria	Leukocyte and leukocyte casts
	Hematuria	RBCs without casts
	Eosinophiluria >1% total white cells	Sensitivity low, specificity moderate, PPV low
	Fractional excretion of sodium	Usually greater than 2%
CBC	Eosinophilia	Variable
	Anemia	Variable
Serum chemistries	Elevated BUN	Varies depending on renal function
	Elevated creatinine	Varies depending on renal function
	Hyper/hypokalemia	Variable based on severity of renal function
	Hyperchloremic metabolic acidosis	Degree of tubulointerstitial injury
Liver function test	Elevated transaminases	Associated with drug-induced liver injury
Miscellaneous	Elevated IgE levels serum	
	ANA, C3, C4, ASO	
Renal biopsy	Gold standard	See pathology section

can be treated symptomatically. Once the diagnosis is suspected or proven by biopsy, if an offending drug agent can be identified, removal of that drug, if possible, is the first intervention. In many situations, there may be several possible offending drugs and those drugs are potentially life-saving for the patient, hence removal may be difficult to actually implement in practice.

Acute renal failure is treated as one would otherwise treat, and is discussed in detail in Chap. 6. The principles of acute renal failure therapy include (1) monitoring for acidosis and hyperkalemia, (2) withdrawing sources of potassium if hyperkalemia is present, (3) using alkaline agents if acidosis is present, (4) using phosphate binders if hyperphosphatemia is present, and (5) monitoring fluid status. Drug dosing should be adjusted for existing level of renal function. Dialysis may be indicated if any of the earlier complications are refractory to other forms of therapy.

The use of pharmacologic therapy to reverse AIN is controversial, both in terms of whether necessary and in timing, since spontaneous recovery is common. Drugs that have been tried to reverse AIN include corticosteroids, cyclophosphamide, and cyclosporine A. The data supporting corticosteroid use originate from small uncontrolled comparison series of less than 30 patients each. In the methicillin era, use of intravenous methyl-prednisolone or oral prednisone led to shorter recovery times, lower serum creatinine values at follow-up, and a higher percentage of complete recovery of serum creatinine value [11, 26]. In these series, corticosteroids were initiated after conservative measures had failed to demonstrate improvement in the first 2 weeks [4, 17]. In contrast, Clarkson et al. performed a relatively larger retrospective single center review of 60 AIN cases over a 12-year period in a relatively modern time period 1988–2001 [5]. Sixty percent of these cases received corticosteroids. The serum creatinine values were not significantly different between the steroid and nonsteroid groups at 1, 6, or 12 months postpresentation. Whether corticosteroids should be started right away is unknown. There are no prospective randomized trials conducted to determine if corticosteroid use would improve outcomes. Successful use of cyclophosphamide or cyclosporine A is documented in even smaller numbers.

The use of pharmacological therapy for AIN, at this time, is recommended for biopsy-proven AIN that is severe, i.e., rapidly rising serum creatinine or diffuse inflammatory involvement on biopsy without significant fibrosis [19].

14.9 What Are the Outcomes?

In most series, the majority of cases make a full recovery, though the incidence of full recovery seems to be diminishing in the modern era, reflecting a different etiology in modern times [26]. Recovery usually takes several weeks. Poor prognostic factors include extent of fibrosis, diffuse nature of inflammation, and >1–6% of neutrophils [14].

Take-Home Pearls

› While the classic presentation of AIN includes fever, skin rash, arthralgias, and eosinophilia/eosinophiluria, this presentation is now seen in less than 10% of cases.
› AIN is a significant cause of unexplained renal failure in the PICU, and thus it should be suspected in such situations.
› Supportive therapy remains the mainstay of management. Corticosteroid therapy is controversial.

References

1. Alon US (2004) Tubulointerstitial nephritis. In: Avner ED, Harmon WE, Niaudet P (eds) Pediatric Nephrology, 5th edn. Lippincott Williams and Wilkins, Philadelphia, PA, pp. 817–34
2. Baker RJ, Pusey CD (2004) The changing profile of acute tubulointerstitial nephritis. Nephrol Dial Transplant 19(1):8 11
3. Bijol V, Mendez GP, Nose V, et al. (2006) Granulomatous interstitial nephritis: a clinicopathologic study of 46 cases from a single institution. Int J Surg Pathol 14(1):57–63
4. Buysen JG, Houthoff HJ, Krediet RT, et al. (1990) Acute interstitial nephritis: a clinical and morphological study in 27 patients. Nephrol Dial Transplant 5(2):94–9
5. Clarkson MR, Giblin L, O'Connell FP, et al. (2004) Acute interstitial nephritis: clinical features and response to corticosteroid therapy. Nephrol Dial Transplant 19(11):2778–83
6. Clive DM, Stoff JS (1984) Renal syndromes associated with nonsteroidal antiinflammatory drugs. N Engl J Med 310(9):563–72
7. Councilman WT (1898) Acute interstitial nephritis. J Exp Med 3:393–422
8. Dharnidharka VR, Rosen S, Somers MJ (1998) Acute interstitial nephritis presenting as presumed minimal change nephrotic syndrome. Pediatr Nephrol 12(7):576–8
9. Farrington K, Levison DA, Greenwood RN, et al. (1989) Renal biopsy in patients with unexplained renal impairment and normal kidney size. Q J Med 70(263):221–33
10. Funaki S, Takahashi S, Murakami H, et al. (2006) Cockayne syndrome with recurrent acute tubulointerstitial nephritis. Pathol Int 56(11):678–82

11. Galpin JE, Shinaberger JH, Stanley TM, et al. (1978) Acute interstitial nephritis due to methicillin. Am J Med 65(5):756–65
12. Greising J, Trachtman H, Gauthier B, et al. (1990) Acute interstitial nephritis in adolescents and young adults. Child Nephrol Urol 10(4):189–95
13. Kapur G, Mattoo TK (2007) Tubulointerstitial nephritis. In: Kher KK, Schnaper HW, Makker SP (eds) Clinical Pediatric Nephrology, 2nd edn. InformaHealthCare, Oxon, pp. 223–34
14. Kida H, Abe T, Tomosugi N, et al. (1984) Prediction of the long-term outcome in acute interstitial nephritis. Clin Nephrol 22(2):55–60
15. Kobayashi Y, Honda M, Yoshikawa N, et al. (2000) Acute tubulointerstitial nephritis in 21 Japanese children. Clin Nephrol 54(3):191–7
16. Kodner CM, Kudrimoti A (2003) Diagnosis and management of acute interstitial nephritis. Am Fam Physician 67(12):2527–34
17. Laberke HG (1980) Treatment of acute interstitial nephritis. Klin Wochenschr 58(10):531–2
18. Markowitz GS, Seigle RL, D'Agati VD (1999) Three-year-old boy with partial Fanconi syndrome. Am J Kidney Dis 34(1):184–8
19. Michel DM, Kelly CJ (1998) Acute interstitial nephritis. J Am Soc Nephrol 9(3):506–15
20. Nasr SH, Koscica J, Markowitz GS, et al. (2003) Granulomatous interstitial nephritis. Am J Kidney Dis 41(3):714–19
21. Neugarten J, Gallo GR, Baldwin DS (1983) Rifampin-induced nephrotic syndrome and acute interstitial nephritis. Am J Nephrol 3(1):38–42
22. Nikolic V, Bogdanovic R, Ognjanovic M, et al. (2001) Acute tubulointerstitial nephritis in children. Srp Arh Celok Lek 129 Suppl 1:23–7
23. Papachristou F, Printza N, Farmaki E, et al. (2006) Antibiotics-induced acute interstitial nephritis in 6 children. Urol Int 76(4):348–52
24. Pettersson E, von Bonsdorff M, Tornroth T, et al. (1984) Nephritis among young Finnish men. Clin Nephrol 22(5):217–22
25. Premalatha R, Phadke KD, Gag I, et al. (2003) Acute renal failure due to acute tubulointerstitial nephritis. Indian Pediatr 40(4):352–5
26. Pusey CD, Saltissi D, Bloodworth L, et al. (1983) Drug associated acute interstitial nephritis: clinical and pathological features and the response to high dose steroid therapy. Q J Med 52(206):194–211
27. Rennke HG, Roos PC, Wall SG (1980) Drug-induced interstitial nephritis with heavy glomerular proteinuria. N Engl J Med 302(12):691–2
28. Rossert J (2001) Drug-induced acute interstitial nephritis. Kidney Int 60(2):804–17
29. Rossert J, Fischer EA (2007) Acute interstitial nephritis. In: Feehally J, Floege J, Johnson RJ (eds) Comprehensive Clinical Nephrology, 3rd edn. Mosby Elsevier, Philadelphia, PA, pp. 681–90
30. Ruffing KA, Hoppes P, Blend D, et al. (1994) Eosinophils in urine revisited. Clin Nephrol 41(3):163–6
31. Sharma A, Wanchu A, Mahesha V, et al. (2006) Acute tubulo-interstitial nephritis leading to acute renal failure following multiple hornet stings. BMC Nephrol 7:18
32. Takahashi S, Kitamura T, Murakami H (2005) Acute interstitial nephritis predisposed a six-year-old girl to minimal change nephrotic syndrome. Pediatr Nephrol 20(8): 1168–70
33. Tokumoto M, Fukuda K, Shinozaki M, et al. (1999) Acute interstitial nephritis with immune complex deposition and MHC class II antigen presentation along the tubular basement membrane. Nephrol Dial Transplant 14(9):2210–15
34. Toto RD (1990) Acute tubulointerstitial nephritis. Am J Med Sci 299(6):392–410

15

The Tumor Lysis Syndrome: An Oncologic and Metabolic Emergency

J. D'Orazio

Contents

Core Messages

> The tumor lysis syndrome (TLS) is a set of metabolic abnormalities caused by widespread tumor cell death and a physiologic inability to maintain adequate clearance rates of tumor metabolites.

> The cardinal metabolic features of TLS are hyperuricemia, hyperphosphatemia (with secondary hypocalcemia), and hyperkalemia.

> TLS-induced renal failure is caused by obstructive uric acid and/or calcium phosphate uropathy and can rapidly promote worsening of TLS by further reducing clearance of TLS metabolites.

> TLS is a life-threatening condition that requires a high level of suspicion, close clinical monitoring, timely therapeutic interventions, and potential involvement of a variety of subspecialty services.

> Early transfer to the Pediatric Intensive Care Unit to allow close monitoring of the fluid and electrolyte status should be considered in children at high risk for TLS.

Case Vignette

A 12-year-old girl presented to her pediatrician with a 2-day history of abdominal pain associated with a rapidly enlarging right upper quadrant mass. Radiologic imaging revealed a large tumor in the portal hepatic region as well as multiple lesions seen throughout both

S.G. Kiessling et al. (eds) *Pediatric Nephrology in the ICU*.
© Springer-Verlag Berlin Heidelberg 2009

kidneys (see Fig. 15.3). Laboratory studies were relevant for elevated serum uric acid (7.3 mg dL^{-1}), LDH (433 U L^{-1}), serum creatinine (1.4 mg dL^{-1}), and serum phosphorus (5.7 mg dL^{-1}). The patient was admitted to the hospital, placed on cardiovascular monitoring, and was aggressively hydrated. Mature B cell (Burkitt's) lymphoma was identified on biopsy. Because of evidence of spontaneous TLS (metabolic derangements even before administration of chemotherapy) as well as extensive renal infiltration by disease, the patient was treated with urate oxidase (rasburicase) along with aggressive hydration before and during the initial days of chemotherapy. Her serum uric acid dropped to <0.5 mg dL^{-1} promptly after rasburicase administration, her serum creatinine slowly returned to normal over the next several days, and her urine output remained brisk. In this vignette, this patient presented with a variety of risk factors predictive of severe TLS (see Table 15.2), including a highly proliferative chemosensitive tumor, bulk disease, anatomic involvement of both kidneys, and baseline elevations of serum LDH, uric acid, and creatinine. Fortunately, this patient maintained adequate renal output throughout the first days of chemotherapy, enjoyed a rapid response to chemotherapy, and had a fine clinical outcome.

15.1 Introduction

It has long been known that patients newly diagnosed with certain types of tumors often have metabolic disturbances that accompany their presentation and that peak during the first few days after the start of chemo- or radiotherapy [28]. The TLS is characterized by the classic pentad of hyperuricemia, hyperkalemia, hyperphosphatemia, hypocalcemia, and renal failure [9]. The diagnosis of TLS in a newly diagnosed oncology patient represents a true medical emergency that if not properly managed can rapidly deteriorate to death. In fact, the severe metabolic disturbances of TLS may represent the most life-threatening aspect of cancer in the first hours-to-days after diagnosis [24, 28]. Appropriate management of TLS requires a high level of suspicion, diagnostic acumen, timely initiation of effective therapeutic measures, and scrupulous attention to clinical condition, electrolyte status, fluid balance, and pharmacologic responses. Importantly, proper management of TLS often involves communication and coordination between oncologists, nephrologists, intensivists, and other subspecialists for optimal patient care. TLS occurs most frequently in the context of high white-cell count leukemias [6, 27] and

Burkitt lymphoma [1, 3, 25, 43], but can occur with a variety of tumors that present with bulky disease and exhibit profound sensitivity to chemotherapy [14, 22, 24, 38, 39, 52, 90].

Mechanistically, TLS is a physiologic consequence of widespread tumor cell death and spillage of intracellular contents – specifically nucleic acids, proteins, potassium and phosphate salts – from dying cells into the interstitial and vascular fluid compartments. This massive release of intracellular elements overwhelms normal physiologic excretory capacity, and metabolites accumulate in the serum and tissues to cause pathology. Because highly proliferative tumors display rapid baseline cell turnover at presentation, TLS may occur even before administration of antineoplastic therapy; this has been termed "spontaneous TLS" [14]. However most often, severity peaks in the first hours to days following administration of therapy to which the tumor is susceptible (either chemo- or radiotherapy). Acute renal failure occurs in TLS because uric acid and calcium phosphate precipitate in renal collecting vessels and cause an obstructive uropathy, which reduces glomerular filtration rate (GFR). This reduction in GFR then worsens TLS because the kidneys are the main excretory route for TLS metabolites, whose serum levels will rise without good renal function. In this manner, a self-amplifying destructive series of interrelated events is established wherein reduced GFR causes serum levels of TLS metabolites to increase, which, in turn, leads to further reduction of renal function. This *vicious cycle* of TLS, if not emergently interrupted, can rapidly result in clinical deterioration and death. Therefore, practitioners must have a high index of suspicion for TLS and must rapidly implement preventive strategies and therapeutic interventions as early as possible in the pathophysiologic cascade of TLS. Effective management of TLS involves frequent and thorough clinical and laboratory assessment, vigilant fluid monitoring with strict attention to urine output and volume balance, and pharmacologic and medical interventions as described in this chapter.

15.2 Definition and Classification

TLS is a constellation of metabolic abnormalities that includes hyperuricemia, azotemia, hyperkalemia, hyperphosphatemia, and hypocalcemia [14]. One group defined TLS as either (1) a doubling of baseline serum creatinine in association with at least one of the following measures: serum phosphate >5 mg dL^{-1}, serum uric acid >7 mg dL^{-1}, or serum potassium >5 meq L^{-1} or (2) elevation of two of these measures regardless of serum creatinine [60]. Cairo and Bishop described a distinction between *laboratory TLS*, which is defined by serologic evidence of TLS in the absence of clinical symptoms, and the more severe *clinical TLS* in which laboratory TLS is accompanied by clinical signs/symptoms [14]. Clinical TLS can be graded based on the severity of clinical findings, with the degree of required medical intervention generally correlating with the severity of TLS grade (Table 15.1).

15.3   Incidence of Risk Factors for TLS

Metabolic complications of malignancy and cancer therapy have been recognized for well over a century by clinicians [73]. In fact, the metabolic

Table 15.1 Definition and clinical grading of TLS

Laboratory TLS

A patient has evidence of TLS if presence of malignancy is suspected or confirmed and at least 2 of the following metabolic abnormalities are found in the serum within 3 days prior to or 7 days after initiation of chemotherapy:

  Uric acid >8 mg dL^{-1} or 25% increase from baseline

  Potassium >6 meq L^{-1} or 25% increase from baseline

  Phosphate >4.5 mg dL^{-1} or 25% increase from baseline

  Calcium <7 mg dL^{-1} or 25% decrease from baseline

Clinical TLS

  A patient has clinical TLS if she meets criteria for laboratory TLS and exhibits one or more of the following:

  Increase serum creatinine (1.5 times upper limit of normal)

  Cardiac arrhythmia or sudden death

  Seizure

	Grade 0	Grade I	Grade II	Grade III	Grade IV	Grade V
Laboratory evidence of TLS	–	+	+	+	+	+
Serum Creatinine	1.5 × ULN	1.5 × ULN	1.5–3 × ULN	3–6 × ULN	>6 × ULN	Death from clinical TLS
Cardiac arrhythmia	None	Nonurgent No medical intervention needed	Nonurgent Medical intervention needed	Urgent Symptomatic Incompletely controlled medically or controlled with a device (e.g., defibrillator)	Life-threatening associated with CHF, hypotension, syncope, or shock	Death from clinical TLS
Seizure	None	None	One brief generalized seizure, controlled by anticonvulsants or infrequent motor seizures not interfering with activities of daily living	Poorly controlled seizures affect consciousness breakthrough despite medical intervention	Prolonged, repetitive, or refractory seizures status epilepticus or intractable epilepsy	Death from clinical TLS

Adapted from [14] and originally modified from [33]

manifestations of TLS can be the first sign of occult malignancy [2, 79]. As effective therapies for tumors developed in the early-to-mid twentieth century, the incidence of therapy-related metabolic complications rose, leading to the syndrome of *tumor lysis* that we know today [10, 11, 23, 28]. Historically, TLS complicates mainly fast-growing, bulky tumors that respond quickly to antineoplastic therapy. Independent of chemo- or radioresponsiveness of the tumor, however, patients at risk for development of TLS can be predicted by various clinical and laboratory criteria (Table 15.2) [24, 33].

The solid tumor most famously associated with TLS is Burkitt's lymphoma. Burkitt's lymphoma is among the fastest growing of all childhood malignancies and often presents with bulky abdominal disease burden, which sometimes compresses or involves renal structures and interferes with normal renal function. It is not uncommon for newly diagnosed Burkitt's lymphoma patients to present with

Table 15.2 Risk factors associated with a high-risk of TLS [7, 14, 20, 37, 39, 60, 71, 82]

Tumor characteristics

Burkitt's lymphoma or acute lymphoblastic leukemia

High proliferative rate (rapid clinical progression, elevated LDH)

Bulky disease, advanced stage of malignancy

Rapid tumor cell turnover

Involvement of abdominal organs

Renal compression or involvement

Leukocytosis (>50,000 per mL)

Exquisite chemosensitivity

Patient characteristics

Elevated uric acid on admission

Low serum calcium on admission

Delayed pharmacologic intervention (hydration, anti-TLS therapy)

Metabolic acidosis

Decreased GFR

Hypovolemic state (dehydration, poor p.o. intake, fever)

Renal involvement by malignancy

Urinary outflow obstruction by tumor

Preexisting renal disease

serum uric acid levels of at least double or triple the upper limit of normal and with reduced GFR as evidenced by elevated serum creatinine and oliguria even before chemotherapy is started [63, 64, 66, 87]. In one study, bulky abdominal disease (especially with external ureteric compression by tumor), elevated pretreatment serum uric acid and lactate dehydrogenase concentrations, and oliguria at presentation all predisposed Burkitt's lymphoma patients to severe TLS once therapy began [17]. Hande and Garrow found through a retrospective analysis that 42% of patients with intermediate- or high-grade non-Hodgkin lymphomas exhibited laboratory evidence of TLS and that 6% were symptomatic from TLS [33]. The frequency of acute renal failure in high-risk patients, especially those with advanced-stage Burkitt leukemia or lymphoma can be as high as 30% [17, 41, 86].

Acute leukemias are the other common cause of TLS in pediatrics, particularly with ALL in which the presenting white blood cell count exceeds 100,000 cells mm^{-3} [26, 57]. Though white cell counts can be very high at the time of diagnosis for either AML or stable-phase CML, it is rarer for TLS to accompany these conditions perhaps because myeloblasts and the mature forms of CML are inherently more stable than lymphoblasts [53, 56, 60, 67]. Other pediatric solid tumors less commonly associated with but capable of causing TLS include Hodgkin's disease [58], large-cell lymphoma [4, 12], neuroblastoma [32, 49, 62], rhabdomyosarcoma [45], medulloblastoma [80], and sporadic carcinomas [7]. CNS tumors and bone tumors typically do not feature TLS as a manifestation of disease, perhaps because they may present earlier and are therefore less bulky or alternatively because they are less sensitive to anticancer therapies than hematologic malignancies. It is important, however, to understand that use of more aggressive therapeutic regimens may cause TLS to emerge in a broader spectrum of malignancies in the future.

Regardless of the particular underlying malignancy, the severity of TLS typically peaks 12–72 h after initiation of the first cycle of antineoplastic therapy. TLS usually does not occur in subsequent chemotherapy cycles, presumably because the greatest amount of cell killing occurs with the initial treatment. TLS can occur, however, with unexpectedly low burden of disease if renal impairment is present [31, 65].

15.4   Pathophysiology of TLS

TLS is ultimately a problem of inadequate physiologic waste clearance mechanisms inundated with metabolites released in the process of widespread tumor cell death (Fig. 15.1). The metabolic by-products of cell lysis can cause TLS before inception of antineoplastic therapy (spontaneous TLS) or after initiation of effective antitumor therapy (*therapy-related TLS*) [21]. In either case, because the kidney represents the primary clearance mechanism for these electrolytes and metabolites, renal function directly influences development and severity of TLS (Table 15.2). Although the pathophysiologic processes of

TLS occur simultaneously and can interact to cause symptomatology, it is useful to consider each metabolic component separately to illustrate mechanistic principles of disease (Table 15.3).

15.4.1   Hyperuricemia

Being highly proliferative by nature, tumor cells are rich in DNA. As they die, DNA is released from cells and is broken down into its basic nucleotide base constituents – the pyrimidines cytosine and thymine and the purines adenosine and guanosine. Catabolism of pyrimidines contributes little to TLS, however, metabolism of purines results in production of uric

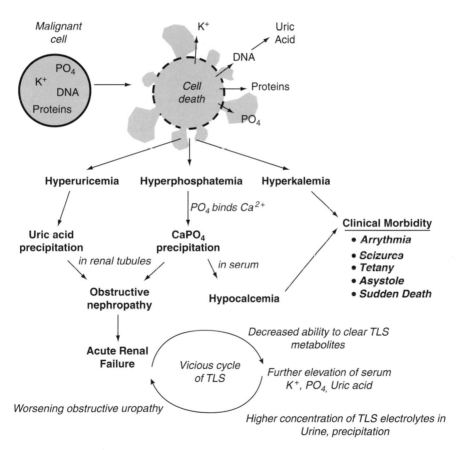

Fig. 15.1 Mechanistic pathophysiology of TLS: Leakage of intracellular metabolites from dying tumor cells in quantities that overwhelm normal excretory mechanisms allow buildup of uric acid, potassium, and phosphate in the serum. These electrolyte abnormalities cause clinical symptoms ranging from mild constitutional complaints to life-threatening sequelae, depending on their severity and rate of development. The kidneys serve as the main organ to clear TLS electrolytes, but become dysfunctional with increasing electrolyte burden. Thus, a vicious cycle is established that if not emergently interrupted medically can lead to significant morbidity and mortality

Table 15.3 Characteristics and clinical consequences of TLS [4, 14, 16, 20, 29, 39, 48, 81, 82]

TLS component	Normal	Critical value[a]	Clinical consequences
Hyperuricemia	Serm uric acid 1.8–5.0 mg dL^{-1}	Serum uric acid > 10 mg dL^{-1}	Renal: precipitation of urate crystals in the renal collecting tubules, blocking urine flow and diminishing GFR, elevation of serum BUN and creatinine; oliguria or anuria possible; hematuria Other: nausea, vomiting, anorexia, edema
Hyperkalemia	Serum potassium 3.2–4.5 mmol L^{-1}	Serum potassium > 6 mmol L^{-1}	Cardiac: arrhythmias, ventricular tachycardia, fibrillation, asystole, cardiac arrest Neuromuscular: weakness, paresthesias, muscle cramps, ascending flaccid paralysis Other: nausea, vomiting, diarrhea, anorexia
Hyperphos-phatemia	Serum phosphate 3.4–6.0 mg dL^{-1}	Serum phosphate > 7 mg dL^{-1}	Renal: precipitation of calcium phosphate crystals that retards or blocks urine flow, decreasing GFR and raising serum BUN and creatinine Other: precipitation of calcium phosphate crystals in soft tissues and circulation, leading to secondary hypocalcemia
Hypocalcemia	Serum total calcium 8.8–10.6 mg dL^{-1} or serum ionized calcium 4.6–5.1 mg dL-1	Total serum calcium 7 (total) or <ionized	Cardiac: hypotension, ventricular arrhythmias, ventricular tachycardia, heart block, ECG changes Neuromuscular: tetany, muscle twitches, cramping, carpopedal spasms, paresthesias, laryngospasm Mental status: confusion, delirium, hallucinations, impaired memory, seizures
Renal failure, uremia	Urine flow > 1–2 mg kg^{-1} h^{-1} Serum creatinine 0.6–1.4 mg dL^{-1} (or age appropriate)	Urine flow < 1 mg kg^{-1} h^{-1} Serum creatinine > 2 × upper limit of normal	Oliguria or anuria, increased serum BUN and creatinine, edema, reduced capacity to excrete TLS metabolites, platelet dysfunction, CNS disturbances

[a] The absolute value wherein an electrolyte imbalance may cause clinical pathology is not the same for every patient. Rate of development of the abnormality and comorbid factors clearly affect outcome. The clinician is strongly encouraged to monitor for symptomatology from a given electrolyte disturbance even before this *critical value* is reached

acid, a chief mediator of TLS. As uric acid accumulates in the serum, it is secreted into the urine by the kidney. With a pKa of 5.4, uric acid tends to remain soluble at physiologic pH but precipitates and crystallizes in solutions of lower pH. Like other salts, the concentration of uric acid increases in solution as water is resorbed, and therefore solute accumulation and precipitation occur predominantly in the distal collecting ducts where urine is less dilute and has an acidic pH [41, 42], leading to microobstructive uropathy. In florid TLS, uric acid precipitation may also occur in deep cortical and medullary blood vessels as a consequence of hemoconcentration and further compromise of GFR. Nonetheless, intraluminal tubular obstruction by uric acid crystals represents the main functional abnormality leading to reduced GFR in uric acid nephropathy [41]. Reduced GFR slows clearance of serum uric acid, worsening hyperuricemia and leading to further uric acid nephropathy. Although the most

important physiologic consequence of elevated uric acid levels is acute renal failure, hyperuricemia can cause a variety of constitutional symptoms including lethargy, nausea, vomiting, arthralgia, and renal colic. Strangely, gout is atypical in TLS, presumably because the intra-arthric urate crystal deposition and inflammation that cause gout are related more to the duration of serum urate elevation rather than the short time that uric acid levels are elevated in most cases of TLS.

Through the activity of deaminases, nucleotidases, and purine nucleotide phosphorylase, uric acid is formed through the metabolic intermediates inosine, hypoxanthine, and xanthine by the purine catabolic pathway (Fig. 15.2). Interestingly, in most mammals, uric acid is further degraded *in vivo* to allantoin via the urate oxidase enzyme. However, humans lack this enzyme because of a universal nonsense mutation in the coding sequence, and are thus unable to terminally convert uric acid into allantoin [88, 89, 91, 92].

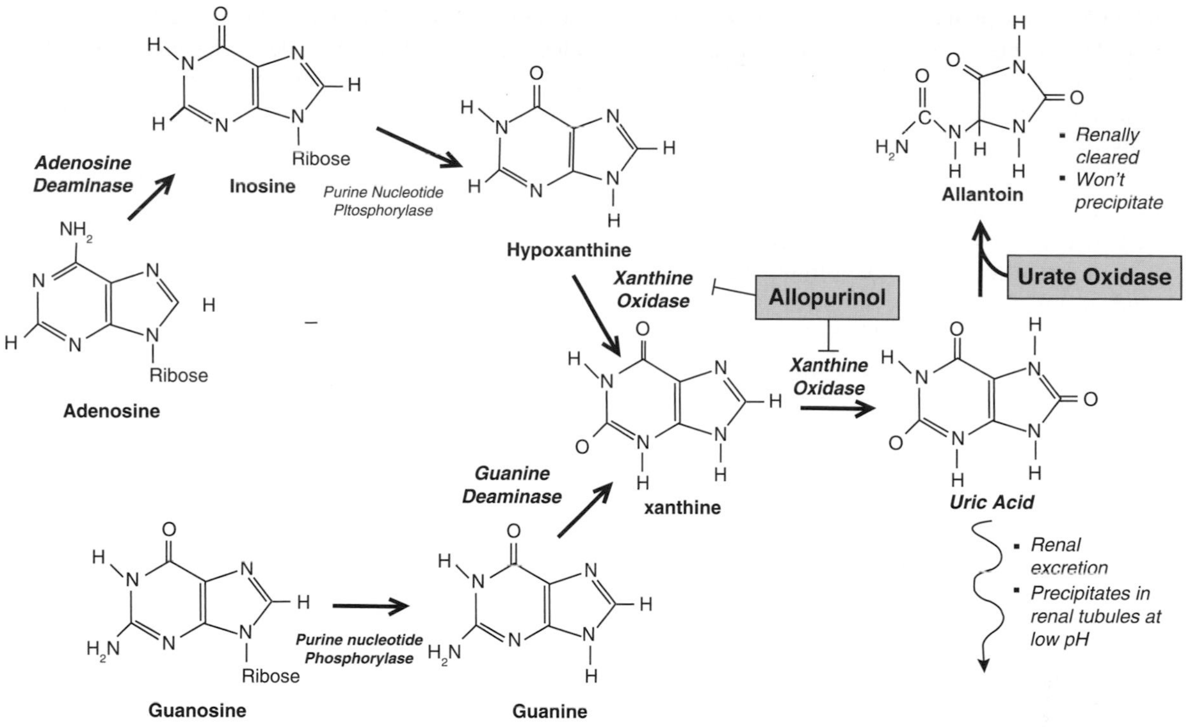

Fig. 15.2 Purine catabolic pathway, generation of uric acid, and biochemical points of pharmacologic intervention: Adenosine and guanosine are metabolized by the purine catabolic pathway, illustrated here in abbreviated form. Through the activity of a variety of deaminases, nucleotidases, and phosphorylases, uric acid is formed through the metabolic intermediates inosine, hypoxan- thine. Urate oxidase, found in other mammals but not in humans, converts uric acid to allantoin, a harmless water-soluble metabolite. Inhibiting xanthine oxidase with allopurinol has been one of the main therapeutic interventions for TLS, though it leads to the buildup of xanthine and hypoxanthine. Rasburicase is a recombinant form of urate oxidase recently introduced into practice

Inhibiting xanthine oxidase with allopurinol has been one of the main therapeutic interventions for TLS, and is still widely used for mild hyperuricemia in TLS. The recent use of recombinant urate oxidase (rasburicase), however, exploits the biochemical fact that allantoin is more water soluble across a range of pH values and is therefore much less prone to precipitation than uric acid. The availability and use of rasburicase has revolutionized the management of TLS in recent years, and patients with TLS treated with rasburicase generally have profound and rapid reversal of hyperuricemia and renal failure. Though much more expensive than allopurinol, rasburicase is fast becoming the treatment of choice for the TLS patient with significant elevation of serum uric acid and renal failure.

15.4.2 Hyperkalemia

Potassium, the principle intracellular cation, freely spills out of cells as the plasma membrane is breached during cell death. In fact, hyperkalemia, defined as a serum potassium >6.0 mmol L^{-1}, is often the earliest laboratory manifestation of TLS, and occult malignancy should be considered in the differential diagnosis of a patient presenting with hyperkalemia of unknown origin. Steady-state concentration of potassium in the serum is a reflection of both influx (from dying cells) and efflux (into the urine); therefore, concurrent impairment of renal function by uric acid or calcium phosphate nephropathy in TLS worsens hyperkalemia by interfering with clearance of potassium. Furthermore, metabolic acidosis, which often accompanies TLS, exacerbates hyperkalemia because normal physiologic compensatory mechanisms are called upon to reduce extracellular acid load function by promoting potassium efflux from normal cells in exchange for hydrogen ions. Simultaneous hypocalcemia in TLS destabilizes cell membrane potential and can exacerbate cardiac symptomatology and other consequences of hyperkalemia. Thus, several interacting biochemical and pathologic pathways may interplay during TLS to affect serum potassium concentration and its effect on tissues [35, 39, 54, 90].

Although clinical complications of hyperkalemia usually do not manifest until serum levels are >6–7 mmol L^{-1}, clinical pathology can certainly be influenced by the rate at which hyperkalemia develops. If hyperkalemia develops rapidly, then clinical symptoms may manifest at lower absolute serum potassium levels due to insufficient time for physiologic adaptive mechanisms to become established. The most feared consequence of hyperkalemia is life-threatening cardiac arrhythmia such as ventricular fibrillation or asystole [40, 55, 78, 84]. It is prudent to monitor ECG status of hyperkalemic patients because subtle changes may predict more significant pathology. Specifically, peaked T waves, flattened P waves, prolonged PR interval, widened QRS complexes, deep S waves, and sine waves must be rapidly diagnosed because they may herald more serious cardiac arrhythmias that develop with ongoing or worsening hyperkalemia. Therapies must be aimed at stabilizing of the myocardial cell membrane and reducing serum potassium to reduce morbidity.

15.4.3 Hyperphosphatemia and Hypocalcemia

TLS-associated hyperphosphatemia occurs because of release of intracellular phosphates and phosphate-rich biomolecules (e.g., nucleic acids and proteins) from dying cancer cells into the circulation. Because lymphoblasts contain up to four times the intracellular phosphate content of normal lymphocytes [83], lymphoid malignancies are especially associated with TLS-associated hyperphosphatemia. The clinical sequelae of hyperphosphatemia are largely benign with one notable exception: when serum phosphate levels reach a certain threshold, soluble calcium interacts chemically with phosphate to precipitate into calcium phosphate. It has been estimated that if the solubility product factor (Ca × P) reaches a level of 60 or more, then calcium phosphate will precipitate [83]. Serum calcium levels will then become depleted as calcium gets incorporated in calcium phosphate crystals and hypocalcemia secondary to hyperphosphatemia results [93]. Calcium phosphate precipitation in the renal collecting tubules, such as uric acid crystallization, retards urine flow and contributes to decreased GFR that, like uric acid nephropathy, worsens TLS. Normal physiologic mechanisms may contribute to the problem. For example, secretion of parathyroid

hormone (PTH) is normally upregulated in the hypocalcemic state. PTH in turn decreases proximal tubular reabsorption of phosphate leading to higher urinary phosphate levels and increased risk of urinary calcium phosphate precipitation [93].

Hypocalcemia can lead to a number of clinical manifestations including spasms, tetany, seizures, and bronchospasm. Furthermore, hypocalcemia contributes to QT interval lengthening, which predisposes patients to ventricular arrhythmia and cardiac arrest particularly in the setting of concurrent hyperkalemia and other electrolyte imbalances. Chvostek and Trousseau signs may be present in the symptomatic hypocalcemic patient and are useful components to test for in the physical examination. Aggressive calcium infusion may, however, cause injury to the patient because it may promote widespread calcification in the face of hyperphosphatemia, including intrarenal calcification that threatens to worsen the renal failure of TLS [90]. Therefore, in the hyperphosphatemic patient, treatment of hypocalcemia should, as a general rule, be reserved only for serious clinical symptomatology directly attributable to low serum calcium.

15.4.4 Uremia and Renal Failure

Intrarenal precipitation of uric acid and calcium phosphate each interfere with the generation and physiologic flow of urine. It is thought that the major cause of TLS-related renal failure prior to chemotherapy is uric acid buildup, whereas calcium phosphate-mediated obstructive nephropathy contributes much more after therapy has begun. Regardless of which crystals actually accumulate in the kidney, however, decreased renal glomerular filtration reduces urine flow, which promotes further crystals to form in static urine. To add to the problem, children presenting with malignancy frequently exhibit some degree of dehydration and prerenal azotemia because of poor oral intake and/or fever at diagnosis. Oliguria from hypovolemia favors intrarenal urate and calcium phosphate precipitation, making timely diagnosis and intervention with intravenous fluids critical to optimal patient care. If the patient has the added misfortune of his/her tumor invading or compressing renal structures, then anatomic obstruction of urine flow will further compromise renal function and predispose the patient to severe TLS [65].

Besides reducing clearance of the electrolytes that cause TLS, a diminished GFR also interferes with clearance of other renally excreted compounds such as urea, creatinine, and free water. Symptoms of uremia include fatigue/weakness, pericarditis, and mental confusion and may interfere with normal platelet function, which is of particular concern in thrombocytopenic patients. As renal function diminishes, signs of volume overload, such as dyspnea, pulmonary rales, edema, and hypertension, may develop. Though the renal failure of TLS is often reversible with appropriate medical intervention aimed at reducing serum uric acid and phosphate levels and reestablishing normal urine output, dialysis or other renal replacement therapy may be required in severe or refractory cases.

15.4.5   Metabolic Acidosis

Large amounts of endogenous intracellular acids are released from dying tumor cells and their buildup in the serum and tissues causes acidosis. Acidemia can worsen the many electrolyte imbalances already present in TLS because normal physiologic compensatory mechanisms aimed at reducing extracellular H^+ concentration in acidemic conditions hinder intracellular K^+ uptake, decrease uric acid solubility, and shift phosphate out of cells. Calcium phosphate solubility, however, improves in acidic conditions; therefore, careful thought must be given as to what degree of acidemia is tolerable for the clinical circumstances. The practice of indiscriminate and universal alkalinization of TLS patients has been called into question in recent years and it should be dictated by clinical condition [14, 22].

15.5   Evaluation of the Patient with TLS

The clinician should attempt to discern the rate of progression of malignancy by history and physical evaluation. Relevant historical information includes time of onset of symptoms referable to the malignancy, pace of growth of a palpable solid tumor, and character and timing of pain or fullness. The patient should be questioned about contributors or symptoms of dehydration including decreased urine output, thirst, dizziness, vomiting, bleeding, and diarrhea. Other pertinent historical components that will help guide clinical decision making include presence of cramps, spasms, tetany, seizures, and alterations in consciousness suggestive of hypocalcemia. On examination, special attention should be given to blood pressure, cardiac rate and rhythm, abnormal masses, degree of lymphadenopathy and hepatosplenomegaly, and presence of pleural or pericardial effusions or ascites. Other useful signs include facial plethora or swelling and head/neck venous congestion, which might suggest superior vena cava syndrome and cough, stridor, and orthopnea that might indicate an anterior mediastinal mass and tracheal compression.

Initial laboratory studies for TLS include a CBC with a manual differential and reticulocyte count (Table 15.4). Critical serum electrolyte studies include a basic electrolyte panel (serum sodium, potassium, chloride, bicarbonate), and serum values for total calcium, phosphorus, magnesium, uric acid, blood urea nitrogen, creatinine, lactate dehydrogenase, and liver function tests. Elevated LDH in particular correlates with high tumor load and may predict a more severe course of TLS [46, 60]. A urinalysis with microscopy will give an indication of specific gravity and may exhibit urate crystals, casts, and/or hematuria. If the serum calcium is low, an ionized calcium and serum albumin should be obtained. If a nonhemolyzed serum potassium is elevated, an ECG is indicated to evaluate for electrocardiographic signs of physiologically significant hyperkalemia (e.g., peaked T waves, QRS widening) or hypocalcemia (e.g., prolonged QT_c interval). If ECG abnormalities are found, the patient should be placed on a cardiac monitor, and therapies should be immediately implemented to restore normal cardiac function.

Because extrinsic compression by tumor can cause renal failure by obstructive uropathy, abdominopelvic imaging (typically ultrasound or CT scan) is useful on any patient with an abdominal or pelvic mass. If kidneys are involved by tumor (see Fig. 15.3 for a clinical example) or if the tumor compresses renal outflow tracts, this places the patient at particular risk of acute renal failure from severe TLS. In such cases, nephrologic and/or urologic consultation may be indicated to determine the need for dialysis and/or urinary stenting/catheterization [59].

It is important to very closely monitor clinical parameters and the relevant serum markers of TLS frequently during the first several hours-to-days of tumor lysis in order to get a sense of the pace of the process and to determine whether alterations need to be made in clinical management. Assessing urine output and fluid balance at least every 6–8 h as well as serum electrolytes, calcium, phosphate, and BUN/creatinine is usually warranted, with intensity and frequency of monitoring governed by clinical status. Keep in mind that severity of TLS often peaks after antineoplastic therapy is initiated.

Table 15.4 Laboratory evaluation for TLS [4, 29, 44, 90]

Serological tests[a]

   CBC with differential (especially in case of leukocytosis)

   Serum electrolytes: sodium, potassium, chloride, and bicarbonate

   Uric acid

   LDH

   Phosphate

   Calcium (total and ionized if indicated)

   Total protein and albumin

   BUN, creatinine

Urine studies

   Urine output (cc kg^{-1} h^{-1})

   Urinalysis: pH, crystals, hematuria

Imaging Studies

   Radiography of the chest is useful to determine the presence of a large tumor, e.g., mediastinal mass

   Ultrasonography or computed tomography scanning of the abdomen and retroperitoneum if mass lesions in the abdomen or renal failure are present; intravenous contrast may be contraindicated in a patient with renal insufficiency

Fluid balance data

   Daily weight

   Daily abdominal girth

Cardiac assessment

   ECG or continuous cardiac monitoring

Begin assessment prior to chemo- or radiotherapy and continues every 6–8 h or more for 48–72 h after treatment induction or as dictated by clinical scenario

[a] Blood should be collected through a wide-bore catheter

15.6 Management of TLS

The keys to successfully managing acute TLS are to (1) maintain a high index of suspicion by promptly identifying patients at risk for TLS, and (2) aggressively institute proactive measures to prevent and/or reduce the severity of the clinical abnormalities associated with TLS [71]. Ideally, antitumor therapy should be delayed until prophylactic TLS measures have been implemented and renal function is restored. However, if delay is not possible (e.g., because of the aggressive nature of their underlying malignancy), then the practitioner must weight the relative risks and benefits of delaying tumor therapy vs. the risk of developing or exacerbating TLS. Patients at risk for TLS should undoubtedly have reliable venous or central access and be treated in an intensive care or oncology unit by well-trained staff familiar with the complications and management of TLS.

15.6.1 Prevention

Patients who present with spontaneous TLS that accompanies initial presentation of malignancy and those at risk of treatment-related TLS should begin prophylactic measures aimed at optimizing hydration and clearance of pathogenic metabolites as soon as possible. This is especially critical in patients with high-risk clinical features (Table 15.2). One or more large-bore peripheral intravenous catheters through which fluids and medications can be administered and from which labs may be drawn is essential. At a minimum, all patients at risk of TLS should be treated with adequate IV hydration to maintain a vigorous urine output. As outlined below, alkalinization of fluids as well as pharmacologic measures to treat hyperkalemia, hyperuricemia, hyperphosphatemia, and hypocalcemia may play valuable roles in tumor lysis prophylaxis and treatment (Table 15.5), but there is

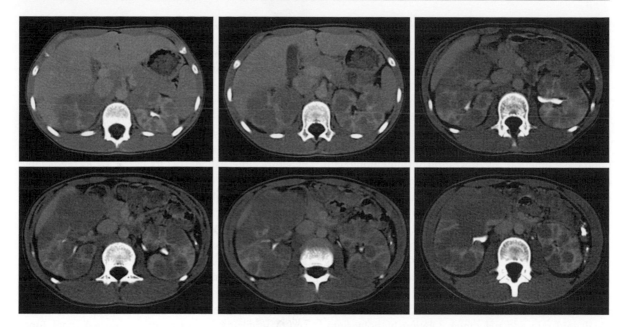

Fig. 15.3 Example of a patient at high risk of developing severe TLS: A 12-year-old girl presented with a rapidly enlarging abdominal mass that was identified as Burkitt's lymphoma on biopsy. As shown in these abdominal CT scan images at diagnosis, there was a large right-sided flank mass as well as extensive involvement of both kidneys by disease. This patient presented with a variety of risk factors predictive of severe TLS (see Table 15.2), including a highly proliferative chemosensitive tumor, bulk disease, anatomic involvement of both kidneys, and baseline elevations of serum LDH, uric acid, and creatinine. Fortunately, this patient maintained adequate renal output throughout the first days of chemotherapy, was treated with rasburicase and nonalkalinized fluids, and had a fine clinical outcome

no universal clinical practice algorhythm appropriate for every TLS patient. Rather, each patient's therapy should be tailored to his/her particular clinical circumstances. Though TLS can often be well-managed pharmacologically, the clinician should keep in mind that debulking or cytoreductive measures (e.g., cytopheresis in leukemias) can be useful antitumor lysis interventions by reducing tumor cell burden before chemotherapy is instituted.

15.6.2 Fluids and Alkalinization

As a general rule, children newly diagnosed with malignancies who are at risk of TLS and who have adequate renal function should be aggressively hydrated [14, 37, 68]. Vigorous fluid therapy maintains urine output, flushes away existing precipitated uric acid or calcium phosphate crystals from renal tubules (thereby reducing obstructive nephropathy), prevents urinary stasis, which favors further crystallization, and reduces metabolic acidosis. Unless acute renal failure or urinary outflow tract obstruction exists at diagnosis, patients should normally be treated with intravenous fluids at a rate of at least twice the daily maintenance requirement ($3 \, L \, m^{-2} \, day^{-1}$ or $200 \, mL \, kg^{-1} \, day^{-1}$ if less than 10 kg in weight). Twice maintenance fluid rate usually promotes a brisk urine output, but fluids can be adjusted up to four times the daily fluid maintenance requirement to optimize urine flow (at least $100 \, mL \, m^{-2} \, h^{-1}$ or at least $3 \, mL \, kg^{-1} \, h^{-1}$ if the patient weighs less than 10 kg). Ideally, urine specific gravity should remain at or below 1.010. Diuretics (mannitol and/or furosemide) may be helpful to achieve this urine output, but should not be used in the setting of acute obstructive uropathy or hypovolemia (Table 15.5) [4, 24, 34, 71]. Historically, the main component of the renal failure associated with TLS has been uric acid nephropathy. Recently, however, hyperuricemic patients who would otherwise be at risk of uric acid nephropathy have been very effectively treated with recombinant urate oxidase, which rapidly and effectively reduces serum uric acid levels and reverses uric acid nephropathy. Consequently, hyperphosphatemia and calcium phosphate nephropathy now represent the main cause of acute renal failure in TLS. Therefore, aggressive alkalinization may do more harm than good when administered to TLS patients effectively treated with urate oxidase and who are at low risk for uric acid nephropathy but who remain at risk for calcium phosphate nephropathy. Careful thought should be given to the need for fluid alkalinization.

If indicated, alkalinization of the urine can be achieved by addition of sodium bicarbonate to intravenous fluids (Table 15.5). An alkaline urine (pH > 6.5) promotes the urinary excretion of uric acid; therefore, if the serum uric acid is only mildly elevated and there is good renal function, alkalinization of fluids along with allopurinol administration remains a viable clinical option for patients with mild TLS. At our institution, we generally add sodium bicarbonate to intravenous fluids for such patients and have had good success in managing TLS by maintaining a brisk urine flow with a urine pH in the 7.0–8.0 range. When alkalinizing and hyperhydrating a patient, each urine void should be dipped and adjustments in the rate and/or amount of sodium bicarbonate should be made to maintain an ideal void rate and pH range. Obviously, potassium, calcium, and phosphate should be withheld from hydration fluids to avoid worsening of hyperkalemia and hyperphosphatemia and to avoid triggering of calcium phosphate precipitation in vivo [5, 14, 41, 75].

15.6.3 Management of Hyperuricemia

15.6.3.1 Allopurinol

Allopurinol is a xanthine analogue with metabolite oxypurinol function in vivo as a competitive inhibitor of xanthine oxidase, the enzyme required to generate uric acid from purines (Fig. 15.2) [47, 77]. Administered either orally or intravenously, allopurinol effectively decreases the formation of new uric acid and has been shown to reduce the incidence of uric acid obstructive uropathy in oncology patients at risk of TLS [17, 61, 85]. Though usually well-tolerated and moderately effective, it has several drawbacks, which should be considered before use: (1) allopurinol does not degrade existing uric acid and should not be expected to result in swift normalization of serum uric acid levels in the markedly hyperuricemic patient, (2) its use leads to predictable accumulation of upstream products of purine catabolism (hypoxanthine and xanthine), which can themselves precipitate in the kidney and block urine flow [51], (3) allopurinol unavoidably decreases metabolism of other purine analogues (e.g., 6-mercaptopurine) whose clearance is xanthine oxidase-dependent, necessitating dose reductions in purine analogues when used simultaneously with allopurinol [8, 23, 50, 77]. In all, allopurinol is useful in the TLS patient with minimal serum uric acid elevation and preserved renal function. If, however, serum uric acid levels are markedly elevated and renal function is significantly impaired, then rasburicase should be considered the treatment of choice to rapidly reverse hyperuricemia and uric acid nephropathy.

15.6.3.2 Recombinant Urate Oxidase (Rasburicase)

Unlike allopurinol that acts by inhibiting formation of new uric acid, urate oxidase (rasburicase) actually breaks down existing molecules of uric acid into harmless water-soluble by-products and can rapidly reverse even the most elevated cases of hyperuricemia. It is

Table 15.5 Pharmacologic management of TLS [22, 41, 71, 74]

Intravenous hydration	5% Dextrose + 0.25–0.5% normal saline
	Add 40–60 meq L^{-1} NaHCO3 if urinary alkalinization is desired (may not be indicated if rasburicase is used)
	Do not add K+ or phosphate to intravenous fluids
	Run fluids at 2–4 × maintenance rate (3–6 L m^{-2} day^{-1}); begin at 200 mL kg day^{-1} if less than 10 kg in weight
	Adjust rate to keep urine output > 100 mL m^{-2} h^{-1} or >3 mL kg^{-1} h^{-1} if the patient weighs less than 10 kg and urine specific gravity is <1.010
Alkalinization	Adding 40–60 meq L^{-1} NaHCO3 to 5% dextrose + 0.25% normal saline generally results in good alkalinization of the urine (pH 7.0–7.5)
	Adjust NaHCO3 concentration in intravenous fluids to maintain urine pH 7.0–7.5
	Consider withholding sodium bicarbonate if rasburicase is used
	Reduce bicarbonate if blood level is >30 meq L^{-1} or urine pH is >7.3
	Consider acetazolamide (5 mg kg^{-1} day^{-1})

(continued)

Table 15.5 (continued)

Uric acid reduction	**Allopurinol**
	$100 \, mg \, m^{-2} \, dose^{-1} \, q8\,h$ ($10 \, mg \, kg^{-1} \, day^{-1}$ divided q8 h) p.o. (maximum $800 \, mg \, day^{-1}$) or 200–$400 \, mg \, m^{-2} \, day^{-1}$ in 1–3 divided doses i.v. (maximum $600 \, mg \, day^{-1}$)
	Reduce dose by 50% or more in renal failure
	Adjust doses of purine analogues and drugs metabolized by P450 hepatic microsomal enzymes with concomitant allopurinol -or-
	Urate oxidase (rasburicase; $0.2 \, mg \, kg^{-1} \, day^{-1} \times 1$–3 days)
	1–3 daily doses usually sufficient
	0.05–$0.2 \, mg \, kg^{-1}$ (round dose to nearest vial size) intravenously over 30 min
	Alkalinization of urine not required when rasburicase is used
	Use with caution in patients with oxidation-sensitive conditions (e.g., G6PD deficiency, unstable hemoglobins)
	Small risk of allergic reaction – have diphenhydramine and epinephrine readily available
	It is necessary to place blood samples immediately on ice in order to follow serum uric acid levels to avoid ex vivo enzymatic degradation
Hyperkalemia	Low potassium diet
	Withhold potassium from all intravenous fluids
	Sodium polystyrene sulphonate (Kayexelate) $1 \, g \, kg{-}1$ with 50% sorbitol orally or via nasogastric tube
	Insulin ($0.1 \, U \, kg{-}1$) + $2 \, mL \, kg^{-1} \, 25\%$ glucose
	Albuterol nebulization
	Potassium-wasting diuretics (furosemide, thiazides)
	Calcium gluconate (100–$200 \, mg \, kg^{-1}$ iv)
Hyperphosphatemia	Low phosphate diet
	Withhold phosphate from intravenous fluids
	Aluminum hydroxide orally or via nasogastric tube $15 \, mL$ (50–$150 \, mg \, kg{-}1$ per 24 h) q6
Hypocalcemia	Asymptomatic – no therapy
	Symptomatic – calcium gluconate 50–$100 \, mg \, kg^{-1}$
	Infusing calcium in the setting of hyperphosphatemia can precipitate calcium phosphate and worsen renal failure
Forced diuresis	Furosemide (0.5–$1 \, mg \, kg^{-1}$)
	Mannitol ($0.5 \, g \, kg^{-1}$ over 15 min every 6–8 h)
	Avoid if patient is hypovolemic
Dialysis (or other renal replacement therapy)	Should be considered if one or more of the following exists:
	Volume overload (pulmonary edema, effusions)
	Renal failure, severe oliguria, or anuria
	Refractory or symptomatic hyperkalemia, hyperphosphatemia, hyperuricemia, or hypocalcemia
	Uncontrolled hypertension
	Severe metabolic acidosis
	Severe uremia with CNS toxicity or bleeding diathesis
	Consultation with nephrology is usually warranted before beginning dialysis or other renal replacement therapies

currently the most effective treatment for the hyperuricemia of TLS [18, 19, 76]. Rasburicase oxidizes uric acid into allantoin, which is readily secreted into the urine and remains soluble regardless of urine pH making alkalinization of the urine unnecessary during rasburicase therapy [19]. Pui et al. initially reported that prophylactic use of rasburicase in 66 children with hematological malignancies at risk of TLS significantly reduced the median uric acid level within 4 h of administration with a therapeutic effect that lasted despite subsequent initiation of chemotherapy [70]. Later, in a randomized trial comparing allopurinol and rasburicase in patients at risk of acute TLS, rasburicase proved far more effective than allopurinol in reducing uric acid levels and overall length of hyperuricemia [30]. Being a recombinant enzyme, however, rasburicase is significantly more expensive than allopurinol, and is therefore generally reserved for patients with very high levels of uric acid and/or clear evidence of acute renal failure due to uric acid nephropathy [15]. Administered intravenously with the dose usually rounded to the nearest vial available in order to minimize waste, rasburicase achieves peak effect within hours of administration and removes existing uric acid without inducing accumulation of xanthine [69]. Usually no more than three daily doses of rasburicase are needed to rapidly reverse hyperuricemia and maintain low-to-normal uric acid levels through the first stages of antineoplastic therapy. Normalization of serum creatinine and GFR often follows within hours after intravenous administration of rasburicase. Some have suggested that in order to reduce therapeutic costs, allopurinol can be safely administered after an initial rasburicase treatment and uric acid reduction [37]. It is important to note that in rasburicase therapy hydrogen peroxide is generated in rasburicase-mediated conversion of uric acid to allantoin; therefore, caution must be used in patients with glucose-6-phosphate dehydrogenase (G6PD) deficiency or other oxidation-sensitive states (e.g., unstable hemoglobins) in order to avoid triggering inadvertent oxidative hemolysis [69]. Because of the minimal but potentially life-threatening risk of allergic reaction elicited by rasburicase administration, appropriate medications (e.g., diphenhydramine, epinephrine) should be available at the bedside during initial administration of rasburicase.

Therefore, in general, patients with grade 0-II TLS (Table 15.1) remain good candidates for allopurinol prophylaxis and fluid alkalinization. However, patients with higher grade TLS are probably best served by rapid administration of at least one dose of rasburicase and hydration.

15.6.4 Management of Hyperkalemia

As hyperkalemia is arguably the most immediate life-threatening aspect of TLS, it must be attentively and rapidly managed. In TLS, serum potassium can rise rather quickly over the span of hours when renal failure accompanies tumor lysis. Therefore, patients with TLS must be closely monitored during the first hours of TLS with particular attention paid to fluid balance, serum potassium, and cardiac status. Clinical manifestations of hyperkalemia usually appear with serum potassium levels above 6.0 mmol L^{-1} and include nonspecific constitutional symptoms (nausea, vomiting, anorexia, and diarrhea) as well as more severe problems such as neuromuscular (weakness, cramping, paresthesias, paralysis) and cardiac abnormalities (conduction disturbances ranging from asystole to ventricular arrhythmias), syncope and sudden death [5, 39, 41]. In general, the degree of pathophysiology correlates with the magnitude of electrolyte imbalance. Often, the first hint of cardiac abnormality due to hyperkalemia can be detected on ECG; therefore, cardiac monitoring is helpful in patients with hyperkalemia.

Management of the hyperkalemic patient begins with optimizing renal function and excluding potassium from all intravenous fluids. In patients who are asymptomatic with only mild elevations of the serum potassium, initial medical treatment may require only sodium polystyrene sulphonate (Kayexelate) administration to absorb potassium in the intestine. In symptomatic patients, however, more vigorous interventions may be required including insulin and glucose infusions, albuterol nebulizations, or even hemodialysis (Table 15.5) Hypocalcemia can worsen physiological consequences of hyperkalemia, thus correcting other metabolic abnormalities can be of great benefit to the hyperkalemic patient.

15.6.5 Management of Hyperphosphatemia and Hypocalcemia

Unlike uric acid that can be markedly elevated at diagnosis even before chemotherapy has begun, hyperphosphatemia usually is not clinically significant until after chemotherapy has begun. Signs/symptoms of severe hyperphosphatemia include nausea, vomiting, diarrhea, lethargy, and seizures. Furthermore, because of tissue and serum precipitation of calcium phosphate, hypocalcemia and calcium phosphate nephropathy can develop [13, 71]. Phosphate should be withheld from all intravenous solutions, and intestinal phosphate binders such as aluminum hydroxide or Sevelamer are useful first-line therapies administered orally or via nasogastric tube that can effectively treat hyperphosphatemia. Like other electrolyte imbalances, however, dialysis may be required in severe refractory cases [36, 41, 72]. Along with hyperkalemia, severe hypocalcemia is one of the most life-threatening aspects of TLS. Signs/symptoms of hypocalcemia include muscle cramps/spasms, paresthesias, tetany, ventricular arrhythmias, heart block, hypotension, confusion, delirium, hallucinations, and seizures. Severe hypocalcemia is manifested by bradycardia, cardiac failure, coma, and rarely death [39, 71]. Aggressive treatment of asymptomatic hypocalcaemia by intravenous calcium infusion, however, is contraindicated in the asymptomatic hypocalcemic hyperphosphatemic patient because of the risk of precipitating calcium phosphate in the urine and worsening of obstructive uropathy. The hypocalcemia of TLS generally resolves as tumor lysis improves; however, symptomatic hypocalcemic patients may require intravenous calcium gluconate or dialysis (Table 15.5) [14, 41].

15.6.6   Dialysis

Despite appropriate and timely pharmacologic intervention, some patients with refractory TLS may require more aggressive therapy. Patients with increasing renal dysfunction and worsening electrolyte abnormalities may benefit from dialysis or hemofiltration [41]. Indications for assisted renal replacement therapies are listed in Table 15.5, and consultation with nephrology is obviously warranted in such cases.

15.7   Conclusions

TLS is a combination of metabolic disturbances caused by inability to sufficiently clear products of cellular degradation as tumor cells rapidly turn over at diagnosis and/or shortly after antineoplastic therapy is begun. It is ultimately a problem of disturbed electrolyte homeostasis, with normal excretory pathways being overwhelmed by an excess of waste products released from dying tumor cells. The specific metabolic imbalances that comprise TLS include hyperuricemia, hyperkalemia, hyperphosphatemia, and hypocalcemia. Improvements in the management of TLS over the last several decades have resulted in much less morbidity and mortality in the first days of therapy for newly diagnosed pediatric oncology patients. In particular, the use of rasburicase has revolutionized the treatment of TLS, making the need for dialysis and other renal replacement measures much less common and overall outcomes much better. Clearly, the management of TLS will evolve

as more therapies are developed. Future prospective studies will help determine which patients are at the highest risk of developing TLS and its complications, and which require rasburicase as first-line therapy vs. which patients only require allopurinol for prophylaxis and/or treatment. Management of newly diagnosed patients at risk of TLS affords a unique opportunity for the oncologist to work hand-in-hand with their nephrology and critical care colleagues to optimize care for this complex life-threatening metabolic disorder.

Take-Home Pearls

> Large tumor cell burden, high rate of malignant cell division, baseline renal failure, renal involvement by tumor and onset of chemo- or radiotherapy are important predictors of severe TLS.
> Recombinant urate acid oxidase (Rasburicase) rapidly reverses hyperuricemia even in the setting of renal failure.
> Aggressive hydration remains a cornerstone therapeutic principle in the management of TLS.
> Alkalinization of intravenous fluids may not be indicated after administration of recombinant urate oxidase and correction of serum uric acid as it risks worsening of calcium phosphate crystallization in renal tubules.
> Though TLS has historically complicated hematopoietic tumors (lymphomas and leukemias), the development of more effective chemotherapeutic agents may herald therapy-related TLS in broader range of malignancies.

References

1. Abou Mourad Y, Taher A, Shamseddine A (2003) Acute tumor lysis syndrome in large B-cell non-Hodgkin lymphoma induced by steroids and anti-CD 20. Hematol J 4(3):222–4
2. Agnani S, et al. (2006) Marked hyperuricemia with acute renal failure: need to consider occult malignancy and spontaneous tumour lysis syndrome. Int J Clin Pract 60(3):364–6
3. Ahamed SM, et al. (2006) Spontaneous tumour lysis syndrome associated with non-Hodgkin's lymphoma – a case report. Indian J Pathol Microbiol 49(1):26–8
4. Alavi S, et al. (2006) Tumor lysis syndrome in children with non-Hodgkin lymphoma. Pediatr Hematol Oncol 23(1):65–70
5. Andreoli SP, et al. (1986) Purine excretion during tumor lysis in children with acute lymphocytic leukemia receiving allopurinol: relationship to acute renal failure. J Pediatr 109(2):292–8
6. Annemans L, et al. (2003) Incidence, medical resource utilisation and costs of hyperuricemia and tumour lysis-syndrome in patients with acute leukaemia and non-Hodgkin's

lymphoma in four European countries. Leuk Lymphoma 44(1):77–83

7. Baeksgaard L, Sorensen JB (2003) Acute tumor lysis syndrome in solid tumors – a case report and review of the literature. Cancer Chemother Pharmacol 51(3):187–92

8. Band PR, et al. (1970) Xanthine nephropathy in a patient with lymphosarcoma treated with allopurinol. N Engl J Med 283(7):354–7

9. Baumann MA, Frick JC, Holoye PY (1983) The tumor lysis syndrome. JAMA 250(5):615

10. Bedrna J, et al. (1929) Harnleiterverschluss nach Bestrahlung chronischer leukamien mit rontgenstrahlen. Med Klin 25:1700–1

11. Bell R, et al. (1979) Complications of tumour overkill when associated with high dose methotrexate therapy. Clin Exp Pharmacol Physiol Suppl 5:47–55

12. Boccia RV, et al. (1985) Multiple recurrences of acute tumor lysis syndrome in an indolent non-Hodgkin's lymphoma. Cancer 56(9):2295–7

13. Boles JM, et al. (1984) Acute renal failure caused by extreme hyperphosphatemia after chemotherapy of an acute lymphoblastic leukemia. Cancer 53(11):2425–9

14. Cairo MS, Bishop M (2004) Tumour lysis syndrome: new therapeutic strategies and classification. Br J Haematol 127(1):3–11

15. Cammalleri L, Malaguarnera M (2007) Rasburicase represents a new tool for hyperuricemia in tumor lysis syndrome and in gout. Int J Med Sci 4(2):83–93

16. Cantril CA, Haylock PJ (2004) Emergency. Tumor lysis syndrome. Am J Nurs 104(4):49–52; quiz 52–3

17. Cohen LF, et al. (1980) Acute tumor lysis syndrome. A review of 37 patients with Burkitt's lymphoma. Am J Med 68(4):486–91

18. Coiffier B, Riouffol C (2007) Management of tumor lysis syndrome in adults. Expert Rev Anticancer Ther 7(2):233–9

19. Coiffier B, et al. (2003) Efficacy and safety of rasburicase (recombinant urate oxidase) for the prevention and treatment of hyperuricemia during induction chemotherapy of aggressive non-Hodgkin's lymphoma: results of the GRAAL1 (Groupe d'Etude des Lymphomes de l'Adulte Trial on Rasburicase Activity in Adult Lymphoma) study. J Clin Oncol 21(23):4402–6

20. Cope D (2004) Tumor lysis syndrome. Clin J Oncol Nurs 8(4):415–16

21. Crittenden DR, Ackerman GL (1977) Hyperuricemic acute renal failure in disseminated carcinoma. Arch Intern Med 137(1):97–9

22. Davidson MB, et al. (2004) Pathophysiology, clinical consequences, and treatment of tumor lysis syndrome. Am J Med 116(8):546–54

23. DeConti RC, Calabresi P (1966) Use of allopurinol for prevention and control of hyperuricemia in patients with neoplastic disease. N Engl J Med 274(9):481–6

24. Del Toro G, Morris E, Cairo MS (2005) Tumor lysis syndrome: pathophysiology, definition, and alternative treatment approaches. Clin Adv Hematol Oncol 3(1):54–61

25. Dhingra K, Newcom SR (1988) Acute tumor lysis syndrome in non-Hodgkin lymphoma induced by dexamethasone. Am J Hematol 29(2):115–16

26. Diamond CA, Matthay KK (1988) Childhood acute lymphoblastic leukemia. Pediatr Ann 17(3):156–61, 164–70

27. Duzova A (2001) Acute tumour lysis syndrome following a single-dose corticosteroid in children with acute lymphoblastic leukaemia. Eur J Haematol 66(6):404–7

28. Fichman M, Bethune J (1974) Effects of neoplasms on renal electrolyte function. Ann N Y Acad Sci 230:448–72

29. Fleming DR, Doukas MD (1992) Acute tumor lysis syndrome in hematologic malignancies. Leuk Lymphoma 8(4–5):315–18

30. Goldman SC, et al. (2001) A randomized comparison between rasburicase and allopurinol in children with lymphoma or leukemia at high risk for tumor lysis. Blood 97(10):2998–3003

31. Hain RD, et al. (1994) Acute tumour lysis syndrome complicating treatment of stage IVS neuroblastoma in infants under six months old. Med Pediatr Oncol 23(2):136–9

32. Hain RD, et al. (1994) Acute tumour lysis syndrome with no evidence of tumour load. Pediatr Nephrol 8(5):537–9

33. Hande KR, Garrow GC (1993) Acute tumor lysis syndrome in patients with high-grade non-Hodgkin's lymphoma. Am J Med 94(2):133–9

34. Haut C (2005) Oncological emergencies in the pediatric intensive care unit. AACN Clin Issues 16(2):232–45

35. Hawthorne JL, Schneider SM, Workman ML (1992) Common electrolyte imbalances associated with malignancy. AACN Clin Issues Crit Care Nurs 3(3):714–23

36. Heney D, et al. (1990) Continuous arteriovenous haemofiltration in the treatment of tumour lysis syndrome. Pediatr Nephrol 4(3):245–7

37. Howard SC, Pui CH (2006) Pitfalls in predicting tumor lysis syndrome. Leuk Lymphoma 47(5):782–5

38. Ikeda AK, et al. (2006) Tumor lysis syndrome. eMedicine from WebMD. Available at http://www.emedicine.com/ped/topic2328.htm

39. Jeha S (2001) Tumor lysis syndrome. Semin Hematol 38(4 Suppl 10):4–8

40. Jona JZ (1999) Progressive tumor necrosis and lethal hyperkalemia in a neonate with sacrococcygeal teratoma (SCT). J Perinatol 19(7):538–40

41. Jones DP, Mahmoud H, Chesney RW (1995) Tumor lysis syndrome: pathogenesis and management. Pediatr Nephrol 9(2):206–12

42. Kanfer A, et al. (1979) Extreme hyperphosphataemia causing acute anuric nephrocalcinosis in lymphosarcoma. Br Med J 1(6174):1320–1

43. Karagiannis A, et al. (2005) Acute renal failure due to tumor lysis syndrome in a patient with non-Hodgkin's lymphoma. Ann Hematol 84(5):343–6

44. Kedar A, Grow W, Neiberger RE (1995) Clinical versus laboratory tumor lysis syndrome in children with acute leukemia. Pediatr Hematol Oncol 12(2):129–34

45. Khan J, Broadbent VA (1993) Tumor lysis syndrome complicating treatment of wide-spread metastatic abdominal rhabdomyosarcoma. Pediatr Hematol Oncol 10(2):151–5

46. Kopecna L, et al. (2002) The analysis of the risks for the development of tumour lysis syndrome in children. Bratisl Lek Listy 103(6):206–9

47. Krakoff IH, Meyer RL (1965) Prevention of hyperuricemia in leukemia and lymphoma: use of allopurinol, a xanthine oxidase inhibitor. JAMA 193:1–6
48. Krimsky WS, Behrens RJ, Kerkvliet GJ (2002) Oncologic emergencies for the internist. Cleve Clin J Med 69(3): 209–10, 213–14, 216–17 passim
49. Kushner BH, et al. (2003) Tumor lysis syndrome, neuroblastoma, and correlation between serum lactate dehydrogenase levels and MYCN-amplification. Med Pediatr Oncol 41(1): 80–2
50. Landgrebe AR, Nyhan WL, Colem M (1975) Urinary-tract stones resulting from the excretion of oxypurinol. N Engl J Med 292(12):626–7
51. LaRosa C, et al. (2007) Acute renal failure from xanthine nephropathy during management of acute leukemia. Pediatr Nephrol 22(1):132–5
52. Lee MH, et al. (2007) Tumour lysis syndrome developing during an operation. Anaesthesia 62(1):85–7
53. Leis JF, et al. (2004) Management of life-threatening pulmonary leukostasis with single agent imatinib mesylate during CML myeloid blast crisis. Haematologica 89(9):ECR30
54. Leonov Y, et al. (1987) Acute tumour lysis syndrome with extreme metabolic abnormalities. Clin Lab Haematol 9(1):85–9
55. Lobe TE, et al. (1990) Fatal refractory hyperkalemia due to tumor lysis during primary resection for hepatoblastoma. J Pediatr Surg 25(2):249–50
56. Lotfi M, Brandwein JM (1998) Spontaneous acute tumor lysis syndrome in acute myeloid leukemia? A single case report with discussion of the literature. Leuk Lymphoma 29(5–6):625–8
57. Macfarlane RJ, McCully BJ, Fernandez CV (2004) Rasburicase prevents tumor lysis syndrome despite extreme hyperleukocytosis. Pediatr Nephrol 19(8):924–7
58. Mahajan A, et al. (2002) Acute tumor lysis syndrome in Hodgkin disease. Med Pediatr Oncol 39(1):69–70
59. Mantadakis E, et al. (1999) Acute renal failure due to obstruction in Burkitt lymphoma. Pediatr Nephrol 13(3):237–40
60. Mato AR, et al. (2006) A predictive model for the detection of tumor lysis syndrome during AML induction therapy. Leuk Lymphoma 47(5):877–83
61. Mihich E, Grindey GB (1977) Multiple basis of combination chemotherapy. Cancer 40(1 Suppl):534–43
62. Milano GM, et al. (2003) Tumor lysis syndrome and neuroblastoma. Med Pediatr Oncol 41(6):592
63. Miyoshi I, et al. (1977) Establishment of an Epstein-Barr virus-negative B-cell lymphoma line from a Japanese Burkitt's lymphoma and its serial passage in hamsters. Cancer 40(6):2999–3003
64. Mohamed AN, et al. (1989) Establishment and characterization of a new human Burkitt's lymphoma cell line (WSU-BL). Cancer 64(5):1041–8
65. Obrador GT, et al. (1997) Acute renal failure due to lymphomatous infiltration of the kidneys. J Am Soc Nephrol 8(8):1348–54
66. Okano M (1997) High susceptibility of an Epstein-Barr virus-converted Burkitt's lymphoma cell line to cytotoxic drugs. Leuk Res 21(5):469–71
67. Przepiorka D, Gonzales-Chambers R (1990) Acute tumor lysis syndrome in a patient with chronic myelogenous leukemia in blast crisis: role of high-dose Ara-C. Bone Marrow Transplant 6(4):281–2
68. Pui CH (2001) Urate oxidase in the prophylaxis or treatment of hyperuricemia: the United States experience. Semin Hematol 38(4 Suppl 10):13–21
69. Pui CH (2002) Rasburicase: a potent uricolytic agent. Expert Opin Pharmacother 3(4):433–42
70. Pui CH, et al. (2001) Recombinant urate oxidase (rasburicase) in the prevention and treatment of malignancy- associated hyperuricemia in pediatric and adult patients: results of a compassionate-use trial. Leukemia 15(10):1505–9
71. Rampello E, Fricia T, Malaguarnera M (2006) The management of tumor lysis syndrome. Nat Clin Pract Oncol 3(8):438–47
72. Sakarcan A, Quigley R (1994) Hyperphosphatemia in tumor lysis syndrome: the role of hemodialysis and continuous veno-venous hemofiltration. Pediatr Nephrol 8(3): 351–3
73. Salkowsky F (1870) Beitrage Zur Kenntins der Leukamie. Virchows Arch Pathol Anat 50:174–7
74. Schelling JR, et al. (1998) Management of tumor lysis syndrome with standard continuous arteriovenous hemodialysis: case report and a review of the literature. Ren Fail 20(4):635–44
75. Silverman P, Distelhorst CW (1989) Metabolic emergencies in clinical oncology. Semin Oncol 16(6):504–15
76. Sood AR, Burry LD, Cheng DK (2007) Clarifying the role of rasburicase in tumor lysis syndrome. Pharmacotherapy 27(1):111–21
77. Spector T (1977) Inhibition of urate production by allopurinol. Biochem Pharmacol 26(5):355–8
78. Stark ME, Dyer MD, Coonley CJ (1987) Fatal acute tumor lysis syndrome with metastatic breast carcinoma. Cancer 60(4):762–4
79. Suh WM, et al. (2007) Acute lymphoblastic leukemia presenting as acute renal failure. Nat Clin Pract Nephrol 3(2):106–10
80. Tomlinson GC, Solberg LA Jr (1984) Acute tumor lysis syndrome with metastatic medulloblastoma. A case report. Cancer 53(8):1783–5
81. Truini-Pittman L, Rossetto C (2002) Pediatric considerations in tumor lysis syndrome. Semin Oncol Nurs 18(3 Suppl 3):17–22
82. Tsimberidou AM, Keating MJ (2005) Hyperuricemic syndromes in cancer patients. Contrib Nephrol 147:47–60
83. Vachvanichsanong P, et al. (1995) Severe hyperphosphatemia following acute tumor lysis syndrome. Med Pediatr Oncol 24(1):63–6
84. Van Der Klooster JM, et al. (2000) Asystole during combination chemotherapy for non-Hodgkin's lymphoma: the acute tumor lysis syndrome. Neth J Med 56(4):147–52
85. Veenstra J, et al. (1994) Tumour lysis syndrome and acute renal failure in Burkitt's lymphoma. Description of 2 cases and a review of the literature on prevention and management. Neth J Med 45(5):211–16
86. Wibe E, et al. (1991) Tumor lysis syndrome. A life-threatening complication during cytostatic treatment of chemosensitive types of cancer. Tidsskr Nor Laegeforen 111(19):2435–7

87. Woo KB, et al. (1980) Analysis of the proliferation kinetics of Burkitt's lymphoma cells. Cell Tissue Kinet 13(6):591–604

88. Wu XW, et al. (1989) Urate oxidase: primary structure and evolutionary implications. Proc Natl Acad Sci USA 86(23):9412–16

89. Wu XW, et al. (1992) Two independent mutational events in the loss of urate oxidase during hominoid evolution. J Mol Evol 34(1):78–84

90. Yarpuzlu AA (2003) A review of clinical and laboratory findings and treatment of tumor lysis syndrome. Clin Chim Acta 333(1):13–18

91. Yeldandi AV, et al. (1992) Localization of the human urate oxidase gene (*UOX*) to 1p22. Cytogenet Cell Genet 61(2):121–2

92. Yeldandi AV, et al. (1992) Molecular evolution of the urate oxidase-encoding gene in hominoid primates: nonsense mutations. Gene 109(2):281–4

93. Zusman J, Brown DM, Nesbit MD (1973) Hyperphosphate-mia, hyperphosphaturia and hypocalcemia in acute lymphoblastic leukemia. N Engl J Med 289(25): 1335–40

Hemolytic Uremic Syndrome

16

S.G. Kiessling and P. Bernard

Contents

Case Vignette

A previously healthy 23-month-old child is admitted to the Pediatric Inpatient Service with pallor, irritability, and decrease in activity as well as urine output. The illness started about 10 days ago with onset of bloody diarrhea, vomiting, and crampy abdominal pain. The diarrhea decreased and the patient improved clinically after 1 week but the family noticed dark urine and irritability on the day of admission. Diapers are less soaked than usual. The parents noted mild periorbital edema and pallor on the morning of presentation.

S.G. Kiessling et al. (eds) *Pediatric Nephrology in the ICU.*
© Springer-Verlag Berlin Heidelberg 2009

> ## Core Messages
>
> › The triad of anemia, thrombocytopenia, and abnormal renal function needs to alert the provider about the possibility of hemolytic uremic syndrome (HUS).
> › Mortality and prognosis of HUS have improved dramatically over the years with improved understanding of the pathophysiology of the disease and advances in fluid and electrolyte management.
> › Early anticipation of and preparation for renal replacement therapy is crucial in the management of oliguric or anuric acute renal failure.
> › Despite the lack of controlled studies, early nutritional support aiming for a positive caloric balance might be an important part of the treatment strategy.

The child was seen in the emergency room, and blood work shows a complete blood count with a hematocrit of 22.3% and a platelet count of 56,000 per mcl. LDH is significantly elevated and the Coombs test is negative. Blood urea nitrogen (BUN) is elevated at 46 mg dL^{-1} with a serum creatinine of 3.2 mg dL^{-1}. There is mild hyponatremia and metabolic acidosis. Peripheral smear confirms schistocytes. Transfer to the Pediatric Intensive Care Unit is arranged as the child becomes clinically more unstable. Twenty-four hours after admission, the child is anuric with progressive anemia and azotemia. A central venous line is placed and preparations for renal replacement therapy are made.

16.1 Introduction

HUS, characterized by the triad of hemolytic anemia, thrombocytopenia, and acute renal insufficiency, is one of the most common causes of acute renal failure in the pediatric age group. It is also known to be associated with a significant risk for the development of chronic renal failure [60]. The disease is known for its unpredictable clinical course and presentation with a wide range of clinical findings, from minimal symptoms to severe involvement of multiple organ systems. Since the first description by Gasser et al. in 1955 [21], the prognosis has improved dramatically; however, given the unpredictable clinical course, hospital admission and transfer to the intensive care unit for management are frequently necessary. Most commonly, HUS presents in the complete form with the triad of a nonimmune, microangiopathic hemolytic anemia (MAHA), thrombocytopenia due to consumption, and oliguric or nonoliguric acute renal insufficiency. The rare incomplete presentation is defined by the combination of either MAHA or thrombocytopenia with acute renal failure. Historically, HUS is associated with significant morbidity and mortality due to the disease itself and therapy-associated complications.

16.2 Classification

HUS is usually divided into a diarrhea positive (D+) and a diarrhea negative group (D−) [18]; this classification is clinically not very useful and often confusing since there is significant overlap between the groups. In this chapter, D + HUS will be used when referral is made to the syndrome being associated with Shiga-toxin-producing *Escherichia coli* 0157:H7, the most common form of HUS in the United States and Europe.

In more than 90% of cases, HUS is caused by Shiga-toxin-producing *Escherichia coli*, first reported by Karmali et al. in 1985, 30 years after the initial report of HUS [29]. Three years prior to that, an association between *E. coli* 0157:H7 and hemorrhagic colitis was reported [43]. HUS can also occur under a variety of other infectious and noninfectious conditions as listed in Table 16.1. Other infectious agents causing HUS include *Shigella dysenteriae* type 1 (also clinically presenting with diarrhea in the majority of cases), *Streptococcus pneumoniae*, and human immunodeficiency virus.

Other types of HUS, clinically not associated with diarrhea as the Shiga-like-toxin-producing *E. coli* or *Shigella dysenteriae*-related forms, are commonly summarized as atypical HUS. This group carries a much higher mortality rate compared with the typical childhood HUS. Some of those forms have a deficiency or defect in Factor H (fH), a glycoprotein,

which is an important component in the regulation of complement, specifically in preventing the production of C5b membrane attack complex and leukotactic C5a by conversion from C3b [6]. The exact role of fH deficiency in the pathogenesis of HUS is unknown but it appears that activation of C3 under those circumstances leads to autoantibody and immunecomplex-mediated glomerular damage. Other, rare forms of atypical HUS are associated with deficiencies in von Willebrand factor-cleaving protease (ADAMTS 13). Von Willebrand factor (VWf), a glycoprotein, forms large multimers able to bridge between platelets and inducing aggregates. This is avoided by ADAMTS 13, a metalloprotease that cleaves VWf before multimeric structures can be formed.

This chapter will focus on the diarrhea positive form of HUS, also frequently referred to as typical HUS.

16.3 Epidemiology of Typical HUS

Enterohemorrhagic *E. coli* (EHEC) are a subclass of *E. coli*, which produce a toxin with the potential to induce hemorrhagic enterocolitis, frequently a clinical prodrome to HUS. It has been estimated in the past that about 5–10% of children infected with Shiga-toxin-producing *E. coli* will progress to HUS [5, 9]. Contributing factors and risk factors leading to progression and ultimately development of the disease have not been clearly identified. This toxin, originally named Verotoxin because of its ability to kill Vero cells (grown from African green monkey kidneys), was renamed Shiga-like toxin because of its close structural relation to the toxin produced by *Shigella dysenteriae* type I, which was detected in 1977.

Shiga-toxin-induced HUS occurs much more commonly during the summer months, mainly June to September. This seems to be at least in part related to the higher incidence of positive fecal cultures for enterohemorrhagic *E. coli* during that time of the year [26]. Since *E. coli* 0157:H7 is frequently colonizing the intestines of cattle, outbreaks have been found to be closely related to contact with beef products [28]. Outbreaks can sometimes be tracked back to a single source of either primarily contaminated beef or unsafe food handling practices [57]. Other risk factors include drinking contaminated water including ingestion of water in swimming pools, handling animal feces, and eating fruit and vegetables fertilized or irrigated with animal manure. Recent outbreaks of *E. coli* 0157:H7 have been widely publicized in

Table 16.1 Classification of hemolytic uremic syndromes in children

1. HUS associated with infection and diarrhea	Shigatoxin-producing EHEC Verotoxin-producing *Shigella dysenteriae*
2. HUS associated with infection	Human immunodeficiency virus *Streptococcus pneumoniae* producing neuraminidase
3. Secondary HUS	SLE and antiphospholipid syndrome
HUS associated with transplantation	Recurrent disease after kidney tranplantation De novo HUS posttransplantation HUS after bone marrow transplantation
HUS associated with drugs	Cytotoxins Calcineurin inhibitors Quinine
Associated with a genetic predisposition	Factor H gene mutations or deficiency von Willebrand factor-cleaving protease deficiency Abnormal Vitamin B12 metabolism
4. HUS of unknown etiology	Autosomal dominant and recessive HUS Idiopathic

conjunction with strawberry and spinach as primary sources. Interestingly, by far the minority of individuals (less than 10%) exposed to *E. coli* 0157:H7 develops the full clinical picture of HUS as shown in a collaborative study by Rowe et al. [47]. Risk factors for progression to typical HUS are unknown, and higher bacterial load does not seem to be correlated with a higher risk to develop disease.

16.4 Pathophysiology

Tsai recently updated our understanding of the molecular biology involved in thrombotic microangiopathies including HUS [55]. The main target of injury in virtually all forms of HUS is the vascular endothelial cell representing the primary step initiating a cascade of events. The Shiga-toxins 1 and 2 produced by *E. coli* are encoded by bacteriophage DNA in contrast to Shiga-toxin from *S. dysenteriae*, a 70-kD protein exotoxin encoded by *S. dysenteriae* DNA. In D + typical HUS, Shiga-toxin, the five B or binding units attached to the A core bind with very high affinity to the glycolipid cell surface receptor globotriaocylceramide (Gb3), inhibiting protein synthesis, leading to cytotoxic injury to target cells including colonic, cerebrovascular, and glomerular epithelial and endothelial cells [55]. The first step in this cascade of events is characterized by intestinal infection of Shiga-toxin-producing *E. coli* in the intestines with consecutive injury to the intestinal epithelial cells inducing bloody diarrhea. The toxin

gains access to the systemic circulation by translocating through the intestinal epithelium [41], binding to Gb3 receptors on endothelial cells in the kidney, brain, and other organs. It also binds to monocytes. Binding to Gb3 on various cell types leads to release of interleukins and chemokines as well as large multimers of vWf secreted by glomerular endothelial cells [38]. Endothelial cell injury leads to release of several intracellular factors including von Willebrand factor and platelet aggregating factor (PAF) [15]. Platelet consumption by formation of hyaline platelet-fibrin microthrombi in areas of endothelial injury leads to consumptive thrombocytopenia [30]. These microthrombi occlude capillaries, in typical HUS, mainly in the kidney. Blood cells passing through injured and (partially) occluded vessels will become dysmorphic and fragmented leading to MAHA and the appearance of schistocytes on the peripheral blood smear. The reticuloendothelial system consecutively removes the fragmented red blood cells (RBCs) from the circulation leading to anemia.

16.5 Clinical Presentation

After a rather short incubation period of only 3–4 days, nine out of ten children present with symptoms of diarrhea. In more than 50% of those cases, the diarrhea becomes bloody within 2–3 days [36, 44]. In typical HUS, the age group at highest risk is between 6 months and 4 years of age with a peak between 12 and 24 months. The diarrhea is often associated with severe, crampy abdominal pain mimicking appendicitis or inflammatory bowel disease. Especially in the early stages of the disease or in the absence of bloody diarrhea, a more aggressive viral gastroenteritis is often the initial working diagnosis. The colitis responsible for the severe diarrhea is often very painful and leads to exhaustion of the child over time. Potential gastrointestinal complications, though rare, include bowel perforation, obstruction, and ischemic infarction. Frequently, the child symptomatically improves with decreased or complete resolution of diarrhea clinically after 5–7 days, at which point irritability and pallor are noted commonly. At that point, most children with typical HUS present with the classic triad of acute renal failure, Coombs-negative hemolytic anemia, and thrombocytopenia leading to the diagnosis. Central nervous system involvement occurs in as many as one-third of children presenting with a variety of clinical findings including seizures, altered level of consciousness, visual and auditory hallucinations, and paresis. Seizures are the most common neurologic finding and are often seen early in the course of the disease. Generalized seizures compared with partial seizures seem to have a better prognosis [16]. In children who require medications for pain control or agitation, a high index of suspicion needs to be kept to differentiate neurologic involvement of HUS from medication effects and side effects. More than 50% of children with typical HUS have a period of oligoanuria for about 1 week, but it can persist for several weeks.

16.6 Diagnosis

The clinical presentation and classic triad of anemia, thrombocytopenia, and renal failure need to alert the provider to include possible HUS in the differential diagnosis. In children with a history of (bloody) diarrhea, anemia, and thrombocytopenia, the diagnosis is normally quite straight forward. In typical HUS, culture of stool within 6 days after onset of the disease on a D-sorbitol-containing McConkey agar yields a positive result in greater than 90% but decreases significantly if sent later in the course [52]. Unfortunately, in the early stages of the disease, the presenting symptoms are commonly unspecific, and *E. coli*-associated diarrhea or HUS is included as a broad range of differential diagnoses. By the time the clinical course becomes more consistent with HUS, the stool culture is frequently

already negative. For that reason, keeping a high index of suspicion early is very important to confirm the diagnosis. Stool should always be sent specifically to assay for *E. coli* 0157:H7 since some children present without abdominal complaints [34].

The anemia is nonimmune mediated and a direct Coombs test is negative. A manual peripheral blood smear usually shows evidence of schistocytes or helmet cells, as well as fragmented RBCs indicating evidence of microangiopathic hemolysis. The fragmentation is thought to occur as RBCs travel through partially occluded areas in the microcirculation causing turbulence and damage to the cells [38]. Thrombocytopenia is usually significant with platelet counts less than 50,000 mm^{-3} but the degree of thrombocytopenia does not necessarily correlate with severity of the disease. Once the diagnosis is suspected, additional laboratory tests are ordered. These include a complete blood count with differential and a reticulocyte count, which is usually elevated indicating an appropriate bone marrow response. Children with *E. coli* 0157:H7 enteritis and an elevated white blood cell count >13,000 per mcl have an up to seven-fold risk to develop HUS but little is known about the effects of initial leukocytosis on prognosis and outcome of typical HUS [6, 13]. A comprehensive metabolic panel with liver function tests, lactate dehydrogenase (LDH), and baseline amylase and lipase should be ordered. Elevation in LDH, abundant in RBCs, is correlated with the degree of hemolysis. A urinalysis to assess for hematuria, hemoglobinuria, and proteinuria should be performed. Microscopic review of a freshly voided urine specimen is very helpful to look for the presence of hyaline, granular and cellular casts, which can be indicative of renal disease but do not necessarily correlate with the degree of injury.

16.7 Differential Diagnosis

HUS, a thrombotic microangiopathy, is usually characterized by the triad of anemia, thrombocytopenia, and acute renal failure. The clinical presentation usually allows differentiation between diarrhea positive and negative forms of HUS, but significant overlap can exist.

Diarrhea secondary to other gastrointestinal infections can potentially present with very similar clinical findings, including amebiasis, Campylobacter, Salmonella, and Shigella gastroenteritis. In cases where diarrhea induces significant dehydration, both the BUN and the creatinine can be elevated mimicking acute renal failure in HUS [2]. In contrast to HUS, the azotemia will improve after proper rehydration and restoration of normal circulating volume.

Thrombotic thrombocytopenic purpura (TTP), another form of MAHA and thrombocytopenia, can present with quite similar clinical symptoms and was in the past thought to be a different presentation of the same disease entity. It was first described by Moschcowitz in 1924 [40]. Both HUS and TTP share the same histological lesions defined by subendothelial space widening and intraluminal thrombi [48]. Whereas platelet-fibrin thrombi are mainly found in the renal circulation in HUS, systemic microvascular aggregation of platelets is causing ischemia to the brain and other organs in TTP. The resulting ischemia to the brain at least partially explains the dominance of neurologic pathology in TTP [38]. Familial forms of TTP in children are caused by a functionally defective metalloprotease called ADAMTS 13, which cleaves large multimers of von Willebrand factor (vWF). This leads to adhesion and aggregation of platelets to vWF multimers ultimately leading to TTP. Other forms of TTP occur in the presence of autoantibodies against ADAMTS 13, transient defects, or abnormal attachment of ADAMTS 13 to endothelial cells [38]. Differentiation of the two entities is very important to decide on appropriate therapies and to optimize outcome. Rarely, patients may present with right lower quadrant pain with preceding diarrhea and be diagnosed with appendicitis [17]. In case reports, appendicitis and HUS have been reported to coexist. Therefore, it is imperative that a high index of suspicion is maintained prior to surgical intervention.

16.8 General Aspects of Management

Given the complexity of the disease and the lack of reliable markers of severity of the clinical course to be expected, inpatient unit admission for further management should be considered in virtually all children once the diagnosis is established. Common reasons for hospital admission or referral to a center experienced in the care of children with HUS include (rapidly) worsening anemia, thrombocytopenia, dec-reased urine output with and without azotemia, electrolyte or acid–base imbalance, and presence of clinically significant blood pressure elevation. The course of HUS is difficult to predict, and children who appear healthy to the treating provider at the initial presentation can worsen within a period of a few hours. For that reason, notifying the pediatric intensivist and planning for early transfer to the ICU have proven to be extremely valuable in our institution. Serial physical exams and blood draws at set intervals to detect changes early are extremely important in the management of the child. A potential diarrhea-induced fluid deficit should be corrected to avoid prolonged prerenal physiology but emphasis needs to be placed on prevention of overcorrection. In other words, once fluid losses have been replaced and perfusion is restored, the strategy needs to be shifted toward replacement of losses to keep fluid balance even and avoid iatrogenic overload. Antibiotics should be avoided in children with evidence of E. coli 0157:H7-induced diarrhea as there is evidence of an increased risk of developing typical HUS [59]. This is thought to be due to increased release of Shiga toxin from bacteria. Also, antimotility drugs appear to increase the risk of progression to HUS in individuals infected with E. coli O157:H7.

Communication with the family is very important. The disease itself and the unpredictable course should be discussed at length initially. Frequent updates will allow the family to better understand potential interventions as they might become necessary at some point during the course of the disease.

16.8.1 Management in the Intensive Care Unit

From a patient care perspective, early transfer of the child to the ICU has several benefits. Common criteria for transfer of care include clinical deterioration and need for closer monitoring, cardiovascular instability, and oligoanuria with impending need for renal replacement therapy. ICU staffing ratios allow close observation and documentation of clinical status with recognition of deterioration of the patient as it occurs rather frequently in HUS. Balancing intake (oral and intravenous fluids) and output (urine, stool, and insensible losses) at set close intervals will allow an accurate assessment of the child's fluid status and early detection of decreased urine output in case of development of oligoanuric acute renal failure. Fluids should be restricted early in cases where volume-related cardiopulmonary effects have been noticed [53]. This is of importance to avoid potential iatrogenic fluid overload. An accurately measured weight of the patient, recorded once or twice per day, can be very helpful to correctly assess the volume status. In edematous patients, either due to severe hypoalbuminemia or a primary vascular leak, the weight on the other hand might not be truly reflecting intravascular or circulating volume status rather than total volume.

Serum electrolytes and acid–base status need to be followed very closely, especially in the setting of decreased urine output. Hyponatremia, most common dilutional, is seen quite frequently in children with HUS and needs to be addressed by minimizing free water excess. Hypotonic fluids should not be administered as the degree of hyponatremia is correlated with the severity of neurologic injury [37]. Intravenous medication infusions should be, if possible, mixed in isotonic saline once hyponatremia is recognized to be progressive. Repeat blood work to assess renal function and serum electrolytes, and progression of anemia will influence the decision to place central venous access or a peritoneal dialysis catheter. Central venous access should be placed early in cases where the clinical course indicates worsening renal function or a progressively positive fluid balance in the setting of decreased urine output. Placement of invasive lines should only be undertaken by experienced professionals as bleeding complications are not infrequently encountered. Early dialysis access placement will avoid difficulties due to marked volume overload and edema and might decrease the risk of procedure-associated complications. Presence of hypertension or respiratory involvement might require the insertion of an arterial line for blood gas and accurate blood pressure monitoring. Also, in most centers, acute forms of dialysis are preferentially performed in the ICU setting, especially continuous renal replacement therapy in the form of CVVH(DF).

16.8.2 Management of Anemia

The potential need for packed red blood cell (PRBC) transfusion in children with HUS has been reported to be as high as 80% [11]. Children with HUS can experience a significant drop in the hemoglobin and hematocrit level within a short period of time, and CBCs need to be followed quite closely, as often as three to four times per day depending on clinical circumstances, to correctly assess the trend. Plasma LDH, an enzyme catalyzing the conversion from pyruvate to lactate, present in abundance in RBCs and released by their breakdown, is a very useful parameter to assess the degree of hemolysis and can be used to assess the potential need for future transfusion. Once dialysis is initiated, its use becomes limited since LDH levels are affected by all forms of renal replacement therapy.

There are no consensus guidelines on when transfusion of packed RBCs becomes an absolute indication. As recently reported by Laverdiere et al. [33], transfusion practices among intensivists vary significantly between centers depending on a variety of factors including type of disease and hemoglobin levels. This does not seem to be different for HUS, and therefore transfusion practices vary depending on experience, provider, and center. Usually, transfusion can be delayed as long as oxygen delivery to the tissue is sufficient and there is no significant cardiovascular or hemodynamic compromise in the patient. On the other hand, a recent study by Grant et al. [25] has shown that in the state of acute anemia, adaptive changes compensate for decreased oxygen delivery. It is unclear if this adaptive state could influence the overall outcome in critically ill individuals.

One of the main risks of blood transfusions is related reactions. Even though it is at times difficult to distinguish between symptoms related to the underlying disease and a true reaction to transfusion, the incidence of transfusion-related reactions has been reported to be as high as 1.6% in a prospective trial [22]. Another important factor to consider when making the decision to transfuse packed red cells is the strong potential of bone marrow suppression in a patient who has an appropriate bone marrow response indicated by an elevated reticulocyte count. Recently, Lacroix et al. [32] recommended a restrictive transfusion strategy and to withhold transfusion in critically ill but stable children until the hemoglobin falls below 7 g dL^{-1}. Serum potassium levels need to be followed closely due to risk of transfusion-related hyperkalemia, especially in the setting of renal dysfunction.

Common criteria for PRBC transfusion include a rapid drop in hemoglobin and hematocrit levels, symptoms associated with anemia, and hematocrit levels less than 18%. Some authors recommend withholding transfusion to even lower hematocrit levels [50]. Frequently, once the decision for transfusion is made, a volume of 10 cc kg^{-1} is transfused over several hours, not faster than at a rate of 2–3 cc kg^{-1} h^{-1} in the hemodynamically stable child. The volume of cells (in cc) can also be calculated by multiplying the estimated blood volume of the child with the desired hematocrit change and by dividing the result by the hematocrit of PBRCs (which is usually around 65%) [12]. Posttransfusion hematocrit levels above 30% (hemoglobin greater than 10 g dL^{-1}) are rarely necessary and carry a significant risk of hypertension, especially in the oligoanuric patient.

16.8.3 Management of Thrombocytopenia

Thrombocytopenia in HUS is secondary to endothelial injury with consumption of platelets in microthrombi [30]. This is a dynamic process, and studies have shown that prolonged thrombocytopenia is associated with an increased risk for long-term renal abnormalities [7]. There are no consensus guidelines on the management of thrombocytopenia in HUS, and the therapeutic approach oftentimes varies significantly depending on the center and the group of treating providers. Limited available data caution treating providers to withhold platelet transfusion given the potential to increase formation of hyaline platelet-fibrin thrombi and worsening of microthrombi by transfusing additional platelets [24, 27]. An absolute indication for platelet transfusion in the setting of documented thrombocytopenia is acute and clinically significant bleeding, which is rarely seen in clinical practice; most centers also agree on platelet transfusion as a prophylactic measure before performing an invasive procedure such as placement of a central venous catheter. Platelets are consumed quite rapidly in the acute phase of the disease; therefore, timing of the transfusion as close to a procedure is possible (or still infusing during the procedure) and appears to be reasonable.

16.8.4 Management of Acute Renal Failure

In the initial stages after the diagnosis of typical HUS has been established, focus is on conservative medical management of acute renal failure. Renal failure can present either in the oligoanuric form or nonoligoanuric form. Accurate fluid management is critical for both groups since renal failure can progress toward oligoanuria at any point in time. A recent study has shown limited evidence of the potential benefit that intravenous fluid expansion very early in the disease might decrease the risk for developing oligoanuric renal failure [1]. Unfortunately, in clinical practice, the diagnosis of HUS is rarely based on the presence of bloody diarrhea early on so that evidence of renal failure in one form or another is already present at the time the correct diagnosis is made. This includes medical management of hyperkalemia and other electrolyte imbalances, acid–base abnormalities, and close documentation of the fluid balance by measuring intake and output including insensible losses $(350–400\,cc\,m^{-2})$; this is important to avoid volume overload, one of the most common indications for initiation of renal replacement therapy. In case of a positive fluid balance and presence of oliguria, it is often useful to consider a trial of diuretics. Loop diuretics are commonly used as first-line agents to increase urine output and to ameliorate fluid overload. There is ongoing debate about the optimal diuretic prescription. It appears that in hemodynamically unstable children continuous intravenous infusion is superior to bolus administration, mainly due to better controlled diuresis and decreased risk for iatrogenic volume depletion with potential for secondary renal injury [31]. A trial of furosemide at a dose of 2–4 $mg\,kg^{-1}\,dose^{-1}$ or as continuous drip should be considered. The addition of a *downstream* thiazide diuretic can potentially further enhance urine output. In a recent meta-analysis of patients with acute renal failure (including critically ill patients), loop diuretics did not affect mortality or the need for renal replacement therapy but shortened the duration of dialysis and improved urine output [3]. However, since the majority of the patients in these studies were not critically ill, conclusions for this particular population are difficult to make.

16.8.4.1 *Indications for Renal Replacement Therapy*

HUS is one of the most common reasons for acute renal failure encountered in the ICU setting. Because of advances in research and clinical experience, the prognosis of acute renal failure in general has dramatically improved over the last 20 years [58]. These advances are due to a combination of several factors, including availability of continuous forms of hemodialysis in children, especially younger children, quality of vascular access, and our improved understanding of the pathophysiology of individual disease entities [35]. Despite optimal conservative management of acute renal failure, as many as 30–50% of children with HUS will require initiation of renal replacement therapy during the course of the disease. Acute renal failure in children has a very high chance of recovery, sometimes even after weeks of oligoanuria, and the majority of children will need renal replacement therapy only for a limited period of time. Preparing the family and child for possible initiation of renal replacement therapy in a timely fashion is crucial in the management of the child with HUS. Several factors need to be taken into consideration, most of all modes of dialysis and early provision of proper access by the pediatric intensivist or pediatric surgeon. Having central venous access available early will avoid difficulties with placement in the setting of volume overload and edema. There is no consensus for the optimal point in time to initiate renal replacement therapy. It is helpful to decide on a mode of dialysis sooner than later so that staff and providers have sufficient time to plan for staffing needs and provision of supplies. Studies have also shown that patients with less volume overload and lower levels of uremia might have an overall better prognosis [23, 46].

The absolute indications for dialysis in children with acute renal failure related to HUS are essentially the same as for any other child suffering from acute renal insufficiency (Table 16.2). It is important to remember that all modalities of dialysis have certain potential risks and that conservative management should be optimized before renal replacement therapy is initiated. This includes fluid restriction for a reasonable period of time and use of a diuretic regimen in the setting of oligoanuria. In the presence of hyperkalemia, diuretics, bicarbonate and potassium binding resins among others (see chapter on hyperkalemia) should be used until proven noneffective and the decision to proceed with dialysis is made. It is important to remember that insulin with glucose and treatment with bicarbonate only lead to a temporary decrease in extracellular potassium levels by intracellular shifting but not decreasing total body potassium. Children with acute renal failure in the intensive care unit are frequently malnourished, often due to a combination of an exhausting primary disease and malabsorption of nutrients [4]. In the past, fluid restriction to avoid a positive fluid balance in a child with oligoanuric renal failure was one of the mainstays of supportive care. Though early dialysis has not been shown to alter the outcome, there is evidence that optimizing nutrition in individuals with acute renal failure leads to a higher rate of recovery. It seems therefore intuitive that early dialysis in oligoanuric children and avoidance of prolonged nutritional restriction might be a reasonable

strategy. Caloric intake should match at least the minimal recommended daily allowance adjusted for age. Assistance by an experienced dietician/nutritionist to optimize the child's nutrition is extremely valuable. Abnormalities in a baseline cholesterol and triglyceride levels might warrant restriction of lipids, which is otherwise not recommended. Need for possible total parenteral nutrition for a period of time in children not tolerating enteral feedings should be assessed early since placement of central venous access can be coordinated with the placement of dialysis access to avoid additional procedural sedation.

16.8.4.2 Choice of Dialysis Modality

Most intensive care units in tertiary care centers will be able to perform all available forms of renal replacement therapy under the direction of the Pediatric Nephrologist and Intensivist. The choice of dialysis mode depends on the individual experience of the treating providers and center. Peritoneal dialysis (PD) is frequently the preferred mode unless abdominal complications, most often serious colitis requiring surgical intervention, pose a contraindication to this form of renal replacement therapy. PD can be learned quite easily and does not require the presence and experience of specialized staff as in the other forms of renal replacement therapy. The peritoneal dialysis catheter can be placed at the bedside or in the operating room and is essentially ready for use immediately after placement. Peritoneal dialysis solutions are available from a number of manufacturers containing 1.5, 2.5, and 4.25% dextrose. An example of an initial PD regimen is hourly exchanges (5-min fill, 45-min dwell, and 10-min drain) with 2.5% dextrose at a fill volume of $10\,cc\,kg^{-1}$ of body weight. Three variables allow adjustment of the ultrafiltration volume and clearance: dextrose content of the solution, fill volume, and frequency of exchanges. Main complications seen in the acute PD setting are leakage around the catheter entry site (since the catheter has no time to heal in), peritonitis, abdominal discomfort, and respiratory compromise.

With advances in filter size, availability of pediatric tubing and improved accuracy of ultrafiltration, continuous forms of hemodiafiltration (CVVHDF) have become available for smaller and younger children, even for infants. Continuous forms of renal replacement therapy are quite gentle and used in the cooperative child but require the presence of experienced personnel. Sedation and potentially intubation might be required for a younger child to successfully perform the procedure, interventions that are rarely necessary

Table 16.2 Indications for renal replacement therapy in typical hemolytic uremic syndrome

1 Need for adequate nutrition
2 Clinically significant volume overload
3 Medically noncontrollable hyperkalemia
4 Metabolic acidosis refractory to conservative therapy
5 Progressive and profound azotemia
6 Need for transfusion of blood products in the setting of oliguria
7 Removal of inflammatory mediators in the critically ill child

with peritoneal dialysis. Advantages of CVVHDF include but are not limited to gentle fluid removal in the hemodynamically unstable child, slow reduction of azotemia, and also easier control of fluid balance compared with both peritoneal and intermittent hemodialysis (IHD). Care must be taken with respect to bleeding complications, clotting of the circuit, and infection. A more detailed discussion of CVVDHF is beyond the scope of this chapter.

Young age and cardiovascular instability of the child frequently limit the potential success of intermittent hemodialysis, the third option in acute renal failure; most centers prefer the other modalities, especially in young children. Despite significant progress and increasing experience with IHD, it remains a challenging procedure to perform especially in young children, who are most commonly affected by D+ HUS. IHD requires nursing staff with experience in hemodialysis that is not readily available in all, even larger institutions. Fluid removal and electrolyte shifting occur over a much shorter time compared with the other forms of dialysis, making this a suboptimal mode of therapy in the hemodynamically unstable patient. Also, it requires careful and advanced planning of fluid removal (ultrafiltration) and fluid balance, both of which can change unexpectedly for a variety of reasons (need for transfusion, intravenous medications, and others). In case the decision to perform IHD is made, treatments should be performed daily given recently supported evidence of improved outcome in a study on adults with acute renal failure [49].

16.8.4.3 Supportive Therapies

The usefulness of plasmapheresis in HUS has been vigorously debated but no consensus approach has emerged so far. Whereas there seems to be a benefit of plasmapheresis in TTP, no clear benefit has been documented in standard-risk HUS [8]. In high-risk HUS on the other hand (atypical HUS, hypertension, and neurologic involvement) and TTP, plasmapheresis has been shown to be beneficial [8, 45].

Antithrombotic agents, thought to have an effect on formation of microthrombi, have been used in clinical trials in the 1980s with no significant difference in the outcome in treatment vs control groups [56]. Moreover, treatment groups had a higher incidence of bleeding.

In the late 1990s Synsorb-Pk, an oral Shiga-toxin binding agent, was used in a controlled clinical study in children with confirmed HUS, but there was no documented difference with regard to mortality [54].

16.8.5 Management of Complications

The spectrum of complications potentially associated with HUS is broad even though the occurrence of serious complications is uncommon. For the clinician, it is important to be familiar with and to be able to differentiate complications from primary disease as opposed to adverse effects of the supportive therapies initiated. This is especially important in the context of neurologic findings. A system-based approach is helpful to organize and manage these issues.

16.8.5.1 Cardiovascular Complications

Hypertension is commonly associated with HUS and can be severe. For that reason, diligent blood pressure monitoring during the acute stage of the disease is mandatory. A detailed discussion on the topic of hypertension can be found elsewhere is this book. In HUS, two major factors have been found to be of significance in the pathogenesis of hypertension: First, hyper expansion of the intravascular volume secondary to an imbalance of fluid needs and inability to excrete and second, activation of the renin–angiotension–aldosterone axis (RAA) due to hypoxic-ischemic pre- and intrarenal injury. In children in the ICU, hypertension is most commonly a combination of both factors. As already outlined, accurate fluid management is crucial to minimize the risk for volume overload and related blood pressure elevation but also to prevent further prerenal injury by preventing volume depletion. Accurate blood pressure readings are extremely important to assess the need for therapy. Especially in very young or uncooperative children, documenting accurate blood pressure readings can be challenging, and placement of an arterial line can be useful. Depending on the severity of the child's illness and degree of blood pressure elevation, either intravenous or oral antihypertensive treatment needs to be considered if elevated blood pressure readings are sustained. The choice of category of the antihypertensive depends on individual preference and route of administration. In the intensive care setting, intravenous therapy is often preferred at least initially and direct vasodilators, beta blockers, or calcium channel antagonists among others can be considered depending on the individual patient.

16.8.5.2 Gastrointestinal Complications

As outlined earlier, gastrointestinal complications of varying severity are rare but have been reported during the acute phase of the disease. Complications involving the colon appear to be the main reason for surgical consultation, mostly due to bowel perforation as shown by Brandt et al. [10]. Pancreatic involvement in HUS is rather common but generally mild, nevertheless severe cases have been reported in the past [42]. Other potential complications include cholelithiasis and rectal prolapse.

16.8.5.3 Neurologic Complications

The brain is the most commonly involved organ in D+ HUS following the intestines and the kidney. Significant neurologic involvement as indicated by the presence of mental status changes, seizures, generalized or focal neurological deficits, or evidence of cerebrovascular events is commonly associated with a poor prognosis and outcome. Any unexplained neurologic symptoms warrant timely and thorough investigation, preferably under the guidance of a pediatric neurologist. This is especially important in cases where the clinical differentiation between HUS and TTP is difficult and plasmapheresis is considered. Magnetic resonance imaging with attention to ischemia as well as electroencephalography to rule out subclinical status epilepticus can be helpful diagnostic tests. It is also important to recognize the myriad of adverse effects of medications used for supportive therapy in HUS, especially in children receiving sedatives to successfully perform renal replacement therapy or other reasons. Minimizing the use of those agents or a trial off might help to differentiate between disease-associated pathology and medication side effects.

16.8.5.4 Other Complications

Pulmonary edema is encountered frequently in HUS. With judicious fluid management and early renal replacement therapy this complication is on the other hand rarely clinically significant. Pancreatic involvement including pancreatitis and transient diabetes mellitus has been reported in 5–15% of individuals [15]. Therefore, close monitoring of serum blood glucose levels and involvement of a pediatric endocrinologist as necessary is recommended.

16.9   Follow-Up and Prognosis

Long-term renal abnormalities are detected in as many as 30–50% of individuals after recovery from HUS [51] despite mortality in the acute phase of the disease dropping to less than 5%. Approximately 5% of patients require long-term dialysis [15]. Since therapy has over the years remained mainly supportive, this

decrease in mortality is primarily due to increased experience and expertise in managing fluid balance and electrolyte abnormalities [15] and improvement of renal replacement therapy. Duration of required renal replacement therapy and risk for chronic renal disease are closely associated. Patients who need dialysis for more than 1 week are at higher risk of chronic renal disease compared with others. Patients requiring renal replacement therapy for more than 1 month and recovering normal renal function after that period of time are the exception. Children with persistent proteinuria, microscopic hematuria, hypertension or those individuals whose level of azotemia do not return to baseline are at highest risk for long-term kidney abnormalities. In a large systemic review by Garg et al. an excellent prognosis was associated with absence of overt proteinuria, predicted creatinine clearance greater than $80\,cc\,min^{-1}$ per $1.73\,m^{-2}$, and normotension greater than 1 year after recovery from the acute event of D + HUS [20]. While renal biopsies are rarely done in modern practice, it appears that cortical necrosis and a greater than 50% disease involvement of glomeruli on histopathology correlate with a poorer prognosis. The clinical course on the other hand might not necessarily predict long-term outcome; renal histology seems to be the best prognostic indicator [19].

Moghal et al. [39] have shown that persistent proteinuria and renal pathology findings on biopsy specimen consistent with hyperfiltration and hyperperfusion injury are closely correlated. Even after apparent full recovery with benign urine sediment, absence of hypertension, and normal renal function on blood work, there is a risk for renal dysfunction to become overt years after the disease and patients need to be followed at set intervals. Conversely, proof of causal relation between HUS and new onset of hypertension or renal damage in the form of proteinuria or hematuria or other pathology years after complete recovery is difficult, and defining true incidence is problematic. Regardless, close follow-up in intervals is of absolute importance for any child after the acute phase of HUS, especially in children who continue to experience signs of persistent renal dysfunction, including hypertension, azotemia, and an abnormal urinalysis with proteinuria or microhematuria.

16.10   Prevention of Typical HUS

Typical D+ HUS is most commonly related to exposure to enterohemorrhagic *E. coli* and therefore, key to disease prevention is to minimize exposure risk and avoidance of bacterial spreading. Proper handling of meat products and preparation of foods, especially ground beef, if cooked to an internal temperature of at least 155 °F can reduce the risk of infection with EHEC. Pasteurization of milk products is also recommended. Early identification of index cases and notification of the local health department to detect the source might help prevent bacterial spread and exposure of other individuals. Even though there are currently no measures to prevent progression of infection with *E. coli* 0157:H7 to the complete form of HUS, early detection of children at risk theoretically could improve management and overall outcome.

Public health outbreaks have been widely publicized in relationship to contaminated swimming water. Local regulations should address pool safety, and swimming pool operators should be encouraged to enforce the use of disposable swim diapers. Some operators now provide these diapers free of charge in response to potential litigation.

Promising basic science development includes intranasal application of the B subunit of *E. coli* Shigatoxin. In a rodent model, rats given the intranasal application showed a neutralizing antibody response [14]. This could be of importance for the development of a vaccine directed against *E. coli* 0157:H7 in the future.

Take-Home Pearls

> Typical HUS is among the most common causes of acute renal failure in children.
> Public education is essential to decreasing the incidence of the disease.
> Early recognition may advert complications such as inadvertent surgical intervention, neurologic involvement, and respiratory failure.
> The decision to transfuse RBCs and platelets should be individualized and based on the severity and stage of the disease as well as associated symptoms.
> Given the overall large percentage of children with chronic renal injury, long-term follow-up is mandatory in the majority of cases.

References

1. Ake JA, Jelacic S, Ciol MA, et al (2005) Relative nephroprotection during Escherichia coli O157:H7 infections: association with intravenous volume expansion. Pediatrics 115:e673–80
2. Amirlak I, Amirlak B (2006) Haemolytic uraemic syndrome: an overview. Nephrology (Carlton) 11:213–8
3. Bagshaw SM, Delaney A, Haase M, et al (2007) Loop diuretics in the management of acute renal failure: a systematic review and meta-analysis. Crit Care Resusc 9:60–8
4. Barletta GM, Bunchman TE (2004) Acute renal failure in children and infants. Curr Opin Crit Care 10:499–504
5. Bell BP, Goldoft M, Griffin PM, et al (1994) A multistate outbreak of Escherichia coli O157:H7-associated bloody diarrhea and hemolytic uremic syndrome from hamburgers. The Washington experience. JAMA 272:1349–53
6. Bell BP, Griffin PM, Lozano P, et al (1997) Predictors of hemolytic uremic syndrome in children during a large outbreak of Escherichia coli O157:H7 infections. Pediatrics 100:E12
7. Bolande RP, Kaplan BS (1985) Experimental studies on the hemolytic-uremic syndrome. Nephron 39:228–36
8. Bosch T, Wendler T (2001) Extracorporeal plasma treatment in thrombotic thrombocytopenic purpura and hemolytic uremic syndrome: a review. Ther Apher 5:182–5
9. Boyce TG, Swerdlow DL, Griffin PM (1995) Escherichia coli O157:H7 and the hemolytic-uremic syndrome. N Engl J Med 333:364–8
10. Brandt ML, O'Regan S, Rousseau E, et al (1990) Surgical complications of the hemolytic-uremic syndrome. J Pediatr Surg 25:1109–12
11. Brandt JR, Fouser LS, Watkins SL, et al (1994) Escherichia coli O 157:H7-associated hemolytic-uremic syndrome after ingestion of contaminated hamburgers. J Pediatr 125:519–26
12. Brunetti M, Cohen J, Hematology. In: Robertson J and Shilkofski N (2005) The Harriet Lane Handbook. Elsevier, Mosby Philadelphia, p 358
13. Buteau C, Proulx F, Chaibou M, et al (2000) Leukocytosis in children with Escherichia coli O157:H7 enteritis developing the hemolytic-uremic syndrome. Pediatr Infect Dis J 19:642–7
14. Byun Y, Ohmura M, Fujihashi K, et al (2001) Nasal immunization with E. coli verotoxin 1 (VT1)-B subunit and a nontoxic mutant of cholera toxin elicits serum neutralizing antibodies. Vaccine 19:2061–70
15. Corrigan JJ Jr., Boineau FG (2001) Hemolytic-uremic syndrome. Pediatr Rev 22:365–9
16. Dhuna A, Pascual Leone A, Talwar D, et al (1992) EEG and seizures in children with hemolytic-uremic syndrome. Epilepsia 33:482–6
17. Edmonson MB, Chesney RW (1978) Hemolytic-uremic syndrome confused with acute appendicitis. Arch Surg 113:754–5
18. Fitzpatrick MM, Walters MD, Trompeter RS, et al (1993) Atypical (non-diarrhea-associated) hemolytic-uremic syndrome in childhood. J Pediatr 122:532–7
19. Gagnadoux MF, Habib R, Gubler MC, et al (1996) Long-term (15–25 years) outcome of childhood hemolytic-uremic syndrome. Clin Nephrol 46:39–41
20. Garg AX, Suri RS, Barrowman N, et al (2003) Long-term renal prognosis of diarrhea-associated hemolytic uremic syndrome: a systematic review, meta-analysis, and meta-regression. JAMA 290:1360–70
21. Gasser C, Gautier E, Steck A, et al (1955) Hemolytic-uremic syndrome: bilateral necrosis of the renal cortex in acute acquired hemolytic anemia. Schweiz Med Wochenschr. 85:905–9
22. Gauvin F, Lacroix J, Robillard P, et al (2006) Acute transfusion reactions in the pediatric intensive care unit. Transfusion 46:1899–908
23. Goldstein SL, Currier H, Graf C, et al (2001) Outcome in children receiving continuous venovenous hemofiltration. Pediatrics 107:1309–12

24. Gordon LI, Kwaan HC, Rossi EC (1987) Deleterious effects of platelet transfusions and recovery thrombocytosis in patients with thrombotic microangiopathy. Semin Hematol 24:194–201

25. Grant MJ, Huether SE and Witte MK (2003) Effect of red blood cell transfusion on oxygen consumption in the anemic pediatric patient. Pediatr Crit Care Med 4:459–64

26. Hancock DD, Besser TE, Kinsel ML, et al (1994) The prevalence of *Escherichia coli* O157.H7 in dairy and beef cattle in Washington State. Epidemiol Infect 113:199–207

27. Harkness DR, Byrnes JJ, Lian EC, et al (1981) Hazard of platelet transfusion in thrombotic thrombocytopenic purpura. JAMA 246:1931–3

28. Hussein HS (2007) Prevalence and pathogenicity of Shiga toxin-producing *Escherichia coli* in beef cattle and their products. J Anim Sci 85:E63–72

29. Karmali MA, Petric M, Lim C, et al (1985) The association between idiopathic hemolytic uremic syndrome and infection by verotoxin-producing *Escherichia coli*. J Infect Dis 151:775–82

30. Karpman D, Manea M, Vaziri-Sani F, et al (2006) Platelet activation in hemolytic uremic syndrome. Semin Thromb Hemost 32:128–45

31. Klinge J (2001) Intermittent administration of furosemide or continuous infusion in critically ill infants and children: does it make a difference? Intens Care Med 27:623–4

32. Lacroix J, Hebert PC, Hutchison JS, et al (2007) Transfusion strategies for patients in pediatric intensive care units. N Engl J Med 356:1609–19

33. Laverdiere C, Gauvin F, Hebert PC, et al (2002) Survey on transfusion practices of pediatric intensivists. Pediatr Crit Care Med 3:335–40

34. Loirat C, Taylor C, Hemolytic Uremic Syndromes. In: Avner E, Harmon W, Niaudet P (2004) Pediatric Nephrology. Lippincott, Williams and Wilkins, pp 887–915

35. Maxvold NJ, Bunchman TE (2003) Renal failure and renal replacement therapy. Crit Care Clin 19:563–75

36. Mead PS, Griffin PM (1998) *Escherichia coli* O157:H7. Lancet 352:1207 12

37. Milford D, Taylor CM (1989) Hyponatraemia and haemolytic uraemic syndrome. Lancet 1:439

38. Moake JL (2002) Thrombotic microangiopathies. N Engl J Med 347:589–600

39. Moghal NE, Ferreira MA, Howie AJ, et al (1998) The late histologic findings in diarrhea-associated hemolytic uremic syndrome. J Pediatr 133:220–3

40. Moschcowitz E (1924) Hyaline thrombosis of the terminal arterioles and capillaries: a hitherto undescribed disease. Proc N Y Pathol Soc 24:21

41. Nataro JP, Kaper JB (1998) Diarrheagenic *Escherichia coli*. Clin Microbiol Rev 11:142–201

42. Rebouissoux L, Llanas B, Jouvencel P, et al (2004) Pancreatic pseudocyst complicating hemolytic-uremic syndrome. J Pediatr Gastroenterol Nutr 38:102–4

43. Riley LW, Remis RS, Helgerson SD, et al (1983) Hemorrhagic colitis associated with a rare *Escherichia coli* serotype. N Engl J Med 308:681–5

44. Robson WL, Leung AK, Kaplan BS (1993) Hemolytic-uremic syndrome. Curr Probl Pediatr 23:16–33

45. Rock GA, Shumak KH, Buskard NA, et al (1991) Comparison of plasma exchange with plasma infusion in the treatment of thrombotic thrombocytopenic purpura. Canadian Apheresis Study Group. N Engl J Med 325:393–7

46. Ronco C, Bellomo R, Homel P, et al (2000) Effects of different doses in continuous veno-venous haemofiltration on outcomes of acute renal failure: a prospective randomised trial. Lancet 356:26–30

47. Rowe PC, Orrbine E, Lior H, et al (1998) Risk of hemolytic uremic syndrome after sporadic *Escherichia coli* O157: H7 infection: results of a Canadian collaborative study. Investigators of the Canadian Pediatric Kidney Disease Research Center. J Pediatr 132:777–82

48. Ruggenenti P, Remuzzi G (1998) Pathophysiology and management of thrombotic microangiopathies. J Nephrol 11:300–10

49. Schiffl H, Lang SM, Fischer R (2002) Daily hemodialysis and the outcome of acute renal failure. N Engl J Med 346:305–10

50. Siegler RL (1995) The hemolytic uremic syndrome. Pediatr Clin North Am 42:1505–29

51. Siegler R, Oakes R (2005) Hemolytic uremic syndrome; pathogenesis, treatment, and outcome. Curr Opin Pediatr 17:200–4

52. Tarr PI, Neill MA, Clausen CR, et al (1990) *Escherichia coli* O157:H7 and the hemolytic uremic syndrome: importance of early cultures in establishing the etiology. J Infect Dis 162:553–6

53. Tarr PI, Gordon CA, Chandler WL, et al (2005) Shiga-toxin-producing *Escherichia coli* and haemolytic uraemic syndrome. Lancet 365:1073–86

54. Trachtman H, Cnaan A, Christen E, et al (2003) Effect of an oral Shiga toxin-binding agent on diarrhea-associated hemolytic uremic syndrome in children: a randomized controlled trial. JAMA 290:1337–44

55. Tsai HM (2006) The molecular biology of thrombotic microangiopathy. Kidney Int 70:16–23

56. Van Damme-Lombaerts R, Proesmans W, Van Damme B, et al (1988) Heparin plus dipyridamole in childhood hemolytic-uremic syndrome: a prospective, randomized study. J Pediatr 113:913–8

57. Vogt RL, Dippold L (2005) *Escherichia coli* O157:H7 outbreak associated with consumption of ground beef, June–July 2002. Public Health Rep 120:174–8

58. Warady BA, Bunchman T (2000) Dialysis therapy for children with acute renal failure: survey results. Pediatr Nephrol 15:11–3

59. Wong CS, Jelacic S, Habeeb RL, et al (2000) The risk of the hemolytic-uremic syndrome after antibiotic treatment of *Escherichia coli* O157:H7 infections. N Engl J Med 342:1930–6

60. North American Pediatric Renal Transplant Cooperative Study Annual Report: renal tranplantation, dialysis, chronic renal insufficiency. (2005) Rockville, MD

Vasculitis

17

James A. Listman and Scott J. Schurman

Contents

Case Vignette

NR was a 9-year-old, previously healthy, girl, who presented with a seven-day history of vomiting, watery diarrhea, weight loss, fever, and lethargy. The gastrointestinal losses were nonbloody, but her urine was dark brown the prior 2 days and was reduced in volume. She also had a rash on her left leg described as the remnants of an infected bug bite she developed 3 weeks prior. This responded well to a 2 week course of antibiotics. She was not taking medications chronically, but she was using acetaminophen for the fever. There was no history of upper or lower respiratory tract problems.

On physical examination, she was pale and appeared moderately ill and dehydrated. She had a temperature of 39 °C, a blood pressure of 133/75 mmHg, and a pulse of 114 beats per minute. The remainder of the examination was only remarkable for a 3 cm red and slightly raised circular lesion on the left lower leg.

S.G. Kiessling et al. (eds) *Pediatric Nephrology in the ICU.*
© Springer-Verlag Berlin Heidelberg 2009

Core Messages

Vasculitis can present with a myriad of signs and symptoms, some of which are classic, but in many instances the presentation overlaps with other diseases (Table 17.1).

The rarity of vasculitis in conjunction with an incomplete presentation may delay diagnosis, potentially increasing morbidity, and mortality.

From a nephrological perspective, nephritis or hypertension typically leads to consultation.

Work-up can be broad and might include laboratory testing, imaging, and biopsy (Table 17.2).

Therapeutic options and aggressiveness are often dictated more by the severity of symptoms than the etiology of the disease:

> Pulse dose steroids should be considered up front as empiric therapy as long as there is reasonable certainty regarding the absence of malignancy or underlying infection.

> Patients with an immediately life-threatening presentation should also be considered for therapeutic plasma exchange, though its benefit is not always clear in all forms of vasculitis.

> Cytotoxic agents have a proven role in most forms of vasculitis.

> IVIG is less well studied (the exception being Kawasaki syndrome), but the literature is full of anecdotal successes with its use.

> Newer immunomodulatory agents are also undergoing evaluation.

The outlook for many contemporary pediatric cases is not as bleak as it once was, particularly if the diagnosis is made early.

Initial laboratory investigations showed normal white blood cell (WBC) and platelet counts, but marked anemia with a hemoglobin of 6.4 g dl^{-1}. The blood smear showed fragmented red blood cells (RBCs) and large platelets. Serum BUN and creatinine

Table 17.1 Differential diagnosis

> Menigiococcal infection
> Malignancy
> Endocarditis
> SLE
> HSP
> Postinfectious GN
> Systemic polyangiitis (Wegener granulomatosis, microscopic polyangitis, polyarteritis nodosa)
> Renal vein thrombosis with pulmonary embolism
> Hemolytic-uremic syndrome/thrombotic thrombocytopenic purpura
> Goodpasture syndrome
> Chronic hepatitis B infection/pneumococcal infection/HIV
> Infiltrative diseases (sarcoidosis, histiocytic proliferative diseases)
> Drug reactions (hypersensitivity angiitis)

Table 17.2 Diagnostic tools for the evaluation of vasculitis

> Blood cultures
> Erythrocyte sedimentation rate/C-reactive protein
> White blood cell count
> Blood smear
> C3, C4, ANA
> Lumbar puncture (CNS involvement)
> Chronic hepatitis/HIV serologies
> Bone marrow aspirate (particularly with FUO or before empiric treatment)
> ANCA
> Anti-glomerular beasement mmbrane antibody
> Renal Ultrasound (including Doppler of renal vessels and inferior vena cava)
> Echocardiogram
> CT/MRI of head (for patients with CNS involvement)
> CTA/MRA or angiogram (if PAN or Takyasu arteritis are suspected)
> Biopsy of diseased tissue

were 80 and 7.5 mg dl^{-1}, respectively, accompanied by mildly disturbed electrolytes. Urinalysis showed dark yellow urine with a specific gravity of 1.020, a pH of 5, 2 + protein, and 25–50 RBCs, 3–10 WBCs, and 0–2 granular casts per high-power field. Renal ultrasound showed enlarged and echogenic kidneys with pulsatile flow in the renal vessels. Chest X-ray was negative.

Blood samples were sent off for the determination of C3 and C4 complement concentrations and antinuclear and antineutrophil antibody titers (ANA, ANCA), and the patient was admitted for hydration, supportive care, and possible dialysis.

Normal complement levels and a negative ANA titer were found on the first hospital day, but the ANCA titer returned strongly positive at 1:2,560, leading to additional testing showing cytoplasmic staining on immunofluorescence (cANCA) and detecting high levels of anti-proteinase 3 (PR 3) antibodies, but no anti-myeloperoxidase (MPO) antibodies. The patient was immediately given pulse-dose steroids and underwent a renal biopsy, which showed 100% of her glomeruli to be globally necrotic on light microscopy. The immunofluorescence and electron microscopy showed no evidence of immune complex disease or linear staining of anti-GBM antibody.

A diagnosis of atypical Wegener's granulomatosis (WG) was made, and no further immunosuppression was used because her kidneys did not appear salvageable. She was placed on chronic kidney disease medications and prepared for renal replacement therapy.

On hospital day 14, she developed dyspnea and fever, followed by hemoptysis and seizure activity, consistent with pulmonary and central nervous system vasculitis. Pulse steroids and cylcophosphamide as well as therapeutic plasma exchange with intermittent IVIG replacement were initiated, eventually leading to stabilization and allowing discharge to home on hospital day 50 on chronic dialysis.

After 6 months, the cyclophosphamide was discontinued and her steroids tapered to a low dose, based on absence of symptoms and AP3 antibody levels that were still slightly above normal but dramatically improved.

After 2 years on dialysis, she received a LRD kidney transplant using standard immunosuppression. The graft remains stable 4 years later, and there has had been no recurrence of her original disease.

17.1 Background

Vasculitic conditions with renal involvement are an anomaly in most pediatric ICU settings where the more common entities one encounters include complications of infection (sepsis and respiratory failure), trauma, or babies with postoperative congenital heart disease. Furthermore, many of the more common forms of vasculitis that the pediatric nephrologist see, e.g., systemic lupus erythematosus (SLE) and Henoch-Schönlein purpura (HSP), will be diagnosed outside the ICU setting, while the more rare forms, e.g. Wegener's granulomatosis (WG), microscopic polyarteritis (MPA), and polyarteritis nodosa (PAN), will primarily be seen in the ICU, probably due to delayed diagnosis because of their rarity and lack of specific diagnostic testing. Pediatric nephrologists often possess unique insights into the management of these diverse diseases because they frequently involve the kidney, require uncommon diagnostic testing (by pediatric standards), and require immunosuppressant therapy. Unfortunately, our treatment plans are often more art than science, as there is a paucity of controlled data for what constitutes optimally effective treatment for many vasculitic diseases, particularly in the maintenance phase of therapy. Therefore, historical outcome data and anecdotal experience form the basis for most management strategies. Exceptions include the treatment of moderately active SLE and WG/MPA, where there exists solid data to support a treatment plan. Newer therapies directed at specific inflammatory mediators are currently undergoing evaluation. Most therapeutic strategies are derived from studies in adult subjects or patients; the exceptions being Kawasaki syndrome or Takyasu's arteritis. Notwithstanding its relative high frequency in the pediatric population, HSP nephritis still has no clear treatment strategy primarily because so many patients improve spontaneously, and the frequency of the more severely-involved patients preclude easy study.

The rapidity at which vasculitis is recognized generally depends on the patients presenting symptoms (Table 17.3). Constitutional symptoms are typically the first signs of more indolent disease, but multiple-organ involvement becomes more apparent with time. In our experience, a CNS presentation (for example seizure) due to hypertensive encephalopathy or microangiopathy oftentimes delays the diagnosis of vasculitis because the initial workup is often directed more toward infectious etiologies or CVA. Furthermore, use of benzodiazepine anticonvulsants and sedatives may obscure significantly elevated blood pressure that might clue the clinician in to renal involvement. Once the elevated blood pressure or hematuria comes to light, a more directed differential diagnosis ensues. In contrast, respiratory disease with hemoptysis and associated hematuria are usually sufficient enough to bring pulmonary/renal syndromes to mind immediately. Vasculitis should also be considered in the differential of a purpuric rash particularly if purpura fulminans is ruled out on clinical grounds. When vasculitis is considered in the differential, rapid diagnostic and therapeutic interventions are warranted and need to be prioritized accordingly. It almost goes without saying that once vasculitis is seriously considered in the differential diagnosis of a critical ill child, high dose corticosteroid therapy should not be withheld as there is minimal

Table 17.3 Signs and symptoms of vasculitis

Feature	Entity	Comment
Fever, chills, night sweats	All	Frequent
Malaise	All	Frequent
Weight loss	All	Weight gain if nephrotic
Myalgias	All	Frequent
Arthralgia/arthritis	Collagen vascular disease, HSP, Wegener's	
CNS (seizure, mental states change)	Potentially all except Bechet's and Kawasaki	Primary CNS involvement or hypertensive
Hypertension	Most syndromes	May present with seizure or CVA
Hematuria	Many (immune complex diseaswes, nectrotizing lesions of smaller vessels)	Less likely in large vessel disease
Dyspnea	Systemic necrotizing vasculitis	Common
Rash	All (includes papules, purpura, nodules, livedo reticularis, necrosis, and Reynaud's)	Classic distributions in immune complex diseases like SLE and HSP
Upper respiratory tract	Systemic necrotizing vasculitis	Common
Eyes	Kawasaki's, Wegener's, and Bechet's syndromes	Common

complications associated its short-term use, and there is sufficient historical evidence that corticosteroid therapy dramatically improves the survival of patients with life-threatening secondary or idiopathic vasculitis. In some instances, it may prove useful to seek assistance from our adult nephrology colleagues who may have considerable more experience with "adult" forms of vasculitis. Bone marrow aspiration for histology and culturing is prudent in patients in whom one is less decisive in declaring a primary diagnosis before using high dose steroids or cytotoxic agents.

17.2   Pathogenesis and Classification

The pathogenesis of vasculitis remains uncertain and controversial. Virtually all components of the immune response are implicated in the pathogenesis of vasculitis. The process probably begins with endothelial activation via induction of adhesion molecules and consequent attachment and transmigration of leukocytes, culminating in the release of proteases and cytotoxic substances [31]. The specific inciting events remain obscure, although several mechanisms have been proposed: Deposition of immune complexes in HSP, superantigen in Kawasaki syndrome, defects in cell-mediated cytotoxicity in PAN, and anti-endothelial antibodies (not to be confused with ANCA) in virtually all forms of vasculitis, including WG [1, 17, 21, 23, 66, 72]. Unfortunately, it remains a nontrivial task to detect anti-endothelial antibodies making their pathogenic relevance in some forms of vasculitis uncertain. SLE can cause vascular injury by a few mechanisms, including immune complex deposition, causing glomerulonephritis (GN) or a rash, or anti-endothelial cell antibodies (e.g., antiphospholipid antibodies) that can cause thrombosis of small or medium-sized vessels. Therapeutic plasma exchange would appear to lend itself well to processes that involve circulating factors, although, the utility of this approach is not uniformly apparent in these diseases.

One of the major hurdles for clinicians remains concise definitions of vasculitic conditions, particularly of the idiopathic variety. Strictly speaking, vasculitis describes and inflammatory lesion of blood vessels. Neutrophil infiltration with necrosis (leukocytoclastic reaction), immune complex deposition, and granuloma formation are some of the more common characteristic findings. Vasculitis may occur as just one manifestation of a more complex disease state (collagen vascular disease or chronic infections like Hepatitis B) or is the defining characteristic of the disease. The secondary forms are generally easier to diagnose because of the availability of sensitive and specific tests. Idiopathic forms of vasculitis may be more difficult to diagnose because of the lack of specific serologic testing. This problem is best illustrated by the pediatric experience with Kawasaki disease in infants who often have a more atypical presentation and are diagnosed at autopsy after succumbing to a catastrophic event. Other examples include clinical situations where disease manifestations are more indolent or develop sequentially over time. HSP, on the other hand, is often easily diagnosed on clinical grounds alone, as are ANCA-associated conditions in the right clinical context.

The most accepted stratifications subdivide vasculitis first by vessel size with further subdivision based upon histologic criteria. Diagnostic tests such as ANCA have previously not been used in the standard classifications, but their diagnostic value is well recognized in the literature. Until recently, classification relied upon criteria set forth in adults only. However, in 2005, several international pediatric organizations with an interest in vasculitic diseases convened for the purpose of establishing a pediatric-specific classification (Table 17.4) [65]. This classification borrows from the standard Chapel Hill criteria that rely upon vessel size to stratify the idiopathic forms of disease, which might fail to detect many patients with idiopathic vasculitis [75]. The main differences are the inclusion of phenotypes encountered primarily in children such as Kawasaki syndrome and the exclusion of those that are extremely rare or never seen in childhood [12]. The classification also includes secondary forms of vasculitis. Furthermore, this group took advantage of newer radiographic and serologic techniques to assist with development of diagnostic criteria for many of the idiopathic forms of vasculitis. Prospective studies to validate these criteria are ongoing.

Hopefully, with time, the pediatric classification will gain acceptance and help categorize patients in a standardized way that will assist future therapeutic trials. Of course, such stratifications do not necessarily shed insight into the pathogenesis of these syndromes. In fact, some argue that stratifying vasculitic diseases has minimal value in terms of treatment because of the considerable overlap in many patients' phenotypes and treatment regimens. Nevertheless, this classification, representing an uniform scheme to support the study

Table 17.4 New classification of childhood vasculitis

	Renal involvement
I Predominantly large vessel vasculitis	
Takayasu arteritis	Yes
II Predominantly medium-sized vessel vasculitis	
〉 Childhood polyarteritis nodosa	Yes
〉 Cutaneous polyarteritis	
〉 Kawasaki disease	Rare
III Predominantly small vessels vasculitis	
(A) Granulomatous	
〉 Wegener's granulomatosis	Yes
〉 Churg-Strauss syndrome	
(B) Nongranulomatous	
〉 Microscopic polyangiitis	Yes
〉 Henoch- Schönlein purpura	Yes
〉 Isolated cutaneous leucocytoclastic vasculitis	
〉 Hypocomplementic urticarial vasculitis	
IV Other vasculitides	
〉 Behcet disease	
〉 Vasculitis secondary to infections (including hepatitis B-associated polyarteritis nodosa), malignancies, and drugs, including hypersensitivity vasculitis	Yes
〉 Vasculitis associated with connective tissue diseases	Yes
〉 Isolated vasculitis of the central nervous system	
〉 Cogan syndrome	
〉 Unclassified	Yes

of these rare disease, is the basis for the more detailed outline presented below of those idiopathic varieties of vasculitis that are likely to include renal involvement.

17.3 Clincopathologic Correlates

17.3.1 Henoch-Schönlein Purpura

HSP is an idiopathic systemic immune complex disease, primarily of the immunoglobulin A (IgA) class, that occurs uncommonly in childhood and even more rarely in adults [71]. It is well described in any general textbook of Pediatrics and Medicine. The most defining and required feature for the diagnosis of HSP is its rash, a palpable purpura generally present in the lower extremities. HSP is generally not a diagnostic dilemma if the classic tetrad of abdominal pain, arthritis/arthralgia, purpuric rash (confined to buttocks and legs), and nephritis

are present (Table 17.5). On many occasions, however, there is limited expression of the disease or staggering of symptoms, resulting in a delayed diagnosis. For example, orchitis is a common but sometimes underappreciated complication in male patients. In contrast, fulminant, and potentially lethal, presentations are also possible, e.g., acute abdomen, CNS vasculitis, or pul-

Table 17.5 Classification criteria for Henoch-Schönlein purpura

Palpable purpura (mandatory criterion) in the presence of at least one of the following four features:

〉 Diffuse abdominal pain

〉 Any biopsy showing predominant IgA deposition

〉 Arthritis[a] or arthralgia

〉 Renal involvement (any haematuria and/or proteinuria)

[a] Acute, any joint

monary hemorrhage. The differential diagnosis includes other forms of vasculitis such as SLE, necrotizing vasculitis, hypersensitivity angiitis, and infection, in particular with pneumoccous. In difficult cases, biopsy of the skin lesions can be diagnostic and shows a leukocytoclastic reaction in small vessel walls staining positive for IgA deposits on immunofluorescence. When HSP afflicts the kidney, the findings mimic the full spectrum of those found in IgA nephropathy.

Despite the risk for severe organ involvement, the reality is that for most patients, HSP follows a relatively benign course, particularly for those with no or minimal renal involvement. However, it is this renal involvement that causes the most morbidity and worry for parents and clinicians [56]. 1.4% of pediatric renal transplants in North America over the past 20 years are done because of end-stage renal disease (ESRD) caused by HSP, and this rate is similar in Europe. Other pediatric patients with HSP are left with a chronic glomerulonephritis (GN) essentially identical to IgA nephropathy and, accordingly, an uncertain fate into adulthood. There is a smaller subset of patients that presents with a rapidly progressive GN, which may well require admission to the ICU, or chronic and relapsing GN that places the nephrologist at a crossroads because there is a paucity of data to guide when or how to treat such patients – all in the face of success treating other vasculitic diseases of the kidney (e.g., SLE or WG) with aggressive immunosuppression.

Evidence of nephritis can be found in 20–50% of children with HSP [77]. There is no correlation between the severity of nonrenal symptoms and the risk of nephritis, and most patients who develop nephritis do so within one month of presentation, although exceptions abound [49, 55, 68, 83]. The most common renal manifestation is microscopic hematuria with or without nonnephrotic proteinuria. Fortunately, most patients with these findings remit spontaneously over the course of several weeks to months [68, 77]. Approximately, one-third of patients with renal involvement will have evidence of a more active nephritis heralded by gross hematuria, hypertension, edema, and/or renal failure. Patients with severe nephrotic syndrome or renal failure are predictably at greatest risk for progression. Their GN may be rapidly or more slowly progressive, with the latter frequently associated with relapsing disease. Other patients may seemingly completely recover. Defining the risk for progression in any individual patient is complicated by epidemiologic data that are mired by center effect. For example, in a series of 275 hospitalized children with

HSP reported by Stewart et al., 20% had any renal manifestation, but only 18% of these had true GN or nephrotic syndrome, and only 1 of 10 patients in this category developed ESRD [77]. This low risk contrasts with the findings of many older case series that generally include only those patients who present with significant renal manifestations and were referred specifically because of their renal involvement (reviewed in [55]). For example, in the classic series of Habib et al., more than half of patients who presented with severe nephrotic syndrome (defined as serum total protein less than $5\,mg\,dl^{-1}$) or renal failure (defined as serum creatinine greater than $2\,mg\,dl^{-1}$ or glomerular filtration rate less than 50% of normal) developed terminal renal failure, despite treatment attempts in at least some of these patients [48]. It is not clear how many of the patients in the Stewart series met the threshold for severe nephrotic syndrome or renal failure because serum protein or severity of azotemia at presentation were not mentioned, but it was probably a very small fraction. The low number of severe cases in the Stewart series also derives from the population base of only 155,000 vs most, if not all, of France for the Habib series.

Renal biopsy may be valuable for prognostication in selected cases. Patients with minor urine abnormalities do not require biopsy because, historically, they recover, and most would show only mesangial proliferation. The findings become more varied with the more advanced cases. Besides mesangial proliferation, one sees variable degrees of endocapillary involvement that may be focal and segmental or diffusely proliferative. This distinction probably has minimal significance as the more worrisome findings are the degree of necrosis and extracapillary crescent formation present. If greater than 50% of glomeruli have crescents, there is an associated 20–50% risk of ESRD within months to several years of presentation [49, 79]. The rate of complete recovery is low, and most patients have residual renal manifestations. This risk of ESRD falls to 5–10% if less than 50% of glomeruli feature crescents. Patients with greater than 80% crescents almost uniformly progress to ESRD, at least if untreated [48]. Thus, biopsy can help coarsely predict a patient's risk for progression or recovery. However, there is a cautionary note here for those with chronic urinary findings and even for those who seemingly completely recover with normal renal function and urinalysis. Two long-term studies have shown that a significant proportion of patients with persistent abnormalities progress to some degree of chronic kidney disease (CKD) or ESRD, and even a minority of patients who completely recover showed progression later on in life, with pregnancy being a particularly notable risk factor for this progression [29, 69]. These authors found that neither clinical nor histologic severity could predict with certainty an individual patient's outcome. They hypothesize that patients who had early complete remission probably sustained significant early nephron loss when younger, followed by chronic hyperfiltration injury with time and growth. Therefore, long-term monitoring for recurrence of proteinuria or hypertension seems prudent for such patients, particularly in women planning a pregnancy.

For the majority of patients, HSP is, as mentioned earlier, a self-limiting disease that waxes and wanes over a few weeks to months. GI complaints and joint pain respond well to brief courses of corticosteroid therapy. However, treatment of HSP nephritis remains controversial because some patients with very active disease spontaneously improve over many months to years. Therefore, each case demands an individualized approach weighing the benefits and risks of treatment. Studies of HSP nephritis treatment fall into two categories: (1) those that treat with corticosteroid therapy at diagnosis of HSP with the goal of preventing nephritis; (2) those that treat after nephritis is diagnosed (generally treating those with the more severe presentations). Previously, most studies concluded that steroid treatment at onset of HSP had no impact on development of renal disease but was beneficial for symptomatic relief of abdominal and joint pain. However, these studies generally used only short courses of therapy (1–2 weeks) and most were probably underpowered. A more recent placebo-controlled study of 171 patients using one month of steroid therapy (starting at $1 \, \text{mg/kda}^{-1} \, \text{day}^{-1}$) showed no difference in risk of developing nephritis compared with placebo, but the severity was less and improved more quickly in the steroid-treated group [68]. The results were particularly striking for subjects over 6 years of age. The treated patients also showed significant improvement in nonrenal manifestations. The risks associated with this relatively modest dosing of steroid therapy were no different than the placebo-treated group. These results suggest that higher risk patients (those over age 6 in this trial) might benefit from such an approach. The main caveat is that if treatment is initiated, it should be for longer duration then many typically use.

When renal disease manifests as nephritic/nephrotic syndromes, biopsy may assist with decisions about treatment, particularly if crescentic GN is present. The rationale to treat is derived historically from the earlier successes using immunosuppression for other vasculitic diseases and is colored by the experience in larger centers were several patients with more severe renal manifestations had progressed to terminal renal failure before dialysis was a viable option [49]. To date, there is only one controlled trial of 56 subjects comparing supportive therapy with treatment using a single agent, oral cyclophosphamide for 42 days, done by the International Study of Kidney Diseases in Children (ISKDC) [79]. This trial showed no benefit of therapy. However, this study, in our view, suffers from small numbers of patients in the highest risk group for progression (≥50% crescents) and, of these most had exactly 50% crescents. Other nonrandomized trials using other strategies suggest a benefit, but also suffer from small patient numbers and the use of historical controls. These include use of various combinations of oral cytotoxic agents with or without steroids [48], pulse-dose steroids followed by oral steroids for several months [60], and pulse steroids followed by daily steroids and daily cyclophosphamide [63]. However, it is hard to ignore these particular data because disease severity in these studies is rather high compared with the ISKDC study, and results compare favorably to historical controls. Figure 17.1 aims to assist with the interpretation of these data, stratified by study, treatment status, and percentage of crescents. One point of clarification here is that the treated and untreated subjects from the ISKDC study are combined in this figure because there was no trend for improvement with treatment. Therefore, the results from this study may serve as historical control for the other studies. The outcomes include complete recovery, partial response (criteria vary by study), and ESRD, and are shown as raw numbers. The one clear message from these data is that patients with less than 50% crescents showed no benefit from treatment regardless of approach. This is because most patients fully recover spontaneously and the risk of ESRD is probably under 10%. Therefore, large numbers of patients would need to be treated to show any potential benefit of therapy in patients with less than 50% crescents. These data become more complex for subjects with ≥50% crescents. Starting with the Levy study, most untreated patients died from terminal renal failure. That trend changed when treatment (mostly chlorambucil and/or steroids) was used, with approximately one-half of the treated patients apparently recovering fully.

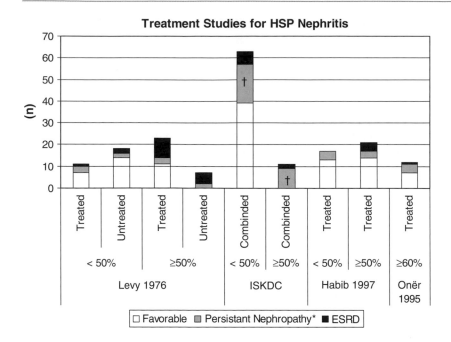

Treatment Studies for HSP Nephritis

Fig. 17.1 Compilation of outcome data from four studies using various therapies for severe HSP nephritis. The studies stratify patients by the indicated percentage of crescents at presentation. The study details are as follows: Levy et al. (1976) reports retrospective outcomes of treated patients compared with historical controls. Most patients were treated with chlorambucil with or without steroids; The ISKDC study is the only controlled trial comparing oral cyclophosphamide to no treatment (results are combined because no difference was found in outcomes between groups); Habib (1997) used pulse-dose steroids and oral steroids and compared with historic controls; Onër used more aggressive therapy with pulse steroids (3 doses), daily cyclophosphamide (for 2 months) and daily maintainance steroids (for 3 months). *Criteria for persistent nephropathy vary between studies. Levy's definition uses proteinuria 0.5 g day^{-1} +/- microsopic hematuria. The ISKDC definition was, more broadly, any urinary abnormalities and included subjects with CKD. Habib's definition was proteinuria >20 mg; kg^{-1} day^{-1} with normal or mild GFR reduction (50–75 ml min^{-1} 1.73 m^{-2}). Onër's definition was any proteinuria. † In the ISKDC study, persistent nephropathy was further segregated: In the group with <50% crescents, most patients had minimal clinical renal findings, while most in the 50% group had heavy proteinuria or CKD. Therefore, these subjects are comparatively more severely affected than the comparable group in the Levy study

The parallel control (combined) group from the ISKDC study had no patient with greater than 50% crescents go on to full recovery, 1/3 of them progressing to ESRD, and most of the remaining having CKD, e.g., at least heavy proteinuria. Although the rate of ESRD was lower in the ISKDC study compared with the untreated patients from the Levy study, it should be recalled that the distribution of histologic severity in the ISCKD study was weighted toward 50% crescents, while the Levy study had more dispersion in this regard. Thus, this difference would portend a better prognosis in the ISKDC study group. Despite this skewing, the treated patients in this category of the Levy study still did better than the ISKDC controls. Habib's 1997 study also shows a favorably outcome when using pulse dose steroids, followed by daily oral steroids (a few patients with ≥80% crescents also received oral cyclophosphamide), with a significant fraction fully recovering. Onër's 1995 study shows even more promise when using more aggres-

sive immunosuppression, including pulse steroids, daily steroids, and daily cyclophosphamide. This was a small study, but disease severity was very high (≥60% crescents), and nearly all patients fully recovered. Even two patients with persistent findings were early in their course and showed a trend toward improvement. The only patient who developed ESRD was lost to follow-up for a time. Finally, plasmapheresis may also be of benefit for patients with severe HSP nephritis [34]. A high proportion (6/9) of patients in this study had complete or nearly complete recovery (normal renal function and normal urinalysis or microhematuria only) following treatment with therapeutic plasma exchange, despite all patients presenting with renal failure, nephrotic syndrome, and most with greater than 50% crescents – historically a group expected to likely have CKD or ESRD. Thus, and while these data are not definitive, there remains a suggestion that treatment is beneficial and perhaps the intensity of immunosuppression or absence of steroid therapy might explain the lack of treatment effect in the ISKDC study.

Despite the uncertainty of the data above, there is room for reason when approaching a patient with HSP nephritis. Certainly, a patient with significant nephrosis but a non-crescentic lesion might benefit from some form of steroid therapy if for nothing else but to hasten recovery. The associated risk of several weeks of steroid use is minimal. Alternatively, one could resort to an angiotensin-converting enzyme inhibitor and diruetics for control of edema while observing clinical trends before intervening with immunosuppression. Those patients with significant or worsening azotemia and ≥50% nonsclerotic crescentic lesions on biopsy are considered by many as candidates for more aggressive therapy with steroids and cytotoxic agents, and one wonders if mycophenolate mofetil could work as well as cyclophosphamide. The rare patient with more immediately life-threatening disease (i.e., pulmonary hemorrhage or CNS involvement) may also benefit from therapeutic plasma exchange [10, 84].

17.3.2 Systemic Lupus Erythematosus

Systemic lupus erythematosus (SLE) is a relatively common disease affecting serosal surfaces, vessel walls, and bone marrow elements. Because these structures exist throughout the body, SLE can present with any number of signs and symptoms. Fortunately, many children (usually adolescent girls) with SLE will present with classic features beginning with the non-healing sunburn of the face with butterfly distribution and eventual onset of malaise and arthritis. Patients with more advanced disease will develop GN with or without nephrotic syndrome. Occasionally, and especially in African-Americans and male patients, SLE may present more dramatically with seizures (either from hypertension or CNS vasculitis), pulmonary hemorrhage, or heart failure from pericarditis. Males in particular may rarely even present only with nephritis and thus not fit the classic diagnostic criteria for SLE, even though a biopsy demonstrates *sine que non* features of lupus nephritis (see below). Because of this heterogeneity, any sick patient presenting with hematuria or, more generally, as a diagnostic dilemma should have a complement C3 level and ANA titers performed as part of their work-up.

The histopathology of SLE nephritis is well documented elsewhere [1, 17, 49, 67]. Most children with evidence of nephritis have either diffuse proliferative GN (World Health Organization class IV) or focal proiferative GN (class III) with immune complexes staining positive for IgG, IgA, C3, C1q, and fibrin ("full house"). Prognosis is poor if untreated and, historically, was improved with liberal use of steroids [13, 76, 78]. However, a significant fraction of patients were still likely to progress to ESRD without the addition of a second immunosuppressant [4]. Induction therapy with pulse steroids followed by oral steroids and pulse Cyclophosphamide given as six monthly IV doses followed by quarterly infusions for a total of 2 years became the standard of care in the late 1980s after the landmark studies from the NIH [3, 7]. To shorten exposure to cyclophosphamide therapy, some advocated abbreviated courses of pulse cyclophosphamide to be replaced by oral azothiaprine or mycophenolate mofetil. Indeed, treatment of SLE nephritis has been revolutionized after more recent controlled trials comparing mycophenolate mofetil to intravenous cyclophosphamide for the induction of remission and the prolongation of renal survival reported equal or superior outcomes with the former [27, 38, 64]. The incidence of side effects was also reduced with mycophenolate mofetil, whose dose may need to be increased to 3 g daily for optimal effect in adults. Mycophenolate mofetil, like calcineurin inhibitors and anti-CD20 monoclonal antibodies, can also serve to salvage patients who fail to adequately respond to standard induction therapy [9, 14, 28, 57, 74, 82].

Most patients will show resolution of systemic symptoms over days or weeks following the start of induction therapy. The serologic markers of disease, including C3 or antidoublestranded DNA will then start to normalize followed by a gradual improvement in the signs of nephritis or nephrotic syndrome with less active urinary sediment, reduction in proteinruia, and increase in serum albumin if the patient was nephrotic. ACE inhibitors and antihypertensives are often required. During this window, the steroids will be tapered. If progress slows or reverses during the steroid taper, one can either increase the dose of the cytotoxic agent or add a salvage drug. The basal level of immunosuppression needed to prevent flares is often individualized, based on the patient's response. Daily low dose prednisone historically was a staple and still may be suitable for patients who presented with less disease activity or who responded quickly to induction therapy. However, compliance is at times a challenge for these patients who are often adolescents, particularly during the transition to independence. Furthermore, a significant proportion of children with

SLE nephritis will experience flares. Vigilance is critical to pick up relapses early. If mild and the inciting cause is known and corrected, a short boost in steroid therapy (1–2 weeks) is generally sufficient to reverse the flare. A common example is a stable patient on maintenance therapy from the Northern latitudes who experience arthralgias, rash, and mildly reduced C3 after a spring break trip to Florida. If the GN flares spontaneously, pulse dose steroids (orally or intravenous), followed by an increase in daily maintenance dosing, is helpful but indicates that the patient will require an increase in basal immunosuppression to maintain remission. In this situation, the addition of one of a calcineurin inhibitor, azathioprine or mycophenolate mofetil should be considered. High risk patients, including African-Americans, males, or those who required salvage therapy, should remain on mycophenolate mofetil, azothioprine, or cyclosporine and may be tapered to alternate day low-dose corticosteroid therapy [11, 58, 62]. The role of therapeutic plasma exchange in SLE GN was addressed in one controlled trial that showed no improvement when pheresis was added to standard therapy with corticosteroids and pulse cyclophosphamide [50]. Other smaller studies have shown more rapid remission of nephritis, but no difference in long-term outcome.

Patients with immediately life-threatening disease involving multiple organs including the CNS should be treated with pulse dose steroids and cyclophosphamide. There may be justification for therapeutic plasma exchange or IVIG to immediately lower the levels of circulating autoantibodies or block low affinity Fc receptors, respectively. If pheresis is entertained, the timing in relation to cyclophosphamide dosing may be critical, based on small trials [15, 16]. Anti-CD20 antibody to reduce numbers of circulating B cells may also be beneficial. One series reports rapid response to therapy in ten patients with CNS manifestations, a group with significant morbidity [81]. Anti-CD20 antibody is currently being investigated for the treatment of SLE GN. Finally, bone marrow transplant has been used with varying degrees of success in patients with severe and unremitting disease [2].

17.3.3 Wegener Granulomatosis and Microscopic Polyangiitis

Wegener granulomatosis (WG) is a vasculitis affecting a broad range of vessels including small to medium-sized arteries, venules, arterioles, and occasionally large arteries [36]. The classic defining feature is the presence of granuloma formation in the larger vessels. The disease tends to start in the respiratory tract (both upper and lower) where it can cause a variety of symptoms including sinusitis, chronic rhinitis (complicated by saddle nose deformity), chronic otitis media, dyspnea, and most notably pulmonary hemorrhage. Constitutional symptoms are common. WG will then classically spread to the kidney and cause RPGN, but it can also affect a number of other organs, including the joints, skin, eyes, and brain. Microscopic polyangiitis (MPA) shares many common clinical features with WG but the pathology is confined to only smaller vessels. MPA usually presents in the reverse order of WG by starting in the kidney and then spreading to the lung or other organs. Many patients present with limited disease to the kidney only (pauci-immune crescentic GN). Both WG and MPA are associated with a positive ANCA, which is typically negative in PAN or other forms of vasculitis. The distinguishing characteristics of MPA are its predilection for small vessels (arterioles, capillaries, and venules), absence of granulomas, and a different pattern of ANCA staining. A positive cANCA test is found in up to 90% or more of adult WG patients [22], and a pANCA is found in most cases of MPA/pauci-immune crescentic GN [61]. In fact, a positive ANCA test is now included as one diagnostic criterion for WG in the pediatric schema shown in Table 17.6. Generally, however, patients with WG or MPA are frequently still lumped together in many clinical trials, cementing the relationship between the two diseases.

WG and MPA are extremely rare in children. Review of cases from one large children's hospital showed that a majority of patients presented with constitutional symptoms and overt pulmonary-renal syndrome (dyspnea and/or hemaptysis with

Table 17.6 Classification criteria for Wegener's granulomatosis

Three of the following six features should be present:
⟩ Abnormal urinalysis[a]
⟩ Granulomatous inflammation on biopsy[b]
⟩ Nasal sinus inflammation
⟩ Subglottic, tracheal, or endobronchial stenosis
⟩ Abnormal chest X ray or CT
⟩ PR3 ANCA or C-ANCA staining

[a] Haematuria and/or significant proteinuria
[b] If a kidney biopsy is done it characteristically shows necrotizing pauciimmune glomerulonephritis

RPGN) [41]. Younger patients are also more likely to develop subglottic stenosis [70]. Adults, in contrast, tend not to develop constitutional symptoms or glomerulonephritis until later in their course [17]. Therefore, it may be easier to diagnosis WG in a pediatric patient. The histopathology shows microvascular necrosis and granulomatous changes in the larger vessels of involved tissues of the respiratory tract. However, renal pathology usually does not show granulomatosis changes, making kidney tissue less useful for diagnostic purposes compared with lung or upper airway biopsy. Renal histology generally shows segmental or global necrotizing lesions of the glomerulus and/or cresentic lesions, similar to what one sees with MPA. Thus, if multiple organs are involved, it is advisable to biopsy nonrenal tissues to confirm the diagnosis of WG. Of course, if readily available, the pattern of ANCA staining can also resolve diagnostics uncertainties. Importantly, immunofluoresent staining will not reveal antibasement membrane Ig deposits in a linear pattern characteristic of Goodpasture syndrome or stain for granular deposits of IgG, IgA, C3, Clq, and fibrin characteristic of SLE GN.

Historically, WG was associated with nearly 100% mortality within a few months of diagnosis [17, 55]. That changed dramatically after uncontrolled studies showed remarkable improvement in survival with use of corticosteroid therapy [36]. Later uncontrolled trials showed even better outcomes with the combination of steroids and cyclophosphamide [18, 19, 36]. Both IV (500–1,000 mg/M2 monthly) and oral cyclophosphamide (2 mg kg^{-1} daily) have been used, and there was anecdotal evidence that oral therapy is more effective [30]. However, the European Vasculitis Study Group (EUVAS) recently completed a controlled trial comparing the two approaches and it appears that there was no difference in outcomes (personnel communication with Dr. Caroline Savage). Furthermore, the IV route probably has less toxicity associated with it [44, 52]. Azothiaprine or methotrexate may also be safely substituted for cyclophosphamide after achieving remission to reduce the risk of toxicity [42, 45]. Patients with severe renal dysfunction also appear to have better outcomes when several courses of therapeutic plasma exchange are used [42]. The typical patient will be treated with cyclophosphamide for 6 months with the dose adjusted to prevent neutropenia (a particular problem in patients with renal failure). This is accompanied by pulse-dose steroids followed by a tapering oral dose. With life-threatening disease,

therapeutic plasma exchange has been reported to be beneficial. Another promising option is the use of mycophenolate mofetil, which was shown in a single center study to have a significantly higher rate of remission compared with cyclophosphamide after 6 months of therapy [37]. The maintenance phase of therapy will include a less toxic cytotoxic agent and low dose corticosteroid therapy. The duration of therapy will be on the order of years for more severe cases of ANCA positive disease. Adults with WG can be successfully weaned from therapy after five years of remission and relatively low ANCA levels [46]. Numerous options are available for salvage therapy or for the treatment of relapsing disease, including IVIG, anti-thymocyte globulin, anti-CD20 antibody, mycophenolate mofetil, high-dose azathioprine, and infliximab [5, 6, 8, 35, 43, 44, 54, 73, 80]. A thorough set of guidelines was recently published by experts in the field from Great Britain and is as a useful clinical tool as of this writing [46].

17.3.4 Polyarteritis Nodosa

PAN is a necrotizing vasculitis of small to medium-sized muscular arteries and adjacent veins [17, 49, 67]. Often insidious at onset, disease activity is segmental and can occur at the bifurcation of vessels in any organ. Histopathology shows fibrinoid necrosis of the entire vessel wall, possibly resulting in aneurysms or vascular occlusion. Constitutional symptoms occur frequently on presentation, and muscle and bone aches as well as rashes are common features. Erythematous and painful nodules in the extremities are characteristic, but livedo reticularis, purpura, and gangrene can also occur. Abdominal pain or an acute abdomen is also frequent. Renovascular hypertension may be the initial presentation, with minimal findings on UA because of only larger vessel involvement, and has historically been a leading cause of death [17, 49, 55]. Mono or polyneuropathy are classic findings, particularly in association with hypertension. CNS symptoms are also relatively common, and pulmonary hemorrhage is possible. Finally, myocardial infarction may be recognized, usually after the patient succumbs. As with most idiopathic vasculitides, there is no diagnostic test specific for PAN. Possible laboratory findings include elevated erythrocyte sedimentation rate, elevated serum immunoglobulin concentrations, and, not infrequently, leukocytosis with eosinophilia. The latter can help distinguish PAN from other necrotizing vasculitides. The diagnosis is confirmed either by biopsy

Table 17.7 Classification criteria for childhood polyarteritis nodosa

A systemic illness characterized by the presence of either a biopsy showing small and mid-size artery necrotising vasculitis OR angiographic abnormalities[a] (aneurysms or occlusions) (mandatory criteria), plus at least two of the following:

> Skin involvement (livedo reticularis, tender subcutaneous nodules, other vasculitic lesions)

> Myalgia or muscle tenderness

> Systemic hypertension, relative to childhood normative data

> Mononeuropathy or polyneuropathy

> Abnormal urine analysis and/or impaired renal function[b]

> Testicular pain or tenderness

> Signs or symptoms suggesting vasculitis of any other major organ system (gastrointestinal, cardiac, pulmonary, or central nervous system)

[a] Should include conventional angiography if magnetic resonance angiography is negative
[b] Glomerular filtration rate of less than 50% normal for age

or more easily with angiography showing the classic aneurysms in the involved organs. MRA angiography is now a suitable substitute to standard angiography for making the diagnosis and is included in the new pediatric classification of PAN (Table 17. 7). PAN can also be secondary to collagen vascular disease, hairy cell leukemia, and chronic hepatitis B infection. Therefore, evidence of these conditions should be sought.

The prognosis of untreated PAN is grim, with most patients dying from myocardial infarction, hypertensive encephalopathy, or renal failure. Five-year survival untreated is only 13%, but treatment has improved this rate to 80% [24, 26]. Steroids are effective in about one half of patients, and addition of a cytoxic agent provides further therapeutic benefit [47]. Therefore, general recommendations are to use corticosteroid therapy initially only for patients with mild disease (constitutional symptoms +/− skin involvement). For children, we recommend $2\,mg\,kg^{-1}\,day^{-1}$ of steroids up to 60–80 mg for at least one month, followed by tapering determined by clinical and inflammatory biomarker response for a total duration of at least 6 months. Treatment of moderately severe disease with solid organ involvement should also include either oral or pulse cyclophosphamide (the latter probably being less toxic but also less convenient), using standard immunosuppressant dosing (oral $2\,mg^{-1}\,kg^{-1}\,day^{-1}$ with a maximum of 100 mg daily or 500–1,000 mg m^{-2} intravenously every month) [25], titrating dosing to response and keeping absolute neutrophil counts

above 1,500. These protocols are generally used for 6 months. Those patients who require prolonged therapy to retain remission may benefit from a switch to a less toxic agent, such as azothiaprine. Patients with immediately life-threatening disease with neurologic complications should also receive pulse dose steroids. Therapeutic plasma exchange has not shown to be effective when added to steroids alone or steroids plus cyclophosphamide in at least two controlled trials [32, 33], although there was a trend for improved survival in both studies, and the sample size may have resulted in a type 2 error. Therefore, in a critically ill patient, we still would consider therapeutic plasma exchange at least in the acute phase of the illness. Finally, newer immunomodulatory agents have been used anecdotally. Several reports have shown a positive outcome of therapy with tumor necrosis factor-alpha blockade in patients with chronic disease that failed to remit with steroid and cytotoxic therapy, including one pediatric patient [20]. Other options include interferon-alpha (particularly for hepatitis B-related PAN), intravenous immunoglobulin, and mycophenolate mofetil, although the efficacy of these agents is circumstantial at this writing.

17.3.5 Takayasu Arteritis

Takayasu arteritis (TA) is strictly a large vessel arteritis that typically involves the major branches of the aorta, especially those coming off the aortic arch. However, it can also affect the aorta's main branches at any level [39, 51], and it may be limited to only the descending thoracic or abdominal aorta in a minority of patients. In the later stages, the pulmonary artery can also be affected. The afflicted region will show mononuclear infiltrates in all layers, with more involved sections containing granulomas with giant cells and central necrosis [67]. Resulting fibrosis will lead to narrowing of the branch orifices (accounting for the past name of pulseless disease). TA tends to afflict younger females and is more prevalent in East Asian populations and South America, but is less frequent in North America. It usually begins with constitutional symptoms and body aches for weeks to months before more significant symptoms occur. Frequently, these will include visual disturbance (Takayasu retinopathy), focal neurologic deficits, claudication, and intestinal angina. Hypertension is common. Of note, blood pressure readings are often lower in the upper extremities compared with the lower extremities (termed reverse coarctation) because of occlusion of

Take-Home Pearls

> ❭ Order a C3 and ANA in any patient with nephritis (even in suspected cases of HSP).
> ❭ Order a renal ultrasound for the evaluation of hematuria even if you think you know the diagnosis.
> ❭ Consider vasculitis in any patient with nephritis and rash.
> ❭ Order an ANCA titer for patients presenting with significant renal dysfunction (and ask for rapid turn-around).
> ❭ You do not always need to wait for the biopsy before treating with pulse steroids when vasculitis is suspected. It will not obscure the histology and has minimal risks.
> ❭ Increase the dose of mycophenolate mofetil to 3 g day^{-1} for older SLE patients who do not seem to be responding.
> ❭ Remember antimicrobial prophylaxis for immunocompromised patients.
> ❭ Remain vigilant: follow the patients who have life-threatening vasculitis regularly even when they are quiescent during the maintenance phase of therapy.

the subclavian arteries. Historically, many patients die from heart failure or sudden death from cerebral vascular accidents or rupture of the aorta. Patients who survive the first few years could only do so with neurologic deficits. Survival depends on the severity of complications at diagnosis, age at onset, and duration of elevated sedimentation rate [40]. In the current era, diagnosis can be made by CT or MR angiography, which can show mural changes at the common aortic sites and, in the case of MRA, thickening of the vessel wall in early stages of the disease [59, 85]. Treatment with immunosuppression, surgery, and stents has dramatically influenced the outcome in affected individuals. There is no consensus for treatment of TA, but corticosteroids are a mainstay, with addition of cytotoxic agents in more severe cases [53]. Surgical intervention or stent placement is necessary in patients with renovascular hypertension or ischemic symptoms.

References

1. Adler SG, Cohen AH, Glassock RJ, Chapter 31: Secondary Glomerular Disease. In: B. M. Brenner (1996) The Kidney. W.B. Saunders Company
2. Alderuccio F, Siatskas C, Chan J, et al. (2006) Haematopoietic stem cell gene therapy to treat autoimmune disease. Curr Stem Cell Res Ther 1:279–87
3. Austin HA, 3rd, Klippel JH, Balow JE, et al. (1986) Therapy of lupus nephritis. Controlled trial of prednisone and cytotoxic drugs. N Engl J Med 314:614–19
4. Balow JE, Austin HA, III, Muenz LR, et al. (1984) Effect of treatment on the evolution of renal abnormalities in lupus nephritis. N Engl J Med 311:491–5
5. Benenson E, Fries JWU, Heilig B, et al. (2005) High-dose azathioprine pulse therapy as a new treatment option in patients with active Wegener's granulomatosis and lupus nephritis refractory or intolerant to cyclophosphamide. Clin Rheumatol 24:251
6. Booth A, Harper L, Hammad T, et al. (2004) Prospective study of TNFalpha blockade with infliximab in anti-neutrophil cytoplasmic antibody-associated systemic vasculitis. J Am Soc Nephrol 15:717–21
7. Boumpas DT, Austin HA, III, Vaughn EM, et al. (1992) Controlled trial of pulse methylprednisolone versus two regimens of pulse cyclophosphamide in severe lupus nephritis. Lancet 340:741–5
8. Brik R, Gepstein V, Shahar E, et al. (2007) Tumor necrosis factor blockade in the management of children with orphan diseases. Clin Rheumatol 26:1783–5
9. Carroll RP, Brown F, Kerr PG (2007) Anti-CD20 antibody treatment in refractory Class IV lupus nephritis. Nephrol Dial Transpl 22:291–3
10. Chen CL, Chiou YH, Wu CY, et al. (2000) Cerebral vasculitis in Henoch-Schonlein purpura: a case report with sequential magnetic resonance imaging changes and treated with plasmapheresis alone. Pediatr Nephrol 15:276–8
11. Contreras G, Tozman E, Nahar N, et al. (2005) Maintenance therapies for proliferative lupus nephritis: mycophenolate mofetil, azathioprine and intravenous cyclophosphamide. Lupus 14 Suppl 1:s33–s38
12. Dillon M, Ozen S (2006) A new international classification of childhood vasculitis. Pediatric Nephrology 21:1219
13. Donadio JV, Jr., Holley KE, Wagoner RD, et al. (1972) Treatment of lupus nephritis with prednisone and combined prednisone and azathioprine. Ann Intern Med 77:829 35
14. Dooley MA, Cosio FG, Nachman PH, et al. (1999) Mycophenolate mofetil therapy in lupus nephritis: clinical observations. J Am Soc Nephrol 10:833–9
15. Euler HH, Schroeder JO, Harten P, et al. (1994) Treatment-free remission in severe systemic lupus erythematosus following synchronization of plasmapheresis with subsequent pulse cyclophosphamide. Arthritis Rheum 37:1784–94
16. Euler HH, Schwab UM, Schroeder JO, et al. (1996) The Lupus Plasmapheresis Study Group: rationale and updated interim report. Artif Organs 20:356–9
17. Fauci AS, The Vasculitic Sydromes. In: A. S. Fauci, E. Braunwald, K. J. Isselbacher, J. D. Wilson, M. J.B., D. L. Kasper, S. L. Hauser and D. L. Longo (1998) Principles of Internal Medicine. McGraw-Hill, New York
18. Fauci AS, Haynes BF, Katz P, et al. (1983) Wegener's granulomatosis: prospective clinical and therapeutic experience with 85 patients for 21 years. Ann Intern Med 98:76–85
19. Fauci AS, Wolff SM (1973) Wegener's granulomatosis: studies in eighteen patients and a review of the literature. Medicine (Baltimore) 52:535–61
20. Feinstein J, Arroyo R (2005) Successful treatment of childhood onset refractory polyarteritis nodosa with tumor necrosis factor alpha blockade. J Clin Rheumatol 11:219–22

21. Finkielman JD, Lee AS, Hummel AM, et al. (2007) ANCA are detectable in nearly all patients with active severe Wegener's granulomatosis. Am J Med 120:643 e9–e14

22. Finkielman JD, Lee AS, Hummel AM, et al. (2007) ANCA are detectable in nearly all patients with active severe Wegener's granulomatosis. Am J Med 120:643.e9

23. Florey OJ, Johns M, Esho OO, et al. (2007) Antiendothelial cell antibodies mediate enhanced leukocyte adhesion to cytokine-activated endothelial cells through a novel mechanism requiring cooperation between Fc γ RIIa and CXCR1/2. Blood 109:3881–9

24. Frohnert PP, Sheps SG (1967) Long-term follow-up study of periarteritis nodosa. Am J Med 43:8–14

25. Gayraud M, Guillevin L, Cohen P, et al. (1997) Treatment of good-prognosis polyarteritis nodosa and Churg-Strauss syndrome: comparison of steroids and oral or pulse cyclophosphamide in 25 patients. French Cooperative Study Group for Vasculitides. Br J Rheumatol 36:1290–7

26. Gayraud M, Guillevin L, le Toumelin P, et al. (2001) Long-term followup of polyarteritis nodosa, microscopic poly-angiitis, and Churg-Strauss syndrome: analysis of four prospective trials including 278 patients. Arthritis Rheum 44:666–75

27. Ginzler EM, Dooley MA, Aranow C, et al. (2005) Mycophenolate mofetil or intravenous cyclophosphamide for lupus nephritis. N Engl J Med 353:2219–28

28. Glicklich D, Acharya A (1998) Mycophenolate mofetil therapy for lupus nephritis refractory to intravenous cyclophosphamide. Am J Kidney Dis 32:318–22

29. Goldstein AR, White RHR, Akuse R, et al. (1992) Long-term follow-up of childhood Henoch-Schonlein nephritis. The Lancet 339:280

30. Guillevin L, Cordier JF, Lhote F, et al. (1997) A prospective, multicenter, randomized trial comparing steroids and pulse cyclophosphamide versus steroids and oral cyclophosphamide in the treatment of generalized Wegener's granulomatosis. Arthritis Rheum 40:2187–98

31. Guillevin L, Dorner T (2007) Vasculitis: mechanisms involved and clinical manifestations. Arthritis Res Ther 9:S9

32. Guillevin L, Fain O, Lhote F, et al. (1992) Lack of superiority of steroids plus plasma exchange to steroids alone in the treatment of polyarteritis nodosa and Churg-Strauss syndrome. A prospective, randomized trial in 78 patients. Arthritis Rheum 35:208–15

33. Guillevin L, Lhote F, Cohen P, et al. (1995) Corticosteroids plus pulse cyclophosphamide and plasma exchanges versus corticosteroids plus pulse cyclophosphamide alone in the treatment of polyarteritis nodosa and Churg-Strauss syndrome patients with factors predicting poor prognosis. A prospective, randomized trial in sixty-two patients. Arthritis Rheum 38:1638–45

34. Hattori M, Ito K, Konomoto T, et al. (1999) Plasmapheresis as the sole therapy for rapidly progressive Henoch-Schonlein purpura nephritis in children. Am J Kidney Dis 33:427–33

35. Hellmich B, Lamprecht P, Gross W (2006) Advances in the therapy of Wegener's granulomatosis. Curr Opin Rheumatol 18:25–32

36. Hoffman GS, Kerr GS, Leavitt RY, et al. (1992) Wegener granulomatosis: an analysis of 158 patients. Ann Intern Med 116:488–98

37. Hu W, Liu C, Xie H, et al. (2007) Mycophenolate mofetil versus cyclophosphamide for inducing remission of anca vasculitis with moderate renal involvement. Nephrol Dial Transplant: doi: 10.1093/ndt/gfm780

38. Hu W, Liu Z, Chen H, et al. (2002) Mycophenolate mofetil vs cyclophosphamide therapy for patients with diffuse proliferative lupus nephritis. Chin Med J (Engl) 115:705–9

39. Ishikawa K (1978) Natural history and classification of occlusive thromboaortopathy (Takayasu's disease). Circulation 57:27–35

40. Ishikawa K, Maetani S (1994) Long-term outcome for 120 Japanese patients with Takayasu's disease. Clinical and statistical analyses of related prognostic factors. Circulation 90:1855–60

41. J. D. Akikusa, Schneider R, Harvey EA, Hebert D, Thorner PS, Laxer RM, Silverman ED (2007) Clinical features and outcome of pediatric Wegener's granulomatosis. Arthritis Care Res 57:837–844

42. Jayne D, Rasmussen N, Andrassy K, et al. (2003) A randomized trial of maintenance therapy for vasculitis associated with antineutrophil cytoplasmic autoantibodies. N Engl J Med 349:36–44

43. Keogh KA, Ytterberg SR, Fervenza FC, et al. (2006) Rituximab for refractory Wegener's granulomatosis: report of a prospective, open-label pilot trial. Am J Respir Crit Care Med 173:180–187

44. Koldingsnes W, Gran JT, Omdal R, et al. (1998) Wegener's granulomatosis: long-term follow-up of patients treated with pulse cyclophosphamide. Br J Rheumatol 37:659–64

45. Langford C, Talar-Williams C, Barron K, et al. (1999) A staged approach to the treatment of Wegener's granulomatosis: induction of remission with glucocorticoids and daily cyclophosphamide switching to methotrexate for remission maintenance. Arthritis Rheum 42:2666–2673

46. Lapraik C, Watts R, Bacon P, et al. (2007) BSR and BHPR guidelines for the management of adults with ANCA associated vasculitis. Rheumatology 46:1615–16

47. Leib ES, Restivo C, Paulus HF (1979) Immunosuppressive and corticosteroid therapy of polyarteritis nodosa. Am J Med 67:941–7

48. Levy M, Broyer M, Arsan A, et al. (1976) Anaphylactoid purpura nephritis in childhood: natural history and immunopathology. Adv Nephrol Necker Hosp 6:183–228

49. Levy M, Gagnadoux MF, Chapter 5: Glomerular Nephropathies in Systemic Disease. In: P. Royer, R. Habib, H. Mathieu and M. Broyer (1974) Pediatric Nephrology. W.B. Saunders Company

50. Lewis E, Hunsicker L, Lan S, et al. (1992) A controlled trial of plasmapheresis therapy in severe lupus nephritis. The Lupus Nephritis Collaborative Study Group. N Engl J Med 326:1373–1379

51. Lupi-Herrera E, Sanchez-Torres G, Marcushamer J, et al. (1977) Takayasu's arteritis. Clinical study of 107 cases. Am Heart J 93:94–103

52. M. Haubitz, et al. (1998) Intravenous pulse administration of cyclophosphamide versus daily oral treatment in patients with antineutrophil cytoplasmic antibody-associated vasculitis and renal involvement: A prospective, randomized study. Arthritis Rheum 41:1835–44

53. M. Vanoli, Daina E, Salvarani C, Sabbadini MG, Rossi C, Bacchiani G, Schieppati A, Baldissera E, Bertolini G; Itaka Study Group. (2005) Takayasu's arteritis: a study of 104 Italian patients. Arthritis Care Res 53:100–7

54. Martinez V, Cohen P, Pagnoux C, et al. (2008) Intravenous immunoglobulins for relapses of systemic vasculitides associated with antineutrophil cytoplasmic autoantibodies: results of a multicenter, prospective, open-label study of twenty-two patients. Arthritis Rheum 58:308–17

55. McLean R, Michael A, Fish A, et al., Chapter 25: Systemic Lupus Erytmatosus, Anaphylactoid Purpura and Vasculitis Syndromes. In: M. I. Rubin (1975) Pediatric Nephrology. The WIlliams and Wilkins Company, Baltimore

56. Meadow SR (1978) The prognosis of Henoch Schoenlein nephritis. Clin Nephrol 9:87–90

57. Mok CC, Tong KH, To CH, et al. (2005) Tacrolimus for induction therapy of diffuse proliferative lupus nephritis: an open-labeled pilot study. Kidney Int 68:813–7

58. Moroni G, Doria A, Mosca M, et al. (2006) A randomized pilot trial comparing cyclosporine and azathioprine for maintenance therapy in diffuse lupus nephritis over four years. Clin J Am Soc Nephrol 1:925–32

59. Nastri MV, Baptista LP, Baroni RH, et al. (2004) Gadolinium-enhanced three-dimensional MR angiography of Takayasu arteritis. Radiographics 24:773–86

60. Niaudet P, Habib R (1998) Methylprednisolone pulse therapy in the treatment of severe forms of Schonlein- Henoch purpura nephritis. Pediatr Nephrol 12:238–43

61. Niles JL, Pan GL, Collins AB, et al. (1991) Antigen-specific radioimmunoassays for anti-neutrophil cytoplasmic antibodies in the diagnosis of rapidly progressive glomerulonephritis. J Am Soc Nephrol 2:27 36

62. Ogawa H, Kameda H, Nagasawa H, et al. (2007) Prospective study of low-dose cyclosporine A in patients with refractory lupus nephritis. Mod Rheumatol 17:92–7

63. Oner A, Tinaztepe K, Erdogan O (1995) The effect of triple therapy on rapidly progressive type of Henoch-Schonlein nephritis. Pediatr Nephrol 9:6–10

64. Ong LM, Hooi LS, Lim TO, et al. (2005) Randomized controlled trial of pulse intravenous cyclophosphamide versus mycophenolate mofetil in the induction therapy of proliferative lupus nephritis. Nephrology (Carlton) 10:504–10

65. Ozen S, Ruperto N, Dillon MJ, et al. (2006) EULAR/PReS endorsed consensus criteria for the classification of childhood vasculitides. Ann Rheum Dis 65:936–941

66. Park MC, Park YB, Jung SY, et al. (2006) Anti-endothelial cell antibodies and antiphospholipid antibodies in Takayasu's arteritis: correlations of their titers and isotype distributions with disease activity. Clin Exp Rheumatol 24: (2 Suppl 41) S10–S16

67. Robbins S, Cotran R, Kumar V, Inflammation - The Vasculitides. In: (1984) Pathologic Basis of Disease. W. B. Saunders Company, Philadelphia

68. Ronkainen J, Koskimies O, Ala-Houhala M, et al. (2006) Early prednisone therapy in Henoch-Schonlein purpura: a randomized, double-blind, placebo-controlled trial. J Pediatr 149:241

69. Ronkainen J, Nuutinen M, Koskimies O (2002) The adult kidney 24 years after childhood Henoch-Schonlein purpura: a retrospective cohort study. Lancet 360:666

70. Rottem M, Fauci AS, Hallahan CW, et al. (1993) Wegener granulomatosis in children and adolescents: clinical presentation and outcome. J Pediatr 122:26–31

71. Saulsbury FT (1999) Henoch-Schonlein purpura in children. Report of 100 patients and review of the literature. Medicine (Baltimore) 78:395–409

72. Savage CO, Pottinger BE, Gaskin G, et al. (1991) Vascular damage in Wegener's granulomatosis and microscopic polyarteritis: presence of anti-endothelial cell antibodies and their relation to anti-neutrophil cytoplasm antibodies. Clin Exp Immunol 85:14–9

73. Schmitt WH, Hagen EC, Neumann I, et al. (2004) Treatment of refractory Wegener's granulomatosis with antithymocyte globulin (ATG): an open study in 15 patients. Kidney Int 65:1440

74. Smith KGC, Jones RB, Burns SM, et al. (2006) Long-term comparison of rituximab treatment for refractory systemic lupus erythematosus and vasculitis: Remission, relapse, and re-treatment. Arthritis Rheum 54:2970–82

75. Sorensen SF, Slot O, Tvede N, et al. (2000) A prospective study of vasculitis patients collected in a five year period: evaluation of the Chapel Hill nomenclature. Ann Rheum Dis 59:478–82

76. Steinberg A, Kaltreider H, Staples P, et al. (1971) Cyclophosphamide in lupus nephritis: a controlled trial. Ann Intern Med 75:165–71

77. Stewart M, Savage JM, Bell B, et al. (1988) Long term renal prognosis of Henoch-Schönlein Purpura in an unselected childhood population. Eur J Pediatr 147:113

78. Sztejnbok M, Stweard A, Diamond H, et al. (1971) Azothioprine in the treatment of systemic lupus erythematosus: a controlled study. Arthritis Rheum 14:639–45

79. Tarshish P, Bernstein J, Edelmann CM, Jr. (2004) Henoch-Schonlein purpura nephritis: course of disease and efficacy of cyclophosphamide. Pediatr Nephrol 19:51–6

80. The Wegener's Granulomatosis Etanercept Trial Research G (2005) Etanercept plus standard therapy for Wegener's granulomatosis. N Engl J Med 352:351–61

81. Tokunaga M, Saito K, Kawabata D, et al. (2007) Efficacy of rituximab (anti-CD20) for refractory systemic lupus erythematosus involving the central nervous system. Ann Rheum Dis 66:470–5

82. van Vollenhoven RF, Gunnarsson I, Welin-Henriksson E, et al. (2004) Biopsy-verified response of severe lupus nephritis to treatment with rituximab (anti-CD20 monoclonal antibody) plus cyclophosphamide after biopsy-documented failure to respond to cyclophosphamide alone. Scand J Rheumatol 33:423–7

83. Wedgwood RJ, Klaus MH (1955) Anaphylactoid purpura (Schonlein-Henoch syndrome): a long-term follow- up study with special reference to renal involvement. Pediatrics 16:196–206

84. Wen YK, Yang Y, Chang CC (2005) Cerebral vasculitis and intracerebral hemorrhage in Henoch-Schonlein purpura treated with plasmapheresis. Pediatr Nephrol 20:223–5

85. Yamada I, Nakagawa T, Himeno Y, et al. (1998) Takayasu arteritis: evaluation of the thoracic aorta with CT angiography. Radiology 209:103–9

Renal Issues in Organ Transplant Recipients in the PICU

18

J. Goebel

Contents

Case Vignette

An 8-year-old, 16-kg boy with multiple medical problems including obstructive uropathy and renal dysplasia leading to end-stage renal disease received a kidney transplant from a living related donor. Two months posttransplant, graft dysfunction developed and was found to be caused by obstruction of the transplant ureter at the level of the bladder anastomosis. A ureteral stent was placed, graft function stabilized (serum creatinine 0.7 mg dL−1), and the patient was transferred to a center with major pediatric urological expertise for more long-term management. There, radiographic and cystoscopic evaluations confirmed a stented, well-draining transplant ureter, a very small bladder, and a solitary dysplastic native kidney with marked hydroureteronephrosis. To confirm the indication for

S.G. Kiessling et al. (eds) *Pediatric Nephrology in the ICU.*

Core Messages

> ❯ Pediatric transplant recipients in the ICU require regular collaborative multidisciplinary care.
>
> ❯ Fluid and electrolyte management in children immediately after receiving a kidney transplant can be very complex and may at times be the main reason for admission to the ICU postoperatively.
>
> ❯ A number of renal problems can occur both in recipients recovering from a renal as well as a nonrenal transplant, including renal hypoperfusion, acute CNI toxicity, and immunosuppressant-associated thrombotic microangiopathy.
>
> ❯ A number of renal problems can occur both in long-term recipients of a renal as well as a nonrenal transplant, including acute kidney injury in the setting of infections or malignancies and chronic kidney dysfunction associated with long-term exposure to CNIs.
>
> ❯ Adjustments and monitoring of immunosuppressant and other drug dosing is a centerpiece of transplant recipients with renal dysfunction readmitted to the ICU.
>
> ❯ Using the *maintenance* fluid concept in the management of patients in the ICU, especially those with renal dysfunction, may be inappropriate.

more definitive intervention, the ureteral stent was removed during the cystoscopy, and the patient was monitored closely for recurrence of graft dysfunction, which occurred within 24 h, as did fever and tachycardia. A percutaneous nephrostomy was placed into the now hydronephrotic transplant, and the patient was transferred to the PICU in uroseptic shock, requiring massive volume resuscitation and pressor as well as ventilator support. Oligoanuric acute kidney injury (AKI, peak creatinine 3 mg dL−1) requiring RRT also developed. With this support, the patient stabilized and eventually recovered, including his graft function, and underwent surgical revision of his transplant ureter.

Children who receive or have received organ transplants require care in the PICU under a variety of circumstances. These circumstances can be categorized into pretransplant (e.g., multiorgan dysfunction in a patient with hepatic failure awaiting liver transplantation), immediately posttransplant (i.e., immediately postoperatively after solid organ transplantation), and later posttransplant (e.g., readmission to the PICU because of infectious, malignant, or other complications). Under all of these circumstances, renal dysfunction can occur, typically requiring complex management tailored to the specific needs of the individual patient. Generally, however, transplant recipients in the PICU are treated in a highly multidisciplinary fashion, usually codirected by a combination of intensivists, pediatric subspecialists, and transplant surgeons and their teams. While the specific logistics of such multidisciplinary care delivery may vary between centers, a highly collaborative and communicative approach appears invariably paramount under these circumstances, e.g., regular multispecialty rounds and consistent discussions, where possible with patients, and with their caregivers.

In this chapter, common problems and general principles in this highly complex and individualized management of pediatric transplant recipients in the ICU will be outlined and reviewed, following the general categorization according to transplant status introduced above.

18.1 Pretransplant Care of Children Awaiting Transplantation

Some children, usually with acute or chronic failure of nonrenal organs such as liver or heart, also have or develop substantial renal dysfunction while awaiting nonrenal organ transplantation (Table 18.1). If this renal dysfunction is advanced and expected to be chronic, it may affect the patient's transplant candidacy significantly, either by presenting a potential contraindication to the desired nonrenal transplantation or by establishing an indication for possible concomitant renal transplantation. Some patients with renal dysfunction prior to nonrenal organ transplantation may be expected to recover kidney function after nonrenal transplantation, likely after an initial worsening immediately posttransplant associated with perioperative instability and virtually unavoidable exposure to substantial amounts of nephrotoxins such as calcineurin inhibitors (CNIs) early after nonrenal transplantation. In these patients, plans for temporary renal replacement therapy (RRT) postoperatively should be implemented pretransplant, e.g., which type of RRT will be used and how access for such therapy will be placed. In recipients of liver or multivisceral transplants, anatomical considerations essentially mandate creation of central vascular access for continuous

Table 18.1 Examples for concomitant renal dysfunction in children awaiting nonrenal organ transplants

Acute kidney injury (AKI) associated with end-stage liver failure

   Multiorgan failure (MOF) in acute intoxications or acute infectious hepatitis with fulminant hepatic failure

   Hepatorenal syndrome (rare in children)

AKI associated with end-stage heart failure

   Acute critical decrease in renal perfusion associated with poor cardiac output

Chronic kidney disease (CKD) in systemic conditions also associated with end-stage liver failure or indication for liver transplantation as enzyme replacement therapy

   Alagille's Syndrome

   Oxalosis

   Tyrosinemia

CKD associated with end-stage heart failure

   Alagille's Syndrome

   Chronically decreased cardiac output with renal hypoperfusion

   Chronic progressive heart and kidney damage from chemotherapeutic regimens for successfully treated malignancies

CKD associated with end-stage lung failure

   Nephrolithiasis or drug toxicity (e.g., **aminoglycosides**) in cystic fibrosis or intermittent hemodialysis and/or -filtration (see chapter 8 and below), while heart recipients may alternatively also benefit from placement of a peritoneal dialysis (PD) catheter. Similarly, plans for early minimization of CNI exposure, complete conversion from CNI-based to non-CNI-containing, e.g., rapamycin-based, immunosuppressive regimens, or even complete avoidance of CNIs could be considered. Such decisions and plans are examples for the aforementioned complex multidisciplinary, individualized, and communicative management approach for these patients and require thorough consideration of medical prognosis, quality of life implications, and other, e.g., psychosocial, factors.

18.2 Immediate Posttransplant Care of Renal and Nonrenal Transplant Recipients

18.2.1 Renal Transplant Recipients

In addition to general perioperative care, which may require efforts at circulatory, respiratory, and nutritional support, postoperative care of the transplant recipient includes often rather unique approaches to fluid and electrolyte management, immunosuppression (IS), hypertension management, and prophylaxis against infection.

18.2.1.1 Fluid and Electrolyte Management

This area of immediate post-kidney transplant care can be challenging and typically consists of replacing insensible losses (calculated as 45 mL per 100 kcal of energy expended, 30) and measured urine output on a volume-for-volume basis. Of critical importance is the realization that the hourly urine output may actually approach the patient's blood volume in some circumstances, particularly when an adult allograft is placed into an infant. This creates a tremendous

opportunity for major fluid and electrolyte, especially sodium, disturbances, which must be anticipated and prevented. At least daily urine sodium measurements can be used to guide the composition of the urine replacement, as fluctuations in serum sodium concentrations can contribute to significant immediate posttransplant morbidity, e.g., seizures [58]. In typically young recipients of a preemptive transplant from a living adult donor, this complication also appears to be driven by dramatic decreases in serum osmolality associated with rapid clearance of uremic toxins from the circulation when renal graft function is excellent right away [54].

Even in older and bigger recipients, the frequency and volume of urine output measurements and replacement adjustments usually require a level of care that can only be delivered in an intensive care or very similar unit. Recovery of tubular abilities to concentrate the urine and reabsorb sodium usually takes several days, over which urine output replacement is gradually transitioned to a more streamlined "maintenance" (see Sect. 18.3.1.3 later) regimen, which may be quite minimal as most kidney recipients can eat and drink soon after transplantation.

Hypophosphatemia and hypomagnesemia can occur quickly posttransplant. The former is largely due to *hungry bones* in the presence of a well-functioning kidney and frequently requires phosphorus supplementation for several months. The latter is associated with CNI, especially tacrolimus, therapy and may also require supplementation, especially if clinical symptoms of hypomagnesemia are present.

18.2.1.2 Immunosuppression (IS)

Table 18.2 outlines Cincinnati Children's Hospital Medical Center's present IS protocol. Generally, immunosuppressive therapy is in constant evolution to achieve the best possible antirejection prophylaxis

Table 18.2 Summary of current peritransplant immunosuppressive protocol used at our institution

Induction (first several weeks and months posttransplant)	Maintenance[a]
Nondepleting (for patients at regular immunological risk[b]) or *depleting* (for all other patients[b]) anti-T-cell antibody	
High-dose *steroids*	Tapered *steroids*
Calcineurin inhibitor (CI), e.g., tacrolimus	Modest-dose *CI*
Antimetabolite, e.g., mycophenolate mofetil	Mycophenolate mofetil

[a] An inhibitor of the mammalian target of rapamycin such as sirolimus (rapamycin) or everolimus can be added or substituted for any one of the three maintenance agents based on center practice

[b] Increased immunological risk is present in recipients of repeat transplants or with panel-reactive antibody titers > 80% and/or other evidence of sensitization (e.g., donor-specific antibodies), in the setting of delayed graft function as evidenced by need for dialysis posttransplant, in any human leukocyte antigen mismatch with a deceased donor, and in African-American recipients

without unacceptably high incidences of over-IS or other drug-related toxicities [28]. In this context, it has become quite clear that immunosuppressive protocols cannot be administered in a *one size fits all* fashion: First-time Caucasian recipients of a living donor kidney who have no evidence of presensitization appear to require less powerful antirejection prophylaxis than recipients of a repeat transplant, especially one from a deceased donor, recipients with evidence of presensitization, or recipients who are African-American [20]. Additionally, the recent discovery of genetic polymorphisms and related phenomena affecting drug metabolism and exposure [7, 15] and immunological responsiveness [2] further undermines the concept of a unified immunosuppressive approach. It therefore likely behooves transplant programs to adapt flexible protocols that can be tailored to each recipient's perceived risk profile. Theoretically, the development of such protocols is augmented by sufficiently powered multicenter studies, but in view of the relatively small number of pediatric kidney transplants performed at any given time and given the increasing number of drugs and drug combinations available, such studies are quite difficult to set up and perform. Of note, the North American Pediatric Renal Trials and Collaborative Studies (NAPRTCS, https://web.emmes. com/study/ped/annlrept/annlrept.html) group has put forth substantial efforts in this area over the past few decades. Nonetheless, additional guidance in the selection of pediatric immunosuppressive regimens is also derived from adult studies and from local practice and experience.

A typical protocol to be used initially in pediatric kidney transplantation currently consists of triple therapy with a CNI, an antiproliferative agent, and steroids, possibly paired with a course of induction with a nondepleting anti-T-cell antibody (Table 18.2). The doses and target levels of these agents are geared toward the recipient's estimated risk for acute rejection, balanced against side effects and other potential disadvantages associated with the use of these agents. Of note, recent efforts by a variety of groups have further broadened the available choices for initial IS: they now include complete steroid avoidance [45], induction with alternative antibody preparations [48], and introduction of a new class of maintenance immunosuppressants, the inhibitors of the mammalian target of rapamycin (mTOR) [29, 32, 45]. This last approach largely aims to reduce or even completely eliminate the use of CNIs, which carries a substantial long-term risk of nephrotoxicity [23, 28]. Similar principles apply to nonrenal transplant recipients [27, 31, 41, 51].

18.2.1.3 Antihypertensive Therapy

Hypertension frequently occurs or worsens in the immediate posttransplant setting for several reasons, including liberal fluid management (see above) and treatment with high doses of corticosteroids. While mild blood pressure elevations above the recipient's pretransplant range may be temporarily desirable to enhance perfusion of the new allograft, more pronounced hypertension, especially if it is causing symptoms, should be treated expeditiously. In this setting, calcium channel antagonists are particularly safe and effective, although attention needs to be paid to the interference of some of these agents, particularly verapamil, diltiazem, amlodipine, and nicardipine with CNI metabolism [20]. Once transplant function has stabilized, the same group of agents may also be particularly beneficial [22, 38], although angiotensin-converting enzyme inhibitors (ACEIs) or angiotensin receptor blockers (ARBs) should also be considered, especially if there is evidence of chronic allograft nephropathy (CAN; see later [8, 13]).

18.2.1.4 Prophylaxis Against Infection

Prophylaxis against bacterial, viral, and fungal pathogens is part of essentially all routine posttransplant medication regimens. Antibiotic coverage is typically provided perioperatively to prevent wound infections and then transitioned to a prophylactic regimen against urinary tract infections and pneumocystis carinii. Specific guidelines have been developed for antiviral prophylaxis in the posttransplant setting [5]. This antiviral prophylaxis is largely directed against cytomegalovirus (CMV) and usually prescribed based on each patient's risk profile, as determined by his or her as well as the donor's history of CMV exposure and by the strength of IS used. Unfortunately, no convincingly effective prophylactic regimens are currently available for the prevention of Ebstein–Barr virus (EBV) infection. Since many pediatric transplant recipients are EBV-naïve and many adult donors carry EBV, primary EBV infection of transplanted children via the graft is a considerable problem, especially because EBV can drive the development of posttransplant lymphoproliferative disorder (PTLD) [24]. Lastly, antifungal prophylaxis is typically provided during the first several months posttransplant, i.e., while the degree of IS prescribed is considerable. Accordingly, a number of centers also *recycle* the full spectrum of infection prophylaxis during and after episodes of acute rejection requiring enhanced immunosuppressive therapy.

18.2.1.5 Other Aspects of Routine ICU Care of Children Immediately After Kidney Transplantation

Gastrointestinal Prophylaxis

Gastrointestinal prophylaxis against steroid-associated gastritis and ulcer disease is typically given in the form of a histamine H2 receptor blocker. At our center, recipients are tried off these agents once they are taking all their medicines by mouth and if they are free of gastrointestinal complaints.

Prophylaxis Against Thrombosis

Graft thrombosis is a significant cause of pediatric transplant loss [49, 56]. Risk factors include hypercoagulopathy (e.g., as seen in chronic nephrotic states), antiphospholipid antibodies (seen in 30–50% of patients with systemic lupus erythematosus), prior thrombosis of a large vein postoperatively (e.g., a renal transplant vein), or thrombosis associated with vascular access (e.g., for dialysis) [36]. Accordingly, hypercoagulability should be corrected before the actual transplant procedure whenever possible. Alternatively, consideration needs to be given to the prescription of anticoagulation during and after the transplant, although controversy exists regarding the routine use of heparin in the perioperative period to reduce the incidence of renal allograft thrombosis. A recent retrospective study showed that young recipient age, young donor age, and increased cold ischemia time were associated with a higher risk for graft thrombosis, but the administration of heparin did not decrease the incidence of early renal allograft thrombosis [39].

18.2.1.6 Early Renal Allograft Dysfunction

Initial Nonfunction

Graft dysfunction immediately posttransplant is suggested by lack or decrease of urine output and by absence of the expected decrease in serum creatinine. Initial nonfunction, i.e., the complete absence of urine production, is very concerning as it could be caused by thrombotic obstruction of arterial blood flow to the graft. Accordingly, initial nonfunction requires immediate diagnostic evaluation and subsequent correction if the transplant is to be salvaged. Many centers therefore perform a Doppler ultrasonographic evaluation or a nuclear scan of the transplant immediately after skin closure or upon arrival in the postoperative care unit, at least if there is no sufficient urine output attributable to the transplant. Along these lines, many recipients still have their native, oftentimes urine-producing, kidneys at the time of transplantation, making the precise determination of the source of urine output – i.e., new transplant vs. old native kidney(s) – immediately posttransplant challenging at times.

If blood flow to the transplant is adequate, acute tubular necrosis should be suspected as alternative cause of initial nonfunction, especially in transplants from deceased donors. In recipients who are not at particularly increased immunological risk, hyperacute rejection is very unlikely. Lastly, the possibility of complete urinary tract obstruction needs to be excluded by ultrasound in this scenario.

Delayed-Onset Graft Dysfunction

In grafts with initially acceptable urine production but a subsequent decrease in output, additional possibilities need to be considered. These include low intravascular volume, rejection, acute CNI toxicity, immunosuppressant-associated thrombotic microangiopathy (TM), and recurrent disease.

Low intravascular volume can be diagnosed if a fluid (crystalloid and/or colloid depending on clinical circumstances) challenge sufficient to raise central venous pressure results in restitution of adequate diuresis, and acute CNI toxicity is suggested by elevated trough levels, e.g., tacrolimus concentrations above 15–20 ng mL^{-1}, in the context of acute renal dysfunction. Both of these complications can obviously also occur after transplantation of nonrenal organs.

Early renal allograft rejection can be difficult to diagnose, as its recognition usually requires a kidney biopsy, which may be risky in a fresh transplant. Moreover, different types of rejection may need to be distinguished as they require different therapeutic responses: Especially in presensitized recipients, acute

Table 18.3 Signs and symptoms of immunosuppressant-associated thrombotic microangiopathy (TM)

Renal dysfunction (decreased urine output, stagnant or rising serum creatinine)
Hypertension
Thrombocytopenia
Hemolytic anemia (fragmented red blood cells, decreased serum haptoglobin, increased serum lactate dehydrogenase)

rejection can not only be cellular but also antibody-mediated, i.e., humoral, necessitating the initiation of plasmapheresis and potentially other specific therapeutic measures instead of treatment for cellular rejection, which consists of steroid pulses or the application of depleting anti-T-cell antibody products. Moreover, cellular and humoral rejection can coexist, and the recognition of humoral rejection requires special studies both on the biopsy material, i.e., staining for C4d, and in the blood, i.e., identification of anti-donor antibody [44].

Immunosuppressant-associated TM causing renal dysfunction can occur early after renal transplantation as well as in recipients of nonrenal organs, especially bone marrow [16, 19, 37]. Characteristic signs and symptoms of this problem are summarized in Table 18.3, but its clinical presentation can be subtle, and many of its signs and symptoms can also be caused by other processes early posttransplant, e.g., acute antibody-mediated rejection [43, 53]. Accordingly, a kidney biopsy may be required to establish the diagnosis and justify subsequent adjustments in IS. Since immunosuppressant-associated TM has historically been associated with the use of CNIs and since most patients are receiving these agents immediately posttransplant, therapeutic options include conversion to a different CNI, e.g., from tacrolimus to cyclosporine, or from CNI-based to mTOR inhibitor-based IS. Recent data indicate, however, that mTOR inhibitors can also be associated with TM [18], although it appears highly unlikely that a given patient would develop this complication both in the context of receiving a CNI and again after conversion to an mTOR inhibitor.

Early renal disease recurrence can be a tremendous diagnostic and therapeutic challenge, typically in recipients with focal segmental glomerulosclerosis (FSGS) who can develop recurrent massive proteinuria within hours or days of transplantation [17, 57]. Since the development of histologic changes proving recurrent FSGS requires several months, and since early therapeutic intervention appears to be an important prognostic factor [17], rapid recognition of nephrotic-range proteinuria (and exclusion of other possible causes of this proteinuria) is of paramount importance. Therapeutic interventions for recurrent FSGS are largely empiric and consist of adjustments in IS (transition to cyclosporine or cyclophosphamide), plasmapheresis, and possibly anti-B-cell antibody therapy [17].

Additional complications resulting in early impairment of graft function are thrombosis of the renal vein or one of its major branches, obstruction of urine flow, e.g., by a blood clot, and urinary leakage, e.g., from an unsatisfactory ureteral anastomosis. Ultrasounds and nuclear scans are useful tools to identify these problems.

18.2.2 Nonrenal Transplant Recipients

Generally, the immediate posttransplant recovery of these patients is highly organ-specific and accordingly driven by very specialized protocols. However, several observations regarding their renal care can be made and applied rather broadly to most areas of nonrenal organ transplantation. As discussed at the beginning of this chapter and summarized in Table 18.1, preexisting acute or chronic renal dysfunction may be a problem *accompanying* children when they receive a nonrenal organ transplant. In these cases, individualized, and ideally proactive, arrangements should be made for the prevention and treatment of worsening renal dysfunction posttransplant, as outlined earlier.

Additionally, the principles regarding IS and its associated complications summarized earlier in Sects. 18.2.1.2 and 18.2.1.6. regarding renal transplant recipients also tend to apply to recipients of nonrenal transplants, as the immunosuppressive protocols used in the latter groups are very similar to those prescribed to the former.

18.3 Readmission of Renal and Nonrenal Transplant Recipients to the ICU

At any given time, ICUs at pediatric transplant centers can be occupied by a substantial cohort of long-term graft recipients readmitted for a variety of issues, e.g., after urgent or elective operations, or because of infectious or malignant complications. Such readmissions pose a number of unique challenges, which are discussed after the following overview.

Transplant recipients may require surgery for many various reasons at some point sooner or later after having received an allograft. Some indications may be entirely unrelated to the patients' posttransplant status, e.g., appendectomies, while others are in some form associated with it. Examples for this latter category range from transplant-related complications, such as intestinal obstruction from adhesions after intra-abdominal transplantation, to more planned operations, such as ileostomy takedowns or other surgical steps after multivisceral/small bowel transplantation or additional parts of complex lower urinary tract revision and reconstruction in children with kidney transplants and underlying complex urologic disease.

Another unique example for such operations is renal transplantation after prior grafting of a non-renal organ. This therapeutic modality is becoming increasingly common as the long-term patient and graft survival rates in nonrenal organ transplantation have continued to improve, at least in part because of the chronic use of CNIs, which, in turn, is associated with chronic nephrotoxicity [41, 51] (also see Sect. 18.3.1.2 later).

Infectious complications are common reasons for admission of transplant patients to the ICU. Both because of their IS and possibly because of their overall medical fragility, these patients are not only at risk for opportunistic infections but also for more morbidity and mortality than the general population from other infections like bacteremia and influenza [25].

Similarly, transplant patients are at increased risk for malignant disease compared with age-matched healthy individuals, at least in part because of their chronic IS [14, 34]. In pediatric transplant recipients, by far the most common malignancy is PTLD, which is often driven by EBV infection and for which therapeutic strategies are still evolving [14, 26] (also see Sect. 18.3.1.1 later).

18.3.1   Unique Challenges and Overriding Principles in the Management of Transplant Recipients Readmitted to the ICU

18.3.1.1   Medication Administration

Especially after surgery involving the gastrointestinal tract or possibly while receiving mechanical ventilation, medications usually given enterally may need to be used parenterally. This can often be achieved with support of dedicated pharmacists who help direct attention in this setting to several important aspects discussed in detail later and broadly categorized in Table 18.4.

Immunosuppression

Solid organ transplant recipients generally require ongoing IS to prevent allograft rejection. Intercurrent problems leading to admission to an ICU, however, often create circumstances in which the immunosuppressive strategy for a particular patient may need to be adjusted in several ways. First, the mere administration of the immunosuppressive agents may need to be adapted as outlined in Table 18.4.

Second, transplant recipients who are in the ICU for infectious or malignant problems may benefit from an overall reduction in the depth of their IS to allow their immune system to better deal with the acute problem at hand. Such a reduction is carefully considered and tailored individually based on the severity of infection or malignancy, the importance of protection of the graft from rejection, and possibly other factors. In kidney transplant recipients, for example, graft rejection may be a more acceptable price to pay in the face of a life-threatening infectious or malignant complication as dialysis is usually available as an alternative. Long-term liver transplant recipients can also lose their need for aggressive ongoing antirejection prophylaxis and may at times do well on minimal or even no IS [11], allowing for such reductions especially in the setting of acute illnesses from which recovery may thus be supported. The risk for rejection in heart and lung transplant recipients, on the other hand, appears higher and

Table 18.4 Conversion to parenteral therapy for transplant recipients readmitted to the ICU and unable to take medications enterally

ROUTINE HOME MEDICATIONS, e.g., immunosuppressants or antihypertensives
Antiproliferative agents and *steroids* can be easily converted to intermittent intravenous administration
CNIs can be converted to a continuous infusion (in consultation with pharmacy)
mTOR inhibitors can not be given parenterally, possibly requiring transition to a CNI
Antihypertensives may be less needed in transplant recipients ill enough to require readmission to the ICU
If needed, *alternative antihypertensive regimens* using intermittent or continuous parenteral dosing can usually be substituted, e.g., *calcium channel blockers* with no or little interaction with CNIs, *labetalol, diuretics*, or a *clonidine* patch, depending on clinical circumstances. *Beta blockers, angiotensin converting enzyme inhibitors*, and *angiotensin receptor blockers* may be less preferable because of their side-effect profile and their limited availability for intravenous administration
NEW MEDICATIONS
Antimicrobials should be chosen and dosed with special attention to possibly present acute and/or chronic renal dysfunction and with consideration of their potential interactions with CNIs (see text)
Similar recommendations should be followed for *other medications*, such as *analgesics* and *sedatives*

leads to significant challenges with regards to balancing ongoing IS with treatment for severe infections or malignancies.

Current guidelines for the management of PTLD illustrate this challenge: the recommended first line of therapy is reduction or even withdrawal of IS, yet additional chemotherapeutic and other protocols are also required, especially for patients who are not considered candidates for minimization of antirejection prophylaxis [26].

Moreover, certain potentially life-threatening opportunistic infections, e.g., CMV disease in kidney transplant recipients, can concomitantly trigger rejection. Accordingly, individualized risk assessments, guided by thorough diagnostic testing and monitoring, should be used to support decisions regarding adjustments in IS for transplant recipients sick enough to require intensive care [25].

While such adjustments typically revolve around reduction or discontinuation of antiproliferative agents (i.e., mycophenolate or azathioprine) or CNIs, the typically relatively modest amount of steroids prescribed chronically as part of antirejection prophylaxis poses a risk factor for adrenal insufficiency and may thus need to be increased to *stress dosing* (50 mg hydrocortisone per m^2 per 24 h) in pediatric transplant recipients in catecholamine-resistant septic shock [21].

mTOR inhibitors such as rapamycin pose several unique opportunities and challenges in transplant recipients who are acutely ill. As they can only be given enterally, their administration may be difficult in patients too sick for this route of administration (see Table 18.4). On the other hand, rapamycin is the only commonly used immunosuppressant that also has beneficial effects against malignancies [6]. Therefore, conversion to this agent should be considered in patients on CNI-based IS who develop malignancies such as EBV-driven PTLD, especially as there is evidence to suggest that rapamycin also has direct antiviral effects [55]. Lastly, rapamycin is associated with significant wound-healing problems [9, 23]. Accordingly, transplant recipients who undergo planned major surgery may benefit from temporary conversion to CNI-based IS before their operation and until most healing has occurred.

Third, intercurrent illnesses requiring ICU admission obviously represent deviations from a transplant recipient's *metabolic steady state*, attributable to a variety of disturbances such as changes in dietary intake, coadministration of new medications that can interfere with immunosuppressant metabolism, and acute dysfunction of organs that are involved in this metabolism. These deviations require close and regular monitoring of those immunosuppressants that can be followed by drug level measurements, e.g., CNIs and mTOR inhibitors.

Other Medications

As already alluded to, the pharmacotherapy of transplant recipients with renal dysfunction is challenging and requires ongoing diligence, essentially for two main reasons: First, the possibility for multiple new drug interactions exists [52]. Second, renal dysfunction in patients in the ICU can quickly get worse or improve, necessitating continuous attention to adjustments in drug dosing based on estimated glomerular filtration rate (GFR). Such estimates can usually be performed reasonably well using the Schwartz formula (as outlined in Chap. 7). Generally, it should be noted that in patients whose renal (dys)function is a *moving target*, pharmacokinetic predictions to guide dosing strategies for potentially nephrotoxic agents or agents excreted renally can at best be made over a very short term and certainly not for 72 or more hours ahead. Instead, daily dose adjustments based on renal status are recommended for these patients. When agents whose blood levels can be measured are used, such as vancomycin or aminoglycosides, trough-level-based dosing is an especially practical strategy, i.e., sequential monitoring of drug levels until they have decreased into the therapeutic trough range, followed by the next dose of the agent and another cycle of drug level measurements.

18.3.1.2   *Renal Function and Renal Reserve*

Not only to guide the selection, dosing, and monitoring of medications needed during an ICU admission of transplant recipients, careful and repeated assessments of the renal function of these patients are of paramount importance. Even in patients who received a nonrenal transplant and who have no history of preexisting kidney problems, at least a subtle degree of renal dysfunction may be present, especially in the context of chronic CNI exposure. This subtle disturbance, referred to as decreased *renal reserve* [1], may then become more apparent during acute illnesses or other stressors.

CNIs are associated with two basic types of renal toxicity [42, 51]. First, each dose of these agents can provide a vasoconstrictive stimulus, leading to a transient reduction in blood flow to the kidneys and other organs. AKI in transplant recipients readmitted to the ICU may accordingly represent excessive acute ischemic injury from this vasoconstriction, even in the absence of substantial elevations of CNI trough levels, and augmented by additional disturbances related to the acute illness on hand and its management. At least equally importantly, patients requiring chronically high CNI target levels to prevent rejection of their transplant or patients with high pharmacogenetic susceptibility to CNI-associated vasoconstriction can develop chronic ischemic changes in their kidneys over time, leading to a characteristic histologic pattern of striped fibrosis (Fig. 18.1). Of note, much of this damage can be compensated by relatively spared areas of the kidneys (*renal reserve,* see above), only to become manifest during acute changes in the patient's overall status, e.g., intercurrent illnesses.

The second mechanism by which CNIs cause renal damage is the induction of transforming growth factor (TGF)-β. CNIs are amongst the most potent inducers of this profibrotic cytokine, and they accordingly drive a process of chronic scarring, again presumably especially in the context of long-term exposure to substantial CNI doses or high pharmacogenetic susceptibility to this complication. In the kidneys, tubulointerstitial fibrosis is the histologic hallmark of this damage [35]. Again, this fibrosis can be substantial and clinically rather silent as long as a patient is doing clinically well, only to become apparent as significant renal dysfunction when this clinical wellness is disturbed.

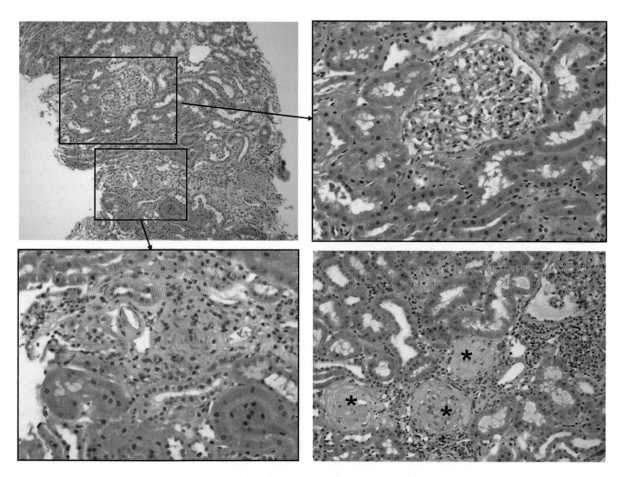

Fig. 18.1 Chronic renal histological changes associated with CNI exposure in a 16-year-old recipient of a liver transplant 4 years earlier. Because of fluctuations in liver function, a diagnostic transplant biopsy was performed, inadvertently yielding renal tissue on one pass. There was no clear history of renal issues and no evidence of renal dysfunction at the time of the biopsy (normal blood pressure, serum creatinine, and urinalysis). *Top left*: Low-power overview of the renal biopsy core. *Top right*: Higher power view of normal area of the biopsy core, featuring a glomerulus with preserved architecture surrounded by healthy appearing tubules. *Bottom left*: High-power view of an area of *striped fibrosis* extending across the biopsy core and featuring loss of structural integrity of the tubulointerstitium. *Bottom right*: High-power view of another biopsy area, demonstrating several sclerotic glomeruli (*asterisks*). The areas featuring tubulointerstitial fibrosis and glomerulosclerosis also contain inflammatory infiltrates of mononuclear cell, which can be seen in chronic CNI toxicity

The cumulative effects of chronic CNI exposure of renal and nonrenal transplant recipients are now well-recognized. In pediatric kidney recipients, CAN, which is increasingly driven by chronic CNI toxicity over time [40], is recognized as the most common cause of graft loss [3]. Similarly, CNI exposure is a risk factor for the development of chronic kidney or end-stage renal disease (CKD, ESRD) in nonrenal transplant recipients, and the substantial incidence of these complications is readily apparent now that more of these patients survive long-term [41, 51].

Figure 18.1 illustrates the scenario described earlier by presenting incidentally detected histological changes of chronic CNI toxicity in a liver transplant recipient with no clear indicators of renal dysfunction in the absence of health status fluctuations but *disproportionate* disturbances in kidney function during such fluctuations.

18.3.1.3 Fluid Management

The frequent absence of renal reserve described above, paired with the potential plethora of other changes associated with an ICU admission that can affect the renal status of a transplant recipient, require special caution when it comes to fluid management. This potentially changed renal status in the ICU may manifest with changes in urine output, i.e., a decrease (oligo- or anuria) or an increase (polyuria) from baseline. Of note, these changes may occur before elevations in serum creatinine are appreciated (see Chap. 7), especially in small children with generous nephron mass after having received a kidney from an adult donor. While many types of AKI seen in the ICU and elsewhere go along with oligo- or anuria, some other types (Table 18.5), as well as recovery from initially oligoanuric AKI, can result in polyuria. Oliguria and polyuria are commonly defined as 24-h urine output per $1.73 \, m^2$ body surface area of less than 500 and more than 3,000 mL, respectively [10, 12]. Polyuria principally occurs when kidney damage predominantly affects the tubulointerstitium and the renal medulla or during recovery from AKI when glomerular filtration returns sooner than tubular concentrating ability and medullary countercurrent function [12].

Other changes in *normal* body fluid homeostasis in the ICU are related to fever and mechanical ventilation with humidified air (respectively, increasing and decreasing insensible losses) as well as ongoing increased sensible losses (e.g., output from the gastrointestinal tract or bleeding) and sensible gains from the administration of multiple medications and blood products.

Table 18.5 Possible causes of polyuric AKI

Drugs and toxins
Lithium
Amphotericin B
Methoxyflurane
Dephenylhydantoin
Aminoglycosides
Preexisting polyuria-prone chronic conditions
Sickle cell nephropathy
Nephronophthisis
Reflux nephropathy
Obstructive uropathy
Nephrogenic diabetes insipidus
Fanconi Syndrome

All of these factors essentially prohibit the use of the *maintenance* fluid concept in many patients in the ICU, especially those with renal dysfunction, because this concept was developed assuming a normal homeostatic state, including normal kidney function [30]. Instead, the fluid status of patients in the ICU should be assessed at least daily based on physical exam (looking at perfusion and for edema), vital signs, recorded intake and output ("ins and outs"), weight, and – if available – central venous pressure and chest X-rays (following heart size and pulmonary vascularity). Based on these parameters, and paired with the anticipated required volume administration ahead (infusions of medications and other therapeutics such as blood products, nutrition), with other therapeutic aspects (e.g., ventilatory needs), and with an estimation of current renal status (e.g., expected urine output), decisions should then be made with regard to overall fluid management in the next 12–24 hours. From a renal standpoint, these decisions specifically involve the possible administration of diuretics (see Chap. 7) and indications for RRT (see Chap. 8 and below). Over the course of the day, this management plan then needs to be reviewed as needed as there are multiple possibilities for unexpected developments in ICU patients, and such developments may require adjustments in the original plan. As mentioned earlier, it is obvious that the development and implementation of such a fluid management strategy is significantly facilitated by a highly collaborative and communicative approach across disciplines, e.g., regular multispecialty rounds.

18.3.1.4 Radiological Studies

Patients in the ICU frequently require radiological studies or interventions, some of which involve the administration of contrast agents. In transplant recipients and other patients with renal dysfunction, caution is required when such administration is considered, as contrast agents invariably represent another potential *nephrotoxin*. Studies requiring the use of such agents should therefore be substituted with alternative diagnostic approaches whenever possible. If contrast agents need to be used, judicious protective strategies, e.g., hydration, should be implemented if at all feasible. In either case, multispecialty communication to develop an optimal management plan may again be very useful. A detailed review of radiocontrast-associated nephropathy is presented in Chap. 7.

18.3.1.5 Renal Replacement Therapy

RRT in the PICU is reviewed in depth in Chap. 8. In transplant recipients, indications and strategies for RRT are no different than in other patients. Specific aspects of RRT in this patient group typically include access and drug dosing and removal. Regarding the former, transplant recipients tend to have had prior central vascular access and, by definition, prior – mostly abdominal – surgeries, which both can affect RRT access placement.

Prior central vascular access may have left stenoses or even thrombi that could impair successful RRT access placement or its use for the typically required rather high blood flow rates in intermittent hemodialysis (IHD) or continuous RRT (CRRT). Planning such access placement in patients with a history of prior central vascular cannulation may therefore include scanning for patency of and flow in the great veins by Doppler ultrasound or magnetic resonance venography.

Prior abdominal surgery, e.g., an intra-abdominal organ transplant, may impair the ability to perform adequate peritoneal dialysis (PD). Unfortunately, there are no reliable diagnostic procedures to accurately predict the feasibility of PD in individual patients with such a surgical history. Generally, *just* having had a kidney transplant usually does not interfere with subsequent PD, but a history of multiple complex abdominal operations may well decrease the likelihood of successful PD. An individualized, detailed discussion with the surgeons knowledgeable of the particular patient's prior surgeries and possible options for PD catheter placement and use may be the most helpful

proactive strategy in this situation. Fortunately, this setting is uncommon in the ICU as acute PD is fraught with several problems, e.g., leakage around a newly placed catheter, which tend to make it a less preferred RRT option than IHD or CRRT, which both require vascular access (see above).

Drug dosing and removal in transplant recipients requiring RRT is no different from other patients receiving RRT but complicated by the IS prescribed to these recipients. Generally, the degree of interference of RRT with immunosuppressant exposure is not very high as these agents are distributed throughout the body in manners that prevent their substantial removal across a dialysis membrane and as they are largely metabolized by the liver. Accordingly, and assuming that hepatic function is not also significantly impaired, dosing adjustments for these agents in the setting of RRT are therefore mostly minor. However, it obviously appears prudent to reassess the need for continued exposure to nephrotoxic immunosuppressive agents in patients who have developed AKI requiring RRT. Specifics regarding drug dosing and removal on RRT largely depend on the details of the RRT administered, e.g., PD vs. intermittent HD or CRRT and, in the case of the latter two, especially on whether or not high-flux filters are used [47]. Individualized assessments of the need for adjusted dosing strategies can therefore be made based on these aspects and typically together with other management team members, e.g., pharmacists.

18.4 Concluding Remarks

The mere success of organ transplantation in children and adults, especially the improvements in the long-term survival of nonrenal organ recipients, has created a growing spectrum of challenges, many of which are related to chronic renal dysfunction in this patient population. In the ICU setting, this chronic renal dysfunction, as well as other unique aspects such as the IS required for these patients, complicates their management, typically requiring individualized, multidisciplinary approaches.

This chapter outlines overriding *nephrological* principles in the ICU care of children with renal and nonrenal organ transplants. While many differences exist between such kidney recipients vs. other organ recipients, their renal care, as outlined earlier, is remarkably similar. In fact, the renal status of recipients of non-kidney solid organs could to some degree be viewed as a human model of chronic CNI exposure.

While many of the principles covered earlier also apply to recipients of a bone marrow transplant (BMT), this patient group differs significantly from solid organ recipients in several ways, including their pretransplant care, their typically only transient exposure to CNIs and even any IS, and the posttransplant dependence on engrafted donor immune system [50]. Especially this last aspect introduces a whole scope of largely BMT-specific issues such as graft-vs-host disease (GVHD), which reach beyond the scope of this chapter. However, it should be noted that some donor immune cells are also introduced into the recipient in solid organ transplantation, and that clinically relevant phenomena such as chimerism, tolerance, and even GVHD are occasionally observed in these patients [4, 33, 46], again exceeding what can be covered in this chapter.

References

1. Ader J, Tack I, Durand D et al (1996) Renal functional reserve in kidney and heart transplant recipients. J Am Soc Nephrol 7:1145–1152
2. Akalin E, Murphy B (2001) Gene polymorphisms and transplantation. Curr Opin Immunol 13:572–576
3. Alexander SI, Fletcher JT, Nankivell B (2007) Chronic allograft nephropathy in paediatric renal transplantation. Pediatr Nephrol 22:17–23
4. Alexander SI, Smith N, Hu M et al (2008) Chimerism and tolerance in a recipient of a deceased-donor liver transplant. N Engl J Med 358:369–374
5. American Society of Transplantation (2004) Cytomegalovirus. Am J Transplant 4(Suppl. 10):51–58.
6. Andrassy J, Graeb C, Rentsch M et al (2005) mTOR inhibition and its effect on cancer in transplantation. Transplantation 80(Suppl. 1):S171–S174
7. Anglicheau DC, Legendre C, Thervet E (2004) Pharmacogenetics in solid organ transplantation: Present knowledge and future perspectives. Transplantation 78:311–315
8. Artz MA, Hilbrands LB, Borm G et al (2004) Blockade of the renin-angiotensin system increases graft survival in patients with chronic allograft nephropathy. Nephrol Dial Transplant 19:2852–2857
9. Augustine JJ, Bodziak KA, Hricik DE (2007) Use of sirolimus in solid organ transplantation. Drugs 67:369–391
10. Barratt TM, Niaudet P, Clinical Evaluation. In: Avner ED, Harmon WE, Niaudet P (2004) Pediatric Nephrology. Lippincott Williams & Wilkins, Philadelphia
11. Benseler V, McCaughan GW, Schlitt HJ et al (2007) The liver: A special case in transplantation tolerance. Semin Liver Dis 27:194–213
12. Bichet DC, Polyuria and Diabetes Insipidus. In: Seldin DW, Giebisch G (2000) The Kidney – Physiology and Pathophysiology. Lippincott Williams & Wilkins, Philadelphia
13. Bostom AD, Brown SS, Chavers BM et al (2002) Prevention of Post-transplant Cardiovascular Disease – Report and Recommendations of an Ad Hoc Group. Am J Transplant 2:491–500
14. Buell JF, Gross TG, Thomas MJ et al (2006) Malignancy in pediatric transplant recipients. Semin Pediatr Surg 15:179–187
15. Cattaneo D, Perico N, Remuzzi G (2004) From pharmacokinetics to pharmacogenomics: A new approach to tailor immunosuppressive therapy. Am J Transplant 4:299–310
16. Chang A, Hingorani S, Kowalewska J et al (2007) Spectrum of renal pathology in hematopoietic cell transplantation: A series of 20 patients and review of the literature. Clin J Am Soc Nephrol 2:1014–1023
17. Choy BY, Chan TM, Lai KN (2006) Recurrent glomerulonephritis after kidney transplantation. Am J Transplant 6:2535–2542
18. Crew RJ, Radhakrishnan J, Cohen DJ et al (2005) De novo thrombotic microangiopathy following treatment with sirolimus: Report of two cases. Nephrol Dial Transplant 20:203–209
19. Daly AS, Xenocostas A, Lipton JH (2002) Transplantation-associated thrombotic microangiopthy: Twenty-two years later. Bone Marrow Transplant 30:709–715
20. Danovitch GM, Immunosuppressive Medications and Protocols for Kidney Transplantation. In: Danovitch GM (2005) Handbook of Kidney Transplantation. Lippincott Williams & Wilkins, Philadelphia
21. Dellinger RP, Levy MM, Carlet JM et al (2008) Surviving sepsis campaign: International guidelines for management of severe sepsis and septic shock: 2008. Crit Care Med. 36:296–327
22. Dudley CRK (2001) Treatment of Posttransplant Hypertension: ACE Is Trumped? Transplantation 72:1728–1729
23. Ekberg H, Tedesco-Silva H, Demirbas A et al (2007) Reduced exposure to calcineurin inhibitors in renal transplantation. N Engl J Med 357:2562–2575
24. Ellis D, Jaffe R, Green M et al (1999) Epstein-Barr virus-related disorders in children undergoing renal transplantation with tacrolimus-based immunosuppression. Transplantation 68:997–1003
25. Fishman JA (2007) Infection in solid-organ transplant recipients. N Engl J Med 357:2601–2614
26. Frey NV, Tsai DE (2007) The management of posttransplant lymphoproliferative disorder. Med Oncol 24:125–136
27. Gras JM, Gerkens S, Beguin C et al (2008) Steroid-free, tacrolimus-basiliximab immunosuppression in pediatric liver transplantation: Clinical and pharmacoeconomic study in 50 children. Liver Transpl 14:469–477
28. Halloran PF (2004) Immunosuppressive drugs for kidney transplantation. N Engl J Med 351:2715–2729
29. Harmon W, Meyers K, Inglefinger J et al (2006) Safety and efficacy of a calcineurin inhibitor avoidance regimen in pediatric renal transplantation. J Am Soc Nephrol 17:1735–1745
30. Hellerstein S (1993) Fluid and electrolytes: Clinical aspects. Pediatr Rev 14:103–115
31. Hingorani S (2006) Chronic kidney disease in long-term survivors of hematopoietic cell transplantation: Epidemiology, pathogenesis and treatment. J Am Soc Nephrol 17:1995–2005
32. Hymes LC, Warshaw BL (2005) Sirolimus in pediatric patients: Results in the first 6 months post-renal transplant. Pediatr Transplant 9:520–522

33. Kawai T, Cosimi B, Spitzer TR et al (2008) HLA-mismatched renal transplantation without maintenance immunosuppression. N Engl J Med 358:353–361

34. Krieger NR, Emre S (2004) Novel immunosuppressants. Pediatr Transplant 8:594–599

35. Liptak P, Ivanyi B (2006) Primer: Histopathology of calcineurin-inhibitor toxicity in renal allografts. Nat Clin Pract Nephrol 2:398–404

36. Manco-Johnson MJ, The Infant and Child with Thrombosis. In: Goodnight SH, Hathaway WE (1999) Disorders of Hemostasis and Thrombosis. McGraw-Hill, New York

37. McLeod BC (2002) Thrombotic microangiopathies in bone marrow and organ transplant patient. J Clin Apher 17:118–123

38. Midtvedt K, Hartmnn A, Foss A et al (2001) Sustained improvement of renal graft function for two years in hypertensive renal transplant recipients treated with nifedipine as compared to lisinopril. Transplantation 72:1787–1791

39. Nagra A, Trompeter RS, Fernando ON et al (2004) The effect of heparin on graft thrombosis in pediatric renal allografts. Pediatr Nephrol 19:531–535

40. Nankivell BJ, Borrows RJ, Fung CL et al (2003) The natural history of chronic allograft nephropathy. N Engl J Med 349:2326–2333

41. Ojo AO, Held PJ, Port FK et al (2003) Chronic renal failure after transplantation of a nonrenal organ. N Engl J Med 349:931–940

42. Olyaei AJ, deMattos AM, Bennett WM (2001) Nephrotoxicity of immunosuppressive drugs: New insight and prevention strategies. Curr Opin Crit Care 7:384–9

43. Ponticelli C (2007) De novo thrombotic microangiopathy. An underrated complication of kidney transplantation. Clin Nephrol 67:335–340

44. Rifle G, Mouson C, Martin L et al (2005) Donor-specific antibodies in allograft rejection: Clinical and experimental data. Transplantation 79:S14–S18

45. Sarwal M, Pascual J (2007) Immunosuppression minimization in pediatric transplantation. Am J Transplant 7.2227–2235

46. Scandling JD, Busque S, Dejbakhsh-Jones S et al (2008) Tolerance and chimerism after renal and hematopoietic-cell transplantation. N Engl J Med 358:362–368

47. Schetz M (2007) Drug dosing in continuous renal replacement therapy: General rules. Curr Opin Crit Care 13:645–651

48. Shapiro R, Ellis D, Tan HP (2007) Alemtuzumab preconditioning with tacrolimus monotherapy in pediatric renal transplantation. Am J Transplant 7:2736–2738

49. Singh A, Stablein D, Tejani A (1997) Risk factors for vascular thrombosis in pediatric renal transplantation: a special report of the North American Pediatric Renal Transplant Cooperative Study. Transplantation 63:1263–1267

50. Starzl TE (2008) Immunosuppressive therapy and tolerance of organ allografts. N Engl J Med 358:407–411

51. Tönshoff B, Höcker B (2006) Treatment strategies in pediatric solid organ transplant recipients with calcineurin inhibitor-induced nephrotoxicity. Pediatr Transplant 10: 721–729

52. Tredger JM, Brown NW, Dhawan A (2006) Immunosuppression in pediatric solid organ transplantation: Opportunities, risks, and management. Pediatr Transplant. 10: 879–892

53. Truong LD, Barrios R, Androgue HE (2007) Acute antibody-mediated rejection of renal transplant: Pathogenetic and diagnostic considerations. Arch Pathol Lab Med 131:1200–1208

54. VanDeVoorde RG, Tiao G, Sheldon C et al (2007) Dysequilibrium syndrome in children after pre-emptive live donor renal transplantation. Pediatr Nephrol 22:1578 (abstract # 674)

55. Vaysberg M, Balatoni CE, Nepomuceno RR et al (2007) Rapamycin inhibits proliferation of Epstein-Barr virus-positive B-cell lymphomas through modulation of cell-cycle protein expression. Transplantation 83:1114–1121

56. Wagenknecht DR, Becker DG, LeFor WM et al (1999) Antiphospholipid antibodies are a risk factor for early renal allograft failure. Transplantation 68:241–246

57. Weber S, Tönshoff B (2005) Recurrence of focal-segmental glomerulosclerosis in children after renal transplantation: Clinical and genetic aspects. Transplantation 80(Suppl. 1): S128–S134

58. Zaltzmann JS (1996) Post-renal transplantation hyponatremia. Am J Kidney Dis 27:599–602

Acute Kidney Injury Following Cardiopulmonary Bypass

19

D.S. Wheeler, C.L. Dent, P. Devarajan, and N.W. Kooy

Contents

Core Messages

> › Cardiopulmonary bypass is a significant risk factor for acute kidney injury (AKI) in children with congenital heart disease.

> › AKI is a significant and independent risk factor for increased morbidity and mortality in critically ill patients.

> › The traditional definitions of acute renal failure that rely on changes in serum creatinine alone are no longer valid, as even small increases in serum creatinine are associated with excess morbidity and mortality in critically ill patients.

> › The concentrations of urinary NGAL, IL-18, and KIM-1, and serum NGAL and cystatin C are emerging as novel, early biomarkers of AKI in children following cardiopulmonary bypass.

> › The treatment of AKI is largely supportive, though early recognition is important. Timing of treatment (i.e., renal replacement therapy) may be crucial to assure the best possible outcome.

Case Vignette

A 3,300 g male infant is delivered by normal, spontaneous vaginal delivery to a 28-year-old Gravida 1, Para 0 female at 38 weeks gestation following a relatively uneventful perinatal course. The pregnancy was complicated by the diagnosis of hypoplastic left heart syndrome at 23 weeks of gestation. The high risk pregnancy team recommended delivery at term, followed by transfer to a tertiary care pediatric center for definitive management. Apgar scores were 8 and 9 at 1 and 5 min, respectively. Umbilical arterial and venous catheters were placed shortly after delivery, and a continuous infusion of prostaglandin E_1 was initiated at $0.03\,\mu g\ kg^{-1}\ min^{-1}$ prior to transfer.

A transthoracic echocardiogram performed on the first day of life confirmed the fetal diagnosis of hypoplastic left heart syndrome (mitral atresia and aortic atresia). The infant was managed on prostaglandin E_1, subambient oxygen (FIO_2 0.18), and dopamine

$5\,\mu g\ kg^{-1}\ min^{-1}$ with baseline oxygen saturations 88%. The infant underwent a stage I Norwood palliation with a 3.5 mm modified Blalock-Taussig shunt (BTS) on day of life 3. The procedure was performed using deep hypothermia, regional low-flow cerebral perfusion, and cardiopulmonary bypass. The infant was subsequently transferred back to the cardiac intensive care unit on epinephrine at $0.05\,\mu g\ kg^{-1}\ min^{-1}$, dopamine at $5\,\mu g\ kg^{-1}\ min^{-1}$, milrinone at $0.5\,\mu g\ kg^{-1}\ min^{-1}$, calcium chloride at 10 mg; $kg^{-1}\ h^{-1}$, and sodium nitroprusside at $1.0\,\mu g\ kg^{-1}\ min^{-1}$. Urine output remained marginal during the first 24 h following surgery with a subsequent peak in serum creatinine on postoperative day 3–2.2 mg dL^{-1} (from a baseline of 0.4 mg dL^{-1}).

S.G. Kiessling et al. (eds) *Pediatric Nephrology in the ICU.*
© Springer-Verlag Berlin Heidelberg 2009

19.1 Introduction

Acute kidney injury (AKI), formerly known as acute renal failure, continues to represent a very common and potentially devastating problem in critically ill children and adults [27, 138, 115, 77, 143]. The reported incidence of AKI in critically ill children and adults varies greatly due to the lack of a standard, consensus definition [106]. For example, Novis et al. [116] performed a systematic review of nearly 30 studies between 1965 and 1989 involving AKI patients undergoing vascular, general, cardiac, or biliary tract surgery. No two studies used the same criteria for AKI. Similarly, a survey of 589 physicians and nurses attending a critical care nephrology meeting noted that nearly 200 different definitions of AKI were used in everyday clinical practice [96]. It is, therefore, not surprising that the reported incidence of AKI varies greatly, affecting anywhere between 5 and 50% of critically ill children and adults [77, 155, 29, 43, 156, 15]. Unfortunately, the mortality and morbidity associated with AKI remain unacceptably high, with mortality rates approaching 80% in critically ill children and adults with multiple organ dysfunction syndrome (MODS). Although this dismal prognosis is partly attributable to other comorbid conditions, recent studies have revealed that AKI may be an independent risk factor for mortality in both critically ill children [15, 126, 5] and adults [39, 108, 14, 93]. In other words, critically ill patients are not just dying *with* AKI, but importantly, in many cases, critically ill patients are dying *from* AKI.

Currently, effective treatments to prevent AKI are lacking [82, 86], and management is largely directed toward reversing the underlying cause (e.g., renal ischemia secondary to hypotension) and providing supportive care. The societal cost of this supportive care represents an enormous financial burden, with annual US medical expenses approaching $8 billion in critically ill adults alone [68, 76]. Supportive care in the pediatric intensive care unit (PICU) has traditionally included optimizing fluid status, avoiding potentially nephrotoxic medications, and maintaining cardiorespiratory stability with vasoactive medications and mechanical ventilatory support. Renal replacement therapy (RRT) is currently the only available, proven therapy for critically ill children with AKI. The experience in critically ill children suggests that early initiation of RRT significantly improves survival in children [61, 101, 62, 59].

The association between cardiopulmonary bypass (CPB) and AKI is well-recognized [2]. The pathophysiology of CPB-induced AKI is multifactorial, and is currently believed to be related to the systemic inflammatory response and renal hypoperfusion secondary to extracorporeal circulation. Nonpulsatile flow during CPB is thought to be an important etiological factor as well, resulting in renal vasoconstriction and ischemia/reperfusion (I/R) injury. Infants and children undergoing CPB for repair or palliation of cyanotic congenital heart disease (CHD) are at especially increased risk for AKI [156, 61, 48, 128, 26, 54, 18, 63, 125, 7, 84, 132], with this risk further exacerbated by the potential development of low cardiac output syndrome during the postoperative period, as in the Case Vignette above. In this chapter, we will briefly review the definition, epidemiology, pathophysiology, early recognition and diagnosis, and management of AKI in children with congenital heart disease following cardiac surgery.

19.2 Definition

In current clinical practice, AKI is typically diagnosed by measuring an acute rise in serum creatinine. However, it is well known that creatinine is an unreliable and insensitive indicator during early, acute changes in kidney function, as serum creatinine concentrations typically do not change until approximately 50% of kidney function has already been lost [114]. Furthermore, the serum creatinine does not accurately reflect kidney function until a steady-state has been reached, which may require several days following an acute insult [114]. Undoubtedly, the lack of an accurate, reliable, sensitive, and specific marker of AKI has greatly contributed to the lack of a consensus definition of AKI, thereby making potential comparisons across studies and populations virtually impossible [106].

The Acute Dialysis Quality Initiative (ADQI) group recently proposed the RIFLE (Table 19.1) criteria for AKI [5, 20]. These criteria have been validated in several different populations [107, 144, 87, 1, 97, 75, 74], including critically ill children [5]. However, recent data suggest that even smaller changes in serum creatinine than those defined by the RIFLE criteria are associated with adverse outcome [107, 88, 127, 37, 65, 64, 133, 94]. Consequently, the Acute Kidney Injury Network has proposed a new, revised classification that defines AKI as an abrupt (within 48 h) reduction in kidney function as measured by an absolute increase in serum creatinine ≥ 0.3 mg dL^{-1}, a percentage increase in serum creatinine $\geq 50\%$, or documented oliguria (<0.5 mL kg^{-1} h^{-1}) for more than 6 h [107]. The RIFLE criteria were, therefore, further modified so that patients meeting the new definition of AKI

Table 19.1 The modified pediatric version of the RIFLE criteria (pRIFLE)

Stage	Estimated creatinine clearance	Urine output
R = Risk for renal dysfunction	eCCl* decrease by 25%	<0.5 mL kg^{-1} h^{-1} for 8 h
I = Injury to the kidney	eCCl decrease by 50%	<0.5 mL kg^{-1} h^{-1} for 16 h
F = Failure of kidney function	eCCl decrease by 75% or eCCl <35 mL/min/1.73 m^2 body surface area	<0.3 mL kg^{-1} h^{-1} for 24 h or anuria for 12 h
L = Loss of kidney function	Persistent failure >4 weeks	
E = End-stage renal disease (ESRD)	Persistent failure >3 months	

Note: eCCl (estimated creatinine clearance) represents the body surface area-corrected glomerular filtration rate (GFR) calculated according to the Schwartz formula [131]:

$$eCCl = GFR = (k \times L)/Pcr$$

where L is length in cm, Pcr is plasma (serum) creatinine, and k is an age-dependent constant (0.33 for premature infants, 0.45 for full-term appropriate for gestational age children less than 1 year of age, 0.55 for older children and adolescent girls, and 0.7 for adolescent boys

Table 19.2 Recent acute kidney injury network definition and staging of AKI

Stage	Serum creatinine criteria	Urine output crite
1	Increase ≥0.3 mg dL^{-1} or increase to more than 150–200% from baseline	<0.5 mL kg^{-1} h^{-1} for more than 6 h
2	Increase to more than 200–300% from baseline	<0.5 mL kg^{-1} h^{-1} for more than 12 h
3	Increase to more than 300% from baseline or increase to ≥4.0 mg dL^{-1} with an acute increase of at least 0.5 mg dL^{-1}	<0.3 mL kg^{-1} h^{-1} for 24 h or anuria for 12 h

could be staged (Table 19.2). This new classification system will require further validation in the critically ill pediatric population, specifically in children with cyanotic CHD following CPB.

19.3 Epidemiology

AKI following CPB is disturbingly common, occurring in as many as 30–50% of adult patients. AKI requiring dialysis occurs in up to 5% of these cases, with reported mortality rates as high as 80% in some series [88, 130, 36]. Similar to other critically ill patients, AKI following CPB in adults is an independent risk factor for mortality [36, 139]. AKI is further associated with increased length of stay and hospital expenditures in this population [102, 100, 99]. As discussed previously, even changes in serum creatinine as small as 0.2–0.3 mg dL^{-1} from baseline are associated with an increase in mortality [88, 139, 157].

AKI also occurs following CPB in children. The association between long-standing cyanotic congenital heart disease and renal dysfunction is well-recognized [48, 47, 78]. Chronic hypoxia associated with cyanotic congenital heart disease leads to glomerular damage by the second decade of life, though evidence of tubular dysfunction may become evident during the first decade of life [3, 10]. Chronic hypoxia may especially predispose these children to AKI following CPB [48]. The presence of congestive heart failure prior to surgery is an additional risk factor [64, 133].

Palliative or corrective surgery under CPB for congenital heart disease is the most common cause of AKI in the pediatric age group in most reported series [77, 156, 15, 84, 132]. AKI affects between 2.7 and 28% of children following CPB [18, 125, 84, 132, 16, 79, 112]. Similar to adults, AKI following CPB is associated with a particularly poor prognosis [8, 32, 117]. Risk factors for mortality include increasing complexity of the congenital heart defect, duration of cardiopulmonary bypass, circulatory arrest, and low cardiac output syndrome in the postoperative period [48, 18, 125, 79, 117, 35].

19.4 Pathophysiology

The pathophysiology of CPB-induced AKI is multifactorial and is currently believed to be related to the systemic inflammatory response and renal hypoperfusion secondary to extracorporeal circulation. CPB elicits a complex host response characterized by activation of the contact system [40], the intrinsic coagulation cascade, the extrinsic coagulation cascade [38], complement [113], the vascular endothelium, and leukocytes [119], resulting in the release of coagulation factors, pro and antiinflammatory mediators, vasoactive substances, proteases, and reactive oxygen and nitrogen species. Further augmenting, this exceedingly complex inflammatory milieu is the secondary release of endotoxin from the gastrointestinal tract [34, 83, 92]. This systemic inflammatory response certainly plays an important role in the organ dysfunction that occurs following cardiac surgery and has been linked with post-CPB AKI [2]. To this end, the duration of CPB appears to be a significant risk factor for AKI in both adults [42, 56, 23] and children [48, 18, 125, 79, 117, 35].

The vascular supply to the renal medulla renders it highly susceptible to ischemia-reperfusion injury. Renal blood flow comprises approximately one- fourth of the total cardiac output, the highest percentage of cardiac output in relation to both the organ weight and regional oxygen consumption in the body. This surplus flow is necessary to establish and maintain optimal glomerular filtration and reabsorption of solute. However, most of the renal blood flow (approximately 90–95%) is directed toward the renal cortex, and the renal medulla receives a relatively small percentage of this surplus blood flow. Within the medulla, the vascular supply is via the vasa recta, which are oriented in a hairpin loop configuration to facilitate maximal concentration of the urine by countercurrent exchange. This anatomic arrangement further compromises oxygen delivery in the medulla. The partial pressure of oxygen in the renal medulla is in fact in the range of 10–20 mmHg, much lower than the partial pressure of oxygen in the renal cortex (approximately 50 mmHg). The osmotic gradients that are necessary to concentrate the urine require the reabsorption of sodium against its concentration gradient, a process that requires ATP and oxygen. Therefore, any process that diminishes renal blood flow places the renal medulla at significant risk for ischemia-reperfusion injury (Fig. 19.1)

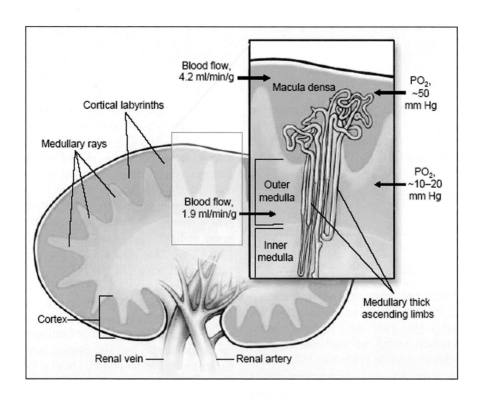

Fig. 19.1 Anatomical and physiologic features of the renal cortex and medulla. The cortex, whose ample blood supply optimizes glomerular filtration, is generally well-oxygenated, except for the medullary-ray areas devoid of glomeruli, which are supplied by venous blood ascending from the medulla. The medulla, whose meager blood supply optimizes the concentration of the urine, is poorly oxygenated. Medullary hypoxia results both from countercurrent exchange of oxygen within the vasa recta and from the consumption of oxygen by the medullary thick ascending limbs. Renal medullary hypoxia is an obligatory part of the process of urinary concentration. Copied with permission from [28]. Copyright © 1995 Massachusetts Medical Society. All rights reserved

[28, 134].The precarious balance between oxygen supply and demand in the renal medulla undoubtedly plays a significant role in the pathophysiology of AKI following CPB. Notably, urinary PO_2 following CPB is highly predictive of AKI in adult cardiac surgery patients [81]. Similarly, medullary PO_2 levels have

been shown to fall to nearly unmeasurable levels in a porcine model of CPB (Fig. 19.2) [134]. In this study, medullary PO_2 gradually increased following cessation of CPB, but remained lower than pre-CPB levels for the duration of the study. Urinary PO_2 correlated directly with medullary PO_2 (Fig. 19.3). Although tissue and urinary oxygen levels have not been measured in children with cyanotic congenital heart disease, it is tempting to speculate that medullary hypoxia could be compounded in this setting.

Renal hypoperfusion, especially when the aorta is cross-clamped during CPB or during periods of deep hypothermic circulatory arrest, is yet another purported mechanism of postoperative AKI [48, 49, 66, 145]. The kidney, along with the brain and heart, has a great capacity for the autoregulation of blood flow. Autoregulation is the intrinsic ability of an organ to maintain a constant blood flow despite changes in perfusion pressure. For example, a decrease in organ

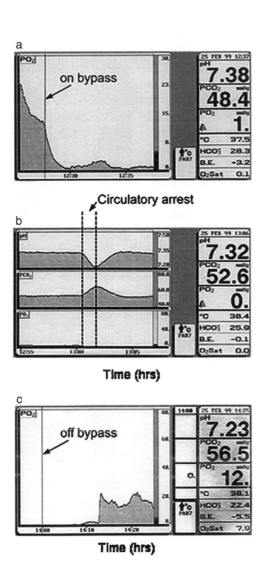

Fig. 19.2 Renal medullary hypoxia is exacerbated during cardiopulmonary bypass. (**a**) Following initiation of CPB, but not sham CPB, medullary PO_2 declined to unmeasurable levels over approximately 15 min while CO_2 and pH remained unchanged. (**b**) In one pig, a brief period of circulatory arrest during CPB resulted in rapid PCO_2 rise and pH decline that corrected with reperfusion. (**c**) After separation from CPB, medullary PO_2 increased, but remained lower than pre-CPB levels, while PCO_2 and pH were unchanged. Copied with permission from [134]. Copyright (©Sage Publications, 2005) by permission of Sage Publications, Ltd

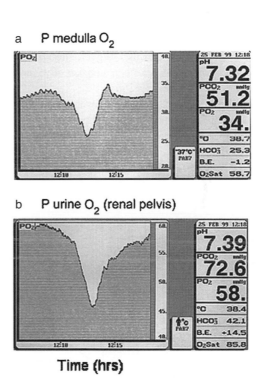

Fig. 19.3 Medullary PO_2 levels correlate with urinary PO_2 levels. Renal pelvis urine PO_2, but not pH or PCO_2, appeared to correlate closely with renal medullary values at all times. The figure demonstrates parallel changes in medullary PO_2 (**a**) and urine PO_2 (**b**) related to a drop from 105 to 70 mmHg systolic blood pressure during aortic cannulation. Copied with permission from [134]. Copyright (©Sage Publications, 2005) by permission of Sage Publications, Ltd

blood flow resulting from a decrease in the perfusion pressure triggers a reflex autoregulatory vasodilation and reduction in vascular resistance, reconciling a return of arterial blood flow to steady state (Fig. 19.4). As the perfusion pressure continues to decrease, however, a point of maximal vasodilation is realized and any further decrease in perfusion pressure results in an uncompensated decrease in organ blood flow. The autoregulatory range of perfusion pressures for the kidney is not known and may be different in infants and young children vs adults. In addition, the effects of CPB on autoregulation in local vascular beds such as the kidney have not been adequately studied.

Although renal hypoperfusion appears to be a plausible mechanism for AKI, several studies have presented contrary findings [146, 89, 9, 90, 91]. For example, Lema et al. [91] measured effective renal blood flow in nine children undergoing CPB. Effective renal blood flow was increased during CPB in this study, though none of these children had complex congenital heart disease. Several pharmacologic interventions to increase renal blood flow (e.g., "renal dose" dopamine, fenoldopam, nesiritide, etc.) have been used in adult patients undergoing cardiac surgery, though none of these interventions have been consistently shown to prevent or ameliorate AKI [66].

The systemic inflammatory response that occurs following CPB results in the generation of reactive oxygen species (ROS) and reactive nitrogen species (RNS), which may contribute to the pathophysiology of AKI. Several therapeutic interventions aimed at reduc-

ing the generation of ROS have been tried, though none have been shown to provide adequate renal protection. For example, N-acetylcysteine (NAC) is a potent antioxidant that reduces oxidative stress during CPB [57, 140]. Several trials of NAC in adults undergoing CPB have been uniformly unsuccessful in preventing AKI [33, 129, 67].

Animal models of AKI have contributed greatly to the mechanistic understanding of AKI and have led to several novel and promising therapeutic approaches for the management of AKI in critically ill patients. Overall, translational research efforts in humans have been greatly disappointing. A major reason for this failure is the lack of early markers for AKI, and hence a delay in initiating timely therapy [27, 138, 52, 135]. Animal models have taught us that while AKI can be effectively prevented and/or treated by several maneuvers, there is an extremely narrow "window of opportunity" to accomplish this, and treatment must be instituted very early after the initiating insult [135]. Unfortunately, the lack of early biomarkers of renal injury in humans has hitherto crippled our ability to launch these potentially effective therapies in a timely manner. Not surprisingly then, clinical studies to date examining a variety of promising interventions have been uniformly unsuccessful, primarily because the treatments were initiated on the basis of elevation of serum creatinine, a late and unreliable measure of kidney function in AKI [27, 138, 115, 52, 135, 51, 118]. The lack of early biomarkers of AKI, akin to troponins or creatine kinase in the acute coronary syndrome, has greatly limited our ability to initiate these potentially lifesaving therapies in a timely manner. Recent translational efforts have, therefore, focused on identifying potential biomarkers of early AKI [70, 142].

19.5 Early Recognition and Diagnosis of AKI

Recent advances in clinical proteomics have allowed significant advances to be made in the identification of biomarkers for AKI. Using this kind of translational research approach, several potential biomarkers of early AKI have been identified (Table 19.3). Neutrophil gelatinase-associated lipocalin (NGAL) is a 25 kDa protein that is highly upregulated in the renal tubules following ischemic stress [137, 109, 46]. NGAL was easily detected in the urine relatively early in mouse and rat models of renal ischemia-reperfusion injury [109]. Subsequent clinical studies have shown

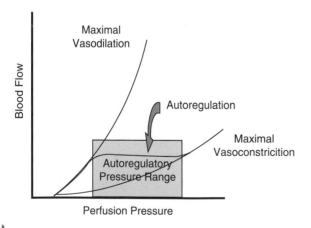

Fig. 19.4 The kidney has a great capacity for autoregulation with consequent preservation of renal blood flow independent of perfusion pressures ranging from approximately 80–180 mmHg in mature kidneys

Table 19.3 Current status of new biomarkers for early detection of AKI in various clinical settings[a]

Biomarker	Source	Cardiopulmonary bypass (CPB)	Contrast nephropathy	Sepsis or ICU	Kidney transplant	Commercial assay
NGAL	Urine	2 h post CPB	4 h post contrast	48 h before AKI	12–24 h posttransplant	ELISA, Abbott[b]
IL-18	Urine	4–6 h post CPB	Not tested	48 h before AKI	12–24 h posttransplant	ELISA
KIM-1	Urine	12–24 h post CPB	Not tested	Not tested	Not tested	ELISA
NGAL	Plasma	2 h post CPB	2 h post contrast	48 h before AKI	Not tested	ELISA, Biosite[b]
Cystatin C	Plasma	12 h post CPB[c]	8 h post contrast	48 h before AKI	Variable	Nephelometry, Dade-Behring

[a] The times indicated are the earliest time points when the biomarker values become significantly elevated from baseline values. The ELISAs are research-based, although clinical platforms for NGAL measurement are nearing completion
[b] In development
[c] Unpublished data

that urine and serum NGAL is a highly sensitive, specific, and highly predictive early biomarker for AKI in a wide range of different disease processes [112, 109, 150, 111, 141, 158]. For example, urine NGAL concentrations greater than 50 µg mL^{-1} reliably predicted AKI in children at 2 h following CPB, with 100% sensitivity and 98% specificity [112]. Although serum NGAL concentrations were not as robust in this study, concentrations greater than 25 µg mL^{-1} had 70% sensitivity, 94% specificity, 82% positive predictive value, and 89% negative predictive value [112]. Of even greater importance to the present discussion, a point-of-care test for NGAL has been developed and is currently undergoing phase II clinical trials (P. Devarajan, *personal communication*). Finally, preclinical studies suggest that exogenously administered NGAL ameliorates ischemia-reperfusion injury in the kidney [110] and may thus not only represent a novel biomarker but also an innovative therapeutic strategy for AKI.

Other biomarkers of AKI have been studied as well. Cystatin C and β_2-microglobulin are low-molecular weight proteins that are freely filtered in the glomerulus. The concentration of these two proteins in the serum is largely determined by the glomerular filtration rate (GFR). Serum β_2-microglobulin and cystatin C have been used as markers of GFR in critically ill patients [73, 4, 11, 71, 72, 103, 104, 149, 153]. Urinary interleukin (IL)-18 [120–123] and Kidney Injury Molecule-1 (KIM-1) [69, 95] also appear to be promising biomarkers in critically ill patients with AKI. On the basis of these studies, there is growing optimism that these biomarkers may allow for early recognition and better prevention and treatment of AKI in critically ill patients [45].

19.6 Approach to Management

As effective, proven treatments to prevent AKI are lacking [82, 86, 148, 80], management of critically ill patients with AKI is largely directed toward reversing the underlying cause and providing supportive care. RRT, including peritoneal dialysis, intermittent hemodialysis, and continuous venovenous hemofiltration (CVVH) is the only available, proven therapy for critically ill patients with AKI. An early, aggressive approach to RRT improves survival in these patients [124, 55, 85, 41, 60, 44, 53, 98, 25, 22]. Although there has been only one prospective, randomized trial of early vs late initiation of RRT in critically ill patients [24], the data suggesting that early treatment is superior to late treatment is encouraging, especially in patients who developed AKI following CPB [44, 53, 22, 17]. More importantly, there is evidence suggesting that early RRT affords critically ill patients with a therapeutic strategy that goes beyond organ support. In other words, RRT may a play a more direct, therapeutic role in ameliorating renal injury and improving the chances of "renal recovery." Renal recovery is variably defined in the literature, though most definitions used include the criterion of freedom from chronic RRT [12, 13]. Similarly, fluid overload adversely affects cardiovascular hemodynamics, and is an independent risk factor for prolonged length of stay in the hospital following CPB [147, 30, 154]. Early and aggressive management of fluid overload with RRT may, therefore, be especially important in this population [19].

Consistent with the adverse effects of fluid overload, a retrospective series of 21 critically ill children receiving CRRT for AKI suggested that the degree of fluid overload at the initiation of CRRT was significantly lower in survivors compared with nonsurvivors, independent of the severity of illness [61]. The authors of this study proposed that the earlier initiation of CRRT, defined as 10% fluid overload vs 25% fluid overload, may prevent morbidity and mortality in critically ill children with AKI by allowing earlier administration of nutritional support and necessary blood products. A larger retrospective series involving 113 children with multiple organ dysfunction syndrome (MODS) [59] confirmed these results – in this study, the median %fluid overload was significantly lower in survivors compared with nonsurvivors, independent of severity of illness. In fact, %fluid overload was independently associated with survival in patients with ≥3 failing organ systems by multivariate analysis. Finally, a multicenter study by the Prospective Pediatric Continuous Renal Replacement Therapy Registry Group involving 116 critically ill children concluded that large fluid requirements from the time of admission to the PICU to the time of initiation of CRRT were independently associated with mortality. These investigators concluded that after initial resuscitation in the PICU, an increased emphasis should be placed upon the early initiation of CRRT, with preferential use of vasoactive medications vs additional administration of fluids [62]. Although these studies generally involved critically ill children with multiple organ failure secondary to septic shock, we believe that the lessons learned may be applied to critically ill children following CPB as well.

Peritoneal dialysis is generally safe and effective in critically ill children with AKI following CPB [84, 35, 152, 105]. Several investigators have suggested that "prophylactic" peritoneal dialysis is effective in children who are at high risk of developing AKI following CPB [50, 6, 136]. Regardless, CRRT modes are generally considered to be superior for solute clearance and fluid removal in this population [79, 58], and surveys of pediatric nephrologists in the United States strongly suggest that CRRT is the preferred modality for treating AKI in the PICU [31, 151, 21].

19.7 Conclusion

The kidney, especially in newborns and infants where it has not reached functional maturity yet, is at risk for injury following cardiopulmonary bypass. The etiology of AKI in this population is multifactorial, though the systemic inflammatory response to bypass and ischemia-reperfusion injury both play a major role. Traditional markers of AKI, most notably serum creatinine, are not very sensitive for AKI in critically ill patients. Several early, sensitive, novel biomarkers of AKI have been validated in critically ill children, and it is likely that these biomarkers will have a significant impact on the management of AKI in the future. Supportive care, avoidance of nephrotoxic agents, and early initiation of RRT, which requires early recognition of AKI with the use of these novel biomarkers, are the mainstays of treatment.

Take-Home Pearls

> AKI following CPB is multifactorial in origin. The systemic inflammatory response to bypass and renal ischemia-reperfusion injury plays major roles.

> Serum cystatin C, serum NGAL, urine NGAL, urine KIM-1 and urine IL-18 are sensitive and early indicators of AKI.

> Supportive care and early use of RRT to prevent fluid overload are the mainstays of management of critically ill children with AKI.

References

1. Abosaif NY, Tolba YA, Heap M, et al (2005) The outcome of acute renal failure in the intensive care unit according to RIFLE: Model application, sensitivity, and predictability. Am J Kidney Dis 46:1038–1048
2. Abu-Omar Y, Ratnatunga C (2006) Cardiopulmonary bypass and renal injury. Perfusion 21:209–213
3. Agras PI, Derbent M, Ozcay F, et al (2005) Effect of congenital heart disease on renal function in childhood. Nephron Physiol 99:10–15
4. Ahlstrom A, Tallgren M, Peltonen S, et al (2004) Evolution and predictive power of serum cystatin C in acute renal failure. Clin Nephrol 62:344–350
5. Akcan-Arikan A, Zappitelli M, Loftis LL, et al (2007) Modified RIFLE criteria in critically ill children with acute kidney injury. Kidney Int 71:1028–1035
6. Alkan T, Akcevin A, Turkoglu H, et al (2006) Postoperative prophylactic peritoneal dialysis in neonates and infants after complex cyanotic congenital heart surgery. ASAIO J 52:693–697

7. Alwaidh MH, Cooke RW, Judd BA (1998) Renal blood flow velocity in acute renal failure following cardiopulmonary bypass surgery. Acta Paediatr 87:644–649

8. Arora P, Kher V, Rai PK, et al (1997) Prognosis of acute renal failure in children: A multivariate analysis. Pediatr Nephrol 11:153–155

9. Asfour B, Bruker B, Kehl HG, et al (1996) Renal insufficiency in neonates after cardiac surgery. Clin Nephrol 46:59–63

10. Awad H, El-Safty I, Abdel-Gawad M, et al (2003) Glomerular and tubular dysfunction in children with congenital cyanotic heart disease: Effect of palliative surgery. Am J Med Sci 325:110–114

11. Baas MC, Bouman CS, Hoek FJ, et al (2006) Cystatin C in critically ill patients treated with continuous venovenous hemofiltration. Hemodial Int 10 Suppl 2:S33–S37

12. Bagshaw SM (2006) Epidemiology of renal recovery after acute renal failure. Curr Opin Crit Care 12:544–550

13. Bagshaw SM (2006) The long-term outcome after acute renal failure. Curr Opin Crit Care 12:561–566

14. Bagshaw SM, Mortis G, Doig CJ, et al (2006) One-year mortality assessment in critically ill patients by severity of kidney dysfunction: A population-based assessment. Am J Kidney Dis 48:402–409

15. Bailey D, Phan V, Litalien C, et al (2007) Risk factors of acute renal failure in critically ill children: A prospective descriptive epidemiological study. Pediatr Crit Care Med 8:29–35

16. Baskin E, Saygili A, Harmanci K, et al (2005) Acute renal failure and mortality after open-heart surgery in infants. Ren Fail 27:557–560

17. Baudouin SV, Wiggins J, Keogh BF, et al (1993) Continuous veno-venous haemofiltration following cardiopulmonary bypass. Indications and outcome in 35 patients. Intensive Care Med 19:290–293

18. Baxter P, Rigby ML, Jones OD, et al (1985) Acute renal failure following cardiopulmonary bypass in children: Results of treatment. Int J Cardiol 7:235–243

19. Bellomo R, Raman J, Ronco C (2001) Intensive care management of the critically ill patient with fluid overload after open heart surgery. Cardiology 96:169–176

20. Bellomo R, Ronco C, Kellum JA, et al (2004) Acute renal failure – Definition, outcome measures, animal models, fluid therapy, and information technology needs: The Second International Consensus Conference of the Acute Dialysis Quality Initiative (ADQI) Group. Crit Care 8: R204–R212

21. Belsha CW, Kohaut EC, Warady BA (1995) Dialytic management of childhood acute renal failure: A survey of North American pediatric nephrologists. Pediatr Nephrol 9:361–363

22. Bent P, Tan HK, Bellomo R, et al (2001) Early and intensive continuous hemofiltration for severe renal failure after cardiac surgery. Ann Thorac Surg 71:832–837

23. Boldt J, Brenner T, Lehmann A, et al (2003) Is kidney function altered by the duration of cardiopulmonary bypass? Ann Thorac Surg 75:906–912

24. Bouman CS, Oudemans-van Straaten HM, Tijssen JG, et al (2002) Effects of early high-volume continuous venovenous hemofiltration on survival and recovery of renal function in intensive care patients with acute renal failure: A prospective, randomized trial. Crit Care Med 30:2205–2211

25. Bouman CS, Oudemans-van Straaten HM, Schultz MJ, et al (2007) Hemofiltration in sepsis and systemic inflammatory response syndrome: The role of dosing and timing. J Crit Care 22:1–12

26. Bourgeois BF, Donath A, Paunier L, et al (1979) Effects of cardiac surgery on renal function in children. J Thorac Cardiovasc Surg 77:283–286

27. Brady H, Singer G (1995) Acute renal failure. Lancet 346:1533–1540

28. Brezis M, Rosen S (1995) Hypoxia of the renal medulla – its implications for disease. N Engl J Med 332:647–655

29. Brivet FG, Kleinknecht DJ, Loirat P, et al (1996) Acute renal failure in intensive care units - causes, outcome, and prognostic factors of hospital mortality: A prospective, multicenter study. French study group on acute renal failure. Crit Care Med 24:192–198

30. Brown KL, Ridout DA, Goldman AP, et al (2003) Risk factors for long intensive care unit stay after cardiopulmonary bypass in children. Crit Care Med 31:28–33

31. Bunchman TE, Maxvold NJ, Kershaw DB, et al (1995) Continuous venovenous hemodiafiltration in infants and children. Am J Kidney Dis 25:17–21

32. Bunchman TE, McBryde KD, Mottes TE, et al (2001) Pediatric acute renal failure: Outcome by modality and disease. Pediatr Nephrol 16:1067–1071

33. Burns KE, Chu MW, Novick RJ, et al (2005) Perioperative N-acetylcysteine to prevent renal dysfunction in high-risk patients undergoing CABG surgery: A randomized controlled trial. JAMA 294:342–350

34. Casey WF, Hauser GJ, Hannallah RS, et al (1992) Circulating endotoxin and tumor necrosis factor during pediatric cardiac surgery. Crit Care Med 20:1090–1096

35. Chan K-L, Ip P, Chiu CSW, et al (2003) Peritoneal dialysis after surgery for congenital heart disease in infants and children. Ann Thorac Surg 76:1443–1449

36. Chertow GM, Levy EM, Hammermesiter KE, et al (1998) Independent association between acute renal failure and mortality following cardiac surgery. Am J Med 104:343–348

37. Chertow GM, Burdick E, Honour M, et al (2005) Acute kidney injury, mortality, length of stay, and costs in hospitalized patients. J Am Soc Nephrol 16:3365–3370

38. Chung JH, Gikakis N, Rao AK, et al (1996) Pericardial blood activates the extrinsic coagulation pathway during clinical cardiopulmonary bypass. Circulation 93:2014–2018

39. Clermont G, Acker CG, Angus DC, et al (2002) Renal failure in the ICU: Comparison of the impact of acute renal failure and end-stage renal disease on ICU outcomes. Kidney Int 62:986–996

40. Colman RW (1984) Surface-mediated defense reactions: The plasma contact activation system. J Clin Invest 73:1249–1253

41. Conger J (1975) A controlled evaluation of prophylactic dialysis in post-traumatic acute renal failure. J Trauma 15:1056–1063

42. Conlon PJ, Stafford-Smith M, White WD, et al (1999) Acute renal failure following cardiac surgery. Nephrol Dial Transplant 14:1158–1162

43. de Mendonca A, Vincent JL, Suter PM, et al (2000) Acute renal failure in the ICU: Risk factors and outcome evaluated by the SOFA score. Intensive Care Med 26:915–921

44. Demirkilic U, Kurulay E, Yenicesu M, et al (2004) Timing of replacement therapy for acute renal failure after cardiac surgery. J Card Surg 19:17–20

45. Devarajan P (2007) Emerging biomarkers of acute kidney injury. Contrib Nephrol 156:203–212

46. Devarajan P, Mishra J, Supavekin S, et al (2003) Gene expression in early ischemic renal injury: Clues towards pathogenesis, biomarker discovery, and novel therapeutics. Mol Genet Metab 80:365–376

47. Dittrich S, Haas NA, Muller C, et al (1998) Renal impairment in patients with long-standing cyanotic congenital heart disease. Acta Paediatr 87:949–954

48. Dittrich S, Kurschat K, Dahnert I, et al (2000) Renal function after cardiopulmonary bypass surgery in cyanotic congenital heart disease. Int J Cardiol 73:173–179

49. Dittrich S, Priesemann M, Fischer T, et al (2002) Circulatory arrest and renal function in open-heart surgery on infants. Pediatr Cardiol 23:15–19

50. Dittrich S, Aktuerk D, Seitz S, et al (2004) Effects of ultrafiltration and peritoneal dialysis on proinflammatory cytokines during cardiopulmonary bypass surgery in newborn infants and children. Eur J Cardiothorac Surg 25:935–940

51. DuBose TDJ, Warnock DG, Mehta RL, et al (1997) Acute renal failure in the 21st century: Recommendations for management and outcomes assessment. Am J Kidney Dis 29:793–799

52. Edelstein CL, Ling H, Schrier R (1997) The nature of renal cell injury. Kidney Int 51:1341–1351

53. Elahi MM, Lim MY, Joseph RN, et al (2004) Early hemofiltration improves survival in post-cardiotomy patients with acute renal failure. Eur J Cardiothorac Surg 26:1027–1031

54. Ellis EN, Brouhard BH, Conti VR (1983) Renal function in children undergoing cardiac operations. Ann Thorac Surg 36:167–172

55. Fischer R, Griffin W, Clark D (1966) Early dialysis in the treatment of acute renal failure. Surg Gynecol Obstet 123:1019–1023

56. Fischer UM, Weissenberger WK, Warters RD, et al (2002) Impact of cardiopulmonary bypass management on post-cardiac surgery renal function. Perfusion 17:401–406

57. Fischer UM, Cox CSJ, Allen SJ, et al (2003) The antioxidant N-acetylcysteine preserves myocardial function and diminishes oxidative stress after cardioplegic arrest. J Thorac Cardiovasc Surg 126:1483–1488

58. Fleming F, Bohn D, Edwards H, et al (1995) Renal replacement therapy after repair of congenital heart disease in children: A comparison of hemofiltration and peritoneal dialysis. J Thorac Cardiovasc Surg 109:322–331

59. Foland JA, Fortenberry JD, Warshaw BL, et al (2004) Fluid overload before continuous hemofiltration and survival in critically ill children: A retrospective analysis. Crit Care Med 32:1771–1776

60. Gettings L, Reynolds H, Scalea T (1999) Outcome in post-traumatic acute renal failure when continuous renal replacement therapy is applied early vs late. Intensive Care Med 25:805–813

61. Goldstein SL, Currier H, Graf JM, et al (2001) Outcome in children receiving continuous venovenous hemofiltration. Pediatrics 107:1309–1312

62. Goldstein SL, Somers MJG, Baum MA, et al (2005) Pediatric patients with multi-organ dysfunction syndrome receiving continuous renal replacement therapy. Kidney Int 67:653–658

63. Gomez-Campdera FJ, Maroto-Alvaro E, Galinanes M, et al (1988–1989) Acute renal failure associated with cardiac surgery. Child Nephrol Urol 9:138–143

64. Gottlieb SS, Abraham W, Butler J, et al (2002) The prognostic importance of different definitions of worsening renal function in congestive heart failure. J Card Fail 8:136–141

65. Gruberg L, Mintz GS, Mehran R, et al (2000) The prognostic implications of further renal function deterioration within 48 h of interventional coronary procedures in patients with pre-existing chronic renal insufficiency. J Am Coll Cardiol 36:1542–1548

66. Haase M, Haase-Fielitz A, Bagshaw SM, et al (2007) Cardiopulmonary bypass-asociated acute kidney injury: A pigment nephropathy? Contrib Nephrol 156:340–353

67. Haase M, Haase-Fielitz A, Bagshaw SM, et al (2007) Phase II, randomized, controlled trial of high-dose N-acetylcysteine in high-risk cardiac surgery patients. Crit Care Med 35:1324–1331

68. Hamel MB, Phillips RS, Davis RB, et al (1997) Outcomes and cost-effectiveness of initiating dialysis and continuous aggressive care in seriously ill hospitalized adults. Ann Intern Med 127:195–202

69. Han WK, Bailly V, Abichandani R, et al (2002) Kidney Injury Molecule-1 (KIM-1): A novel biomarker for human renal proximal tubule injury. Kidney Int 62:237–244

70. Han WK, Bonventre JV (2004) Biologic markers for the early detection of acute kidney injury. Curr Opin Crit Care 10:476–482

71. Herget-Rosenthal S, Marggraf G, Husing J, et al (2004) Early detection of acute renal failure by serum cystatin C. Kidney Int 66:1115–1122

72. Herget-Rosenthal S, Pietruck F, Volbracht L, et al (2005) Serum cystatin C–a superior marker of rapidly reduced glomerular filtration after uninephrectomy in kidney donors compared to creatinine. Clin Nephrol 64:41–46

73. Herrero-Morin JD, Malaga S, Fernandez N, et al (2007) Cystatin C and beta2-microglobulin: Markers of glomerular filtration in critically ill children. Crit Care 11:R59

74. Hoste EA, Kellum JA (2006) RIFLE criteria provide robust assessment of kidney dysfunction and correlate with hospital mortality. Crit Care Med 34:2016–2017

75. Hoste EA, Clermont G, Kersten A, et al (2006) RIFLE criteria for acute kidney injury are associated with hospital mortality in critically ill patients: A cohort analysis. Crit Care 10:R73

76. Hoyt DB (1997) CRRT in the area of cost containment: Is it justified? Am J Kidney Dis 30:S102–S104

77. Hui-Stickle S, Brewer ED, Goldstein SL (2005) Pediatric ARF epidemiology at a tertiary care center from 1999 to 2001. Am J Kidney Dis 45:96–101

78. Inatomi J, Matsuoka K, Fujimaru R, et al (2006) Mechanisms of development and progression of cyanotic nephropathy. Pediatr Nephrol 21:1440–1445

79. Jander A, Tkaczyk M, Pagowska-Klimek I, et al (2007) Continuous veno-venous hemofiltration in children after cardiac surgery. Eur J Cardiothorac Surg 31:1022–1028

80. Jones D, Bellomo R (2005) Renal-dose dopamine: From hypothesis to paradigm to dogma to myth and, finally, superstition? J Intensive Care Med 20:199–211

81. Kainuma M, Yamada M, Miyake T (1996) Continuous urine oxygen tension monitoring in patients undergoing cardiac surgery. J Cardiothorac Vasc Anesth 10:603–608

82. Kellum JA, Leblanc M, Gibney RT, et al (2005) Primary prevention of acute renal failure in the critically ill. Curr Opin Crit Care 11:537–541

83. Khabar KS, el Barbary MA, Khougeer F, et al (1997) Circulating endotoxin and cytokines after cardiopulmonary bypass: Differential correlation with duration of bypass and systemic inflammatory response/multiple organ dysfunction syndromes. Clin Immunol Immunopathol 85:97–103

84. Kist-van Holthe tot Echten JE, Goedvolk CA, Doornaar MB, et al (2001) Acute renal insufficiency and renal replacement therapy after pediatric cardiopulmonary bypass surgery. Pediatr Cardiol 22:321–326

85. Kleinknecht D, Jungers P, Chanard J, et al (1972) Uremic and non-uremic complications in acute renal failure: Evaluation of early and frequent dialysis on prognosis. Kidney Int 1:190–196

86. Komisarof JA, Gilkey GM, Peters DM, et al (2007) N-acetylcysteine for patients with prolonged hypotension as prophylaxis for acute renal failure (NEPHRON). Crit Care Med 35:435–441

87. Kuitunen A, Vento A, Suojaranta-Ylinen R, et al (2006) Acute renal failure after cardiac surgery: Evaluation of the RIFLE classification. Ann Thorac Surg 81:542–546

88. Lassnigg A, Schmidlin D, Mouhieddine M, et al (2004) Minimal changes of serum creatinine predict prognosis in patients after cardiothoracic surgery: A prospective cohort study. J Am Soc Nephrol 15:1597–1605

89. Lema G, Meneses G, Urzua J, ct al (1995) Effccts of extracorporeal circulation on renal function in coronary surgical paticnts. Ancsth Analg 81:446–451

90. Lema G, Urzua J, Jalil R, et al (1998) Renal protection in patients undergoing cardiopulmonary bypass with preoperative abnormal rcnal function. Ancsth Analg 86:3–8

91. Lema G, Vogel A, Canessa R, et al (2006) Renal function and cardiopulmonary bypass in pediatric cardiac surgical patients. Pediatr Nephrol 21:1446–1451

92. Lequier LL, Nikaidoh H, Leonard SR, et al (2000) Preoperative and postoperative endotoxemia in children with congenital heart disease. Chest 117:1706–1712

93. Levy EM, Viscoli CM, Horwitz RI (1996) The effect of acute renal failure on mortality. A cohort analysis. JAMA 275:1489–1494

94. Levy MM, Macias WL, Vincent JL, et al (2005) Early changes in organ function predict eventual survival in severe sepsis. Crit Care Med 33:2194–2201

95. Liangos O, Perianayagam MC, Vaidya VS, et al (2007) Urinary N-acetyl-beta(D)-glucosaminidasc activity and kidney injury molecule-1 are associated with adverse outcomes in acute renal failure. J Am Soc Nephrol 18:904–912

96. Liano F, Junco E, Pacual J, et al (1998) The spectrum of acute renal failure in the intensive care unit compared with that seen in other settings. The Madrid Acute Renal Failure Study Group. Kidney Int Suppl 66:S16–S24

97. Lin CY, Chen YC, Tsai FC, et al (2006) RIFLE classification is predictive of short-term prognosis in critically ill patients with acute renal failure supported by extracorporeal membrane oxygenation. Nephrol Dial Transplant 21:2867–2873

98. Liu KD, Himmelfarb J, Paganini E, et al (2006) Timing of initiation of dialysis in critically ill patients with acute kidney injury. Clin J Am Soc Nephrol 1:915–919

99. Loef BG, Epema AH, Smilde TB, et al (2005) Immediate postoperative renal function deterioration in cardiac surgical patients predicts in-hospital mortality and long-term survival. J Am Soc Nephrol 16:195–200

100. Lok CE, Austin PC, Wanh H, et al (2004) Impact of renal insufficiency on short- and long-term outcomes after cardiac surgery. Am Heart J 148:430–438

101. Lowrie LH (2000) Renal replacement therapies in pediatric multi-organ dysfunction syndrome. Pediatr Nephrol 14:6–12

102. Mangano CM, Diamondstone LS, Ramsay JG, et al (1998) Renal dysfunction after myocardial revascularization: Risk factors, adverse outcomes, and hospital resource utilization. The multicenter study of perioperative Ischemia research group. Ann Intern Med 128:194–203

103. Mazur MJ, Heilman RL (2005) Early detection of acute renal failure by serum cystatin C: A new opportunity for a hepatologist. Liver Transpl 11:705–707

104. McDougal WS (2005) Early detection of acute renal failure by serum cystatin C. J Urol 174:1024–1025

105. McNiece KL, Ellis EE, Drummond-Webb JJ, et al (2005) Adequacy of peritoneal dialysis in children following cardiopulmonary bypass surgery. Pediatr Nephrol 20:972–976

106. Mehta RL, Chertow GM (2003) Acute renal failure definitions and classification: Time for change? J Am Soc Nephrol 14:2178–2187

107. Mehta RL, Kellum JA, Shah SV, et al (2007) Acute Kidney Network: Report of an initiative to improve outcomes in acute kidney injury. Crit Care 11:1–8

108. Metnitz PG, Krenn CG, Steltzer H, et al (2002) Effect of acute renal failure requiring renal replacement therapy on outcome in critically ill patients. Crit Care Med 30:2051–2058

109. Mishra J, Ma Q, Prada A, et al (2003) Identification of NGAL as a novel urinary biomarker for ischemic injury. J Am Soc Nephrol 14:2534–2543

110. Mishra J, Mori K, Ma Q, et al (2004) Amelioration of ischemic acute renal injury by neutrophil gelatinase-associated lipocalin. J Am Soc Nephrol 15:3073–3082

111. Mishra J, Mori K, Ma Q, et al (2004) Neutrophil gelatinase-associated lipocalin: A novel early urinary biomarker for cisplatin nephrotoxicity. Am J Nephrol 24:307–315

112. Mishra J, Dent C, Tarabish R, et al (2005) Neutrophil gelatinase-associated lipocalin (NGAL) as a biomarker for acute renal injury after cardiac surgery. Lancet 365:1231–1238

113. Moat NE, Shore DF, Evans TW (1993) Organ dysfunction and cardiopulmonary bypass: The role of complement and complement regulatory proteins. Eur J Cardiothorac Surg 7:563–573

114. Moran SM, Myers BD (1985) Course of acute renal failure studied by a model of creatinine kinetics. Kidney Int 27:928–937

115. Nolan CR, Anderson RJ (1998) Hospital-acquired acute renal failure. J Am Soc Nephrol 9:710–718

116. Novis BK, Roizen MF, Aronson S, et al (1994) Association of preoperative risk factors with postoperative acute renal failure. Anesth Analg 78:143–149

117. Otukesh H, Hoseini R, Hooman N, et al (2006) Prognosis of acute renal failure in children. Pediatr Nephrol 21:1873–1878

118. Paller MS (1998) Acute renal failure: Controversies, clinical trials, and future directions. Semin Nephrol 18:482–489

119. Paparella D, Yau TM, Young E (2002) Cardiopulmonary bypass induced inflammation: Pathophysiology and treatment. An update. Eur J Cardiothorac Surg 21:232–244

120. Parikh CR, Jani A, Melnikov VY, et al (2004) Urinary interleukin-18 is a marker of human acute tubular necrosis. Am J Kidney Dis 43:405–414

121. Parikh CR, Abraham E, Ancukiewicz M, et al (2005) Urine IL-18 is an early diagnostic marker for acute kidney injury and predicts mortality in the intensive care unit. J Am Soc Nephrol 16:3046–3052

122. Parikh CR, Jani A, Mishra J, et al (2006) Urine NGAL and IL-18 are predictive biomarkers for delayed graft function following kidney transplantation. Am J Transplant 6:1639–1645

123. Parikh CR, Mishra J, Thiessen-Philbrook H, et al (2006) Urinary IL-18 is an early predictive biomarker of acute kidney injury after cardiac surgery. Kidney Int 70:199–203

124. Parsons F, Hobson S, Blagg C, et al (1961) Optimum time for dialysis in acute reversible renal failure. Lancet 277:124–129

125. Picca S, Principato F, Mazzera E, et al (1995) Risks of acute renal failure after cardiopulmonary bypass surgery in children: A retrospective 10-year case-control study. Nephrol Dial Transplant 10:630–636

126. Plotz FB, Hulst HE, Twist JW, et al (2005) Effect of acute renal failure on outcome in children with severe septic shock. Pediatr Nephrol 20:1177–1181

127. Praught ML, Shlipak MG (2005) Are small changes in serum creatinine an important risk factor? Curr Opin Nephrol Hypertens 14:265–270

128. Rigden SP, Barratt TM, Dillon MJ, et al (1982) Acute renal failure complicating cardiopulmonary bypass surgery. Arch Dis Child 57:425–430

129. Ristikankare A, Kuitunen T, Kuitunen A, et al (2006) Lack of renoprotective effect of i.v. N-acetylcysteine in patients with chronic renal failure undergoing cardiac surgery. Br J Anaesth 97:611–616

130. Rosner MH, Okusa MD (2006) Acute kidney injury associated with cardiac surgery. Clin J Am Soc Nephrol 1:19–32

131. Schwartz GJ, Brion LP, Spitzer A (1987) The use of plasma creatinine concentration for estimating glomerular filtration in infants, children, and adolescents. Pediatr Clin North Am 34:571–590

132. Skippen PW, Krahn GE (2005) Acute renal failure in children undergoing cardiopulmonary bypass. Crit Care Resusc 7:286–291

133. Smith GL, Vaccarino V, Kosiborod M, et al (2003) Worsening renal function: What is a clinically meaning-ful change in creatinine during hospitalization with heart failure? J Card Fail 9:13–25

134. Stafford-Smith M, Grocott HP (2005) Renal medullary hypoxia during experimental cardiopulmonary bypass: A pilot study. Perfusion 20:53–58

135. Star RA (1998) Treatment of acute renal failure. Kidney Int 54:1817–1831

136. Stromberg D, Fraser CDJ, Sorof JM, et al (1997) Peritoneal dialysis: An adjunct to pediatric postcardiotomy fluid management. Tex Heart Inst J 24:269–277

137. Supavekin S, Zhang W, Kucherlapati R, et al (2003) Differential gene expression following early renal ischemia-reperfusion. Kidney Int 63:1714–1724

138. Thadhani R, Bonventre JV (1996) Acute renal failure. N Engl J Med 334:1448–1460

139. Thakar CV, Worley S, Arrigain S, et al (2005) Influence of renal dysfunction on mortality after cardiac surgery: Modifying effect of preoperative renal function. Kidney Int 67:1112–1119

140. Tossios P, Bloch W, Huebner A, et al (2003) N-acetyl-cystein prevents reactive oxygen species-mediated myo-cardial stress in patients undergoing cardiac surgery: Results of a randomized, double-blind, placebo-controlled clinical trial. J Thorac Cardiovasc Surg 126:1513–1520

141. Trachtman H, Christen E, Cnaan A, et al (2006) Urinary neutrophil gelatinase-associated lipocalin in D + HUS: A novel marker of renal injury. Pediatr Nephrol 21:989–994

142. Trof RJ, Di Maggio F, Leemreis J, et al (2006) Biomarkers of acute renal injury and renal failure. Shock 26:245–253

143. Uchino S (2006) The epidemiology of acute renal failure in the world. Curr Opin Crit Care 12:538–543

144. Uchino S, Bellomo R, Goldsmith D, et al (2006) An assessment of the RIFLE criteria for acute renal failure in hospitalized patients. Crit Care Med 34:1913–1917

145. Undar A, Masai T, YAng SQ, et al (1999) Effects of per-fusion mode on regional and global organ blood flow in a neonatal piglet model. Ann Thorac Surg 68:1336–1343

146. Urzua J, Troncoso S, Bugedo G, et al (1992) Renal func-tion and cardiopulmonary bypass: Effect of perfusion pressure. J Cardiothorac Vasc Anesth 6:299–303

147. van Dongen EI, Glansdorp AG, Mildner RJ, et al (2003) The influence of perioperative factors on outcomes in children aged less than 18 months after repair of tetralogy of Fallot. J Thorac Cardiovasc Surg 126:703–710

148. Venkataraman R, Kellum JA (2007) Prevention of acute renal failure. Chest 131:300–308

149. Villa P, Jimenez M, Soriano MC, et al (2005) Serum cysta-tin C concentration as a marker of acute renal dysfunc-tion in critically ill patients. Crit Care 9:R139–R143

150. Wagener G, Jan M, Kim M, et al (2006) Association between increases in urinary neutrophil gelatinase-associ-ated lipocalin and acute renal dysfunction after adult car-diac surgery. Anesthesiology 105:485–491

151. Warady BA, Bunchman T (2000) Dialysis therapy for children with acute renal failure: Survey results. Pediatr Nephrol 15:11–13

152. Werner HA, Wensley DF, Lirenman DS, et al (1997) Peritoneal dialysis in children after cardiopulmonary bypass. J Thorac Cardiovasc Surg 113:64–70

153. Westhuyzen J (2006) Cystatin C: A promising marker and predictor of impaired renal function. Ann Clin Lab Sci 36:387–394

154. Wheeler DS, Dent CL, Manning PB, et al (in press) Factors prolonging length of stay in the cardiac intensive care unit following the arterial switch operation. Cardiol Young In Press

155. Wilkins RG, Faragher EB (1983) Acute renal failure in an intensive care unit: Incidence, prediction and outcome. Anaesthesia 38:628–634

156. Williams DM, Sreedhar SS, Mickell JS, et al (2002) Acute kidney failure: A pediatric experience over 20 years. Arch Pediatr Adolesc Med 156:893–900

157. Zakeri R, Freemantle N, Barnett V, et al (2005) Relation between mild renal dysfunction and outcomes after coronary artery bypass grafting. Circulation 112:I270–I275

158. Zappitelli M, Washburn KK, Arikan AA, et al (2007) Urine neutrophil gelatinase-associated lipocalin is an early marker of acute kidney injury in critically ill children: A prospective cohort study. Crit Care 11: R84

Contrast-Induced Nephropathy   20

V.M. Kriss and S.G. Kiessling

Contents

Core Messages

> › Any child in the intensive care unit undergoing diagnostic imaging using contrast material should be considered to be at risk to develop contrast-induced nephropathy (CIN).
> › The risk for CIN is increased in children with preexisting renal dysfunction
> › Direct communication with the pediatric radiologist to minimize the dose of contrast material as possible and optimize timing of the study might be valuable.
> › Preventative strategies of CIN should be discussed and evaluated ahead of time by the ICU team and the nephrologist, especially in children at high risk.

Case Vignette

A term infant was admitted to the neonatal intensive care unit with respiratory distress and congestive heart failure due to a hemangioendothelioma. This highly vascular hepatic mass encompassed most of the infant's right lobe of his liver. The baby continued to deteriorate, and the decision was made to proceed to angiography with the hope to at least partially embolize the lesion. Angiographic embolization of the hemangioendothelioma was successful. A total of 20 mL of nonionic, low osmolar contrast material was utilized in the procedure, resulting in a patient dose of 7 mL kg^{-1}. Because of the heart failure, the infant was fluid restricted prior to and after the procedure.

Within 24 h after the procedure, the baby's serum creatinine rose from 0.6 to 0.9 mg dL^{-1} indicating a significantly decreased glomerular filtration rate. He developed oligoanuria. Plain radiographs of the abdomen demonstrated bilateral, persistent nephrograms. By postprocedure day 4, however, the infant's creatinine and urine output had normalized. The child experienced no further renal compromise.

20.1   Introduction

Iodinated contrast material is a common adjunct to radiographic procedures. It can be used in the gastrointestinal or genitourinary tract in children with virtually no adverse reactions. Intravascular use of iodinated contrast material can be seen with angiography, which requires intra-arterial injection of contrast material. Far more common is intravenous use of contrast material for computed tomography (CT). Iodinated contrast material is a crucial component in computed tomography for delineating anatomic structures and enhancing infection or tumor. However, the injection of intravascular iodinated contrast can result in a number of complications ranging from anaphylaxis to renal failure. The latter is much more commonly seen in adults than in children. Hence, virtually all of the data on CIN are found in the adult realm and comprehensive reviews are available in the adult literature [39].

Nephrotoxicity of radio contrast material and acute kidney injury (AKI) were first described in the 1960s

S.G. Kiessling et al. (eds) *Pediatric Nephrology in the ICU.*

with an increasing incidence due to more common use of radio contrast studies over the years.

A transient mild rise in serum creatinine following contrast administration is a common phenomenon [53]. The vast majority of these patients rapidly recover normal renal function with no long-term problems. Some patients, however, experience a significant decline in renal function following contrast administration, raising the question of a CIN once all other possible etiologic factors are ruled out.

A true CIN is broadly defined as acute renal failure with a 25% increase in serum creatinine over baseline (or a rise of 0.5 mg dL^{-1} from baseline) that occurs within 48 h of contrast administration in the absence of any other known causes [42, 48]. Fortunately, most cases of CIN are mild and reversible and only rarely advance to oliguric or anuric acute renal failure. Following onset of CIN, serum creatinine usually peaks in 3–5 days with a return to normal renal function within an average time of 7–21 days [22, 31]. However, long-term morbidity remains a concern; up to 30% of adult patients with CIN will develop some permanent renal impairment, including 1% who will require dialysis [1, 11] Clearly, it is this latter group that contributes to the prolonged hospital stay and increased medical costs of CIN that are estimated at $32 million annually [38].

20.2 Risk Factors

In this era of ever-increasing medical procedures (particularly, CT examinations) CIN is said to be the third most common cause of hospital-acquired acute renal failure after surgery and hypotension [17]. How common is CIN? An incidence of 14% has been quoted in all patients; a number that drops to less than 2% in the general population without any known risk factors [4, 37]. The incidence of CIN, however, dramatically rises with the presence of known risk factors. Preexisting renal dysfunction appears to be a primary risk factor. In patients with serum creatinine levels in excess of 2 mg dL^{-1}, the incidence of CIN rose up to 50% in patients who received intravascular contrast material [43, 50]. Diabetes mellitus with associated renal insufficiency is also included as a known risk factor for CIN, yet the presence of diabetes, alone, was not found to be a significant risk factor [33, 43].

A reduction in intravascular or effective circulating volume is another key risk factor for CIN. Dehydration, congestive heart failure, and prolonged hypotension all contribute to a prerenal reduction of renal perfusion, which can markedly enhance the toxicity of contrast material [5, 45, 59]. Generalized sepsis with an impairment of circulation and potential bacterial toxin damage of renal tubules can also accentuate CIN [10]. Similarly, diuretic usage (especially loop diuretics such as furosemide) has also been implicated as a risk factor for CIN. Preexisting administration of nephrotoxic drugs such as cyclosporine A, cisplatin, aminoglycosides, and amphotericin B has been recognized as a factor in the higher incidence of CIN, as these renal toxic agents may render the kidney more vulnerable to CIN. Even nonsteroidal anti-inflammatory drugs (NSAIDs) have been implicated, possibly because of inhibition of local renal vasodilatory effects of prostaglandins [27, 41].

Another important factor to consider in CIN is the contrast material, itself. The route of administration is relevant. Angiography with an intra-arterial injection is more nephrotoxic, probably because a higher intrarenal concentration is achieved as compared with an intravenous route as used for CT examinations [17]. Osmolarity of the contrast material is also a crucial consideration, particularly in high-risk patients. The use of low-osmolarity contrast agents clearly reduces the incidence of CIN in patients with preexisting renal insufficiency as compared with using high osmolar agents. Such an obvious reduction in CIN, however, was not demonstrated in patients with normal renal function when using the low-osmolarity agents [3, 51].

Most important is the actual dose (volume) of contrast received within a fixed period of time. Clearly, patients receiving angiographic/interventional procedures receive far more contrast material volume than those receiving contrast for diagnostic purposes only (such as CT examination). Aiming for the lowest contrast dose possible to achieve the desired result is always the goal. Definitive cut-off numbers have not been rigorously established, but the following numbers can be a practical guide. Diagnostic procedures (such as CT examination) can be done with a 2 mL kg^{-1} dose or less in children, which is considered a relatively safe dose [9]. Angiographic/interventional procedures can reach 4 mL kg^{-1} dose with 5 mL kg^{-1} considered a level at which CIN becomes a clear concern [9, 57]. Prudence also dictates a waiting period of at last 72 h if at all possible between different procedures that require contrast material to allow the kidney to *recover* and help decrease the potential appearance of CIN [17].

20.3 Pathophysiology

The exact mechanism of CIN is still a mystery. It is likely that CIN is actually a combination of pathologic factors. Plausible theories such as direct renal tubular epithelial cell toxicity (possibly by oxygen-free radicals) have been described as well as mechanisms related to altered renal hemodynamics that result in renal ischemic change [2, 60]. The latter is particularly convincing given that laboratory animals only acquired CIN when the systemic or renal circulation was compromised [6, 13, 44]. Although contrast material does initially cause a vasodilatory effect for the first hour or two, it soon launches into a prolonged vasoconstrictive period with a subsequent decrease in renal blood flow. As a result, renal medullary ischemia can now occur, a stress that is difficult to tolerate for a kidney already compromised by factors such as diabetes or renal failure. Margulies et al. also discussed microshowers of atheroemboli to the kidneys as well as atheroemboli-induced renal vasoconstriction as important pathophysiologic factors [36].

Classic radiographic features can be seen in the presence of CIN. Following contrast administration, the presence of a persistent nephrogram (outline of the kidneys easily seen on plain radiograph or CT scout image) is very worrisome for CIN. The nephrogram is a visible sign of contrast material that has entered the renal cortical glomerular apparatus following intravascular injection, but cannot be filtered out into the collecting system due to the acute renal failure that has ensued.

Asymptomatic (nonoliguric) transient rise in creatinine mentioned earlier is a common early clinical presentation suggestive of a benign course. Once oliguria is present, however, morbidity rises significantly. Urinary findings such as epithelial cell casts, urate and calcium crystals have been described, but are nonspecific [55]. Similarly, low urinary sodium has been reported with CIN, but has not proven to be a convincing sign [14, 24].

20.4 Preventative Strategies

Extensive studies have been done investigating potential preventative strategies for CIN. Undoubtedly, there are several simple principles for the clinician to consider and some obvious questions to ponder:

› Is the study that utilizes contrast material really needed for the child's care?

› Are there other imaging studies that do not utilize contrast material that might be used as a substitute?

› Is it the time to initiate potential nephroprotective therapies?

› Can the study be delayed until renal function is improved (in situations with reversible acute renal injury)?

Sonography and MRI are both superb imaging studies that render excellent images, often providing even superior information compared with the results a CT examination could offer, particularly in infants. There is also an even safer alternative to angiography, namely CO_2 angiography that can be used in visceral, noncardiac imaging [28].

Once the decision is made to administer intravascular contrast, however, several preventative measures can be considered. Hydration is a crucial preventative strategy that is also the most efficacious in the prevention of CIN [12, 49]. Known high-risk patients, in particular, need to benefit from hydration, both pre and postcontrast administration. Although oral hydration is always an acceptable option, IV hydration clearly works best [54]. An appropriate protocol is 0.45% saline administered at $1-1.5\,\mathrm{mL\ kg^{-1}\ h^{-1}}$ beginning 6–12 h before contrast bolus and continuing up to 12 h following contrast administration [11]. Interestingly, recent data discusses the superiority of sodium bicarbonate hydration in the prevention of CIN. These authors contend that the bicarbonate ion is inhibitory toward free radical formation due to its increasing pH effects, and their data showed a decrease in CIN with sodium bicarbonate hydration as opposed with sodium chloride hydration [40].

Many pharmacologic agents have been used in experimental attempts to reduce CIN. Avoidance of nephrotoxic drugs such as cyclosporine A, aminoglycosides, and even NSAIDs for at least 24 h prior to contrast administration, if possible, is always a prudent move. The antioxidant drug N-acetylcysteine (adult dose of 600 mg administered twice the day before and the day of contrast administration) has been shown to be efficacious in the reduction of CIN, presumably due to its ability to prevent direct oxidative tissue damage following contrast administration. These benefits have been particularly noted in high-risk patients with renal insufficiency [47, 52]. Nevertheless, the results of clinical studies have shown significant variation as recently reviewed by Fishbane [16].

Other pharmacologic agents have been suggested in the prevention of CIN, but their true efficacy is questionable. These drugs include fenoldopam (a dopamine agonist that produces vasodilation of peripheral, mesenteric, and renal arteries), theophylline/aminophylline (adenosine antagonist to counteract adenosine's known vasoconstrictive role in CIN), and calcium channel blockers (vasodilation of afferent arterioles in the nephron) [8, 21, 23, 32, 46, 56]. Because of the conflicting evidence (some experimental trials showing efficacy while others show no statistical advantage), none of the aforementioned agents can clearly be recommended.

Newer preventative therapies for CIN are still being suggested. Usage of angiotensin-converting enzyme (ACE) inhibitors and even prostaglandin E1 (to counteract the vasoconstrictive properties seen in CIN) is enticing, and early pilot studies do show some promise [19, 26]. Without a doubt, more experimental data are required before these agents can be definitively added to the recommended preventative regiment for CIN.

Hemodialysis immediately postcontrast administration is an attractive idea: rapid removal of the offending contrast agent could limit renal exposure to its *toxic* effects. Unfortunately, studies have shown that hemodialysis had no effect on incidence of CIN as compared with saline hydration alone [29]. Interestingly, those who did receive hemodialysis postcontrast administration actually had a deleterious outcome with increasing decline of renal function [58]. Hemofiltration of administered contrast, however, was controversial. Encouraging results were published in 2003, yet critical evaluations of this work are mixed and hemofiltration cannot be recommended at this time [30, 35].

Hence, a realistic preventative regimen for CIN (especially in high-risk patients) would involve the following steps [17]:

1. Identify and discontinue any nephrotoxic drugs at least 48–72 h prior to contrast administration.
2. Request that nonionic, iso- or low osmolar contrast material be used.
3. Begin IV hydration with either 0.45%/0.9% sodium chloride or 150 meq sodium bicarbonate in 1 L of 5% dextrose/water IV at $1\,mL\,kg^{-1}\,h^{-1}$ for 6–12 h prior to the procedure and then continue for 12–24 h after the procedure.
4. Six-hundred milligram of *N*-acetylcysteine (adult dose) twice daily administered the day before and the day of the procedure.

Once contrast material has been administered, consideration can be given to serum creatinine and urine output monitoring for at least 72 h postprocedure to ascertain the emergence of CIN.

In addition to prevention of CIN, early recognition has become a prominent focus in recent years. With a rise in serum creatinine, the most commonly used indicator for CIN, generally occurring later in the course, efforts have been made to identify other markers allowing earlier recognition of CIN. The clinical impact of a reliable predictor of CIN could be significant. Patients at risk could be observed more closely and timely intervention be initiated, potentially ameliorating the disease course; also, avoidance of additional renal insults including administration of nephrotoxic medications and suboptimal fluid status could be minimized. Hirsch et al. [20] recently reported in a pilot study promising results of neutrophil gelatinase-associated lipocalin (NGAL) as a potential early marker of CIN.

20.5 Treatment

Once CIN has actually occurred, very little in the way of treatment regimen can be done. Certainly continued hydration and optimization of the extracellular volume is a prudent step. This requires close monitoring of the fluid balance as hydration needs to be decreased in the setting of oliguria to avoid iatrogenic volume overload. Diuretics to enhance urine flow are not recommended as they might increase contrast-induced diuresis and add to the renal toxicity [61]. Serum creatinine and serum electrolyte should be monitored in intervals (the latter to prevent hyperkalemia, hyponatremia, hyperphosphatemia, hypocalcemia, hypermagnesemia, and the metabolic acidosis associated with acute renal failure). In general, then, treatment for CIN is limited to general supportive therapy for the patient in nonspecific acute renal failure [15]. Time is clearly a factor: the vast majority of CIN will spontaneously resolve in a few days regardless of treatment regimen, particularly in the child without preexisting risk factors.

As for prevention, focus in therapy of CIN should also be placed on the avoidance of additional risk factors for nephrotoxicity, especially antibiotics and NSAIDs [61].

20.6 Gadolinium (MRI Contrast) Complications

MRI is often cited as an excellent alternative imaging modality to replace contrast CT. Contrast material is often not needed for MRI with its outstanding tissue differentiation and multiplanar ability. Occasionally,

MRI contrast material (gadolinium) is beneficial in imaging acuity, particularly with vascular, neoplastic, or infectious work-ups. For years, gadolinium was considered *safe* with virtually no recognizable or reproducible complications with its usage. Anaphylactic reaction was virtually unheard of and more importantly, renal function (even in those patients with preexisting renal disease) was not compromised following gadolinium administration. Hence, MRI, even with contrast administration, was considered a safe, viable alternative to CT in patients with preexisting renal disease. Recent research on adult patients, however, has introduced a new association with gadolinium usage. In patients with preexisting ESRD (end-stage renal disease), the administration of gadolinium has resulted in an increased incidence of nephrogenic systemic fibrosis (a rare, multisystemic fibrosing disorder, primarily involving the skin). A possible mechanism to explain the etiology is the dissociation of the organic chelate binding the gadolinium, resulting in the release of a toxic ion because of the inability of the kidneys to adequately clear the original gadolinium contrast in a timely fashion. As a result, avoidance of contrast MRI with gadolinium usage in the face of preexisting renal disease has been advocated [7, 18, 25, 34].

Take-Home Pearls

> Transient mild rise in serum creatinine following iodinated contrast administration is common. CIN is defined as acute renal failure with a 25% increase in serum creatinine levels over baseline that occurs within 48 h of iodinated contrast administration. The vast majority of children recover with no long-term renal sequelae.
> Risk factors for CIN include the following:
> - Dehydration
> - Preexisting renal disease
> - Nephrotoxic drugs
> - High-dose of contrast material (exceeding 5 mL kg^{-1})
> Preventative strategies for CIN include the following:
> - Discontinue any nephrotoxic drugs at least 48–72 h prior to contrast administration
> - Request nonionic, iso, or low osmolar contrast material
> - IV hydration 6–12 h prior to the procedure and then continue for 12–24 h after the procedure
> - Administration of N-acetylcysteine twice a day administered the day before and the day of the procedure
> Especially in infants, alternative imaging studies avoiding the use of contrast should be considered and discussed.

References

1. Asif A, Epstein M (2004) Prevention of radiocontrast induced nephropathy. Am J of Kidney Dis 44:12–24
2. Bakris GI, Lass N, Gaber AO, et al. (1990) Contrast media induced decline in renal function: a role for oxygen free radicals. Am J Physiol 258:115–120
3. Barrett BJ, Carlisle EJ (1993) Meta analysis of the relative nephrotoxicity of high and low osmolarity iodinated contrast media. Radiology 188:171–178
4. Berg KJ (2000) Nephrotoxicity related to contrast media. Scan J Urol Nephrol 34:317–322
5. Berns J, Ridnick M (1992) Contrast associated nephrotoxicity. Kidney 24:1–5
6. Brezis M, Rosen AS (1995) Hypoxia of the renal medulla: its implications for disease. N Engl J Med 332:647–655
7. Broome DR, Girguis MS, Baron PW, et al. (2007) Gadolinium associated nephrogenic systemic fibrosis: why radiologists should be concerned. AJR 188:586–592
8. Chamsuddin AA, Kowalik KJ, Bjarnason H, et al. (2002) Using a dopamine type 1A receptor agonist in high risk patients to ameliorate contrast associated nephropathy. AJR Am J Roentgenol 179:591–596
9. Cigarroa RG, Lange RA, Williams RH, et al. (2001) Dosing of contrast material to prevent CIN. Am J Med 111:692–698
10. Cochran ST, Wong WS, Roe DJ (1983) Predicting angiography induced acute renal function impairment: clinical risk model. AJR 141:1027–1033
11. Cox CD, Tsikouris JP (2004) Preventing contrast nephropathy: what is the best strategy? J Clin Pharmacol 44:327–337
12. Eisenberg RL, Bank WO, Hedgock MW (1981) Renal failure after major angiography can be avoided with hydration. AJR 136:859–861
13. el Sayed AA, Haylor JL, el Nahas AM (1991) Haemodynamic effects of water-soluble contrast media on the isolated perfused rat kidney. Br J Radiol 64:435–439
14. Fang L, Sirota R, Ebert T, et al. (1981) Low fractional excretion of sodium with CIN acute renal failure. Arch Intern Med 141:1652–1656
15. Finn WF (2006) The clinical and renal consequences of contrast induced nephropathy. Nephrol Dial Transplant 21:2–10
16. Fishbane S (2008) N-Acetylcysteine in the prevention of contrast-induced nephropathy. Clin J Am Soc Nephrol 3:281–287
17. Gleeson TG, Bulugahapitiya S (2004) CIN. AJR 183:1673–1689
18. Grobner T (2006) Gadolinium—a specific trigger for the development of nephrogenic systemic fibrosis? Nephrol Dial Transplant 21:1104–1108
19. Gupta RK, Kapoor A, Tewari S, et al. (1999) Captopril for prevention of CIN in diabetic patients. Indian Heart J 51:521–526
20. Hirsch R, Dent C, Pfriem H, et al. (2007) NGAL is an early predictive biomarker of contrast-induced nephropathy in children. Pediatr Nephrol 22:2089–2095
21. Huber W, Ilgmann K, Page M (2002) Effect of theophylline on CIN in patients with chronic renal insufficiency. Radiology 223:772–779
22. Katholi R (2006) CIN: update and practical clinical applications. US Cardiovasc Dis 2:73–80

23. Katholi RE, Taylor GJ, McCann WP, et al. (1995) Nephrotoxicity from contrast media: attenuation with theophylline. Radiology 195:17–22

24. Katzberg RW (1997) Urography in the 21st century. Radiology 204:297–312

25. Khurana A, Runge VM, Narayanan M, et al. (2007) Nephrogenic systemic fibrosis: a review of 6 cases related to gadolinium injection. Invest Radiol 42:139–145

26. Koch JA, Plus J, Grabensee B, et al. (2000) Prostaglandin E1: a new agent for the prevention of renal dysfunction in high risk patients caused by contrast media? Nephrol Dial Transplant 15:43–49

27. Kolonko A, Wiecek A (1998) CIN: old clinical problem with new therapeutic options. Nephrol Dial Transplant 13:803–806

28. Kriss VM, Cottrill C, Gurley JC (1997) CO2 angiography in children. Pediatric Radiol 27:807–810

29. Lehnert T, Keller E, Condolf K, et al. (1998) Effect of hemodialysis after contrast administration in patients with renal insufficiency. Nephrol Dial Transplant 13:358–362

30. Lin J, Bonventre JV (2005) Prevention of radiocontrast nephropathy. Curr Opin Nephrol Hypertens 14:105–110

31. Maddox TG (2002) Adverse reactions to contrast material: recognition, prevention and treatment. Am Fam Physician 66:1229–1234

32. Madyoon H, Croushore L, Weaver D, et al. (2001) Use of fenoldopam to prevent CIN in high risk patients. Cathet Cardiovasc Interv 53:341–345

33. Manske CL, Sprafka JM, Strony JT, et al. (1990) Contrast nephropathy in azotemic diabetic patients. Am J Med 89:615–620

34. Marckmann P, Skov L, Rossen H, et al. (2006) Nephrogenic systemic fibrosis: suspected etiological role of gadolinium used for contrast enhanced MRI. J Am Soc Nephrol 17:2359–2362

35. Marenzi G, Marana I, Lauri G, et al. (2003) The prevention of CIN by hemofiltration. N Engl J Med 349:1333–1340

36. Margulies K, Schirger J, Burnett J Jr (1992) Radiocontrast induced nephropathy: current status and future prospects. Int Angiol 11:20–25

37. McCullough PA, Wolyn R, Rocher LL, et al. (1997) Acute renal failure after coronary intervention incidence, risk factors and relationship to mortality. Am J Med 103:368–374

38. McCullough PA, Sandberg KR (2003) Epidemiology of CIN. Rev Cardiovasc Med 4:3–9

39. McCullough PA, Soman SS (2005) Contrast-induced nephropathy. Crit Care Clin 21:261–280

40. Merten GJ, Burgess WP, Gray LV, et al. (2004) Prevention of CIN with sodium bicarbonate: a randomized trial. JAMA 291:2328–2334

41. Morcos SK (1998) CIN: questions and answers. Br J Radiol 71:357–365

42. Murphy SW, Barrett BJ, Parfrey PS (2000) Contrast nephropathy. J Am Soc Nephrol 11:177–182

43. Parfrey PS, Griffiths SM, Barrett BJ (1989) Contrast material induced renal failure in patients with diabetes, renal insufficiency or both. N Engl J Med 320:143–153

44. Prasad PV, Proatna A, Spokes K, et al. (2000) Changes in intrarenal oxygenation as evaluated by BOLD MRI in a rat kidney model for CIN. J Magn Reson Imaging 13:744–747

45. Rudnick M, Berns J, Cohen R, et al. (1994) Nephrotoxic risks of angiography: a critical review. Am J Kidney Dis 24:713–727

46. Shammas NW, Kapalis MJ, Harris M, et al. (2002) Aminophylline does not protect against CIN in patients undergoing angiographic procedure. J Invasive Cardiol 13:738–740

47. Shyu KG, Cheng JJ, Kuan P (2002) Acetylcysteine protects against acute renal damage in patients with abnormal renal function undergoing coronary procedure. J Am Coll Cardiol 40:1383–1388

48. Solomon R (1998) Contrast medium induced acute renal failure. Kidney Int 53:230–242

49. Solomon R, Werner C, Mann D, et al. (1994) Effects of saline, mannitol and furosemide on acute diseases in renal function induced by radiocontrast agents. N Engl J Med 331:1416–1420

50. Stevens MA, McCullough PA, Tobin KJ, et al. (1999) A randomized trial of prevention measures in patients at high risk for CIN. J Am Coll Cardiol 33:403–411

51. Taliercio CP, Vlietstra RE, Ilstrup DM, et al. (1991) A randomized comparison of the nephrotoxicity of iopamidol and diatrizoate in high risk patients. J Am Coll Cardiol 17:384–390

52. Telep M, van der Giet M, Schwarzfeld C, et al. (2000) Prevention of CIN by acetylcysteine. N Engl J Med 343:180–184

53. Tommaso C (1994) Contrast induced nephrotoxicity in patients undergoing cardiac catheterization. Cathet Cardiovasc Diagn 31:316–321

54. Trivedi HS, Moore H, Nasr S, et al. (2003) A randomized prospective trial to assess the role of saline hydration on the development of contrast nephrotoxicity. Nephron Clin Pract 93:29–34

55. Tublin ME, Murphy ME, Tessler FN (1998) Current concepts in CIN. AJR 171:933–939

56. Tumlin JA, Wang A, Murray PT, et al. (2002) Fenoldopam blocks reduction in renal blood flow after contrast infusion. Am Heart J 143:894–903

57. Vlietstra RE, Nunn CM, Narvarte J, et al. (1996) Contrast nephropathy after coronary angioplasty in chronic renal insufficiency. Am Heart J 132:1049–1050

58. Vogt B, Ferrari P, Schonholzer C, et al. (2001) Prophylactic hemodialysis after contrast administration in patients with renal insufficiency is potentially harmful. Am J Med 111:692–698

59. Waybill MM, Waybill PN (2001) CIN: identification of patients at risk and algorithms for prevention. J Vasc Interv Radiol 12:3–9

60. Weisberg LS, Kurnik PB, Kurnik BR (1992) CIN in humans: role of renal vasoconstriction. Kidney Int 41:1408–1415

61. Wong GT, Irwin MG (2007) Contrast-induced nephropathy. Br J Anaesth 99:474–483

Intoxications

21

P. Bernard

Contents

Case Vignette

A 4-year-old female is seen in the emergency department for an accidental overdose. She has taken her mother's lithium pills. In the emergency room, lithium blood level returns at 5 mmol L^{-1}. The emergency room physician reviews available written references and con-

S.G. Kiessling et al. (eds) *Pediatric Nephrology in the ICU.*
© Springer-Verlag Berlin Heidelberg 2009

Core Messages

› Poisonings, intoxication, and medication overdoses are leading causes for admission to the pediatric intensive care unit.

› In the care of the intoxicated patient in which the substance is unknown, a reasonable starting point is trying to identify a specific toxidrome.

› Perhaps the greatest role for the nephrologist (and the kidney) in the management of the poisoned pediatric patient is the preservation of renal function and enhancement of toxin elimination via the kidneys.

› Regardless of the ingestion, importance must be given to the relative risks of renal replacement therapy vs. a more conservative approach.

sults with poison control. Recommendations are to begin hemodialysis for any patient with a blood level equal to or greater than 4 mmol L^{-1}, regardless of the symptomatology. After consultation with the pediatric intensivist and the pediatric nephrologist, the child is admitted to the pediatric intensive care unit. During the admission, the physicians weigh the evidence supporting extracorporeal elimination of lithium vs. a conservative approach. They elect to monitor the child closely with neurologic monitoring and attention to any symptoms of toxicity. Normal saline was administered to preserve and enhance renal flow. The lithium blood level decreased with conservative management and hemodialysis was never instituted. The patient was discharged after an uneventful stay of 48 h following admission.

21.1 Introduction

Poisonings, intoxications, and medication overdoses are the leading causes for admission of pediatric patients to the intensive care unit. However, the vast majority of these admissions have no significant adverse sequelae. In fact, pediatric fatalities from ingestion remain constant at approximately 20–30 deaths per annum in the USA [25]. In some circumstances, altering of the acid–base status or augmentation of urine output may reduce the morbidity and mortality of a toxin. In even rarer circumstances, extracorporeal removal of the toxin may be helpful. One must constantly assess the risks vs. benefits of invasive therapy. To achieve excellent outcomes, close communication between the intensivist and nephrologist is vital, especially in circumstances when initiation of renal replacement therapies is considered. Close collaboration with a poison control center as well as vigilant monitoring are essential components to the management of any patient with a significant intoxication.

21.2 Identifying the Intoxication

In the care of the intoxicated patient in which the substance is unknown, a reasonable starting point is trying to identify a specific toxidrome. This is defined as a constellation of signs and symptoms, a syndrome typical for a specific kind of poisoning. Key to the treatment of any pathology is the identification of the syndrome and the offending agent (Table 21.1).

It is important to differentiate the multitude of potential pharmacologic toxins, which can contribute to or be exclusively responsible for renal injury. Most of these agents lead to toxicity as part of the unintended result of treatment for an underlying condition while receiving appropriate medical care. As the majority of those agents (including aminoglycosides, nonsteroidal anti-inflammatory drugs, contrast material [see previous chapter]) are readily appreciated as a potential source of iatrogenic renal failure they will therefore not be included in this monograph.

The use of newer techniques such as thin-layer chromatography and gas chromatography-mass spectrometry has greatly simplified the definitive identification of unknown substances in the blood and urine. We recommend close consultation with the laboratory to specify what substances are possible based on the history, physical and laboratory analysis available at presentation.

21.3 The Role of the Kidney in Intoxications

Elimination of a toxin is primarily through the metabolism of the substance through the liver and elimination or clearance of the substance through the kidneys.

Table 21.1 The majority of intoxications can be clinically suspected or identified due to a specific toxidrome

Toxin	Toxidrome
Alcohols	Slurred speech, desinhibition, ataxia, hypothermia, confusion, memory loss
Salicylates	Nausea, vomiting, abdominal pain, increased respiratory effort, hyperthermia, coma
Lithium	Vomiting, diarrhea, vertigo, confusion, hyperreflexia, coma
Anticholinergics	Fever, tachycardia, dry skin, urinary retention, mydriasis, choreoathetosis, seizures, coma
Opioids	Hypotension, hypoventilation, pulmonary edema, miosis, bradycardia, unresponsiveness, coma
Cyclic antidepressants	Tachycardia, drowsiness, hypotension, insomnia, agitation, cardiac arrhythmia

The toxin can either be eliminated unchanged (as in ethanol poisonings) or through its active and inactive metabolites. It has been estimated that toxins contribute to renal failure in up to 20% of patients.

It is useful from the start to have an accurate picture of the toxin's pharmacokinetics. Many toxins in high concentrations deviate from their published half-lives and therefore plotting out the concentration of the drug with serial levels can be useful. As for most pharmacologic processes involving resorption, distribution, and elimination, most toxins also follow first-order kinetics as outlined in Fig. 21.1.

The practical result of this time of elimination is rapid decreases in toxicity over time as the patient quickly returns to nontoxic concentrations. However, some drugs such as ethanol exhibit zero-order kinetics, and the pathways for its metabolism become saturated quickly. The velocity of those reactions is independent of the dose of the toxin and a linear decrease in the amount of toxin is seen when concentration is plotted against time (Fig. 21.2). These toxins take much longer to clear to nontoxic levels.

Chronic renal failure involves not only decreasing toxin clearance of renal-eliminated toxins but also decreased hepatic clearance. Major clearance systems,

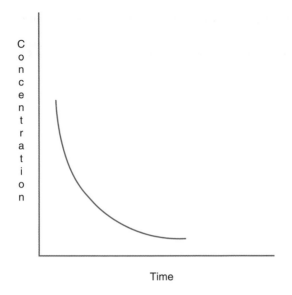

Fig. 21.1 First-order kinetics. The majority of drug metabolism takes place with first-order kinetics (the velocity of the elimination reaction is dependent on the concentration of the toxin)

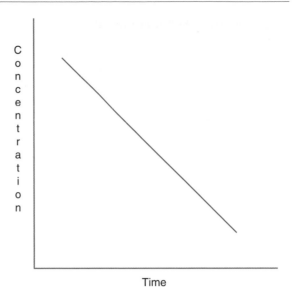

Fig. 21.2 Zero-order kinetics. The classic example of a zero-order kinetic elimination is ethanol intoxication

such as the hepatic cytochrome P450 system, are downregulated in renal failure [32].

The pediatric nephrologist and the intensivist share a common appreciation for acid–base disturbances. For the intensivist, the acid–base status is an important clue in the detective work that goes into identifying the toxin the child has been exposed to. In addition, acid–base disturbances markedly alter patient's toxicity, binding to serum proteins, and availability to the kidneys for clearance.

21.3.1 Kidneys as a Therapeutic Agent

Perhaps the greatest role for the nephrologist (and the kidney) in the management of the poisoned pediatric patient is the preservation of renal function and enhancement of toxin elimination via the kidneys. This is especially important if there is evidence of acute renal injury related to an acute intoxication or in the presence of documented nephrotoxicity without systemic involvement. Cases of increased pigment load (i.e., rhabdomyolysis, heme-pigment-induced acute tubular necrosis) are believed to be the result of decreased volume status and the formation of intratubular casts. Maintenance of intravascular volume status is essential to decrease precipitation of the pigments. Volume loading with $20\,mL\,kg^{-1}$ of isotonic solution and maintenance fluids at $3{,}000\,mL\,m^{-2}$ to maintain urine output greater than $2\,mL\,kg^{-1}\,h^{-1}$ in children with normal renal function seems a widely

used approach. Theoretically, urine alkalinization should decrease the toxic effects of a myoglobinuria. The proposed mechanisms are by decreasing the precipitation of hemoglobin [22]. However, recently this concept has come under scrutiny with a number of published reports [9, 19] questioning the necessity of alkalinization in the face of adequate volume expansion. Alkalinization may be accomplished by giving $1–2\,meq\,kg^{-1}$ of sodium bicarbonate intravenously over 30 min. This alkalinization may be continued by preparing a solution of D5W with $80\,meq\,L^{-1}$ of sodium bicarbonate running as maintenance fluids. Repeated urine pH's should be performed to keep the pH > 7.5 [33]. Potential complications from alkalinization of the urine include local tissue infiltration with resulting tissue necrosis as well as hypokalemia. Given the relative minimal risks, the authors recommend alkalinization with severe crushing injuries.

Alkalinization may also be useful for the enhanced elimination of toxin. Alkalinization is likely to be most effective if a toxin is eliminated by the kidneys essentially unchanged, has a small volume of distribution, is minimally bound to protein, and is a weak acid (pK_a > 5). Essentially, a toxin has increased elimination from the renal tubules if it crosses the renal tubular lumen and cannot readily diffuse across the renal epithelium. Alkalinization may have a role in the treatment of poisonings such as phenobarbital, methotrexate, chlorpropamide, and fluoride. However, only salicylate poisoning has convincing evidence supporting the routine use of alkalinization to enhance elimination [33].

21.3.2 Monitoring the Patient in the ICU

Pediatric ICU admission should be considered in virtually all children with an acute intoxication. Despite the availability of newer, safer antidepressants, tricyclic antidepressants (TCA) continue to be a frequent source of admission to the pediatric intensive care unit and monitoring will be discussed related to this specific intoxication. Those medications are nowadays frequently used in a variety of situations unrelated to the traditional indication of major depressive disorder, such as sleep aids, migraine prevention, and neuropathic pain treatment.

Admission to the ICU allows for close observation of the patient and rapid initiation of renal replacement therapies in case necessary. Favorable patient/nursing ratio, cardiovascular as well as fluid monitoring, and documentation of changes in patient exam facilitate early intervention if necessary.

The most concerning effect of TCA overdoses is its cardiotoxicity. TCA poisons the fast-acting sodium channels on the myocyte, leading to QRS prolongation, increasing the possibility of ventricular tachycardia [27]. The inhibition of these sodium channels can be blocked in an alkaline environment; however, some believe that the effects may be largely the result of the increasing sodium concentration that occurs with the large volume administration of sodium bicarbonate [31]. Regardless, in order to achieve reduction in toxicity of a TCA overdose, serum pH must be raised. This cannot be accomplished by dilute quantities of bicarbonate.

Patients admitted to the pediatric intensive care unit with TCA overdose require diligent telemetry to monitor for signs of cardiotoxicity. To adequately achieve treatment in the setting of cardiotoxicity, sodium bicarbonate (1 meq mL^{-1}) should be given through a large-bore IV followed by an infusion of sodium bicarbonate. The authors use D$_5$ ¼ NS with 80 meq L^{-1} of sodium bicarbonate running at maintenance rates. Caution should be undertaken when administered through a small-bore intravenous catheter, as extravasation can be associated with significant local tissue necrosis.

21.4 Role of Renal Replacement Therapy in Intoxications

The decision to start dialysis is a child with intoxication is based on a variety of factors. Regardless of the type of ingestion, importance must be given to the relative risks of renal replacement therapy vs. a more conservative approach. As mentioned before, death from a pediatric ingestion is a relatively uncommon occurrence [25]. The risks of hemodialysis are well described and include hypotension, dialysis disequilibrium syndrome, and hemorrhage [36]. In addition, the pediatric population is particularly problematic with regard to vascular access. Even in the most ideal situation, under generalized anesthesia, success rates are guarded [3]. Complications are frequent, even in the most experienced hands [13]. The mortality from pediatric central line insertion is not inconsequential [4]. Continuous renal replacement therapy may require blood product transfusions, and complications including life-threatening bleeding and hypocalcemia [8]. Therefore, the decision to start a patient on hemodialysis or other renal replacement therapy must be an overwhelming one.

21.5 Specific Intoxications

Entire texts are dedicated to the field of toxicology. Later, the most common indications for involvement of the Pediatric Nephrology Service in the intoxicated pediatric patient will be discussed in more detail.

21.5.1 Ethylene Glycol

Ethylene glycol is an alcohol ideally suited for use in antifreeze solutions. Although most commonly found in a relatively pure form in antifreeze, it is a component of common household cleaners, break fluid, and deicing solutions [6]. Its combination of sweetness and odorless nature make it an ideal candidate for consumption by toddlers. A common presentation is the accidental ingestion of ethylene glycol stored in a container that originally held potable consumables, such as a milk carton.

Ethylene glycol consumption is characterized at first by inebriation and altered mental status. Like ethanol, ethylene glycol is metabolized in the liver by the enzyme, alcohol dehydrogenase. Its final metabolite, oxalic acid is converted to calcium oxalate crystals. The calculi can be the identifying factor in establishing the cause of the renal failure in an unidentified poisoning [20].

Traditionally, ethylene glycol is thought to have three phases. In the first phase, the patient experiences euphoria, intoxication, and central nervous system (CNS) involvement. In the second phase, the ethylene glycol is metabolized down a cascade to glycoaldehyde, glycolic acid, glyoxylic acid, and oxalic acid. As the metabolism takes place, the patient develops a metabolic acidosis with ensuing hypertension and tachycardia. The third phase occurring is renal failure, induced by calcium oxalate calculi.

Conventional treatment is as follows: by slowing the metabolism of ethylene glycol, the acidosis may be prevented and renal failure may be avoided. Ethanol, given either intravenously or via the enteral route, competes for the enzyme ethanol dehydrogenase. The toxic metabolites can then be eliminated without development of adverse events. During the period of ethanol infusion, extreme care must be taken to maintain a patent airway and prevent the patient from hurting himself while intoxicated. For the younger patient or combative patient, the practitioner may consider intubation and mechanical ventilation in order to provide adequate sedation.

With its introduction in 1986, fomepizole, a more effective and safer blocker of the ethanol dehydrogenase, care of the patient with known or suspected ethylene glycol ingestion has eased greatly. Fomepizole has a significantly lower side-effect profile than ethanol [7]. The dosing of fomepizole is straightforward and does not require frequent readjustment [10]: 15 mg kg^{-1} loading dose intravenous over 30 min, followed by 10 mg kg^{-1} every 12 h for four doses, then 15 mg kg^{-1} every 12 h.

In addition, fomepizole has no effect on the CNS; therefore, patients will not experience the intoxication that accompanies therapeutic administration of ethanol. Also, hypoglycemia is not associated with fomepizole administration. These advantages are specifically valuable in children, where the risk of hypoglycemia may be more influential on the developing brain. Adverse effects from inadequately sedated children can be devastating.

Regardless of antidote used, hemodialysis has been essential in the presence of a metabolic acidosis or in the presence of elevated levels of ethylene glycol. Hemodialysis can achieve clearance of ethylene glycol and its metabolites approximately seven times greater than native kidney function. However, recent results have called the traditional indications for hemodialysis into question [29]. In a study of the efficacy of fomepizole, Borron et al. treated 11 patients with ethylene glycol poisoning. No patient experienced renal insufficiency in the seven patients that presented with normal renal function. One patient died; however, this patient presented with multiple organ system failure. Prospective randomized trials are needed to conclusively answer the question of who needs hemodialysis with the new availability of fomepizole. In the author's opinion, such randomized trials are unlikely to occur. We continue to recommend hemodialysis for any patient with a significant metabolic acidosis.

21.5.2 Methanol

Methanol is also a member of the alcohol family. Traditionally known as wood alcohol, today methanol is found in a variety of solvents. Frequent intoxications occurred in the course of drinking "moonshine" during the prohibition era. However, methanol ingestions still occur today [1]. Methanol is a by-product of distillation in the production of ethanol; however, it has a lower boiling point than ethanol. This fraction of methanol could be eliminated by throwing out the head or first fraction to be collected. The moonshiners would maximize their profit and neglect this step. Unfortunately, methanol looks and smells of ethanol, thereby making it difficult to distinguish the two. In the United States, denatured alcohol is sold without taxation for consumption. In this process, ethanol is made undrinkable, i.e., toxic, by the process of adding methanol or another toxic agent.

Unfortunately, the toxicity associated with methanol is profound as it is completely and rapidly absorbed after oral ingestion. Toxicity is associated with blindness, severe metabolic acidosis, and death. Methanol is converted to formaldehyde by alcohol dehydrogenase and then further converted to formic acid or formate. Formate has a direct toxic effect on the CNS, specifically the optic nerve. Clinically, a latent period is frequently observed as the toxicity occurs secondary to formate accumulation. The inebriation may have passed, and the metabolic acidosis and visual changes are yet to come.

Physical exam findings are unspecific and new onset of visual disturbance after a relatively asymptomatic interval is quite helpful in making the diagnosis. Metabolic acidosis, a positive serum osmolar gap (in the early stages before methanol is metabolized), and an increased anion gap are useful diagnostic tests.

Treatment is much as described earlier for ethylene glycol. Fortunately, methanol ingestion is frequently coingested with ethanol, which competes for the enzyme ethanol dehydrogenase. However, as discussed earlier, dosing with fomepizole is a much simpler process. Fomepizole has a much greater affinity for ethanol dehydrogenase and its dosing is predictable [30]. Other therapies include the administration of intravenous bicarbonate and gastric drainage especially if the ingestion was recent.

Hemodialysis should be promptly considered in the presence of therapy refractory metabolic acidosis, visual impairment, or evidence of end-organ failure. Ingestion of greater than 50 mL of pure methanol, and serum levels greater than 50 mg dL^{-1} are also indications for the initiation of renal replacement therapy [5]. This recommendation is made despite questions over whether hemodialysis alters the half-life of the active metabolite, formate. Clearly, hemodialysis does remove formate. In addition, the correction of acid–base disturbances (i.e., promoting an alkaline environment) may lead to enhanced elimination of formate, both through decreased reuptake of formate in the proximal tubules as well as increasing active transport formate/chloride ion channels [23]. In addition, fomepizole dosing should be increased during hemodialysis as fomepizole is dialyzable.

21.5.3 Ethanol

Alcohol intoxications are frequently encountered in children and young adults and can lead to organ dysfunction including hypotension, cardiac arrhythmias, respiratory depression, and asphyxia with possible death as the worst outcome. Recently, this topic has received increased attention in Europe due to the rising number of adolescents showing binge-drinking behavior [35]. Fortunately, most children can be treated supportively. This includes management with intravenous fluids and close attention to serum electrolytes including glucose. Use of extracorporeal therapies including hemodialysis and hemo(dia)filtration should only be considered in severely intoxicated children.

21.5.4 Theophylline

Theophylline is a methylxanthine; the mechanism of action is inhibition of the cyclic nucleotide phosphodiesterase, thereby increasing intracellular cyclic AMP and producing smooth muscle relaxation. Theophylline has an exceedingly narrow therapeutic index, with toxic side effects commonly seen in serum concentrations greater than 25 mg L^{-1} [21]. Seizures, tachyarrhythmias, as well as the more common gastrointestinal effects are noted. Rhabdomyolysis and acute renal failure can also occur. Although theophylline use has declined remarkably [16], it is still in use for selected patients.

Theophylline is approximately 60% protein bound. The traditional indications for hemoperfusion are intractable seizures, cardiac arrhythmias, or emesis. Oral charcoal is equally as effective as hemoperfusion and

therefore the authors suggest levels not to be used as an absolute indicator of need for hemoperfusion. The goal of treatment should be to achieve levels less than 60 mg L^{-1} in acute cases vs. 40 mg L^{-1} in chronic overdoses or until symptoms abate. Charcoal hemoperfusion is preferred to traditional dialysis. While drug clearance rates (185.1 mL kg^{-1} h^{-1} – hemodialysis vs. 294.8 mL kg^{-1} h^{-1} – hemoperfusion) are much greater with hemoperfusion [38], hemoperfusion is not readily available in many institutions.

21.5.5 Carbamazepine

Carbamazepine is one of the most frequently used antiepileptic medications for children, inhibiting voltage-dependent sodium channels. Zhang et al. have shown in preliminary studies in mice that some of the toxicity may be induced via the GABA$_A$ pathway [41]. Despite its frequent use, fatalities due to overdose are rare. Intentional overdose in more common in teenagers, whereas accidental ingestion occurs predominantly in young children. Carbamazepine has a number of side effects, which contribute to its toxicity. CNS depression including seizures, coma, anticholinergic effects exerted through blockade of muscarinic and nicotinic receptors, and cardiovascular effects including ventricular arrhythmias have been reported in overdose [18].

Traditional treatment of carbamazepine toxicity is oriented toward management of the CNS effects and cardiorespiratory compromise. Benzodiazepines are effective therapy for seizure activity as a result of carbamazepine toxicity. In rare cases, midazolam or barbiturate infusions may be indicated for the management of refractory status epilepticus [39]. Catastrophic cardiovascular compromise has been reported in large overdoses [26], but the majority of ingestions have mild cardiovascular effects [2].

Carbamazepine is bound by approximately 80% to protein. Because of the large binding to protein, activated charcoal via the enteral route is the treatment of choice. In addition, carbamazepine has a relatively large volume of distribution and the concept of a rebound phenomenon is possible [28]. Therefore, multiple dosing of activated charcoal has been studied with a reduction in the carbamazepine half-life from 27.88 ± 7.36 to 12.56 ± 3.5.

No published guidelines exist that specifically state when extracorporeal removal of toxin is appropriate. Mortality resulting from acute carbamazepine toxicity is rare [25]. Clearly in the minority of cases, the CNS effects with or without cardiovascular involvement are significant enough to consider extracorporeal removal of toxin. This dilemma may be compounded by carbamazepine's intrinsic gastrointestinal hypomotility [14]. Based on the large volume of distribution as well as the high percentage of protein-bound drug, hemoperfusion as the first line treatment continues to be the recommendation of choice if the practitioner feels that extracorporeal removal of carbamazepine and its metabolites is necessary. Absolute indications in this author's opinion for hemoperfusion include refractory status epilepticus, refractory hypotension requiring vasopressor support, and unstable cardiac arrhythmias.

Theoretically, routine hemodialysis is unlikely to be of value given the drug's high protein binding, large volume of distribution, and insolubility in water. However, published reports exist of up to 50% decreases in carbamazepine levels within 2 h of hemodialysis initiation and positive outcome in children [12, 40]. In the absence of readily available hemoperfusion, conventional hemodialysis should be considered as an option based on literature case observations.

21.5.6 Lithium

Lithium, available in various salt forms, is one of the oldest commonly used medications available. Its primary use is in the treatment of bipolar disorder. Serum levels between 0.7 and 1.2 meq L^{-1} are considered therapeutic. Lithium has a very narrow therapeutic range and drug level monitoring is essential. As a cation, lithium is distributed throughout the intracellular space. Acutely, children experience gastrointestinal symptoms but with higher doses may express neurologic involvement including lethargy and hypertonia. Severe poisonings may progress to seizures and coma. In addition, chronic administration of lithium can cause renal impairment including diabetes insipidus.

While lithium does not bind to protein, it is distributed throughout the intracellular and extracellular space. It is quickly removed via the kidneys essentially intact. As the excretion depends on the glomerular filtration rate, dose reduction is necessary in patients with abnormal renal function; unfortunately, the half-life is ~24 h due to its large amount stored in the tissues. However, lithium will be reabsorbed similarly to sodium if the patient is volume-contracted. Hemodialysis should be considered in patients with chronic toxicity and serum levels greater than 4 meq L^{-1} as well as unstable patients with levels greater than 2.5 meq L^{-1}.

Hemodialysis readily decreases serum lithium levels; however, following dialysis levels may rebound secondary to redistribution into the intravascular space. On this basis, some authors have proposed use of continuous hemodiafiltration. Numerous authors have proposed hemodialysis criteria on the basis of experience with limited number of patients.

Clearly, enhanced elimination is warranted in the setting of renal insufficiency or chronic toxicity, where the incidence of sustained morbidity is higher.

21.5.7 Salicylate

Salicylates have been used in healthcare extensively since the introduction of aspirin in 1900. Originally used as an analgesic, its usage in pediatrics today is largely due to its anti-inflammatory and anticlotting properties. While fairly well tolerated at large doses (80–100 mg kg^{-1} day^{-1}), doses of 500 mg kg^{-1} can be fatal.

Symptomatology includes gastrointestinal upset, tinnitus, and hyperventilation with respiratory alkalosis. As the toxidrome progresses, metabolic acidosis ensues, with convulsions and coma leading to death. Hypotension and renal failure are also present as the condition worsens. Pulmonary edema is also seen, more commonly in children than in adults.

Plasma levels may be beneficial. Levels less than 20 mg dL are unlikely to have significant morbidity Oral activated charcoal may be effective early. However, if the patient is showing signs of severe toxicity (plasma levels > 45 mg dL^{-1}), urinary alkalinization is warranted (see earlier discussion). With severe intoxication (levels > 70 mg dL^{-1}), hemodialysis is effective. Salicylates are rapidly cleared with correction of acid–base abnormalities. An excellent algorithm for salicylate poisoning is presented by Chapman et al. [11].

21.5.8 Hyperammonemia

Even though hyperammonemia is not an exogenous intoxication, it is included in this chapter as pediatric nephrologists and intensivists are universally involved in the care of those children with hyperammonemia. Some of the most difficult patients in the pediatric intensive care unit carry the range of diagnoses in the realm of inborn errors of metabolism. This broad spectrum of diseases is challenging both in terms of diagnosis as well as management. The differential diagnosis of hyperammonemia includes valproate ingestion, liver dysfunction, urea cycle defects, organic acidemias, as well as transient hyperammonemia of the newborn. Care should be undertaken in a multidisciplinary environment using pediatric intensivists, nephrologists, and metabolic specialists. For a comprehensive review, the reader is referred to references that discuss the diagnosis and management of conditions leading to hyperammonemia [15, 37].

The provision of renal replacement therapy can rapidly reverse extreme metabolic acidosis and hyperammonemia. Concurrent therapy must be undertaken to treat the underlying cause of the metabolic derangement. Current therapy options include peritoneal dialysis, traditional hemodialysis, as well as CVVHD. The majority of newborns and infants with a serious inborn error of metabolism will need renal replacement therapy. In our institution, hemodialysis is the initial method of choice. A suggested approach to hemodialysis in children with hyperammonemia was recently published by Kiessling et al. [24].

21.6 Novel Modes of Extracorporeal Removal of Toxin

The improvement in vascular access, technique, and safety measures incorporated into today's renal replacement devices allows new approaches to intoxication as well as other forms of renal involvement in the pediatric intensive care unit. A recent review by Goodman and Goldfarb provides an excellent discussion of published articles incorporating CRRT and intoxication [17]. The authors outline little use for CRRT in this patient population. However, as noted earlier in the detailed indications for hemodialysis, the major indication for extracorporeal removal of toxin is hemodynamic instability. In cases such as these, the practitioner may choose to use continuous extraction of toxin rather than risking further hemodynamic compromise.

While the use of extracorporeal elimination for fulminant hepatic failure is beyond the scope of this chapter, the concepts for elimination of protein-bound toxins apply. There are both theoretical as well as case reports of the use of albumin-enhanced dialysis to facilitate the elimination of protein-bound toxins [34]. Sauer et al. compared the use of the molecular adsorbent recirculation system (MARS) to single-pass albumin-enhanced dialysis (SPAD) to continuous veno-venous hemodiafiltration (CVVHDF). Both the MARS and SPAD systems add albumin to the dialysate. In addition, the MARS recirculates the albumin by running it against a charcoal filter and anion filter after dialyzing the albumin against standard CVVHDF. The investigators found that CVVHD continued to have the greatest elimination of water-soluble substances such as ammonia and urea. However, they were able to show significant removal of protein-bound toxin using bilirubin as a prototypical solution in both the molecular adsorbent recirculation system.

Take-Home Pearls

› Intoxications and ingestions are a common admitting diagnosis to the pediatric intensive care unit.
› Pediatric ingestions rarely cause long-term morbidity or mortality.
› Most intoxications should at least initially be managed conservatively.
› Pediatric nephrologists and intensivists need to weigh the risks and benefits of extracorporeal therapy in the removal of toxins.

References

1. Ahmad K (2000) Methanol-laced moonshine kills 140 in Kenya. Lancet 356:1911
2. Apfelbaum JD, Caravati EM, Kerns Ii WP, et al. (1995) Cardiovascular effects of carbamazepine toxicity. Ann Emerg Med 25:631–635
3. Arain SR, Ebert TJ (2002) The efficacy, side effects, and recovery characteristics of dexmedetomidine versus propofol when used for intraoperative sedation. Anesth Analg 95:461–466
4. Bagwell CE, Salzberg AM, Sonnino RE, et al (2000) Potentially lethal complications of central venous catheter placement. J Pediatr Surg 35:709–713
5. Barceloux DG, Bond GR, Krenzelok EP, et al. (2002) American Academy of Clinical Toxicology Ad Hoc Committee on the treatment guidelines for methanol poisoning. Clin Toxicol 40:415–446
6. Brent J (2001) Current management of ethylene glycol poisoning. Drugs 61:979–988
7. Brent J, McMartin K, Phillips S, et al. (1999) Fomepizole for the treatment of ethylene glycol poisoning. N Engl J Med 340:832–838
8. Brophy PD, Tenenbein M, Gardner J, et al. (2000) Childhood diethylene glycol poisoning treated with alcohol dehydrogenase inhibitor fomepizole and hemodialysis. Am J Kidney Dis 35:958–962

9. Brown CV, Rhee P, Chan L, et al. (2004) Preventing renal failure in patients with rhabdomyolysis: do bicarbonate and mannitol make a difference? J Trauma 56:1191–1196

10. Casavant MJ (2001) Fomepizole in the treatment of poisoning. Pediatrics 107:170–171

11. Chapman BJ, Proudfoot AT (1989) Adult salicylate poisoning: deaths and outcome in patients with high plasma salicylate concentrations. QJM 72:699–707

12. Chetty M, Sarkar P, Aggarwal A, et al. (2003) Carbamazepine poisoning: treatment with haemodialysis. Nephrol Dial Transplant 18:220–221

13. Citak A, Karaböcüo lu M, Ucsel R, Uzel N (2002) Central venous catheters in pediatric patients – subclavian venous approach as the first choice. Pediatr Int 44:83–86

14. Deshpande G, Meert KL, Valentini RP (1999) Repeat charcoal hemoperfusion treatments in life threatening carbamazepine overdose. Pediatr Nephrol 13:775–777

15. Fernandes J, Saudubray JM, Van den Berghe G (2000) Inborn metabolic diseases: diagnosis and treatment. Springer, Berlin, pp xii, 467

16. Goodman DC, Lozano P, Stukel TA, et al. (1999) Has asthma medication use in children become more frequent, more appropriate, or both? Pediatrics 104:187–194

17. Goodman JW, Goldfarb DS (2006) The role of continuous renal replacement therapy in the treatment of poisoning. Semin Dialysis 19:402–407

18. Hojer J, Malmlund HO, Berg A (1993) Clinical features in 28 consecutive cases of laboratory confirmed massive poisoning with carbamazepine alone. J Toxicol Clin Toxicol 31:449–458

19. Homsi E, Leme Barreiro MFF, Orlando JMC, et al. (1997) Prophylaxis of acute renal failure in patients with rhabdomyolysis. Renal Failure 19:283–288

20. Huhn KM, Rosenberg FM (1995) Critical clue to ethylene glycol poisoning. CMAJ 152:193–195

21. Jacobs MH, Senior RM, Kessler G (1979) Clinical experience with theophylline – relationship between dosage, serum concentration, and toxicity. JAMA 235.1983–1986

22. Kapur G, Valentini RP, Mattoo TK, et al. (2008) Ceftriaxone induced hemolysis complicated by acute renal failure. Pediatr Blood Cancer 50(1):139–142

23. Karniski LP, Aronson PS (1985) Chloride/formate exchange with formic acid recycling: a mechanism of active chloride transport across epithelial membranes. Proc Natl Acad Sci USA 82:6362–6365

24. Kiessling SG, Somers MJG (2005) Hemodialysis in children. In: Nissenson AR, Fine R (eds) Clinical dialysis. McGraw-Hill, New York, 293–308

25. Lai MW, Klein-Schwartz W, Rodgers GC, et al. (2006) 2005 Annual report of the American Association of Poison Control Centers' national poisoning and exposure database. Clin Toxicol 44:803–932

26. Leslie PJ, Heyworth R, Prescott LF (1983) Cardiac complications of carbamazepine intoxication: treatment by haemoperfusion. Br Med J (Clin Res Ed) 286:1018

27. Liebelt EL, Francis PD, Woolf AD (1995) ECG lead aVR versus QRS interval in predicting seizures and arrhythmias in acute tricyclic antidepressant toxicity. Ann Emerg Med 26:195–201

28. Low CL, Haqqie SS, Desai R, et al. (1996) Treatment of acute carbamazepine poisoning by hemoperfusion. Am J Emerg Med 14:540–541

29. Mégarbane B, Borron SW, Baud FJ (2005) Current recommendations for treatment of severe toxic alcohol poisonings. Intensive Care Med 31:189–195

30. Mycyk MB, Leikin JB (2003) Antidote review: fomepizole for methanol poisoning. Am J Ther 10(1):68–70

31. Pentel P, Benowitz N (1984) Efficacy and mechanism of action of sodium bicarbonate in the treatment of desipramine toxicity in rats. J Pharmacol Exp Ther 230:12–19

32. Pichette V, Leblond FA (2003) Drug metabolism in chronic renal failure. Curr Drug Metab 4:91–103

33. Proudfoot AT, Krenzelok EP, Vale JA (2004) Position paper on urine alkalinization. J Toxicol Clin Toxicol 42:1–26

34. Sauer IM, Goetz M, Steffen I, et al. (2004) In vitro comparison of the molecular adsorbent recirculation system (MARS) and single-pass albumin dialysis (SPAD). Hepatology 39:1408–1414

35. Schoeberl S, Nickel P, Schmutzer G, et al. (2008) Acute ethanol intoxication among children and adolescents. Klin Padiatr. DOI: 10.1055/s-2007–984367

36. Schulman G, Himmelfarb J (2004) Hemodialysis. Saunders, Philadelphia, PA

37. Scriver CR (2001) The metabolic and molecular bases of inherited disease. McGraw-Hill, New York, pp 4 v (xlvii, 6338, 6140)

38. Shannon MW (1997) Comparative efficacy of hemodialysis and hemoperfusion in severe theophylline intoxication. Acad Emerg Med 4:674–678

39. Spiller HA, Carlisle RD (2002) Status epilepticus after massive carbamazepine overdose. J Toxicol Clin Toxicol 40:81

40. Yildiz TS, Toprak DG, Arisoy ES, et al. (2006) Continuous venovenous hemodiafiltration to treat controlled-release carbamazepine overdose in a pediatric patient. Pediatr Anaesth 16:1176–1178

41. Zhang Z-J, Postma T, Obeng K, et al. (2002) The benzodiazepine partial inverse agonist Ro15–4513 alters anticonvulsant and lethal effects of carbamazepine in amygdala-kindled rats. Neurosci Lett 329:253–256

Index